DATE DUE

DEMCO 38-296

Space Biology and Medicine

Joint U.S./Russian Publication in Five Volumes

Series edited by

Arnauld E. Nicogossian, Stanley R. Mohler (U.S.)
Oleg G. Gazenko, Anatoliy I. Grigoryev (Russia)

Co-Editors

United States

L. F. Dietlein
C. L. Huntoon
S. R. Mohler
J. D. Rummel
F. M. Sulzman

Russia

V. V. Antipov
S. A. Bugrov
A. M. Genin
A. I. Grigoryev
A. A. Gurjian
M. V. Ivanov
V. A. Kotelnikov
I. D. Pestov

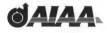

Published and distributed by
**American Institute of
Aeronautics and Astronautics**
Washington, DC

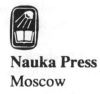

Nauka Press
Moscow

American Institute of Aeronautics and Astronautics, Inc.
370 L'Enfant Promenade, SW, Washington, DC 20024-2518

Library of Congress Cataloging-in-Publication Data

Space biology and medicine.
Simultaneously published in Russian.
Includes bibliographical references and index.
Contents: v. 1. Space and its exploration / editors, J.D. Rummel
and V.A. Kotelnikov, M.V. Ivanov--
v. 2. Life support and habitability.
1. Space medicine. 2. Space biology. I. Nicogossian, Arnauld E.
RC1135.S62 1993   616.9'80214   93-26189
ISBN 1-56347-061-6 (v. 1)
ISBN 1-56347-082-9 (v. 2)

Data and information appearing in this book are for informational purposes only. AIAA is not responsible for any injury or damage resulting from use or reliance, nor does AIAA warrant that use or reliance will be free from privately owned rights.

ISBN 1-56347-082-9

This series is dedicated to the men and women who have devoted their lives to the exploration and conquest of space.

Series Preface

The appearance of this work has an entire history behind it. As early as the mid 1960s Hugh L. Dryden and Dr. Anatoliy Arkadevich Blagonravov signed a number of agreements on collaboration in space research between the National Aeronautics and Space Administration of the U.S. and the U.S.S.R. Academy of Sciences. One of them was an agreement to publish a joint scientific work—"Foundations of Space Biology and Medicine"—in both Russian and English.

The material in that book, published in 1975, was based on the results of observations and research that had been conducted mainly on short-term flights of approximately 50 manned spacecraft carrying more than 70 crew members, and also of dozens of space flight experiments conducted on dedicated biosatellites or "hitch-hiking" on unmanned spacecraft. The 1975 edition was generally well received by readers and reviewers, and for some time satisfied the need for information in space biology and medicine.

However, since that time, human space flight has made extensive use of space shuttle systems and long-term orbital space stations. New empirical data—the results of numerous, often unique flight and simulation experiments—have accumulated rapidly. The scope of biological experiments in space has expanded significantly. Thus by the mid 1980s it had become clear that it was time to summarize and analyze the knowledge we have gleaned in this area.

In 1987 a new intergovernmental agreement, Concerning Cooperation in the Exploration and Use of Outer Space for Peaceful Purposes, was signed (the first one was signed in 1971). Item 16 of the Addendum to this Agreement stipulated publication of a new edition of the joint U.S./U.S.S.R. scientific work, "Foundations of Space Biology and Medicine." A joint editorial board was formed to implement this project within the framework of the U.S./U.S.S.R. Joint Working Group on Space Biology and Medicine.

After considering the complexity of preparing and publishing a work covering the knowledge and experience acquired by both countries, the editorial board concluded that given the enormous amount of new material, and the new set of authors who would be preparing the chapters, the new edition would not simply be an updated version of the 1975 book, but in essence a whole new work. The goal of this new work would be to provide access for specialists, physicians, biologists, and engineers involved in space flight planning and management and the general scientific community to concise and systematic information about space biology and medicine that has accumulated during the last 25-30 years.

The five-volume work will be published in authenticated Russian and English versions. The editors of Volume 1, *Space and Its Exploration*, are Dr. J. D. Rummel of the U.S. and Academicians V. A. Kotelnikov and M. V. Ivanov of the Russian Federation. This volume covers the history of space exploration, the space environment, life in the universe, and spacecraft technology.

Volume II, *Life Support and Habitability*, has two parts: Part 1—*The Spacecraft Environment*, and Part 2—*Life Support Systems*. The editors are Dr. F. M. Sulzman of the U.S. and A. M. Genin of the Russian Federation. This volume addresses major issues and requirements for safe habitability and work beyond the Earth's atmosphere.

Volume III, *Humans in Space Flight*, is edited by Dr. C. L. Huntoon of the U.S. and Professor V. V. Antipov and corresponding member of the Academy of Sciences, A. I. Grigoryev of the Russian Federation. This volume has two books, which provide in-depth discussions of physiological adaptation to the space environment.

Volume IV, *Crew Health, Performance, and Safety*, is edited by Dr. L. F. Dietlein of the U.S. and Professors I. D. Pestov and S. A. Bugrov of the Russian Federation. This volume presents a concise description of systems and preventive measures necessary to assure crew health.

Volume V, *Reference Material*, is edited by Professor S. R. Mohler of the U.S. and Dr. A. A. Gurjian of the Russian Federation. This volume includes extensive reference material relevant to the major topics discussed in the previous volumes.

With only a few exceptions, volumes are being written by chapter authors who did not contribute to the 1975 version, and the editors had to devote considerable effort to ensure the consistent organization of the book as a whole, avoid contradictions, and link individual chapters. Nevertheless, we are aware that in spite of all our efforts, we have not been able to produce a work that is homogeneous with respect to consistency of presentation, being written by scientists of two countries.

Thus, this five-volume edition represents another successful completion of a collaborative project between the Russian Academy of Sciences and the U.S. National Aeronautics and Space Administration in the area of space biology and medicine. We hope that this work will be a useful reference to the reader. We would like to officially express our gratitude for the efforts of the Joint Editorial Board and the many individuals who provided invaluable help in the preparation of this work for publication.

In addition, on behalf of the Joint Editorial Board we wish to express our sincere appreciation to the publication staff.

Arnauld E. Nicogossian, U.S.
Oleg G. Gazenko, R.F.
Editors-in-Chief

Foreword

The National Aeronautics and Space Administration and the Russian Academy of Sciences are once again pleased to introduce a joint work devoted to "Space Biology and Medicine."

The first such work, "Foundations of Space Biology and Medicine," appeared in both English and Russian versions in 1975 on the eve of the historic first international space mission, the Apollo-Soyuz Test Project. This classic work provided an exhaustive overview of fundamental and applied knowledge in space medicine, biology, exobiology, radiobiology, and environmental medicine, written by leading experts, and acquired painstakingly by the scientists of both countries over the first 15 years of space exploration. For many years this edition provided sound reference material to the serious students and specialists involved in the exploration of the final frontier—space.

Since that time, many changes have occurred in space exploration. New discoveries have been made, new spacecraft and laboratories have been flown. More men and women have flown in space, some for extended periods of time in low Earth orbit. Robotic spacecraft landed on Mars, ventured beyond the solar system, and opened windows on worlds never before seen so closely. Many of the engineering and medical advances in space biology and medicine have found application in the practice of terrestrial medicine and public health.

The joint U.S. and Russian editorial board, established under the 1987 Agreement between the United States of America and the Union of Soviet Socialist Republics Concerning Cooperation in the Exploration and Use of Outer Space for Peaceful Purposes, has made significant efforts to bring the reader this up-to-date treatise, renamed "Space Biology and Medicine." Significant revisions and rewrites occurred in the process of reviewing the first treatise. This second edition, in essence, can be considered a totally new publication.

Daniel S. Goldin
Administrator
U.S. National Aeronautics
   and Space Administration

Yuriy S. Osipov
President
Russian Academy of
   Sciences

Космическая Биология и Медицина

Совместное российско-американское издание в пяти томах

под общей редакцией

Олега Г. Газенко, Анатолия И. Григорьева (РФ)
Арнольда Е. Никогоссяна, Стенли Р. Молера (США)

ТОМ II

ОБИТАЕМОСТЬ КОСМИЧЕСКИХ ЛЕТАТЕЛЬНЫХ АППАРАТОВ

Редакторы

А.М. Генин (РФ)
Ф. М. Салзман (США)

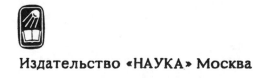

Издательство «НАУКА» Москва

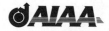

Американский Институт
Авиации и Космонавтики
Вашингтон, ОК

Volume II

Life Support and Habitability

Editors

F. M. Sulzman (U.S.) and A. M. Genin (Russia)

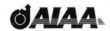

Published and distributed by
**American Institute of
Aeronautics and Astronautics**
Washington, DC

Nauka Press
Moscow

Acknowledgments for Volume II

The authors and editors would like to thank all of the U.S. and Russian scientists and engineers who provided invaluable aid in preparing this volume. The names of these individuals, as well as those of the translators, are cited in a footnote to each chapter.

The translation of English chapters into Russian was performed by L. B. Burakova, A. I. Dyachenko, and V. P. Nikolayev. Editorial assistance was supplied on the Russian side by E. F. Panchenkova and T. B. Kasatkina, and V. V. Kiselev provided valuable technical help. For the English version, Lydia Razran Stone was responsible for translating, editing, and coordinating with authors and editors. The following individuals made valuable contributions to the production of the English volume: Karen Gaiser, Mary Anne Frey, Mary Lou Burnell, Ronald Teeter, Galina J. Tverskaya, Carla J. Howard, Glenn Ferraro, Vladimir Fishel, and Edward J. Stone. The editors express their appreciation to all of these individuals.

Finally, we would like to acknowledge the contribution of Natalie Karakulko (1940–1994). A highly proficient interpreter and translator, she facilitated virtually every aspect of U.S./U.S.S.R. and U.S./Russian space cooperation since the Apollo-Soyuz Test Project. Her integrity, commitment, human understanding, and warmth gained her the respect and affection of everyone—on both sides of the Atlantic—who worked with her. She is missed.

Frank M. Sulzman and A. M. Genin

Introduction to Volume II:
Life Support and Habitability

The most notable characteristic of manned space flight is the prolonged habitation of humans in a pressurized, closed space that isolates them from the life-threatening effects of the harsh environment of space. Thus, all manned spacecraft must be equipped with oxygen, water, and food, as well as an artificial environment with optimal conditions for the health, well-being, and performance of the spacecraft crew.

Creating an appropriate artificial living environment requires information about optimal and acceptable levels of certain physical and chemical substances. Also essential are data on the needs of individuals engaging in various forms of activity and about optimal strategies for accommodating these needs in routine and emergency conditions. Unfortunately, the goal of maximal satisfaction of human needs can conflict with limitations imposed by the technical capabilities of the life support system. For space missions to be completed successfully, life support systems must meet demands for minimal weight, space, and energy, while retaining maximum reliability. Frequently, it is not possible (and sometimes not even rational) to exactly reproduce conditions on Earth, and so the standards set for habitability conditions on space flights must inevitably represent a compromise between the ideal and the technologically feasible.

Volume II of the "Space Biology and Medicine" series, *Life Support and Habitability*, is devoted to these issues. The volume comprises two parts, "The Spacecraft Environment" and "Life Support Systems."

The authors of chapters in Volume II are specialists in the United States and Russian Federation with a great deal of experience working to support manned space missions. In two of the chapters, Chapters 1 and 11, authors were also contributors to the earlier joint U.S./U.S.S.R. work, "Foundations of Space Biology and Medicine," published in 1975. In these cases, their chapters are similar in content and structure to those of the earlier work. The remaining chapters are new.

The volume editors have attempted to standardize the style of presentation to the extent possible; however, this was difficult, since each author had his own ideas about how his or her material should be presented. The greatest difficulties arose in writing and editing chapters written by U.S. and Russian coauthors. However, it would seem that these chapters also best serve the goals of a joint work; that is, they most fully represent the achievements of both nations.

The volume editors requested that the authors present their material in either a problem-oriented manner or in chronological order, and they complied in the majority of cases. However, some chapters are structured around a comparison of U.S. and Soviet scientific, methodological, and engineering solutions. Evidently, the authors preferred this structure, and we did not think it appropriate to pressure them to do otherwise.

As a result of the efforts of NASA and the Russian Federation Academy of Sciences and Ministry of Health, the editors had the opportunity to discuss the chapters in person or using modern communications technology. However, the geological distance between our countries and the pressure of other tasks inevitably limited opportunities for joint work, and each editor naturally devoted somewhat more attention to the chapters in which his countrymen were the sole or first authors.

We hope that the audience for Volume II will be rather broad. It is intended for the use of students at various levels, who are majoring in biomedical and technical subjects and intending to specialize in space sciences; engineers developing life support systems; and physicians and scientists formulating medical specifications for habitability conditions onboard spacecraft and monitoring compliance with them. The extensive references provided for the majority of chapters will also be useful for scientists.

Frank M. Sulzman, *Washington, DC*
A. M. Genin, *Moscow*

Table of Contents

Volume II
Life Support and Habitability

Acknowledgments

Introduction

Part I:

The Spacecraft Environment

Chapter 1

Barometric Pressure and Gas Composition of Spacecraft Cabin Air

V. B. Malkin

The normal atmospheric conditions required to enable humans to live and work in space are achieved through the use of regenerative pressurized cabins, which establish and maintain an artificial atmosphere throughout a flight. Such an atmosphere is essential for humans, animals, and plants on spacecraft—not only for life support but also for the protection of living organisms against many of the hostile effects of space, especially the extremely hazardous effects of low barometric pressure.

Because of the need for an artificial atmosphere in the spacecraft cabin, scientists (biologists, physiologists, and physicians) and engineers have been compelled to examine the physiological, hygienic, and technical criteria such an atmosphere must meet with respect to total barometric pressure, composition, diluent gases, acceptable ranges of fluctuation in partial pressure of oxygen (PO_2), partial pressure of carbon dioxide (PCO_2), temperature, and other parameters.

The problem of generating an optimal artificial atmosphere can be solved only if the complex interactions among many physiological and technical factors are taken into account. In other words, the problem requires a compromise between biomedical and technical approaches. The goal of the former is to create hygienic conditions that are as comfortable as possible; the latter goal constrains efforts to achieve this by compelling designers to confront technical difficulties, such as the need to limit the weight and size of equipment and to prevent explosions, fires, and various other emergency situations. The need to avert disaster forces designers of artificial atmospheres to consider the possibility of cabin decompression. They must also remember that a mission may require crewmembers to leave the spacecraft for extravehicular activity (EVA) or to land on another celestial body that has virtually no atmosphere (the Moon), an extremely rarefied atmosphere (Mars), or a high-density atmosphere (Venus). Clearly, the designers of artificial atmospheres must also contend with the structural characteristics (particularly pressure level) of space suits, descent modules, and living quarters to be used on such missions.

This chapter deals with the biomedical aspects of designing artificial atmospheres for spacecraft cabins. It focuses on human responses to decreases in barometric pressure, changes in the chemical composition of the atmosphere, decreases and increases in PO_2 and PCO_2, the total absence of nitrogen and inert gases from the atmosphere, and the use of inert gases (other than nitrogen) as diluents.

It should be noted that this chapter does not discuss such important atmospheric parameters as temperature, humidity, acceptable concentrations of toxic compounds, or the nature and electrical charges of aerosols. These issues are covered in Chapters 2 and 3 of the current volume.

I. Barometric Pressure

Thirty years of experience with space flight have demonstrated that acceptable levels of barometric pressure in inhabited spacecraft cabins can vary widely (from a fraction of an atmosphere to 1–1.2 atm), depending on spacecraft design.

When evaluating barometric pressure as a critical parameter of cabin atmosphere during normal spacecraft operation and under emergency conditions, we must consider that this parameter is closely linked with others, especially PO_2. This can be seen in Fig. 1, which depicts three zones of PO_2 associated with different levels of oxygen supply to the body:

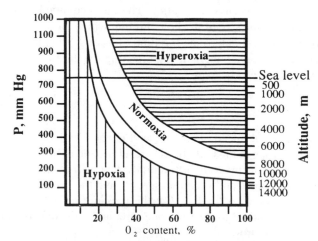

Fig. 1 PO_2 of an artificial atmosphere as a function of barometric pressure.

The English version of this chapter was translated by Galina Tverskaya and Lydia Razran Stone. Dr. Michael R. Powell acted as technical editor of the English version.

hypoxia; normal or near-normal oxygen supply; and elevated PO_2, which is unacceptable because of the toxic effects of elevated levels of O_2.

In a subsequent section, we focus on the physiological effects of diminished and elevated partial oxygen pressure in an artificial atmosphere. Here it should be noted that normal supply of oxygen to the body is possible only when barometric pressure remains no lower than 190–200 mm Hg, as shown in Fig. 1.

Oxygen supply is not the sole limiting factor. When barometric pressure drops significantly, to levels of 200–350 mm Hg, the possible development of dysbarism becomes a problem, even if the composition of the atmosphere ensures normal oxygen supply.

A. Explosive Decompression

Dysbarism is caused by diminished atmospheric pressure. The greatest danger comes from a rapid and large drop in pressure, which can ultimately result in explosive decompression (ED).

Currently, there is no universally agreed upon definition of ED. Attempts by several authors to develop quantitative physical criteria to distinguish it from ordinary depressurization[1–3] have not been widely accepted. Since the occurrence of pulmonary overpressure is the most significant effect of ED, all instances where a sharp drop in cabin pressure creates pulmonary overpressure of more than 20–30 mm Hg can be considered to entail ED.[3] However, the probability of ED occurring in space is usually associated with the risk of being hit by a meteorite, which is comparatively low. Furthermore, the importance of ED is relatively slight compared to other dangers of cabin decompression for the crew, such as injury from being struck by fragments of the cabin walls, the mechanical effects of air escaping from the cabin, and the effects of low pressure. This does not mean, however, that ED should be neglected in developing and evaluating artificial atmospheres. The damage done by ED is largely a function of the pressure level of the artificial atmosphere and, to a far lesser extent, its gas composition. The cabin volume V (cubic meters) and the size of the hole through which gas escapes S (square meters) determine the time t (seconds) and force of ED. The time characteristic t_c, reflecting the duration of ED in the cabin, can be expressed as

$$t_c = V/S \cdot C$$

where C is the speed of sound (see Fig. 2).

Responses of the body to ED are a function of three major parameters: the pressure differential ΔP, which is equal to the difference between initial pressure P_i and the final pressure P_f in the cabin ($\Delta P = P_i - P_f$); the pressure ratio P_i/P_f, the ratio of the initial to the final pressure; and t, the duration of the pressure drop.

Because ED generally occurs during space flight when the external environment is under extremely low pressure, the

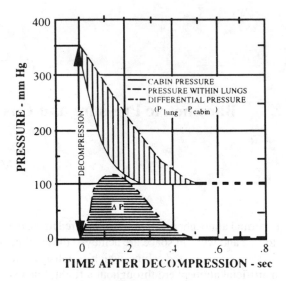

Fig. 2 Dynamics of pulmonary overpressure (pressure differential) during rapid decompression in an artificial atmosphere.[15,25]

associated damage will depend primarily on P_i and the duration of decompression. The latter, in turn, is a function of V and S. Physiological responses will also be affected by the gas volume in the lungs V_l (i.e., the respiration phase during which decompression occurs) and the resistance to airflow in the respiratory tract. Elevated air volume and resistance to airflow are factors that can aggravate the effects of ED.

In ED, the volume of gas in the hollow organs (lungs, gastrointestinal tract, middle ear, and nasal sinuses) increases rapidly. Because the cavities within these organs are connected with the external atmosphere by relatively small orifices, pressure in them reaches ambient pressure slowly, and there is overpressure for some period of time. This leads to tissue distension, which can result in injury, such as rupture. Animal experiments have shown that rupture of the pulmonary alveoli and vessels presents the greatest danger from ED.[4–7] Significant pulmonary damage is associated with shock and gas embolism of vessels and has been found to lead to death of experimental animals.[6–10]

In order to evaluate the damage caused by ED, we should know the value of the pressure differential ΔP_l that is associated with rupture of pulmonary alveoli. This value is not known for the lungs of a healthy human. The majority of authors (arguing from the results of Adams and Polak and Benzinger) maintain that, at $\Delta P_l = 80$ mm Hg, lungs can be injured in the absence of protective tightening of the stomach and chest muscles to limit pulmonary distension.[2,3,11,12] Some authors, however, claim this value to be 50 mm Hg.[13–17]

Thus, the value of the pressure differential is important in predicting damage from decompression. This motivated a number of attempts to calculate ΔP_l as a function of the conditions under which ED occurs. It should be noted that all of the authors who performed this calculation assumed that lung distension was uniform.

When the glottis is closed in an individual exposed to ED,

Table 1 Pulmonary overpressure in humans (DP_l) in ED as a function of external atmospheric pressure in a spacecraft cabin (with closed   glottis)

V_i/V_{max}	Cabin pressure before explosive decompression (P_i)			
	760 mm Hg	362 mm Hg	268 mm Hg	191 mm Hg
1.0	760	362	268	191
0.55	439	220	169	121
0.25	225	126	102	83

ΔP_l can be derived from the following equation:

$$\Delta P_l = [V_i/V_{max}(P_i - 47)] + 47 - P_f$$

where V_i is lung volume before ED, V_{max} is the maximum volume of undamaged lungs, P_i is cabin pressure before ED, and P_f is final cabin pressure. (This expression is derived from the Boyle-Mariotte law with the inclusion of a correction for PH_2O at body temperature.)

The above equation can be used to calculate the pressure differential during ED for different values of P_i in the spacecraft cabin and for different lung volumes.

Table 1 provides an idea of the value of ΔP_l in ED when the glottis is closed. When the glottis is open the pressure differential for the lungs will be substantially lower than when it is closed. Differential pressure with the glottis open as a function of time after decompression is graphed in Fig. 2.

Violette,[2] in a seminal work on the effects of ED on humans, showed that lung volume begins to change only 7.5 ms after the onset of decompression. If the duration of decompression is 7.5 ms or less, the lungs behave like a rigid vessel with constant volume.

To calculate the actual value of the pressure differential for the lungs in ED, Violette proposed the following equation and confirmed it experimentally.

$$\Lambda P_l = (P_i - P_f) \cdot ch[K_c \ (S/V) \ (P_a/\rho_a)/(2t_0 - t)]$$

where P_i is the initial pressure in the cabin, P_f is the final pressure, ch is the cosine in hyperbolic functions, K_c is the experimental equivalent of the flow compression coefficient, S/V is the ratio of the area of the hole through which gas is escaping to the cabin volume (i.e., the coefficient of gas escape from the cabin), ρ_a is gas density at pressure P_a, t_t is the total duration of decompression, and t is the time elapsed since the onset of decompression.

Violette believed that the ratio of initial cabin pressure to final pressure was critical with regard to the risk of ED. He argued that if this ratio was below 2.3, the risk that ED would mechanically damage the lungs could be considered negligible.

J. Boyle attempted to calculate ΔP_l in a way that included both the constant volume phase and the phase of air escape from the lungs (in which lung volume changes). Based on a series of simulations and animal experiments, he was able to calculate ΔP_l for certain ED conditions.[18] Boyle proposed a relatively simple equation for calculating the maximum value of pressure differential for the lungs during ED:

$$\Delta P_l = \{[(P_i - 47)V_i/V_{max}] + 47 - P_f\} \ (1 - t_{cc}/l_c)$$

The first term is essentially the expression used by Luft to calculate ΔP_l for ED with the glottis closed and thus without gas escape from the lungs.

The new second term ($l - t_{cc}/l_c$) allows for gas escape from the lungs in ED. The ratio t_{cc}/l_c is a dimensionless factor reflecting the different rates of decompression of the cabin t_{cc} and the lungs l_c.

It should be noted that the proposed equation for calculating the maximum value of ΔP_l assumes that this value occurs at the point in time when cabin pressure is equilibrated with ambient pressure. This is not always true because, for small values of P_f, the maximum pressure differential for the lungs may occur before cabin pressure reaches equilibrium with ambient pressure.

We now turn to the results of animal experiments that have made it possible to evaluate (albeit only approximately) the danger associated with ED as a function of its physical parameters.

Kolder[19] demonstrated that, when rats were exposed to ED with ΔP_l of 662 mm Hg and P_i/P_f on the order of 10, only 10 percent of the animals died if V/S was 3.3 m^3/m^2; 50 percent died if V/S was 1.2 m^3/m^2; and 100 percent died if V/S was 0.12 m^3/m^2 (where V/S is the inverse of the gas escape coefficient). If the lungs were protected from distension by bandaging the animals' bodies, the negative effects of ED were markedly attenuated. According to Violette,[2] and Kolder,[19] lung hemorrhages developed only when lung volume increased by a factor of 2.3–2.5; and significant pulmonary ruptures occurred only after the volume had increased by a factor of 3 or more. Various studies[4,8,20] have shown that the deleterious effects of ED on animals can be attenuated by drugs (atropine and anesthetics), suggesting that reflex mechanisms are involved in the development of severe

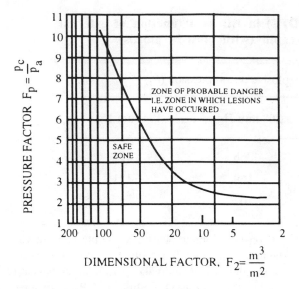

Fig. 3 Curve derived from data of Violette,[2] defining zones of safety and probable danger in explosive decompression.[21] (Reproduced from: Fryer, D.J. Failure of the pressure cabin. In: Gillies, J.A., Ed. _A Textbook of Aviation Physiology_, 1964, London, Pergamon Press, Ltd., 1965)

pathologies in response to ED.

Thus, significant pulmonary distension (which is nonuniform because of regional ventilation characteristics) leading to pulmonary injury is the primary source of the damage associated with ED. In addition, because of the danger of embolism, damage from ED can also be affected by atmospheric composition.

Violette used the results of animal experiments to establish the approximate danger and safety zones for ED with regard to the magnitude of pressure decrease and the gas escape coefficient $F = S/V$, i.e., the ratio of the area of the hole through which gas escapes from the cabin to the cabin volume.[2] Fryer[21] has argued persuasively that the curve in Fig. 3 delineates two zones. The first can be considered to be absolutely safe. While the second area has not yet been mapped accurately, it is clear that some part of it is dangerous. Given the curve in Fig. 3, we can assume that when $P_i/P_f < 2.3$, there will be no damage to the lungs. This is also true whenever the escape coefficient S/V at a given rate of decompression does not exceed 0.01 m^2/m^3. This rate of escape provides enough time for pressure in the lungs to become partially equilibrated with ambient pressure so that the critical level is not exceeded. For this reason, it is important to understand the principles underlying the escape of gas from the lungs during ED. Luft and Bancroft[17] used an esophageal probe equipped with a sensor to record transthoracic pressure in human subjects. They showed that, in humans, pulmonary pressure increases as a function of both the pressure ratio P_i/P_f and the pressure differential (ΔP). In addition, the temporal characteristics of the lungs and respiratory tract in subjects exposed to ED at the end of expiration were equiva-

lent to cabin decompression with $S/V = 0.005$ m^2/m^3. These data are in full agreement with results obtained by Hitchcock,[5] who observed no signs of damage in subjects who were exposed to significant levels of ED for 1 s and those of Kuznetsov et al., who did not observe any injuries associated with ED lasting 0.5 s in duration with pressure drops of 300–400 mm Hg.[22,23]

Experiments with humans revealed only isolated instances of lung damage occurring only when the glottis was closed at the moment ED occurred.[12,24]

When evaluating the effects of ED, it should be remembered that even in cases where no morphological damage occurs, the physiological status and work capacity of humans are certain to be diminished. At the moment of exposure to ED, one has the sensation of a blow to the chest and of air being forced from the lungs, as if through a deep and powerful exhalation. The normal pattern of respiration is disturbed, particularly when ED occurs during inhalation. Subjects exposed to ED, especially for the first time, stop whatever they are doing and fail to respond to conditioned stimuli. This dazed state typically lasts 3–5 s but is shorter in subjects previously exposed to ED.[22,24]

ED produces emotional stress and, thus, a higher heart rate and corresponding motor reactions. In such situations, subjects tend not to notice decreases in ambient temperature and may attribute the fog that forms in the cabin as a result of water vapor condensation to fire. This suggests that it would be beneficial to prepare spacecraft crews (through the use of films) for the conditions arising during ED.[22,26] In planning future long-term interplanetary flights through regions with high meteor density, we should prepare crews for the contingency of ED and flight in a depressurized cabin.

B. High-Altitude Flatulence and Other Manifestations of Dysbarism

Studies performed on human subjects have shown that ascents to high altitudes occasionally evoke complaints of unpleasant or painful sensations in the stomach. These sensations are associated with flatulence and, x-rays have shown, are a function of the amount of gas initially in the intestine, its location, and its route of escape. This implies that, to prevent high-altitude flatulence, which (through pain and reflex reactions) may disturb cardiovascular functioning (causing extrasystoles, bradycardia, and collapse), diets should exclude foods that increase gas formation in the intestines. The induction of severe pathologies by high-altitude flatulence is infrequent. According to data summarized by Berry,[27] of 4259 cases of abdominal pain at high altitude, severe disorders occurred in only 12 cases. Differential diagnosis is important with severe cases, since similar symptoms may be signs not only of high-altitude flatulence but also of decompression sickness. In either case, the affected person should be moved to an environment with normal barometric pressure as soon as possible.

In addition to flatulence, dysbarism may manifest itself as

pain in the ears and nasal sinuses, or as a toothache. The latter is usually associated with latent pulpitis and is probably caused by expansion of gas in and impaired gas escape from the dental pulp.[1,3,26]

C. Altitude Decompression Sickness

On actual space flights or during preparation for them, the entry of crewmembers into an artificial atmosphere with low barometric pressure can give rise to altitude decompression sickness. Altitude decompression sickness occurs not only in emergency situations (such as when a low-pressure space suit is donned after cabin depressurization) but also, in some instances, during the transition from a high- to a low-barometric-pressure atmosphere, if the diving table is inadequate or the subject has not complied with it. For example, such a situation might have arisen when cosmonauts moved from the normobaric, mixed gas atmosphere of the Soyuz spacecraft to the hypobaric, oxygen atmosphere of the Apollo spacecraft if special measures had not been taken.[28,29]

Altitude decompression sickness, like caisson disease, develops as a result of gas bubbles forming in the body.[30–34] Some authors prefer to use the term decompression disorders rather than altitude decompression sickness, because they claim that symptoms associated with the bends, such as joint and muscle pain, are not produced by a true disease, which would be associated with relatively stable morphological changes.[20,22]

1. Formation and Growth of Bubbles

When ambient pressure drops, blood and tissues become supersaturated with gases. According to E. N. Harvey[35] and others,[33,36,37] gas bubbles develop from the gas nuclei constantly being formed in the body as a by-product of various physiological processes. Bubble nuclei may evolve in blood at points of vessel constriction or bifurcation, where there is turbulent blood flow, and in muscles during contraction as the result of a local decrease in hydrostatic pressure.[3,36] Sharp movements cause the hydrostatic pressure to become negative in extended muscles or body fluids, with negative pressure peaking at -100 atm and even more.[33,35,36] During these short time intervals, the affected tissues or fluids become supersaturated with gas. A cavity develops; and, because of "local boiling," first fluid vapors and then gas molecules diffuse into the cavity. When pressure returns to its initial level, the cavity contracts, but some traces remain in the fluid.

The formation of gas nuclei and bubbles can be facilitated by lyophobic surfaces since, for some geometric shapes, their surface tension generates sites of low pressure. For this reason, gas nuclei and gas bubbles persist on lyophobic surfaces for a long period of time.

The presence of gas nuclei is essential to the formation of free gas bubbles in body tissue under conditions of exposure to diminished barometric pressure. In experiments with biological fluids and tissues, the outstanding American biophysicist E. N. Harvey demonstrated that plasma, whole blood, and intact tissues that contain no bubble nuclei remain free from gas bubbles even during decompression from 1000–1 atm.[35]

It has been empirically demonstrated that gas bubbles do not form in animals under conditions that severely limit gas nuclei formation; e.g., in hibernating susliks (ground squirrels), when they are raised to high altitudes.[36]

A gas bubble capable of sustained growth can form only when its initial size exceeds a critical value; i.e.,

$$R > 2\delta/Pb - H$$

where R is the radius of the bubble (centimeters); Pb is the pressure inside the gas bubble, which is the sum of partial pressures of the gases and water vapor it contains (dynes/cm^2); H is the hydrostatic pressure of fluid, which in most cases is essentially equal to the ambient pressure (dynes/cm^2); δ is the coefficient of surface tension at the interface between the bubble and its environment (dynes/cm^2). A bubble that meets this criterion can form only when P_i in the area of formation is extremely high.[33,36]

Thus, for gas bubbles to form in the body, it is not sufficient merely for the tissues to be supersaturated with gases. There are additional conditions facilitating disruption of the metastable state of the supersaturated solution that must be met. It should be noted, however, that these additional conditions are continually created as a by-product of normal physiological processes, particularly motor activity. However, in different individuals, and even within the same individual, the extent to which they are met varies as a function of a number of factors. This is the major source of individual differences in susceptibility to altitude decompression sickness.[38–40]

2. Evolution of Gas Bubbles in the Body

The gas bubbles that form in the body after decompression exert pressure on the surrounding tissues, distorting and disrupting them, which, in turn, may produce pain. The interaction of bubbles forming in blood or tissue with their environment can be described by the equation

$$Pb = H + 2\delta/R + DR$$

where H is the hydrostatic pressure of the tissue (blood), which is the sum of ambient pressure A and tissue turgor pressure T or blood pressure (dynes/cm^2); DR is deformation pressure produced by the bubble and is a function of its size and the elasticity of the tissue (dynes/square centimeter).

Gas bubbles can be divided into two categories: 1) autochthonous bubbles, the evolution of which is governed solely by gas exchange with the surrounding tissues through diffusion; 2) bubbles that grow not only as a result of diffusion but also as a result of merging with one another.

It appears that the majority of the relatively immobile extravascular, interstitial bubbles should be included in the first category. They probably play an important role in the development of osteoarticular pain (the bends), the most common form of altitude decompression sickness. The more mobile intravascular bubbles generally should be included in the second category. Their occurrence is associated with the most severe forms of altitude decompression sickness. However, intravascular bubbles that lodge in the capillaries should be included in the first category.[33]

The evolution of autochthonous (type 1) bubbles depends primarily on the rate of gas exchange between them and their environment. The evolution of type 2 bubbles is determined by the same factors; i.e., the value of ΔP in the medium surrounding the bubble. However, it is virtually impossible to determine the maximum size and true rate of growth or resorption of mobile bubbles, since they merge or split on a purely random basis. Bubble movement modifies the distribution of inert gas in the body. In tissues where bubbles tend to form, the total level of inert gas exceeds the average value and its washout is delayed. Bubbles in poorly perfused tissues are resorbed very slowly. Thus, bubble migration, in association with inert gas redistribution, facilitates the formation of slowly resorbing bubbles in certain tissues. This may be the reason why, in some cases, treatment of altitude decompression sickness by recompression to the initial pressure has not worked, whereas treatment with hyperbaric oxygenation has been successful. This may also account for the higher incidence of altitude decompression sickness during repeated ascents.

In summary, it should be reiterated that structural, physiological, and biochemical characteristics of the living organism are important factors determining rate of bubble growth and bubble size and, thus, are symptoms of altitude decompression sickness.

3. Clinical Picture of Altitude Decompression Sickness

As early as 1906,[3,17] Schroetter described pains in his joints when he "ascended" to an altitude of 9000 m in a barochamber; however, he failed to attribute this effect to decompression. In 1908, Haldane and Boycott (and Henderson in 1917) postulated that caisson disease developed in individuals who ascended to high altitudes in a barochamber.[31]

In 1929, Jongbloed served as his own experimental subject and described the development of altitude decompression sickness at an altitude of 10,000–12,000 m as taking the form of pain in the ankles and knees. Subsequently, this observation was confirmed by a number of studies.[41,42] However, a long period elapsed before gas bubbles were detected in association with development of these symptoms. Gradually, with the increasing use of x-ray and then ultrasonic methods,[17,40,43] gas bubbles began to be detected by a number of observers. They were also found following decompression in persons who did not develop symptoms of altitude decompression sickness.[39,45]

At present, flight surgeons and physiologists believe that the clinical course and severity of altitude decompression sickness are largely a function of the quantity, size, and location of gas bubbles, as well as their rates of growth and resorption.[17,26,33,46]

The large variations in the possible locations of gas bubbles in vessels and tissues make for heterogeneous clinical symptoms of altitude decompression sickness. Many years of experience with ascents (primarily by flight personnel breathing oxygen in barochambers at simulated altitudes of 6000–12,000 m, as well as flying to altitudes of 5500–11,000 m) show that pain in the bones and joints (bends) is the most common form of altitude decompression sickness, occurring in more than 90 percent of all cases.[22,29,44] Less frequently, decompression sickness induces dermatological symptoms, such as itching, rashes of the urticaria type, edema, and local color changes of the skin. It has been observed that, in approximately 10 percent of the cases, dermatological symptoms precede severe altitude decompression sickness leading to collapse.[17,41,47,48]

Fortunately, severe forms of altitude decompression sickness occur very rarely, in less than 1 percent of cases. This is because of the use of prolonged oxygen prebreathing to eliminate nitrogen prior to barochamber ascents and the immediate descent to normal barometric pressure when early signs of decompression sickness, usually the bends, occur. Because it is more difficult to utilize such prophylactic and therapeutic measures in flight, the percentage of more severe forms of decompression sickness is higher than in barochamber tests. Severe forms include attacks of choking (the chokes), often preceded by coughing and substernal pain; cardiovascular disorders, including vasomotor collapse; and severe central nervous system disorders, including loss of consciousness, clonic spasms, hemiparesis, and other symptoms of local injury to various centers of the brain and spinal cord.[3,17,41,49]

In 1938, Apollonov and Mirolyubov[41] made an attempt to classify various forms of altitude decompression sickness. They identified three levels of severity. The first or mild form included joint and bone pain, varying in severity, that disappeared entirely during descent from 7000–8000 m. The second, more serious, form was also characterized by joint pain, but in these cases the pain intensified rapidly and spread to the tissue surrounding the joints. In such cases, joints were still painful to palpation 2–3 h after descent, and slight edema of soft tissues surrounding the affected joint persisted. The third or most severe form included all cases where the subjects manifested severe joint pain, substernal pain, and other symptoms, accompanied by radical deterioration of general state.

Currently, the classification of various forms of altitude decompression sickness has been improved and extended. According to Gray[50] and others, pain in the bones and joints (associated with the bends) can be divided into three types: mild, moderate, and severe. The mild type is characterized by mild pain that arises primarily upon movement and frequently disappears during continued exposure to high altitudes or in response to the compression of tissue surrounding the affected joint. The second type involves moderate pain, in some cases increasing in intensity, that always disappears completely during descent. The third type is characterized by intense pain, sometimes intolerable, causing drastic deterioration of general state.

The mild forms of altitude decompression sickness include cases where pruritus and paresthesia are the only symptoms. Experience has shown that these symptoms sometimes precede more serious pathologies.

The pulmonary form of altitude decompression sickness is particularly dangerous, since it is frequently accompanied by impending collapse or collapse. Symptoms include coughing and choking attacks induced by the formation of large numbers of gas bubbles in vessels of the pulmonary circulation tract and possibly also in lung tissues. According to Fryer et al.,[13,17] subjects who develop choking attacks initially experience chest pain on deep inhalation and, after a short period of time, a dry cough and fits of choking. In severe cases, coughing and choking culminate in loss of consciousness or collapse. In some cases, choking attacks persist for several hours after descent.

One of the most dangerous forms of decompression sickness is neurocirculatory. Severe cases may lead to loss of consciousness caused by vasomotor collapse. Multiple gas embolisms in vessels of the systemic and pulmonary circulation tracts probably are the cause of collapse and the decrease in plasma volume that frequently accompanies it. In less severe cases, neurocirculatory decompression sickness involves hypotension and cardiac arrhythmia. Some cases also develop marked hyperventilation with its typical symptoms of vertigo, muscle tension, and (occasionally) tetanic spasms.[15,24,27] The neurologic form of decompression sickness is marked by general malaise, headache, clonic spasms, and various symptoms typical of local injury to the brain and spinal cord, such as hemiparesis, monoparesis, scotoma, various aphasias, and hyperthermia.[17,24,40,51]

The classification of forms of altitude decompression sickness inevitably involves a degree of oversimplification. Manifestations of this condition are extremely varied, and symptoms frequently suggest the presence of mixed forms. For example, dermatological symptoms can accompany choking, and mild joint pain can be followed by vasomotor collapse.[3,24] For proper classification, it is important to have a correct understanding of the course of altitude decompression sickness.

Most authors believe that, if an individual displaying early, mild symptoms of altitude decompression sickness remains at a high altitude (descent being impossible or undesirable for some reason), there is a high risk that he or she will develop a severe form of the condition. It should be noted that the course of decompression sickness may include periods of remission, in which symptoms rapidly disappear following descent and the patient feels fine. However, some time later, his/her condition may suddenly deteriorate, with more serious cases leading to coma and/or loss of consciousness. In several cases, such delayed syncopes have been followed by death. As was noted above, these symptoms are caused by multiple gas embolisms in the small vasculature of the brain, producing edema. Some authors argue that fat and bone marrow emboli may also contribute to these pathologies.[24,52]

A study of the etiology and pathogenesis of altitude decompression sickness demonstrates persuasively that this condition results from the occurrence of gas bubbles in blood and tissues, whereas it is doubtful that fat embolism is a leading factor. Evidently, only in rare cases are fat embolisms important in aggravating the course of altitude decompression sickness. The high effectiveness of hyperbaric therapy in severe cases of altitude decompression sickness (as demonstrated by a number of authors) indirectly demonstrates that fat embolisms generally do not play an essential role in the pathogenesis of this disorder.

4. Treatment of Altitude Decompression Sickness

Descent from high altitude, or recompression, is a highly effective method of treating altitude decompression sickness. Many authors have found that muscle and joint pain occurring at an altitude of 12,000–10,000 m has disappeared entirely on recompression to 250–300 mm Hg. An important factor in the efficacy of such treatment of decompression sickness (by recompression to normal barometric pressure) is the time elapsed between the onset of the first symptoms and the beginning of descent. As a rule, the sooner descent is begun, the faster the symptoms disappear. In rare instances, symptoms may reappear after a short interval (usually 1–3 h). Since the further course of the condition in such cases is severe, medical surveillance of patients for several hours after symptoms of altitude decompression sickness have disappeared is indicated.

In all severe cases of altitude decompression sickness, it is necessary not only to treat the symptoms but also to subject the patient to recompression.[3,17,24] In recompression chambers, oxygen pressure is usually increased to 3 atm, with the duration of exposure limited by oxygen toxicity. In the symptomatic treatment of severe cases of altitude decompression sickness, particularly with signs of serious brain involvement, such as loss of consciousness and/or coma, it is especially important to prevent brain edema. Drugs that stabilize osmotic pressure in brain cells have been recommended for this purpose.[24,40,49,53]

5. Factors Influencing the Probability of Altitude Decompression Sickness

The factors that determine the probability of altitude decompression sickness include 1) physical parameters such as the altitude attained, rate of ascent, and pressure ratio; 2) duration of exposure to high altitude; 3) temperature and chemical composition of the atmosphere; and 4) age, body build, and physiology of the test subject. In addition, since the formation of gas bubbles after decompression is a function of the level of tissue supersaturation with dissolved gases, many

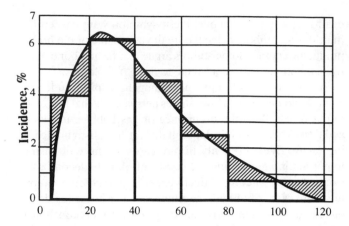

Fig. 4 Rate of development of altitude decompression sickness symptoms during a 2-h exposure to an altitude of 10,500 m.[46]

authors have tried to identify the role of this factor in the occurrence of altitude decompression sickness.[30,33,42]

Haldane ascertained empirically that decompression sickness, which is very similar to altitude decompression sickness in etiology, was observed in divers only at depths greater than or equal to 13 m. On this basis, he proposed, as a safety criterion, that the ratio between the initial and final pressure should equal 2.3. Many subsequent observations in aviation medicine have supported the conclusion that the same factor can be applied to altitude chamber ascents. Today, Haldane's approach is being revised.[30,33]

In theory, free gas bubbles could appear in tissues when barometric pressure drops to a value slightly below the saturation level of venous blood and tissues; for example, when pressure drops from 760–700 mm Hg. Fortunately, however, altitude decompression sickness occurs only at much greater pressure differentials[17,43,54] (see Fig. 5).

The probability of altitude decompression sickness increases with altitude attained and pressure ratio. Following ascent to an altitude of 8000 m (256 mm Hg, pressure ratio approximately 3.0), altitude decompression sickness develops not only in exercising subjects (15–25 percent of cases) but also in resting subjects (3–5 percent of cases).[17,54] Following ascent to 11,500–12,000 m, the incidence of altitude decompression sickness increases to 25–48.5 percent at rest and to 62–93 percent during exercise.[17,20,25,43,54] Various authors have derived very different estimates of the probability of altitude decompression sickness at altitudes of 8000–10,000 m and 12,000 m. The variance can be attributed to many factors, such as differences in rates of ascent and the inhomogeneity of test subjects in terms of age, weight, activity, and different durations of exposure.

Altitude decompression sickness largely depends on rate of decompression; i.e., the higher the rate, the greater the probability of altitude decompression sickness at a high altitude.

In the Everest II study, the slow ascent of mountaineers to an altitude of 8500 m did not induce altitude decompression sickness, whereas the rapid ascent of observers to the same altitude did, in some instances, even though the affected individuals were breathing 100 percent oxygen.

According to Hitchcock et al., a slow ascent (at a rate of 20–30 m/s) to an altitude of 11,600 m and a subsequent stay at that altitude for 90 min induced altitude decompression sickness in 62 percent of cases, whereas a rapid ascent (total of 1 s) induced it in 88 percent of cases (all other conditions, including exertion level, being identical).[5]

Following ascents to altitudes of 8000–12,000 m, altitude decompression sickness very rarely occurs during the first 3–5 min. This may be explained by the fact that it takes time for gas bubbles to form. Many authors have found the maximum incidence of altitude decompression sickness to occur within 20–40 min of exposure. The incidence of sickness decreases after 1 h at high altitude and becomes very low after 2 h.[17,22,40,42]

The distribution of occurrences of altitude decompression sickness over time resembles a Poisson distribution with a peak at the 20th–40th minute (see Fig. 4).

Ambient temperature also has an effect on the occurrence of altitude decompression sickness. A decrease in ambient temperature sufficient to produce sensations of cold facilitates the development of altitude decompression sickness.[42,56–58] Other data suggest that increase in ambient temperature accelerates denitrogenation, thus reducing the probability of altitude decompression sickness.[27,33]

The effects of atmospheric composition on gas bubble formation and, thus, on the development of altitude decompression sickness have not been adequately studied. There are works indicating that an increase in PCO_2 in an artificial atmosphere facilitates the development of altitude decompression sickness.[20,36,57,59] Following decompression to 200–145 mm Hg, experimental animals maintained in an atmosphere with PCO_2 equal to 22–45 mm Hg developed altitude decompression sickness more frequently and showed more gas bubbles in their blood than control animals exposed to the same pressure but previously maintained in a normal atmosphere.[20]

It is known that prolonged (several days') pre-exposure of humans to an altitude of 3000–4000 m, despite hypoxia (which should, in itself, foster altitude decompression sickness), significantly diminished incidence of altitude decompression sickness following ascents to 11,500 m. This is attributed to partial washout of nitrogen from the body.

When designing artificial atmospheres, one should know the potential contribution of the components of biologically inert gases to the development of altitude decompression sickness. The physical and biophysical parameters of nitrogen and other inert gases used as diluents should be considered in the comparative evaluation of the probability of altitude decompression sickness.

Following decompression, the formation of gas bubbles depends primarily on two parameters: gas solubility in vari-

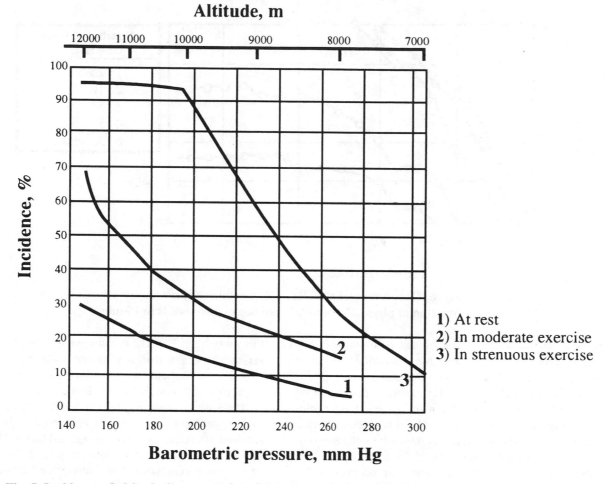

Fig. 5 Incidence of altitude decompression sickness at altitudes of 12,000–7,000 m at rest and exercising.[3,17] (Reproduced from: Fryer, D., and Roxburgh, H.L. Decompression sickness. In: Gillies, J.A., Ed. *A Textbook of Aviation Physiology*. London, Pergamon Press, Ltd., 1965.)

ous tissues (such as fat, muscle, and blood) and its diffusivity across cell membranes.

With respect to the probability of altitude decompression sickness, possible diluent gases can be arranged in ascending order of risk as follows: neon, helium, nitrogen, hydrogen, argon, krypton, and xenon.[33] Unfortunately, results of experiments with humans do not provide sufficiently convincing data in support of this sequence. It should be added that the difference between helium, neon, and nitrogen will diminish at low space cabin pressures.[27,60,61] At a cabin pressure of 380 mm Hg in a 50 percent oxygen atmosphere, the probability of altitude decompression sickness during EVA in a space suit (with a working pressure of 230–290 mm Hg) is so low that there is essentially no difference between helium, neon, and nitrogen.

Many authors maintain that obese people are more susceptible to altitude decompression sickness.[3,58] They also report that obese individuals, more frequently than those of normal weight, suffer from severe forms of altitude decompression sickness. This higher incidence of severe forms of decompression sickness is normally ascribed to the higher solubility of nitrogen in the adipose tissue and the lower level of blood supply to such tissue, leading to a higher probability of bubble formation in fat and, in the event of tissue rupture, to penetration of fat globules and gas bubbles into the bloodstream.

It has been assumed that the incidence of altitude decompression sickness increases with age.[17,33,63] Fryer and Roxberg have reported observations of 2633 servicemen, ages 17–36, who ascended to an altitude of 8500 m and remained there for 2 h breathing 100 percent oxygen. The incidence of altitude decompression sickness in different age groups, at rest, was 0.78, 1.67, 4.98, 7.43, 5.99 percent in subjects of age 17–20 yr, 21–23 yr, 24–26 yr , 27–29 yr, and 30–35 yr, respectively.[17] Factors that may influence the age-related incidence of altitude decompression sickness are weight (which normally increases with age) and circulation changes that can reduce the rate of denitrogenation.

Physical exercise fosters the development of altitude decompression sickness, and a direct correlation has been established between the level of exertion and incidence of this disorder.[17,55,62] This is clearly shown in Fig. 6, which presents data from test subjects doing deep knee bends at a high altitude.[54] The nature of the exercise performed also influ-

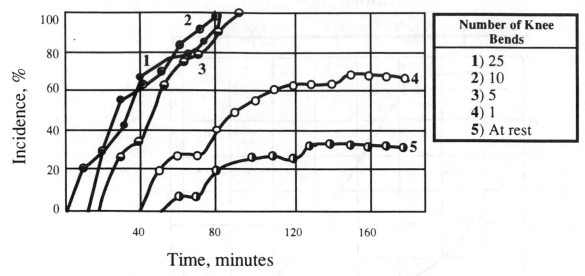

Fig. 6 Occurrence of altitude decompression sickness as a function of physical loading,[54] number of knee bends in 15 min.

ences the localization of joint and muscle pain during development of decompression sickness. Many authors[22,43,54] have reported pain in the joints and muscles that are directly involved in the physical exercise; for example, pain occurred in the knee joint during its flexion or in the shoulder joint when the arms were raised repeatedly. It has been reported that high levels of exertion reduces the altitude threshold of altitude decompression sickness by 1000–1500 m.[3,17,62–65]

Finally, factors other than physical exertion may induce or facilitate intensive formation of gas nuclei and, thus, altitude decompression sickness. It is known that repeated ascents (at an interval of several hours), and underwater dives (to relatively small depths), as well as the use of alcohol and tobacco, may also increase the likelihood of altitude decompression sickness.[20,26,58]

6. Prevention of Altitude Decompression Sickness

In space flight, altitude decompression sickness can be prevented effectively by using equal or similar pressures in the spacecraft cabin and space suit. However, this approach presents serious technical problems. At high suit pressures, the performance of cosmonauts diminishes because their movement is impeded; at low cabin pressures, the percentage of O_2 must be elevated, increasing the fire hazard.

Methods of preventing altitude decompression sickness involving washout of nitrogen or other inert gases in the artificial atmosphere are highly effective. Washout can be achieved either by slowly reducing cabin pressure or having crewmembers prebreathe 100 percent oxygen under normal or diminished barometric pressure. During preparations for EVA, cosmonauts and astronauts have prebreathed 100 percent oxygen to prevent altitude decompression sickness. Many authors have performed experimental studies of the time course of nitrogen washout and identified factors affecting

this process.[30,66–69] The denitrogenation curve reflects differing rates of nitrogen elimination from different tissues.[30,69,70] Washout rates are a function of the solubility of nitrogen in different tissues and in the blood supply.

The washout rate is very high during the first min of breathing 100 percent oxygen because nitrogen is removed primarily from the respiratory tract, lungs, and blood. Then, 10–20 min later, the rate becomes noticeably lower because nitrogen is being eliminated from muscles and internal organs. Within the first hour of 100 percent oxygen breathing, almost 50 percent of dissolved nitrogen is eliminated from the body (see Figs. 7 and 8).

After 2–3 h of oxygen breathing, denitrogenation slows down, and the completion of the process takes many hours.

Aviation and space flight have made it necessary to develop highly effective and rapid methods of nitrogen washout. These include voluntary hyperventilation, exercise, and drugs (e.g., caffeine and aspirin).[67,68] Ardashnikova[67] noted that the nitrogen washout rate increased during voluntary hyperventilation with oxygen. Next, she investigated the effects of adding 3–5 percent carbon dioxide to the oxygen, anticipating enhanced effects of involuntary hyperventilation. However, although the addition of carbon dioxide to the oxygen enhanced pulmonary ventilation, it decreased the denitrogenation rate by 10–15 percent. The reason for this was redistribution of blood flow as a result of the vasoconstrictive effect of carbon dioxide in many areas of the body. Exercising during oxygen breathing significantly accelerates nitrogen and helium elimination, as Figs. 7 and 8 clearly show.

It is known that breathing 100 percent oxygen at normal barometric pressure leads to vasoconstriction and reduced blood supply to many tissues. It was expected that this would have an adverse effect on denitrogenation. To avoid this, some researchers investigated the effect of breathing 100 percent oxygen at various altitudes on denitrogenation. Apollonov

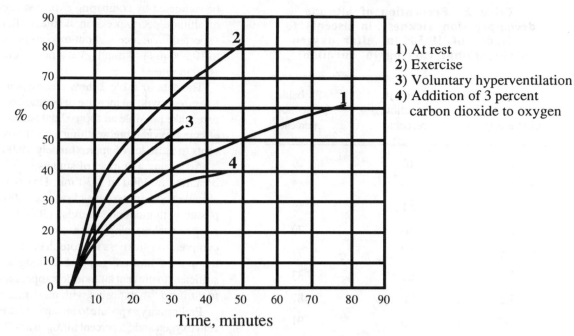

1) At rest
2) Exercise
3) Voluntary hyperventilation
4) Addition of 3 percent
carbon dioxide to oxygen

Fig. 7 Rate of nitrogen washout during oxygen breathing under different conditions.[66-68]

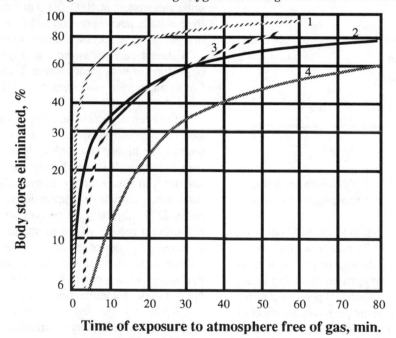

**Fig. 8 Rate of nitrogen (3,4) and helium (1,2) washout at sea level
during oxygen breathing at rest (2,4) and during exercise (1,3).**[25,57]

and Shik[66] demonstrated that the total amounts of nitrogen eliminated as a result of 1 h of oxygen breathing at a normal pressure and at 8000 m were almost the same. However, the amount of nitrogen removed during the first 10–15 min was larger, and the rate of nitrogen washout 20 min later was slower at high altitude than at sea level. This observation may help clarify the factors responsible for the lower protective effect of denitrogenation when 100 percent oxygen prebreathing occurs at reduced barometric pressure.

According to Marbarger et al.,[45] the protective effect pro-

duced by 2 h of oxygen breathing prior to ascent to 11,600 m decreased with the altitude at which denitrogenation was carried out, beginning at 3600 m. Altitude decompression sickness occurred in 6.1 percent of cases following ascent to 11,600 m when normobaric oxygen was prebreathed, in 15 percent of individuals prebreathing oxygen at 3600 m, and in 21 percent of those prebreathing oxygen at 6700 m. After ascent to 11,500 m without oxygen prebreathing, altitude decompression sickness occurred in 48.5 percent of the subjects.[3] These observations can be explained by the fact that,

Table 2　Prevention of altitude decompression sickness in ascents to altitudes of 10,500 m after oxygen prebreathing, varying in duration[61]

Duration of O_2 prebreathing, hr	Minimal protection, percent	Probable protection, percent
0.5	16	26
1.0	29	45
1.5	41	59
2.0	50	70
2.5	58	77
3.0	61	83
3.5	70	87
4.0	75	91
4.5	79	–
5.0	82	–
5.5	85	–
6.0	86	–
6.5	89	–
7.0	91	–

during denitrogenation at altitudes of 3600–6700 m, nitrogen washout is impeded because of the formation of nitrogen-containing bubbles.[33]

Several days' exposure to an altitude of 3000–4000 m, during which all tissues lose about 35 percent of their nitrogen, has a greater protective effect during subsequent ascents to 10,000–11,500 m than 1 h of oxygen prebreathing under normal barometric pressure, when about 50 percent of nitrogen is lost. These data suggest that the prophylactic effect of denitrogenation is a function not only of the amount of nitrogen lost but also of the tissues from which it is eliminated. It is important that inert gas be eliminated from tissues with slow washout rates.

From a practical standpoint, it is important to evaluate how different periods of oxygen prebreathing at normal pressures affect prevention of altitude decompression sickness. The magnitude of the predicted protective effect may be rated as minimal, moderate, or maximal.

From data obtained by Jones,[69] Roth[14] computed the protective effect of duration of oxygen prebreathing when followed by exposure to reduced pressure (179 mm Hg) while exercising moderately. Roth argues that, when ages and weights of subjects are not known, prophylactic effects may be estimated by comparing expected decrease in incidences of altitude decompression sickness after prebreathing with expected incidence without oxygen prebreathing for ascents to 10,500 m (179 mm Hg) at a rate of climb of no more than 1000 m/min.[14]

The data in Table 2 show a consistent increase in protective effects with an increase in duration of prebreathing. These data make possible an approximate estimate of the protective effect of oxygen prebreathing for various periods prior to ascents to altitudes of approximately 10,000–11,000 m.

According a number of studies,[3,29,71] 2 h of oxygen prebreathing at 4500 m (430 mm Hg) is sufficient to prevent altitude decompression sickness at 7000 m during a 5-h exposure with moderate exercise (300–400 kcal/min); without oxygen prebreathing, these conditions induced altitude decompression sickness in more than 10 percent of cases. Furthermore, 5 h of oxygen prebreathing at 4500 m has proved sufficient to prevent altitude decompression sickness at 10,000 m during a 5-h exposure with moderate exercise.

Preliminary exposure to an atmosphere comprising 45 percent oxygen and 55 percent nitrogen at 4500 m for 10 h yielded a beneficial effect. However, preliminary exposure to this same atmosphere at 4000–5000 m for 4–6 h proved ineffective; altitude decompression sickness symptoms developed in 9 out of 30 subjects when they were taken to 11,000 m.[72]

It should be emphasized that oxygen prebreathing must be performed with great caution, because the probability of fire in an oxygen environment is 5 times that in ordinary air.[73,74]

It has been suggested that, to prevent altitude decompression sickness during space flight, those individuals who are found to be highly susceptible should be eliminated during crew selection. It is well known that substantial individual variations in susceptibility do exist. According to Fryer and Roxburth,[17] altitude decompression sickness developed in 71 out of 2273 subjects (3.12 percent) exposed to 8500 m for 2 h. During a second ascent to the same altitude, symptoms occurred in 47 out of the 2202 subjects (2.13 percent) who did not suffer from altitude decompression sickness in the first ascent. Of a group of 60 of the subjects who had developed altitude decompression sickness on the first ascent, 13 (21.7 percent), showed symptoms on the second ascent. Heightened susceptibility to altitude decompression sickness has been found in subjects who are overweight or who have scar tissue.[3]

7. Vapor Formation in the Body

At barometric pressure below the saturated vapor pressure of water at body temperature (47 mm Hg), body fluids begin to vaporize, complicating the course of decompression disorders.

Vapor formation in various tissues and body cavities depends on ambient temperature, tissue elasticity, presence of gas nuclei, etc. If a person is wearing a partial pressure suit, local intratissue vapor formation may still occur in unpro-

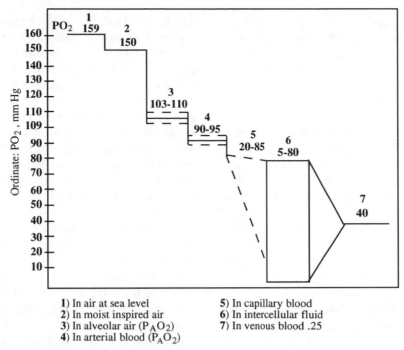

1) In air at sea level
2) In moist inspired air
3) In alveolar air (P_AO_2)
4) In arterial blood (P_AO_2)

5) In capillary blood
6) In intercellular fluid
7) In venous blood .25

Fig. 9 Normal PO$_2$ values at different stages of oxygen transport.

tected parts of the body (most often, the hands) when he or she is exposed to depressurization at an altitude over 18,000 m; this may cause decompression emphysema.

Subcutaneous emphysema of the hands of subjects wearing altitude gear without gloves has been reported at barochamber altitudes of 20,000–40,000 m.[22,39,61,75–77]

Experimental data show that emphysema fails to occur during the first 1–3 min after ascent, even when altitude chamber pressure is decreased 8 mm Hg, as well as in in some subjects who are exposed to a pressure equivalent of 20,000–30,000 m for 15 min and longer. This can be explained by the effect of turgor in the tissues, which helps them to withstand distension and rupture. Thus, the absence of subcutaneous emphysema during the first minutes of exposure and individual variations in symptoms may be ascribed to differences in turgor.[22] It may be added that gas nuclei, which act as a source of decompression bubbles, may also contribute to individual variations in emphysema, because vaporization of water inside the gas bubble may affect the early stage of its development. Altitude emphysema occurs only when the sum of intratissue pressure (Pt – turgor) and barometric pressure Pb is lower than 47 mm Hg ($Pt + Pb < 47$ mm Hg).

The first few minutes of emphysema involve no deterioration in well-being or general state. This makes it possible to study its time course. Emphysema often occurs in only one hand, starting on the back of the hand between the first and second fingers; then, it gradually spreads to the entire hand. The first unpleasant sensations—sensations of skin tightening, prickling, and pain—have been reported 3–5 min after onset. In some cases, no pain was reported, even when the emphysema was so pronounced that the hand was swollen into a spherical shape.[22,39] After a rapid descent, gas always remains in the radiocarpal joint. Some x-rays have

also shown that very small "light" bands in the soft tissues of hands were affected by emphysema.

II. Oxygen Concentration

Support of PO$_2$ in an artificial atmosphere at a level biologically equivalent to that of normal air is one of the main objectives of cabin atmosphere design and an important safety factor. Unfortunately, in space, the possibility of emergency situations, such as cabin depressurization, breakdown of the air regeneration system, or failure of an oxygen breathing unit, leading to hypoxia or hyperoxia, can never be completely precluded. This implies that an understanding of the effects of hypoxic hypoxia of varying degrees is of key importance for space medicine.[1,79,80]

A. Acute Hypoxia

Normal cell functioning requires that PO$_2$ in the intercellular fluid be maintained at a certain level, 1–5 mm Hg for cerebral cells, which are the most sensitive to oxygen deficit.[81,82] A drop of the PO$_2$ of intercellular fluid below this level (termed the critical level) results in reduced oxygen uptake; i.e., true hypoxia of the cell.

Oxygen is supplied to the tissues primarily through the process of diffusion. The efficiency of this physical process depends on the concentration gradient during different stages of oxygen transport. The normal values of PO$_2$ gradients for the main stages of oxygen transport are shown in Fig. 9.

When the percentage concentration of oxygen in the cabin atmosphere or ambient barometric pressure decreases, PO$_2$ in inhaled air will diminish in accordance with Dalton's law. This will ultimately lead to a lower intake of oxygen by the tissues; i.e., development of hypoxia. The first to suffer are the cells located the maximum distance from the capillaries, since oxygen diffusion to them is the most diminished. As hypoxia increases, the number of cells suffering hypoxia continues to grow, which clearly is important in the occurrence of various symptoms of hypoxia.

The pathogenesis of oxygen deficiency is associated with the direct effects of hypoxia on cellular metabolism, as well as with the indirect effects of adaptive changes that stimulate the cardiorespiratory system. Increased pulmonary ventilation in hypoxia maintains partial oxygen pressure in alveolar air (P_AO_2), but simultaneously leads to hypocapnia and alkalosis; i.e., a new disruption of homeostasis. In acute forms of oxygen deficiency (e.g., in rapid ascents to altitudes of 10,000 m or above) severe pathologies develop rapidly—within 1–2 min. In such cases, there is no time for significant hyperventilation to develop and the cerebral effects of oxygen deficiency are decisive.

P_AO_2 and partial oxygen pressure in arterial blood (P_aO_2), which are close in value, are the parameters indicative of the severity of hypoxia. Thus, it is important to measure these parameters at various altitudes and when oxygen levels vary in an artificial atmosphere. An approximate formula for calculating P_AO_2 as a function of barometric pressure was first proposed in 1880 by Sechenov,[83] who analyzed the cause of death of two French aeronauts who had reached an altitude of 8600 m in the balloon *Zénith*. Sechenov also believed that a decrease in P_AO_2 to 20 mm Hg for even a short period of time is fatal. Later, the calculation of P_AO_2 as a function of PO_2 in ambient air was refined; in particular, a correction was introduced to allow for the respiratory quotient RQ.[3,80] P_AO_2 can be computed from the formula:

$$P_AO_2 = (B - PH_2O) \cdot C - P_ACO_2 [1 - C(1 - RQ)/RQ]$$

where B is the barometric pressure; PH_2O is the partial pressure of water vapor in the lungs, which is a function only of temperature and is equal to 47 mm Hg at a body temperature of 37 °C; P_ACO_2 is the partial pressure of carbon dioxide in alveolar air; C is the oxygen concentration in the ambient air by volume; and RQ is the respiratory quotient.

Subsequently, the critical value of P_AO_2 was also revised based on empirical observations. According to different authors, it varies from 27–33 mm Hg,[27,81,84] and the critical value of PO_2 in mixed venous blood is 19 mm Hg.[85]

Even a relatively short exposure to a significant and rapid decrease of ambient PO_2 leads to acute hypoxia, which provokes pathologies of varying severity in healthy individuals who have not been pre-adapted. In real life, such situations occur after rapid ascent to 4000–5000 m and higher without oxygen or when the oxygen supply is suddenly cut off during high-altitude flights.

Extensive experimental data on the effects of acute hypoxia on animals were first collected by Bert in 1878.[86] He demonstrated that in barochamber ascent to high altitudes, animals developed pathologies, the severity and outcome of which were a function of the decrease in PO_2 in inhaled air and the duration of exposure to the rarefied atmosphere. Animals displayed disorders of cerebral origin, such as convulsions and loss of postural tone, followed by permanent impairment of respiration and circulation.

The effects of hypoxia on the central nervous system are probably associated with both the direct consequences of an oxygen deficit in the blood on neurons, and indirect effects mediated by chemoreceptors. At an early stage of hypoxia, the stimulation of chemoreceptors of the sinocarotid and aortal zones activates the reticular formation of the brain stem, which then involves other higher brain structures, including the cerebral cortex.[93,94]

During this early stage of hypoxia, adaptive reactions, such as increases in pulmonary ventilation, heart rate, and cardiac output, develop and serve to enhance oxygen transport. On electroencephalograms (EEGs), this stage is marked by activation of β-rhythms.[3,87–89] As hypoxia continues, the second stage develops, during which severe disruption of brain function (total inhibition of conditioned reflexes, loss of postural tonus, and clonic and tonic convulsions) occur.[3,81,90] On EEGs, θ- and Δ-rhythms prevail, with the subsequent gradual inhibition of cerebral bioelectric activity.[3,81,85] Emergence of Δ-waves is accompanied by partial or complete inhibition of neuronal impulses. Some neurons do not recover their bioelectric activity after return to normal oxygen supply, suggesting that they have died.

Central nervous system disorders in humans exposed to acute hypoxia include deterioration of mental performance; failures of short- and long-term memory; inability to concentrate; sensory, especially visual, disturbances; loss of fine motor coordination (handwriting illegibility); mood changes such as lethargy, sleepiness, or, conversely, euphoria, which sometimes leads to inappropriate responses to the environment.[84,85,89,91,92]

Symptoms of an uncompensated hypoxic state can be classified as belonging to two syndromes. The first one is typical of impending collapse or collapse and includes bradycardia, a drop in blood pressure, and hyperhydrosis, as well as pallor or hyperemia and lethargic and apathetic behavior. At this stage, changes in brain bioelectric activity are relatively slight: first, depression of α-rhythm; and, then, the appearance of low-amplitude θ- and Δ-waves with the continuation of β-waves. These symptoms occur in relatively moderate hypoxia, following ascents to 5000–6000 m. They are accompanied by complaints of malaise, including sensations of weakness, burning in the head, vertigo, nausea, grayout, etc. Oxygen breathing for 5–10 min fails to have immediate effects on restoring well-being or correcting functional disorders; e.g., sinus arrhythmias on EKGs.[3,22] This suggests that hypocapnia may be involved in the genesis and development of this pathology.

The second syndrome is typical of high-altitude syncope. It includes: deterioration of mental performance; inappropriate responses to the environment and oneself; impaired coordination (deterioration of handwriting); clonic convulsions that begin with the writing hand muscles (writer's cramp); and disturbances of consciousness (including syncope). These central nervous system disorders are accompanied by increased pulmonary ventilation, sinus tachycardia, and some blood pressure elevation. θ- and Δ-waves predominate on the EEG.[85,92,93]

Many researchers have found that changes in brain bioelectric activity are an objective parameter that reflects the time course variations of hypoxia-induced central nervous system disorders. The appearance of the first changes in handwriting and lethargy coincide with isolated waves and short volleys of waves with elevated amplitudes on EEG records. Convulsions and severe disorders of consciousness coincide with high amplitude θ- and Δ-waves on EEGs.[3,85,94–96]

When θ- and Δ-waves predominate in EEGs, acoustic signals, light signals, or spoken commands may temporarily improve performance and general state. A lack of response to external stimulation in the presence of θ- and Δ-waves generally indicates severe central nervous system impairment.[22,85,89,94–96]

The development of such severe impairments of central nervous system functioning often go unremarked by subjects. In many instances, they are incapable of appropriately evaluating their own condition and—even immediately prior to loss of consciousness—report that they feel fine.

Numerous examples can be cited here. Before an ascent to 7000 m, subjects were instructed to don an oxygen mask and inhale oxygen as soon as any signs of oxygen deficit occurred. Out of 16 subjects, only 2 complied with the instructions. Two others made a note that they needed oxygen, but did not use the mask in front of them, whereas the remaining 12 subjects reported that they felt fine throughout the study, although they showed severe impairment of nervous activity (disorders of consciousness and convulsions).

A similar effect of hypoxia has also been observed on flights in which pilots developed hypoxia because of misuse or failure of the oxygen breathing system.

Descent or provision of oxygen to subjects leads to rapid recovery (10–20 s) of normal physiological and psychological status. Some subjects have been found to display retrograde amnesia; they often have been unable to recall the events that preceded loss of consciousness and only guess at them using indirect evidence.[1,3,22,91]

Acute hypoxia in flight is always hazardous, since failure of the oxygen supply, even at relatively low altitudes (5200–6000 m) may cause death.[1,3,91] Moreover, subjects often do not recover fully from acute hypoxia involving prolonged or repeated loss of consciousness. Changes in membrane permeability and disorders of fluid-electrolyte metabolism are implicated in the mechanism responsible for the pathologies associated with hypoxia. Increases in the permeability of blood-tissue barriers, primarily blood-brain and blood-alveolar barriers, lead to severe and dangerous pathologies, such as brain or lung edema. Hypoxia-induced brain edema may be the major cause of such serious complications as encephalopathy or persistent deterioration of memory and

mental performance.[3,26,84]

In aerospace medicine, great importance is placed on data pertaining to the duration of the period during which a person can retain consciousness and performance capacity at exposure to various high altitudes without oxygen breathing. This problem was investigated before World War II, mainly in the U.S.S.R. and Germany. The concept of "reserve time" refers to the time interval before complete loss of performance capacity at high altitudes in the absence of oxygen breathing.[98,99] The term "time of useful consciousness" is used for the same concept in American and British literature.[45,90]

Figure 10 depicts data on reserve time or time of useful consciousness in humans at various altitudes. The value of this parameter depends primarily on the altitude and the individual's susceptibility to hypoxia. It can be seen from Fig. 10 that, as altitude increases, individual differences in time of useful consciousness decrease and disappear entirely at an altitude over 9000 m.[1,3,98,104,107] At altitudes of 15,000 m and higher, the time of useful consciousness is negligibly small (8–10 s). After a rapid ascent (1–2 s) to this altitude, subjects fainted without any precursory symptoms in 12–15 s, whether they were breathing air or 100 percent oxygen.[3,22,98] When they were exposed for no more than 8–10 s and then rapidly returned to sea level, they fainted in 5–7 s during descent, because it took their oxygen-impoverished blood 5–7 s to reach the vessels of the brain after the descent began.[16,85] The nearly complete absence of a period of useful consciousness and failure of oxygen breathing to have a protective effect can be explained by the fact that, at an ambient pressure of 87 mm Hg (which is equivalent to 15,200 m), PO_2 in the lungs reaches zero even if 100 percent oxygen is used. This occurs because the partial pressure of water vapor $P_A H_2O$ at normal body temperature (37 °C) in alveolar air is equal to 47 mm Hg, and the partial pressure of carbon dioxide in alveolar air $P_A CO_2$ under normal conditions is close to 40 mm Hg. Therefore, the total pressure ($P_A CO_2 + P_A H_2O$) is 87 mm Hg. For this reason, with respect to the hypoxia factor, the altitude of 15,200 m (at which barometric pressure is 87 mm Hg) is regarded as equivalent to the vacuum of space.

After cabin depressurization during space flights, unsuited crewmembers have an extremely short time (5–8 s) to evaluate the situation, make a decision, and act on it. In acute hypoxia, severe pathologies develop very rapidly. In a famous instance in 1875, two Frenchmen, Croce-Spinelli and Sivel, flew the balloon *Zénith* to an altitude of 8000 m and died from hypoxia.

Another tragic death occurred in the U.S.S.R. during altitude suit tests on November 1, 1962. P. I. Dolgov, wearing a space suit, left the gondola of the Volga stratostat at an altitude of 25,485 m. During egress, he broke his helmet and died in the air from acute hypoxia. This was also the cause of death of three Soyuz 11 crewmembers: G.T. Dobrovolskiy, V.N. Volkov, and V.I. Patsayev. They died on June 30, 1971, as a result of depressurization of the descent module. Only one of the cosmonauts (who was closest to the valve that had

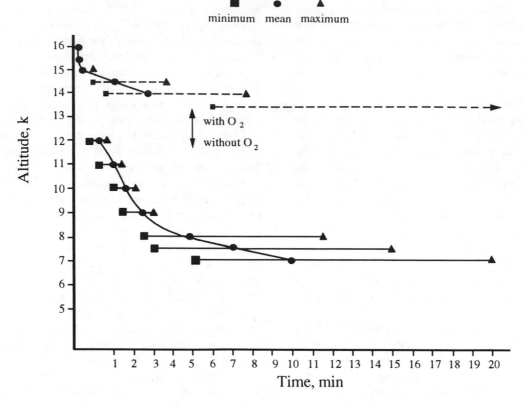

Fig. 10 Time to unconsciousness at altitudes of 7,000–12,000 m (without additional oxygen) and at altitudes of 13,000–16,000 m (with oxygen breathing).[89,92,98]

malfunctioned) managed to unfasten his belt, whereas the other two did not have time to respond to depressurization.

B. Chronic Hypoxia

The chronic effects of hypoxia have been investigated in great detail in mountain climbing expeditions and barochamber experiments. These studies have established that, during prolonged exposure to a moderate oxygen deficit at 2000–3000 m, humans develop adaptive reactions allowing prolonged residence at 6000–7000 m with retention of relatively high-performance capacity. These adaptive responses can be divided into two categories.

1) Reactions that serve to increase oxygen transport: hyperventilation; increased cardiac output; enhanced regional circulation in the lungs and in tissues that are especially sensitive to oxygen deficit (e.g., the brain); increased blood oxygen capacity (because of a higher red-blood-cell count and more hemoglobin, as well as an increase in the oxygen-binding properties of hemoglobin); increase in number of functioning capillaries; and modified membrane permeability resulting in enhanced oxygen diffusion.[84,91,100,101]

2) Responses that are related to metabolic changes, including intensified glycolysis. The role of glycolytic processes in adapting to hypoxia is not likely to be great, because of their low energy efficiency. Glycolytic breakdown of one molecule of glucose to yield two molecules of pyruvate produces only two molecules of adenosine triphosphate (ATP). Some au-

thors have noted that, during adaptation to hypoxia, mitochondrial capacity to extract oxygen from oxygen-impoverished intercellular fluid increases and have attributed this to higher activity or concentration of cytochromes.[102,103] The occurrence of this type of adaptation is, however, still open to question.

Meyerson has emphasized the importance of increased synthesis of nucleic acids and protein in adaptation to chronic hypoxia. He believes that adaptation of the brain to hypoxia is highly dependent on this mechanism because, when synthesis of nucleic acids is inhibited by injecting animals with actinomycin, they fail to adapt and many die of hypoxia.[103] It has long been known that, in chronic hypoxia, erythropoiesis intensifies; the synthesis of hemoglobin increases; and the heart, especially the right ventricle, increases in size. These observations suggest that protein synthesis is stimulated in hyperfunctioning organs. Such responses are obviously adaptive. When evaluating this adaptation pathway, one should note that, although synthesis of nucleic acids and protein increases in the vital organs (the heart and brain), it decreases in other organs (e.g., the reproductive organs). This may explain the decrease in the reproductive capacity and weight loss of people exposed to altitudes of 4000–5000 m and higher for long periods.

Studies of settlements at high altitudes suggest that adaptation of the native population to hypoxia is limited to altitudes on the order of 4500 m. This seems to be the natural limit of adaptation. An attempt of mountaineers to acclimate themselves to hypoxia at an altitude of 5800 m in the Himalayas over a period of several months proved unsuccessful. Although the group included highly experienced mountaineers (e.g., Hillary, who, with Tensing, was the first to reach the summit of Mount Everest in 1953),[84] its members developed chronic altitude sickness.

Altitude sickness may develop in the course of adaptation to moderate hypoxia (or be a sign of failure of adaptation). Its acute forms are characterized by discomfort: headache, vertigo, dyspnea, nausea, intestinal disorders, loss of fine motor coordination, tendency to tire easily even after mild exertion, sleepiness, occasional euphoria, deterioration of mental performance, and increased irritability. Chronic altitude sickness involves increasing malaise, diminished performance capacity, progressive weight loss, sometimes erythrocythemia, pulmonary hypertension, and cardiac hypertrophy.[26,86,91,100] This suggests that the designers of cabin atmospheres should take measures to counteract altitude sickness. Specifically, it is important to identify the lower limit of acceptable PO_2 and to know how long it will take for symptoms of altitude sickness to develop when partial oxygen pressure decreases gradually.

Most experts believe that, if normal barometric cabin pressure is maintained, the lowest acceptable level for PO_2 is 120–110 mm Hg. This conclusion is based on many observations at high altitudes that have shown that discomfort, especially during physical exertion, and symptoms of altitude sickness occur in newcomers to the mountains at an altitude of about 2000–3000 m.[3,80,84,100]

A study of the effects of different depressurization rates, in simulations of gas escape from a cabin, has demonstrated that, at a rate of approximately 0.1 m/s, symptoms of acute altitude sickness occur at an altitude of 4500–5000 m (i.e., 8–13 h after the beginning of gas escape). When oxygen concentration decreases at a rate of 1 percent per hour in a cabin simulator with a normoxic pressure, subjects continue to perform adequately for as long as 48 h. When PO_2 reaches 75–90 mm Hg, many subjects display acute symptoms of altitude sickness.[84,100]

It can, therefore, be concluded that individuals who have not been preadapted to hypoxia can work satisfactorily for 2–3 days when they are in an atmosphere equivalent to 3000–3500 m in terms of PO_2. In space flight, PO_2 should not be lower than it would be at 2000 m, because of the additional strain imposed by the need to perform physical work in a weightless state, with its adverse cardiovascular and vestibular effects.

Methods for increasing adaptation to the prolonged effects of hypoxia include pre-exposure to hypoxia in an altitude chamber or at high altitudes,[100,102,104–107] addition of carbon dioxide to the cabin atmosphere if there is an oxygen deficit, and the use of drugs (e.g., acetazolamide, ammonium chloride, and ascorbic acid).[30,107,108]

It has long been known that adding carbon dioxide to the breathing mixture has a positive effect in acute hypoxia at 7000–8000 m.[3,104,116] An experiment in a cabin simulator at normal barometric pressure and PO_2 = 75–90 mm Hg showed that the addition of 2–3.5 percent carbon dioxide prevented acute hypoxia and helped maintain adequate performance for 2 days. This effect was produced by a significant enhancement in pulmonary ventilation, which increased the oxygen saturation of arterial blood and partially eliminated hypocapnia. If ambient PO_2 falls to a level two-thirds to one-half normal, an increased concentration of carbon dioxide (PCO_2 = 15–25 mm Hg) should be maintained.[107]

It has long been known that pre-exposure to an altitude chamber or actual high altitude can increase tolerance to high altitudes and exercise capacity.[3,108–110] The magnitude of the effect attained is a function of exposure duration and schedule and altitude. Whether this type of pre-exposure should be recommended before space flights is currently under discussion.

The desire to facilitate adaptation within a short period of time has led to the development of short-term protocols (2–8 h nightly high-altitude exposure while sleeping, for a period of 2–3 days), which have proved effective.[106,110]

Figure 11 graphs physiological status and performance as a function of PO_2 and P_AO_2. These data provide a general estimate of the severity of hypoxic hypoxia at different altitudes.

C. Hyperoxia: Oxygen Toxicity

Because the PO_2 in a spacecraft cabin atmosphere may be higher than that of normal air, the study of the toxic effects of oxygen is an important area of space biology and medicine.

Elevated PO_2 is employed in an effort to use a technically simpler one-gas environment, to prevent altitude decompression sickness, and to provide a reserve in case of gas leakage. Examples include the atmospheres of the Mercury, Gemini, and Apollo spacecraft, where PO_2 was 258 mm Hg. At certain flight stages (for instance, during crew transfer to an atmosphere with a lower pressure), PO_2 can be increased to wash out nitrogen or other inert gases. Aside from intentional use of elevated PO_2, oxygen pressure may be high as a result of the malfunctioning of the oxygen regeneration system.[3,14]

Priestley, the discoverer of oxygen, knew or suspected its toxic effect. In 1775, he wrote, "...although dephlogisticated air can prove highly useful as a medicine, it nonetheless would not be wholly suitable for us when we are healthy: just as a candle burns faster in dephlogisticated air than in ordinary air, we would live too fast and our vital forces would be expended too rapidly in this purified air" (cited from Ref. 3).

In 1878, Bert published his conclusion[86] that oxygen in high concentrations acts as a "general protoplasmic" poison, exerting a toxic effect on plant and animal cells. Many later investigations supported this hypothesis.[111–116,123] However, the mechanism of oxygen toxicity responsible for various symptoms of oxygen intoxication has not yet been studied in sufficient detail.

Many authors maintain that oxidation of enzymes and coenzymes containing SH groups (thiol groups) is important in

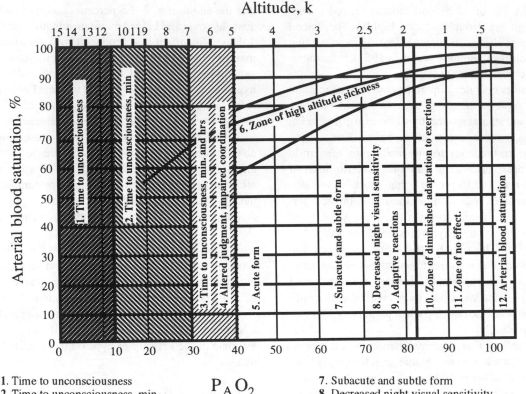

1. Time to unconsciousness
2. Time to unconsciousness, min
3. Time to unconsciousness, min. and hrs
4. Altered judgment, impaired coordination
5. Acute form
6. Zone of high altitude sickness

$P_A O_2$

7. Subacute and subtle form
8. Decreased night visual sensitivity
9. Adaptive reactions
10. Zone of diminished adaptation to exertion
11. Zone of no effect.
12. Arterial blood saturation

Fig. 11 Effects of different altitudes on humans previously unadapted to hypoxia (time to unconsciousness measured in resting subjects).[25] (Reproduced with permission from: McFarland, R.A. *Human Factors in Transportation.* **McGraw-Hill Book Company, copyright 1953.)**

the mechanism of the toxic effects of oxygen at the cellular level. In particular, they associate this mechanism with the damage to cell membranes occurring in hyperoxia.

It has been established experimentally that elevated PO_2 inactivates enzymes containing SH groups (e.g., succinate dehydrogenase) in vitro; however, this may not always occur in vivo because most enzymes are probably protected against the toxic effect of oxygen by their substrate-coenzymes and other compounds in the cells.[112,115,116] It is still unclear whether the mechanism of oxygen toxicity is associated with oxygen molecules, as such, or with other free radicals produced during hyperoxia.

Some authors believe that oxygen toxicity can be caused by free radicals forming hydrogen peroxide and organic peroxides by breaking the intramolecular bonds of enzymes containing SH-groups.[111,113,115] This hypothesis is based on data showing, on the one hand, enhanced formation of free radicals in hyperoxic animals and, on the other, reduced oxygen toxicity (e.g., protection of the erythrocyte membrane) in response to antioxidants that inhibit free radicals [e.g., mexamine (5-methoxytryptamine hydrochloride) and tocopherol (vitamin E)].[113,117–119]

In order to understand oxygen toxicity, it is important to understand the effects of hyperoxia on different physiological systems.

Animal and human experiments have shown that oxygen toxicity is a function of the level of PO_2, the duration of hyperoxic exposure, and the susceptibility of the species and individual. The latent period of oxygen toxicity, also a function of PO_2, is different for various tissues.

Three ranges of PO_2 can be distinguished on the basis of differences in associated symptoms of oxygen toxicity:

1) For $PO_2 = 1500–2000$ mm Hg, central nervous system effects predominate: nausea, dizziness, visual impairments, local or generalized clonic convulsions, and cardiorespiratory pathologies. Wood et al.[120] exposed animals to hyperbaric hyperoxia and detected a drastic increase in blood pressure, probably of neurogenic origin; cardiac insufficiency; and an increase in pressure in pulmonary circulation, which could be a cause for initial damage to lung capillaries and subsequent acute pulmonary edema.

2) For $PO_2 = 400–1500$ mm Hg, oxygen toxicity leads to respiratory problems: irritation of the upper respiratory tract, development of bronchitis, and later pneumonia and pulmo-

nary edema. Hyperoxia, like hypoxia, strongly affects blood-tissue barriers.

3) For $PO_2 = 280$–400 mm Hg, oxygen toxicity may cause changes in the respiratory organs, blood, and lymphoid tissue.[112,116,120–123]

To ensure the safety of manned space missions, it is necessary to determine the maximally acceptable limits of PO_2 to preclude oxygen toxicity in cabin atmospheres. This value can be found through animal and human experiments using different levels of PO_2. Animal studies have shown that exposure to a pure-oxygen environment at normal barometric pressure causes death from pneumonia.

Experiments with white rats, which are highly sensitive to oxygen, have revealed a sequence of morphological changes developing in the lungs after exposure to hyperoxia of different durations. At $PO_2 = 1$ atm, experimental animals exhibit the following symptoms: after 1 h, atelectasis; after 3–6 h, changes in capillary structure and permeability; after the first 24 h, lung edema, enlargement of alveolar membranes, engorgement of capillaries, and diapedetic hemorrhages; after 36 h, marked lung hyperemia and areas of inflammation; after 48–60 h, further development of pneumonia resulting in lung hepatization and death.[123–125]

In hyperoxia, development of atelectasis is associated with damage to the alveolar surfactant, called surfactant-dependent atelectasis.[122] After prolonged (24-day) exposure of rats to 32–37 percent oxygen, a large number of membrane formations of mature surfactant and osmiophilic bodies appeared inside the alveolar lumens, suggesting surfactant disintegration on their surface.[123] One of the potential mechanisms responsible for this is disruption of surfactant synthesis. Another possibility is that oxygen has an indirect effect on the alveolar surfactant—by altering the permeability of the air-blood barrier—causing intra-alveolar edema.[122]

Many authors assume that hyperoxia-induced pneumonia inevitably leads to hypoxia and, finally, to the death of experimental animals.[116] However, Genin et al. detected high oxygen tension in the brains of such animals, although they developed severe hyperoxic toxicosis and pneumonia,[121] suggesting that hypoxia develops only at late stages of oxygen poisoning.

The time of onset of pathological changes in rat lungs is a function of the PO_2 level in the breathing medium. At $PO_2 = 760$ mm Hg (100 percent oxygen), inflammation was seen after 2–3 days from the start of exposure; at $PO_2 = 570$ mm Hg (75 percent oxygen), it was detected only after 2–3 weeks; and, at $PO_2 = 380$–450 mm Hg (50–60 percent oxygen), no lung changes were observed after 30 days of exposure.[124–126] Some researchers have noted that the primary pathological effect of a relatively slight increase of PO_2 is pulmonary atelectasis.

Atelectasis has also developed in humans breathing 100 percent oxygen,[128,129] because of mucous blockage of the smaller bronchial tubes. This causes oxygen to diffuse rapidly from the alveoli of obstructed bronchi into the blood. The rate of alveolar collapse depends on the chemical properties of the gases in them; collapse is very slow in the presence of nitrogen and other inert gases. DuBois et al. attributed the individual differences in susceptibility to atelectasis that they observed in humans to differing patency in the respiratory tract.[129]

These results do not support the conclusion that the development of pulmonary atelectasis is induced by oxygen toxicity. Rather, it should be attributed to the lack of an inert gas in the alveoli. When ambient PO_2 is elevated, the addition of small amounts of a biologically inert gas to the atmosphere prevents pulmonary atelectasis, which as has been demonstrated experimentally.[3,24,112,129,130,133]

In animals, oxygen toxicity may lead to oxidative hemolytic anemia, which develops as a result of accelerated breakdown of red blood cells and simultaneous inhibition of hemopoiesis.

Morphological analyses of the blood of humans and animals exposed to hyperoxia (revealing inhibited erythropoiesis and acanthosis) suggest that damage to the erythrocyte membrane and inhibition of erythropoiesis may result from oxygen toxicity. The administration of antioxidants (e.g., vitamin E and vitamin C) prevents such damage.[131,132,147] These observations seem to be supported by human data; i.e., the peripheral blood of Gemini 4, 5, and 7 astronauts showed a decrease of red blood cells and hemoglobin after flight.[27,134]

Data also suggest that a slight increase in PO_2 (300 mm Hg) leads to immune suppression, producing pathological changes in lymph organs.[135,136]

Despite the establishment of maximum acceptable concentrations of oxygen, the acceptable upper limit of PO_2 in a breathing mixture for long-duration exposures of humans and animals has not yet been determined. Before a hyperoxic atmosphere ($PO_2 = 258$ mm Hg) was accepted for use in spacecraft cabins, U.S. investigators carried out detailed studies of the effects of such atmospheres.[127,137–139] These studies, one of which lasted 8 months, supported a conclusion that exposure to an atmosphere with $PO_2 = 258$ mm Hg did not cause serious pathologies in experimental animals. However, it could not be concluded that the treatment produced no adverse effects, because certain morphological changes were detected in internal organs. The same conclusion was drawn from experiments with mice, in which animals were maintained for 23 days at $PO_2 = 260$–280 mm Hg, with a total pressure of 720 mm Hg, and then were exposed to a hyperbaric environment with 98 percent oxygen at 4 atm. The experimental animals in the hyperbaric environment died significantly more rapidly than did equivalent controls, showing acute hyperemia and pulmonary edema at autopsy.[123]

However, there is also evidence suggesting the possibility of adaptation to hyperoxia. In order to investigate evidence for adaptation in a hyperoxic environment, animals were first exposed to elevated PO_2 and then to nearly pure oxygen at 760 mm Hg for a long period of time. These experiments did not yield unambiguous results. Some authors reported an increase in the longevity of pre-exposed animals, whereas others found no significant effect or even greater toxic effects of

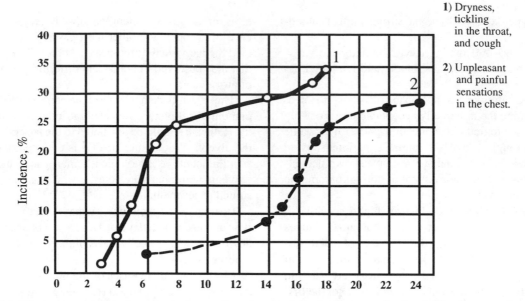

1) Dryness, tickling in the throat, and cough

2) Unpleasant and painful sensations in the chest.

Fig. 12 Time course of various symptoms of oxygen toxicity in humans during 24 h of oxygen breathing (number of complaints expressed as a percentage of number subjects, listed in ascending order).[121]

oxygen in pre-exposed animals. On the other hand, experiments performed on tissue cultures suggest the possibility of adaptation to hyperoxia at a cellular level.[140]

To summarize the data in the literature, it may be concluded that although animals and humans may have some ability to adapt to normobaric hyperoxia, the range of this adaptation is limited.

Information about the toxic effects of hyperoxia on humans is critical from the standpoint of cabin atmosphere design. This important problem cannot be solved easily, because precise criteria for oxygen toxicity at PO_2 as high as 400 mm Hg are lacking. Individual susceptibility to hyperoxia can vary widely and may be modified by other flight factors.

The physiological and pathophysiological mechanisms of hyperoxic effects must be understood if we are to develop adequate criteria for oxygen toxicity. Human responses to hyperoxia are diverse; and some of them should be considered adaptive, since they tend to reduce oxygen transport. These include decreases in pulmonary ventilation, heart rate, and cardiac output, as well as the narrowing of cerebral vessels. Such reactions evolve during the first minutes of hyperoxia.[112,121,141] Some of them, such as lowered heart rate and reduced circulating blood volume, persist for almost the entire period of exposure to elevated PO_2, whereas others gradually disappear.

Many investigators point out that a decline in vital lung capacity in hyperoxia is a significant symptom for early diagnosis of oxygen toxicity. A 20–30 percent or greater decrease in vital capacity undoubtedly is an indicator of the toxic effect of oxygen. However, such marked decreases generally occur either immediately prior to substernal pain or when chest pains are experienced during deep inhalation; i.e., when the clinical oxygen poisoning has already developed.[112,116,121,139] The most common clinical symptoms of oxygen poisoning are cough, dryness in the mouth, or unpleasant or painful sen-

sations in the chest. The occurrence of such symptoms, especially chest pain, has usually been taken as a signal to terminate human experiments. This is because chest pain has continued to increase, followed by intercostal pain, dyspnea, and deterioration of general state.[121,139,141] The mechanism underlying the development of chest pain and substernal discomfort is evidently related to the occurrence of atelectasis and, probably, bronchial spasms. Edema of bronchial mucosa is also likely to be present.

Chest pain is often preceded by irritation of the upper respiratory tract; i.e., dryness in the mouth, tickling sensation in the nasopharynx, and cough; 6–12 h after termination of a study (i.e., removal from the hyperoxic environment), these symptoms disappear completely, as do the chest pains. These symptoms should be taken seriously, since they have been known to precede development of acute tracheobronchitis and pneumonia.[121,142]

In human studies with elevated PO_2 (1 atm), DuBois found significant individual differences in sensitivity to oxygen toxicity.[129] He reported that, under conditions of 24 h of exposure to elevated PO_2, clinical symptoms occurred in only some subjects and the times of onset varied. Figure 12 contains data on the incidence and time of onset of symptoms of upper respiratory irritation and chest pain.[129]

Individual differences in symptoms of oxygen toxicity seem to explain discrepancies in the literature concerning the limits of oxygen tolerance. For instance, Genin et al. detected no symptoms of oxygen toxicity in a 30-day exposure to PO_2 = 290–280 mm Hg,[130] whereas Welch[139] reported pulmonary atelectasis during shorter exposure to PO_2 = 200 mm Hg. Such individual differences in sensitivity to hyperoxia make it difficult to determine the maximally acceptable concentrations of oxygen in cabin atmospheres for long-term space flights.

Figure 13 presents data on the time parameters and nature

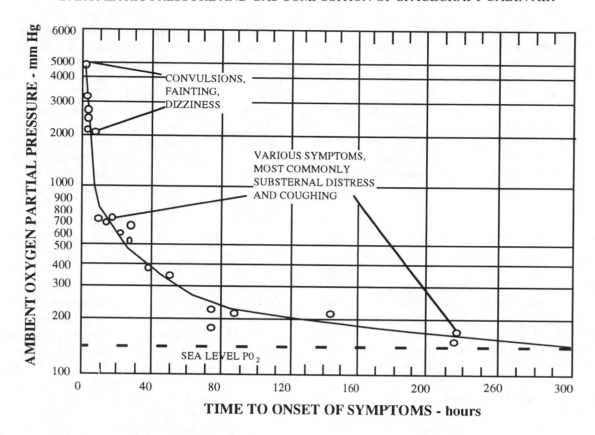

Fig. 13 Time of onset of symptoms of oxygen toxicity as a function of PO_2 in the atmosphere.[25,61,139]

of oxygen toxicity at various PO_2 values in an artificial atmosphere.

Since some individuals are highly sensitive to oxygen toxicity, an atmosphere with PO_2 significantly exceeding that of normal air is hardly suitable for long-term flights. The factors responsible for the large differences in individual sensitivity to hyperoxia have not been studied adequately. We currently possess neither reliable criteria for selecting highly sensitive individuals nor reliable means to increase human tolerance.

The upper limit of acceptable PO_2 in a cabin atmosphere for long-term flights has been decreased repeatedly and, at present, is tentatively set to correspond to 200 mm Hg in alveolar oxygen.

On space flights passing through high-radiation zones or other sources of crew exposure to ionizing radiation, elevated PO_2 would be undesirable. This conclusion is based on the results of the many experiments that demonstrate increased sensitivity of animals to ionizing radiation when exposed to hyperoxia. The above effect is usually explained by the similarity between the effects of hyperoxia and those of ionizing radiation.[68]

To date, the modifying effect of weightlessness on human sensitivity to elevated oxygen concentrations has not been considered. However, there are grounds to assume that weightlessness may modify sensitivity to hyperoxia, because both factors can induce redistribution of blood and circulation.

III. Hypercapnia: Toxic Effects of Carbon Dioxide

In space flight, there is no way to completely preclude emergencies that compromise the efficiency of the air regeneration system. If this occurs, carbon dioxide concentration could increase to a significant level at a variety of rates. Furthermore, it is technically difficult to maintain low carbon dioxide concentrations. Hence, higher than normal carbon dioxide concentrations in cabin air are virtually inevitable.

In a pressurized cabin, humans themselves are the major sources of carbon dioxide, since this gas is one of the main end products of metabolic reactions. At rest, a human produces about 400 liters of carbon dioxide per day; and the rate of generation is even higher during exertion. In addition, carbon dioxide is generated constantly during the processes of fermentation and decay. Carbon dioxide gas is colorless and has a faint odor and sour taste. In spite of these properties, humans cannot detect carbon dioxide at concentrations of several percent, since its smell and taste are only detectable at very high concentrations.

Breslav demonstrated that test subjects who were allowed "free choice" of an atmosphere would reject a gas medium only when its PCO_2 exceeded 23 mm Hg. At this level, their reactions were associated with detectable physiological effects of carbon dioxide—an increase in pulmonary ventilation and a decline of physical work capacity.[143]

The Earth's atmosphere contains a small amount of carbon dioxide (0.03 percent) resulting from the biological and geophysical cycles. A tenfold increase of carbon dioxide in inspired air (0.3 percent) does not have a marked effect on human physiological functions or work capacity.[30,144,145] Humans can live in such an environment for a very long time, maintaining good health and high performance. A substantial increase of PCO_2 in the atmosphere, however, produces changes in the central nervous system, respiration, and circulation, as well as acid-base equilibrium and mineral metabolism. The nature of the changes evoked by hypercapnia is a function of the level of PCO_2 and the duration of exposure.

A. Acute Hypercapnia

The severe pathologies found in animals confined in unventilated environments for long periods of time are induced by elevated carbon dioxide levels. The mechanisms of the physiological and pathological effects of carbon dioxide have been investigated experimentally, primarily using animals.

It should be noted that, during prolonged exposure to PCO_2 = 60–70 mm Hg, physiological responses, especially those of the central nervous system, change drastically; i.e., the stimulating effect of hypercapnia gives way to an inhibitory effect or a narcotic state that develops rapidly at PCO_2 = 100 mm Hg and above.

Hyperventilation is the most important adaptive reaction to hypercapnia. Increased pulmonary ventilation at PCO_2 = 10–15 mm Hg is supported by at least two mechanisms: stimulation of the respiratory center by chemoreceptors of the vascular areas, particularly the carotid sinus; and stimulation of the respiratory center and central chemoreceptors. The efficacy of this reaction diminishes as PCO_2 increases, because P_ACO_2 continues to increase despite the enhancement of pulmonary ventilation.

The stimulating effect of carbon dioxide on the vasomotor center and the sympathetic nervous system induces vasoconstriction and increased peripheral resistance, heart rate, and cardiac output. It also has a direct effect on the walls of blood vessels, fostering dilation. The interaction of these antagonistic effects ultimately determines the reactions of the cardiovascular system to hypercapnia. The state of collapse that has been observed in animals in experiments involving significant increases in carbon dioxide levels can be concluded to result from drastic decreases in the central vasoconstrictive effects of hypercapnia.[152]

At high PCO_2, narcosis develops, followed by a pronounced decrease in metabolism. This response can be viewed as adaptive, because it leads to a strong decrease of carbon dioxide production in a situation where the transport and buffer systems of the blood can no longer sustain P_ACO_2, the most important constant of the internal milieu, at a near-normal level.

Human physiological reactions to various levels of PCO_2 in inspired air have been studied in detail.[146–148] During relatively short-term exposure to PCO_2 > 10 mm Hg, no serious physiological changes occur, despite slight respiratory acidosis. Human subjects exposed to this environment for several days maintain a normal mental capacity and voice no complaints about indisposition. At PCO_2 = 15 mm Hg, some subjects report a decline of physical performance, especially at heavy levels of exertion. At PCO_2 = 20–30 mm Hg, subjects display respiratory acidosis and increased pulmonary ventilation. A relatively short-lived improvement on rate of mental task completion is followed by deterioration of performance. Physical work capacity declines markedly. Subjects also exhibit sleep disturbances, headaches, dizziness, dyspnea, and a sensation of lack of air during strenuous exercise.

At PCO_2 = 35–40 mm Hg, subjects show a threefold increase in pulmonary ventilation, tachycardia, and a rise in blood pressure. Even after brief exposure, they complain of headaches, dizziness, visual impairment, loss of spatial orientation, fatigue, and acute dyspnea when performing light physical exercise. They also show deterioration of mental work capacity, as measured by test performance.

At PCO_2 = 45–50 mm Hg, acute hypercapnia-induced disorders develop very rapidly; i.e., within 10–15 min.[26,128,148]

Human tolerance to hypercapnia is also a function of the rate at which PCO_2 increases. When placed in a cabin atmosphere with a high PCO_2 or given a carbon-dioxide-enriched breathing mixture, humans experience a rapid rise of P_ACO_2 and acute hypercapnic disorders that develop much faster than with slow increases in PCO_2. Because of the large cabin volume in space flight, PCO_2 increases are likely to be slow if they result from a malfunction in the air regeneration system. However, if a similar malfunction occurs in the air regeneration system of a space suit, the resulting PCO_2 increase will be rapid.

When the ranges of PCO_2 associated with qualitatively different manifestations of carbon dioxide toxicity are delineated, it is important to take into consideration that there is a stage of "initial adaptation," the duration of which increases with carbon dioxide concentration.[146]

Levels of human endurance at various concentrations of PCO_2 are shown in Fig. 14.

It has been established that human tolerance to carbon dioxide toxicity declines as physical exertion increases. Therefore, it is important to understand carbon dioxide toxicity at various levels of exercise. Unfortunately, there is little relevant information in the literature, and the issue is in need of further study. Nonetheless, based on the available data,[26,30,56,144,146,148] it is possible to provide an approximate idea of the duration and level of exercise that can be performed by humans as a function of PCO_2. These data are summarized in Table 3.

The best way to eliminate the adverse effects of acute hypercapnia is to return the patient to normal air. However, many experiments have shown that rapid transfer of subjects long exposed to increased PCO_2 to a pure-oxygen or air atmosphere often results in a deterioration of their general state. This phenomenon was first observed in animal experiments by Albitskiy,[149] who termed it the "CO_2 reverse effect." Pa-

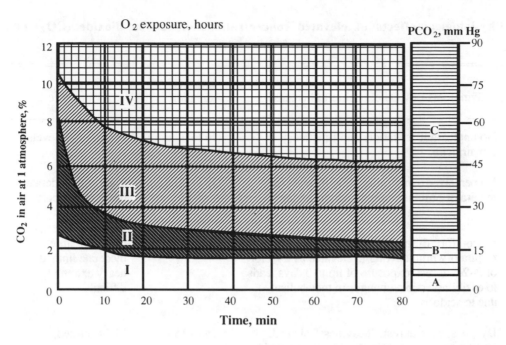

I) No effect
II) Minor perceptive change
III) Distracting discomfort
IV) Severe disorders, loss of consciousness

A =0.5% CO_2; no effects
B = 0.5 to 3.0% CO_2 adaptive biochemical changes noted
C >3.0% CO_2 pathological changes noted

Fig. 14 Symptoms common to most subjects exposed for various times to CO_2 air mixtures at 1 atmosphere. (Reproduced from: King, B.G., High concentration, short-time exposures and toxicity. *Journal of Industrial Hygienic Toxicology*, 1949, vol. 31, pp. 365-375.)

tients developing the hypercapnic syndrome should be removed from the carbon-dioxide-enriched medium slowly.[26,14,144] Attempts to counteract the hypercapnic syndrome by using Tris-buffer, soda, or other alkalis were found to partially normalize blood pH but failed to produce a stable improvement.[26]

Of practical importance is the study of the general state and work capacity of humans in response to a simultaneous decrease of PO_2 and increase of PCO_2, such as would be caused by a failure of the air regeneration system.

Haldane and Priestley[30] found that a high rate of increase of carbon dioxide and a corresponding rate of decrease of oxygen in a small enclosed environment led to a drastic decline in physiological status. This occurred at CO_2 = 5–6 percent in the breathing mixture (PCO_2 = 38–45 mm Hg), even though the absolute decrease in oxygen was small and in itself would not have induced significant problems. When hypercapnia and hypoxia develop slowly, physiological status and work capacity begin to decline significantly at PCO_2 = 25–30 mm Hg and PO_2 = 110–120 mm Hg. According to data presented in a review by Roth,[61] subjects' performance declined considerably as a result of a 3-day exposure to an atmosphere containing 3 percent carbon dioxide (22.8 mm Hg) and 17 percent oxygen. These observations are inconsistent with data indicating only slight changes in performance in response to significant variations of oxygen (12 percent

decrease) and carbon dioxide (3 percent increase).[107]

When hypercapnia and hypoxia develop simultaneously, the main symptom of their toxic effect is dyspnea. Marked increase in pulmonary ventilation results from the elevation of carbon dioxide sensitivity of the respiratory center associated with hypoxia; thus, the effects of excess carbon dioxide and deficient oxygen should potentiate each other. The fact that the combined effects of diminished P_AO_2 and elevated P_ACO_2 on pulmonary ventilation are synergistic suggests that this is the case.

B. Chronic Effects of Hypercapnia

Study of the effects of prolonged exposure to elevated levels of PCO_2 in humans and animals suggests that clinical symptoms of chronic carbon dioxide toxicity are preceded by regular changes in acid-base equilibrium, specifically respiratory acidosis leading to metabolic disorders. This is followed by shifts in mineral metabolism, which appear to be adaptive, since acid-base equilibrium is maintained. These changes are reflected in variations in calcium levels in the blood and in levels of calcium and phosphorus in bone. As P_ACO_2 increases, the amount of carbon-dioxide-bound calcium in bone increases. Shifts in mineral metabolism facilitate renal calculus formation. This is confirmed by rodent studies in which kidney stones were detected after prolonged

Table 3 **Physiological effects of elevated concentrations of carbon dioxide (CO_2) in an artificial atmosphere**

PCO_2, mm Hg	Symptoms of CO_2 exposure in humans	Exposure duration	Exercise performance	Mental performance
Up to 7.5	No unpleasant sensations, no functional impairments	Up to 3–4 months	Possible (all levels)	Possible
Up to 15	No perceived symptoms; some increase in respiratory minute volume; slight acidosis	Up to 30 days	Light and moderate; heavy is difficult	Possible
Up to 25–30	Discomfort; dyspnea, especially on exertion; respiratory minute volume elevated by a factor of 2–2.5 at rest; exposure of up to 3 days leads to easily reversible changes in metabolism due to acidosis	Up to 7 days	Light possible; moderate limited; heavy extremely difficult	Possible, if well-learned
Up to 35–40	Dyspnea, even at rest, "heaviness" of head, vertigo; respiratory minute volume elevated by a factor of 3–4; parameters of cardiovascular function relatively stable; respiratory acidosis; impaired cerebral functioning; sleep disorders	Up to 15 h	Light limited; moderate extremely difficult	Limited, even for familiar tasks
Up to 50	Dyspnea, headache, vertigo, visual impairments, sleep disorders; respiratory minute volume elevated by a factor of 4–5, respiratory acidosis; marked changes in cardiovascular function; tachycardia, elevated blood pressure; disruption of central nervous system function	Up to 3–4 h	Light difficult, moderate and heavy impossible	Difficult
Up to 60	Drastic worsening of symptoms	Up to 1 h	All types impossible	Impossible
Over 60 (but no greater than 75)	Drastic worsening of symptoms	–	Precluded	Precluded

exposure to PCO_2 = 21 mm Hg.[150]

Metabolic changes produced by moderate gas acidosis were noted in humans exposed to PCO_2 exceeding 7.5–10 mm Hg for a long period of time, although these subjects maintained good health and high performance.

During "Operation Hideout," subjects spent 42 days in a submarine with an atmosphere containing 1.5 percent carbon dioxide (PCO_2 = 11.4 mm Hg). Their vital signs and weight remained essentially unchanged. However, their respiration, acid-base equilibrium, and calcium and phosphorus metabolism showed adaptive variations. Blood and urine pH measurements showed that, from day 24 of their exposure to 1.5 percent carbon dioxide, the subjects developed uncompensated gas acidosis.[145] Young male subjects who remained for 30 days at 1 percent carbon dioxide displayed no changes in blood pH despite a slight increase in P_ACO_2 and an 8–10 percent increase in pulmonary ventilation, which indicated slight, compensated gas acidosis.[105]

Exposure of subjects for 30 days to 2 percent carbon dioxide led to pH decreases, P_ACO_2 increases, and 20–25 percent enhancements of pulmonary ventilation. The subjects felt well when at rest, but some complained of headaches and rapid development of fatigue when they exercised strenuously.[105]

In a 3 percent carbon dioxide atmosphere (PCO_2 = 22.8 mm Hg), most subjects reported deterioration of their general state. Blood pH changes suggested rapid development of uncompensated gas acidosis. Although it is possible to remain in such an environment for many days, there will always be discomfort and a progressive decline in work capacity.

From these studies, it was inferred that prolonged exposure (many months) of humans to PCO_2 exceeding 7.5 mm

Hg is highly undesirable because of chronic carbon dioxide toxicity.[105]

Evaluating the effects of chronic hypercapnia, we follow Schaeffer,[148] who believes it is useful to distinguish three main levels of increased PCO_2 associated with different human responses to hypercapnia.

1) When $PCO_2 = 4$–6 mm Hg, no notable physiological effects on humans are apparent.

2) When $PCO_2 = 11$ mm Hg, vital physiological functions do not undergo serious changes; however, respiration responses, acid-base equilibrium, and electrolyte balance do change slowly, and pathological shifts are possible.

3) When $PCO_2 = 22$ mm Hg and higher, results include decline in performance, pronounced physiological changes, and acute pathologies developing after different time intervals.

Thus, PCO_2 in space cabins, submarines, and other vehicles where humans are confined for long periods of time should not be exceed 4 mm Hg and can be allowed to increase only for very short intervals (see Table 3).

IV. Artificial Atmospheres

It is generally believed that the idea of generating an artificial atmosphere to protect man in high-altitude flights and underwater diving was first advanced by the famous French science-fiction writer, Jules Verne. Without trying to detract from Verne's reputation, it should be noted that the first truly scientific treatments of this idea were presented by the French physiologist, Paul Bert,[86] and the Russian chemist, D. I. Mendeleyev,[151] who were the first to propose the use of pressurized cabins with air pressure higher than ambient pressure in high-altitude flights. Later and independently, K. E. Tsiolkovskiy[152] justified the need for an artificial atmosphere in spacecraft cabins.

This idea found practical implementation in the design of a flying vehicle cabin in the early 1930s, when (first in Switzerland, and then in the U.S.S.R. and United States) stratonauts made balloon flights to altitudes of 15,500–22,000 m. On May 27, 1931, two Swiss stratonauts, A. Piccard and M. Kinfer, reached an altitude of 15,780 m; and, in 1933, Soviet stratonauts, G. A. Prokofiev, E. K. Birnbaum, and K. D. Godunov, reached an altitude of 19,000 m flying the SSSR-1 balloon. In 1934, P. F. Fedoseyenko, A. B. Vasenko, and I. D. Usyskin, ascended to an altitude of 22,000 m on a balloon, but died during the descent.

In preparing for these flights, scientists tested different types of atmosphere and conducted human experiments in cabin simulators.[3,45,105] These studies furnished important data, not only about methods of atmosphere regeneration but also about such physiological parameters as oxygen consumption and carbon dioxide production by crewmembers.

It is noteworthy that U.S.S.R. and U.S. investigators drew similar conclusions from their studies. They decided to reduce the weight of a stratospheric balloon to maintain cabin pressure at 550–450 mm Hg, and to increase the oxygen concentration to ensure normal PO_2. At that time, both U.S.S.R. and U.S. researchers rejected the idea of using pure oxygen or liquid oxygen because of the high risk of fire.[29,45,74,109]

The short duration of stratospheric balloon flights (no more than several hours) greatly simplified the solution to this problem. For space flights, particularly long-term flights, the solution was much more difficult. However, the above efforts should be noted, since they were the first to produce useful information.

A. Normobaric and Hypobaric Atmospheres

The simplest approach to developing atmospheres for early spacecraft was to reproduce the Earth's atmosphere at sea level (total pressure = 760 mm Hg, $PO_2 = 160$ mm Hg, and $PCO_2 < 4$ mm Hg). It was not necessary to carry out any special studies of the physiological effects of prolonged confinement in such an atmosphere.

However, reproduction of the Earth's normal atmosphere cannot be considered ideal for missions of different types because of its obvious disadvantages: 1) High partial pressure of nitrogen (500 mm Hg) requires extended denitrogenation to prevent altitude decompression sickness prior to EVA operations in a space suit with pressure = 0.3–0.4 atm; 2) High cabin pressure = 1 atm requires thick cabin walls, which may increase the launch weight of the spacecraft; 3) At a pressure of 1 atm, gas leakage from the cabin may be much higher than at a lower pressure (this is especially important during the opening and closing of airlocks); and 4) High gas density increases the power requirements for cabin ventilating fans.

An alternative to a terrestrial atmosphere is a one-component oxygen medium with pressure intermediate between normoxia and that which causes the appearance of the initial symptoms of hypoxia (200–250 mm Hg). Both alternatives ensure normal gas exchange; do not stress adaptive mechanisms; and, thus, do not deplete the adaptive reserves of the human body.[29,153] Since both alternatives have disadvantages, scientists and engineers are continuing their efforts to develop optimal solutions for different spacecraft and flight profiles.

Many U.S.S.R. and U.S. authors have noted that a compromise, a two-component atmosphere equivalent to normal air in gas composition, but with lower barometric pressure and higher concentration of oxygen, can frequently be used in spacecraft cabins.[73,74,128,154]

In our discussion of two-component oxygen and nitrogen atmospheres, we will consider only four levels of reduced pressure: 526, 405, 308, and 267 mm Hg, which correspond to altitudes of 3000, 5000, 7000, and 8000 m, respectively.

Ivanov et al. tested three of the above levels—526, 405, and 308 mm Hg—in laboratory experiments.[155] They did not study lower pressures because 1) there is a risk of altitude decompression sickness after transfer to this pressure, starting at 7500–8000 m; and 2) there is an increased risk of fire in atmospheres with higher percentages of oxygen.

These studies showed that a 30-day exposure to an atmosphere with oxygen content equivalent to normal air, at a pressure corresponding to an altitude of 3000–7000 m, produced no adverse effect on humans. All three of the atmosphere variants studied proved physiologically equivalent. Physiological changes observed in subjects (e.g., 10–15 percent decline in oxygen consumption; increase of heart rate, especially during stand tests; diurnal variations in the EEG frequency spectrum and an increased number of slow waves in the daytime) were independent of atmospheric composition and pressure and were induced by hypokinesia and changes in the work, rest, and sleep schedules.

This line of research was continued by Kuznetsov et al.,[156] who studied human subjects exposed to a total pressure of 308 mm Hg for 2 months. The physiological changes displayed by these subjects were attributable solely to hypokinesia.

It is not surprising that U.S. and U.S.S.R. scientists have devoted considerable attention to artificial atmospheres with a total pressure of about 300 mm Hg.[73,155,156] Some authors maintain that this pressure is optimal because it is high enough to prevent altitude decompression sickness, thus eliminating the need for denitrogenation for oxygen-nitrogen atmospheres. This pressure level is also desirable when a low-pressure space suit is used because, again, it precludes altitude decompression sickness, which could arise in rare cases of accidental depressurization during the first hours of flight. From an engineering point of view, the use of a two-component atmosphere with a pressure of 300 mm Hg is desirable, since it allows reductions in cabin weight and fire risk (see Table 4).

Now, let us consider artificial atmospheres with a total pressure of 260 mm Hg. It is noteworthy that, as early as 1940, Spasskiy recommended such atmospheres for high-altitude aircraft.[157] Since the differences between this atmosphere and one at 308 mm Hg are slight, we will not consider them in detail here. We will note only that an atmosphere at 260 mm Hg has some slight, primarily technical advantages compared to one at 308 mm Hg, but these cannot compensate for its disadvantages. At 260 mm Hg, there is a high probability of altitude decompression sickness and a reduction in time of useful consciousness if there is leakage of gas from the cabin.

The potential use of helium-oxygen (heliox) atmospheres is worthy of discussion. Before considering the advantages and disadvantages of replacing nitrogen with helium, we must determine whether nitrogen is required in an artificial atmosphere and whether it is of any biological significance, since animals and humans have adapted to it in the course of their evolution.

At present, there is a large body of data indicating that animals and humans can live normally in a nitrogen-free atmosphere.[158–162] It appears that the physiological function of nitrogen is to fill the cavities in the human body—primarily the lungs—to maintain their volume and prevent atelectasis. Evidently, other inert gases, including helium, can also fulfill this function.[13,161,163]

There is evidence that helium has no adverse physiologi-

cal effects on animals or humans and, therefore, can be used as a component of an artificial atmosphere. Physiological studies of humans and animals exposed to an atmosphere in which helium replaced nitrogen at normal and elevated pressures have demonstrated that helium has no toxic effects and proved it, like nitrogen, to be a biologically inert gas.[161,163–166] It should be mentioned here that Epperson et al.[166] noted higher oxygen intake, lower red-blood-cell count and hemoglobin level, and a related increase of iron consumption by rats in a heliox environment. Dianov[167] described changes in the resistance of animals to hypoxia in a heliox atmosphere. These physiological changes are associated with the thermal and physical properties of helium.

Having proved that helium can replace nitrogen in an atmosphere, we must determine how desirable such a replacement is. Those who favor this substitution argue that helium decreases the probability of altitude decompression sickness and particularly its severe forms, which may develop after exposure to a low barometric pressure environment. This is associated with the fact that the Bunsen coefficient of solubility in fat is approximately four times higher for nitrogen than for helium.

In addition, washout time for helium is much shorter than for nitrogen because of the low solubility of helium and its high coefficient of diffusion. However, as we have already noted, U.S. authors[60] have reported a higher incidence of the joint-pain form of decompression sickness in a heliox atmosphere, although incidence of severe forms of altitude decompression sickness in this atmosphere has not been determined. A heliox atmosphere probably would be associated with increased tolerance of hypercapnia, strenuous exercise, and other factors significantly increasing pulmonary ventilation. This is because, during forced inhalation, resistance in the respiratory tract is lower in the heliox mixture than in normal air due to the low density of helium. In normal respiration at rest, this effect is virtually undetected, since resistance in the respiratory tract is mainly a function of gas viscosity, and the viscosities of helium and nitrogen are not effectively different at low pressures.[167,168]

One of the arguments in favor of substituting helium for nitrogen is the high resistance of helium atoms to different forms of radiation, including cosmic radiation. Furthermore, when helium is used, no secondary radiation occurs. In an oxygen-nitrogen atmosphere, ionizing radiation may induce the formation of excited nitrogen atoms and ions. These react with oxygen to produce toxic compounds; e.g., nitric oxide, nitrous oxide, and nitrogen dioxide. Heliox mixtures also have the technical advantage that the density of helium is approximately one-seventh the density of nitrogen, so that the use of heliox mixtures in space cabins reduces launch weight and the weight of gas stores for replenishment of escaped gas. However, this advantage of heliox mixtures is not always fully realized because of the high fluidity of helium. This causes the reserve time associated with gas leakage to be shorter for a heliox atmosphere, which is certainly a disadvantage of replacing nitrogen with helium. Another point is that the use of

Table 4 Comparative evaluation of artificial atmosphere variants[23,61,73,156]

Symptoms	P=760 mm Hg O2=21% N2=79%	P=760 mm Hg O2=21% He=79%	P=405 mm Hg O2=42% N2=59%	P=405 mm Hg O2=42% He=43%	P=308 mm Hg O2=57% N2=43%	P=308 mm Hg O2=100% He=43%	P=258 mm Hg O2=100%	P=258 mm Hg O2=100%
Adverse effects: atelectasis of the lungs, hemolysis of erythrocytes, etc.	−	−	−	−	−	−	±	±
Risk of altitude decompression sickness:								
a) At launch	−	−	±	±	−	−	+	+++
b) In flight, using suits with pressure (170–250 mm Hg)	+++	+++	±	±	−	−	−	−
Need for washout of inert gas								
a) At launch	+++	+++	±	±	−	−	+	+++
b) In flight on EVAs	−	−	−	−	−	−	+	+++
c) Prebreathing time	6–8 h	2–3 h	?	?	−	−	4 h	6–8 h
Risk of injury from explosive decompression	++++	+++	++	++	+	+	+	+
Risk during gas escape from cabin (time of useful consciousness)	±	++	+	+++	++	++++	+++	++++
Risk of fire and explosion	±	±	+	+	++	++	++++	+++
a) Generation of toxic by-products	+	−	++	−	+	−	−	−
b) Rate of combustion of tissues and plastic	±	+	+	+	++	+++	++++	+++
Weight of atmosphere weight and power of fan	++++	+++	+++	++	++	+	+	−

Key: −, none; ±, very slight; +, slight; ++, moderate; +++, high; ++++, very high.

helium instead of nitrogen saves power required for cabin ventilation. In spite of the advantages of heliox mixtures, there are relatively few experimental studies on the effects of such mixtures on humans.

Dianov[162,167] investigated heliox mixtures at normal barometric pressure (1 atm). He did not find any significant changes in the health status, behavior, or work capacity of his subjects. However, replacement of nitrogen with helium induced changes in heat exchange, speech, and respiration. Temperatures that are comfortable in normal air (18–24 °C) were perceived as cold in the heliox atmosphere. For example, at 21°C in the heliox mixture, the subjects rapidly began to feel unpleasantly cool. The weighted mean skin temperature dropped by almost 2° C within 2 h. In the heliox mixture, the zone of thermal comfort was displaced in the direction of higher temperatures and fell between 24.5 and 27.5 °C in the daytime. It should be noted here that, in the heliox mixture, the thermally comfortable zone was narrowed (by 3 °C) compared to normal air. This effect is related to the high thermal conductivity of helium.[167,169,171]

The use of helium in the atmosphere alters human speech. The spectrum shifts by about 0.7 octave in the direction of high frequencies. Speech intelligibility deteriorates but returns to normal immediately after transition to normal air. Computations show that the speed of sound propagation in a heliox mixture at a pressure of 1 atm and a temperature of 27°C is 1.85 times greater than in air, and this is what causes speech distortions in a heliox atmosphere.[170]

Respiratory changes occurring in a heliox atmosphere include an increase in maximum pulmonary ventilation[167,168] because of diminished resistance in the respiratory tract.

Thus, experimental results in which nitrogen was replaced by helium suggest that the use of a heliox mixture is practical.

U.S. scientists have conducted experimental studies of heliox atmospheres with total pressures of 258, 360, and 380 mm Hg.[163,164,166,169,171] Results suggest that prolonged confinement (up to 56 days) in a heliox atmosphere has no adverse effects on metabolism, respiration, circulation, or functioning of the central nervous system. The pathological changes that were observed were attributed to factors other than helium. For instance, Zeft et al.[169] observed conjunctivitis caused by the low moisture level in the atmosphere (at 380 mm Hg), and this problem disappeared when humidity was increased. One subject also suffered from orthostatic intolerance that was, as in most confinement studies, produced by hypokinesia.

Dryness of the mucous membranes and conjunctivitis observed during a 56-day exposure to a heliox atmosphere at a total pressure of 258 mm Hg ($PO_2 = 175$ mm Hg, partial pressure of helium $PHe = 74$ mm Hg, and partial pressure of nitrogen $PN_2 = 2$ mm Hg) were produced by low humidity.[169] Subjects also reported abdominal pain and flatulence, which should be attributed to factors other than helium, possibly a poor diet. Only speech distortion and skin temperature changes during exercise were associated with helium. However, these effects are not very significant, since speech distortions can be eliminated easily by using technical devices, and unpleasant thermal sensations can be remedied by raising the ambient temperature.

In conclusion, it should be said that, whereas the advantages of using heliox mixtures for deep sea diving have been demonstrated, it has yet to be established whether such cabin atmospheres should be recommended for space flights.

U.S. and U.S.S.R. scientists have demonstrated that it would be possible for humans to live in a nearly pure-oxygen atmosphere (with $PN_2 < 10$ mm Hg), at a pressure of 190–200 mm Hg for long periods of time[137,138,144,168] These works showed that experimental animals exposed to a one-component atmosphere with the oxygen equivalent to normal air developed pulmonary atelectasis. This pathology caused the death of some mice during the first 48 h of exposure, although most animals tolerated the entire 59-day exposure without any physiological or behavioral changes.[168]

The effect on the human body of a one-component atmosphere at a total pressure of 190–200 mm Hg has been investigated by U.S. and U.S.S.R. researchers.[130,139,172] These works established that, whereas a pure-oxygen atmosphere can be used if necessary, breathing this atmosphere may induce adverse effects. For example, Welch et al.[139] reported that, with ambient $PO_2 = 176$ mm Hg, chest pain developed in one subject, which could have been associated with lung atelectasis. (The painful sensations disappeared when pressure was increased.) Several developed ear atelectasis, and all showed symptoms of dehydration.

Morgan et al.[138] detected rale in six subjects, joint pain in one, and a slight (to 90 percent baseline) decrease in $P_{A}O_2$ in two test subjects.

In another study,[23] subjects showed good tolerance of a 30-day exposure to an oxygen atmosphere (with nitrogen = 5–10 percent), maintaining high mental and physical work capacity. This may have been attributable to regular exercise and the fact that nitrogen content was higher than in the Welch study.[139,172] This study also revealed some disadvantages of a pure-oxygen environment, particularly the necessity of extended denitrogenation before the experiment began. In nearly all cases, when the period devoted to denitrogenation was shorter than 3 h, subjects developed symptoms of altitude decompression sickness.

In summary, studies with humans have shown that a nearly pure-oxygen atmosphere with total pressure of 200 mm Hg can be used in space, provided that precautions are taken (i.e., oxygen prebreathing prior to transfer to this atmosphere, the use of exercise to prevent lung atelectasis, and fire safety measures).

From an engineering perspective, a one-component atmosphere is advantageous because it simplifies and increases the reliability of life support system regulation and decreases the weight of both the air regeneration system and the cabin. In addition, because the low pressure in the cabin decreases the risk of altitude decompression sickness, this atmosphere allows the use of a low-pressure space suit in emergencies.

Table 5 Pressure and gas composition of AGA in U.S. and U.S.S.R. space cabins

Spacecraft	Pressure		Oxygen, percent	Nitrogen, percent
	mm Hg	psi		
Vostok, Voskhod	760	14.7	19–32	66–78
Soyuz, Salyut, and Mir	(730–890)			
Mercury	258	5.0	100	
Gemini	258	5.0	100	
Apollo (command and lunar modules)	258	5.0	100	
Skylab	258	5.0	70	30
Space Shuttle and Spacelab	760	14.7	21	79
Apollo-Soyuz Test Project				
Soyuz-19	760	14.7		
During transfer	520–30		35–40	
In special Apollo tunnel	258	5.0		

Nevertheless, there are serious disadvantages associated with a pure-oxygen atmosphere. The most important of these is the high risk of fire associated with the high concentration of oxygen and the absence of diluent gases (nitrogen, helium, or neon), that reduce the combustion rate of various materials. Increased fire hazard limits the choice of construction materials and requires stringent fire safety measures.

All the factors described above made the selection of an atmosphere for early spacecraft very difficult. The cabins of the U.S. Mercury, Gemini, and Apollo were supplied with pure oxygen at a pressure of 260 mm Hg.

In the U.S.S.R., the possibility of using a cabin atmosphere with a total pressure of 400 mm Hg, $PO_2 = 160$ mm Hg, and $PN_2 = 240$ mm Hg was considered for the Vostok. However, it was concluded that, given the design of the Vostok cabin, such an atmosphere had no significant advantages over a normal atmosphere with 21 percent oxygen, which was ultimately adopted. This decision was based primarily on the desire to reduce fire hazard. It was greatly influenced by a tragic accident in February 1961, occurring while a candidate cosmonaut, Bondarenko, was in a barochamber with diminished pressure and high oxygen level. An ethanol-soaked cloth caught fire, which immediately spread throughout the cabin, causing fatal burns. As a result, Soviet researchers selected a cabin atmosphere that, in its major parameters (i.e., pressure and gas composition), was close to normal air.

In the United States, a single-component, pure-oxygen atmosphere, at a pressure of 258 mm Hg, was used for more than 20 yr. The use of this atmosphere led to a great tragedy: three U.S. astronauts—V. Grissom, E. White, and R. Chaffee—died on January 27, 1967, as a result of a fire during an Apollo training exercise.

This tragedy led U.S. experts to abandon the use of pure oxygen in spacecraft cabins. Nevertheless, it is widely used in EVA suits and can be recommended for use in situations where there is no danger of fire. However, the artificial atmospheres used in existing spacecraft and space stations and those designed for use in the near future are composed of two gases (nitrogen and oxygen) at normobaric pressure.

The major data concerning the pressure and composition of the atmospheres of U.S. and U.S.S.R. spacecraft are presented in Table 5.

B. Active Artificial Atmospheres

When considering various types of artificial atmospheres, most researchers have agreed that the more biologically inert they are, the better. This point of view is not without its critics. Opponents assert that a cabin atmosphere that could stimulate adaptive responses to the adverse effects of extended flights would prevent deconditioning in cosmonauts on long-term flights. Such an atmosphere is referred to as active.[3,24,173]

It is very important to note that, in almost all studies of extended exposure to an artificial atmosphere, regardless of what variant was used, deconditioning resulting from diminished motor activity has been observed. Such deconditioning included reduced performance capacity and orthostatic tolerance, as well as diminished tolerance of acceleration, hypoxic hypoxia, and other effects.[130,154,155,175] It should be added here that, on long-term space flights, the adverse effects of reduced activity can be expected to be aggravated by microgravity. This is confirmed by the results of water immersion and bedrest studies, which simulate the physiological effects of microgravity. Subjects in these experiments show significant disruptions of circulation, declines in orthostatic tolerance, impairment of motor control, and changes in the musculoskeletal system and in protein and mineral metabolism.

In light of these results, Soviet[154,174,175] and U.S.[173,176] authors have advanced the idea of using a controlled atmosphere to prevent deconditioning on extended space flights. Lamb[173] demonstrated that the biochemical and physiological changes developing during adaptation to moderate hypoxic hypoxia would ameliorate certain negative effects of microgravity. This led him to propose a hypoxic cabin atmosphere, and this idea was implemented in studies by Lynch et al.[176] and Stevens et al.,[177] who exposed subjects undergoing bed rest to two schedules of increasing hypoxia.

Soviet scientists also conducted barochamber studies on subjects undergoing bedrest. They showed that 6 h of daily conditioning involving ascents to increasing altitudes of 2500–4500 m alleviated symptoms characteristic of hypokinesia, although the hypoxia itself did evoke short-term discomfort. In particular, this conditioning prevented decreases in tolerance to acceleration and slightly increased tolerance to acute hypoxia. It was postulated that deconditioning can be prevented by using a cabin atmosphere with a gas composition that varies cyclically. This hypothesis was advanced because exposure to such an atmosphere should not produce stable adaptation to an altered gas environment. At the same time, the composition of the atmosphere could be selected in such a way as to increase performance capacity. It should also be noted that an atmosphere of this type may, in the future, prove useful for maintaining the normal biological rhythms of physiological responses, especially on long-term flights.[174]

Cabin atmospheres with nonstationary barometric pressure and gas composition may be important on future manned space flights. Thus, it is critical to develop programs that determine how levels of atmospheric parameters should vary as a function of flight profile.

The first step in this direction involves a procedure for modifying atmospheric parameters prior to EVAs by Space Shuttle astronauts. This procedure stipulates that 24 h before EVA, the cabin barometric pressure should be decreased gradually from 760–528 mm Hg to prevent altitude decompression sickness. At the same time, the atmosphere is enriched with oxygen to 27 percent as the nitrogen content is diminished to maintain normal respiration. After 24 h at 528 mm Hg, astronauts breath pure oxygen for 40 min before EVA to provide additional denitrogenation. Crewmembers perform EVA in space suits with a low pressure of 222 mm Hg.

In conclusion, space missions of many months to many years in duration impose new requirements on the quality of cabin atmospheres. In the future, we will need to evaluate atmospheric quality using not only traditional physiological and hygienic parameters but also long-term biological parameters that reveal the effects of the atmosphere on longevity, aging rate, reproductive capability, etc.

References

[1]Armstrong, H.G. Aerospace Medicine, Baltimore, Williams & Wilkins, 1961.

[2]Violette, F. *Étude Experimentale at Théorique de la Décompression Explosive et de ses Effets Physiologiques.* Paris, Serv. Doc. Inf. Tech. Aeronaut. (France, Min. de L'Air. Bull. Serv. Tech., No. 118), 1955.

[3]Malkin, V.B. Barometric pressure, gas composition. In: Calvin, M., and Gazenko, O.G., Eds. *Foundations of Space Biology and Medicine.* Washington, D.C., NASA, vol. II, book 1, 1975, pp. 3–64 (in Russian).

[4]Pozhariyskiy, F.I.; Rozenblyum, D.Ye.; and Khazen, I.M. Analysis of changes in the respiration and circulatory functions during rapid shifts of atmospheric pressure. In: *Abstracts of Papers presented at a Conference on the Physiology and Pathology of Respiration, Hypo- and Hyperoxia, and Oxygen Therapy.* Moscow, 1935 (in Russian).

[5]Hitchcock, F.A. Physiological and pathological effects of explosive decompression. *Journal of Aviation Medicine,* 1954, vol. 25, pp. 578–586.

[6]Kemph, J.P.; Burch, B.H.; Beman, F.M.; and Hitchcock, F.A. Further observations on dogs explosively decompressed to an ambient pressure of 30 mm Hg. *Journal of Aviation Medicine,* 1954, vol. 25, no. 2, pp. 107–112.

[7]Kolder, H.J., and Stockinger, L. Small structural changes in the lungs after explosive decompression and compression. *Arch. Pathol. Pharmakol.,* 1957, vol. 231, pp. 23–33 (in German).

[8]Lyle, C.B., Jr., and Dahl, E.V. Protection of rapidly decompressed rats by pharmacologic and physical means. *American Journal of Physiology,* 1961, vol. 201, no. 5, pp. 759–761.

[9]Sweeney, H.M. Explosive decompression. *Air Surgeon's Bulletin,* 1944, vol. 1, pp. 1–4.

[10]Vail, E.G. Forces produced in the thorax by explosive decompression. *Journal of Aviation Medicine,* 1952, vol. 23, no. 6, pp. 577–583.

[11]Adams, B.H., and Polak, I.B. Traumatic lung lesions produced in dogs by simulating submarine escape. *U.S. Naval Medicine Bulletin,* 1933, vol. 31, pp. 18–20.

[12]Benzinger, T. Explosive decompression. In: USAF Surgeon General. *German Aviation Medicine in World War II.* Washington, D.C., U.S. Government Printing Office, 1950, vol. 1, pp. 395–408.

[13]Roth, E.M. Selection of space cabin atmospheres. *Space Sciences Review,* 1967, vol. 6, no. 2, pp. 452–492.

[14]Roth, E.M., Ed. Compendium of human responses to the aerospace environment, vols. I, II, III, IV (NASA-CR-1205). Washington, D.C., NASA, 1968.

[15]Luft, U.C. Physiological aspects of pressure cabins and rapid decompression. In: Booth, W., Ed. *Handbook of Respiratory Physiology.* Brooks AFB, Texas, USAF School of Aviation Medicine, 1954.

[16]Luft, U.C. Principles of adaptation to altitude. In: Yousef, M.K.; Horvath, S.M.; and Bullard, R.W., Eds. *Physiological Adaptations. Desert and Mountain.* New York and

London, Academic Press, 1972, p. 143.

[17]Fryer, D., and Roxburgh, H.L. Decompression Sickness. In: Gillies, J.A., Ed. *A Textbook of Aviation Physiology*. Oxford, Pergamon Press, 1965, pp. 122–151.

[18]Boyle, J. Theoretical trans-respiratory pressures during rapid decompression. *Aerospace Medicine,* 1973, vol. 2, no. 44, pp. 153–162.

[19]Kolder, H.J. Explosive decompression following a drop in pressure. *Sitzungsber. Akad. Wiss.* (Wien), 1956, vol. 165 pp. 358–419 (in German).

[20]Gramenitskiy, P.M. *Decompression Disorders. Problems of Space Biology, Volume 25*. Moscow, Nauka, 1974 (in Russian).

[21]Fryer, D.J. Failure of pressure cabins. In: Gillies, J.A., Ed. *A Textbook of Aviation Physiology*. Oxford, Pergamon Press, 1965, pp. 187–206.

[22]Malkin, V.B. The efficacy of positive oxygen pressure in the lungs in maintaining man's work capacity at altitudes of 13,000–30,000 m. Dissertation for degree of Doctor of Medical Sciences, 1963 (in Russian).

[23]Zharov, S.G.; Kustov, V.V.; Seryapin, A.D.; and Fomin, A.G. Artificial atmosphere in spacecraft cabins. In: Yazdovskiy, V.I., Ed. *Space Biology and Medicine. Biomedical Problems of Space Flights*. Moscow, Nauka, 1966, pp. 285–298 (in Russian).

[24]Busby, D.E. Clinical space medicine. A prospective look at medical problems from hazards of space operations. NASA-CR-856, Washington, D.C., NASA, 1967.

[25]Billings, C.E. Barometric pressure; Atmosphere. In: Parker, J.F., Jr., and West, R.W., Eds. *Bioastronautics Data Book*. NASA-SP-3006, Washington, D.C., NASA, 1973, pp. 1–63.

[26]Ivanov, D.I., and Khromushkin, A.I. *Human Life Support Systems in High Altitude and Space Flights*. Moscow, Mashinostroyeniye, 1968 (in Russian).

[27]Berry, C.A.; Coons, D.O.; Catterson, A.D.; and Kelly, G.F. Man's response to long-duration flight in the Gemini spacecraft. In: *Gemini Mid-Program Conference*. NASA-SP-121, Washington, D.C., NASA, 1966, pp. 235–261.

[28]Vorobyov, Ye.I.; Gazenko, O.G.; Gurovskiy, N.N.; Nefedov, Yu.G.; Yegorov, B.B.; Spitsa, I.I.; Biryukov, Ye.N.; Bryanov, I.I.; Yeryomin, A.V.; and Yegorov, A.D. Apollo-Soyuz Test Flight. Preliminary biomedical results of Soyuz-19 flight. *Kosmicheskaya Biologiya i Aviakosmicheskaya Meditsina*, 1976, vol 10, no. 1, pp. 19–22 (in Russian).

[29]Nicogossian, A.E., and Parker, J.F. *Space Physiology and Medicine*. NASA SP-447, Washington, D.C., NASA, 1982, pp. 108–124.

[30]Haldane, J.S., and Priestley, J.G. *Respiration*. 2nd ed. New Haven, Yale University Press, 1935.

[31]Henderson, J. Effect of altitude on aviators. *Aviation and Aeronautical Engineering,* 1917, vol. 2, no.3, pp. 145–147.

[32]Rozenblyum, D.E. Caisson sickness at altitude. *Problemy Sovestskoy Fiziologii, Biokhimii i Farmakologii,* 1949, vol. 2, pp. 632–633 (in Russian).

[33]Nikolayev, V.P. Prediction of decompression safety based on mathematical models of gas bubble formation and growth in the body. Dissertation for degree of Doctor of Medical Sciences, Moscow, 1990, pp. 38 (in Russian).

[34]Streltsov, V.V. Effect of low barometric pressure and acceleration on the human body. Dissertation for degree of Doctor of Medical Sciences, Moscow, 1938, p. 241 (in Russian).

[35]Harvey, E.N. Physical factors in bubble formation. In: Fulton, J.F., Ed. *Decompression Sickness*. Philadelphia, Saunders, 1951, p. 108.

[36]Genin, A.M. On the etiology and pathogenesis of decompression sickness. *Voyenno-Meditsinskiy Zhurnal*, 1948, no. 8, pp. 48–51 (in Russian).

[37]Evans, A.D., and Walder, D.N. Significance of gas micronuclei in the aetiology of decompression sickness. *Nature,* 1969, vol. 222, pp. 251–252.

[38]Waligora, J.M.; Horrigan, D.J.; and Concin, J. The effect of extended O_2 prebreathing on altitude decompression sickness and venous gas bubbles. *Aviation, Space, and Environmental Medicine,* 1987, vol. 58, no. 9 (Suppl.), pp. A110–A112.

[39]Ivanov, P.N.; Kuznetsov, A.G.; Malkin, V.B.; and Popova, Ye.O. Decompression disorders in man exposed to extremely low barometric atmospheric pressure. *Biofizika,* 1960, vol. 5, no. 6, pp. 704–709 (in Russian).

[40]Chernyakov, I.N., and Malkin, V.B. Altitude decompression disorders. In: Rudnyi, N.M.; Vasilyev, P.V.; and Gozulov, S.A., Eds. *A Handbook of Aviation Medicine*. Moscow, Meditsina, 1986, pp. 43–56 (in Russian).

[41]Apollonov, A.P., and Mirolyubov, V.G. The effect of altitude on pilots. *Voyenno-Sanitarskoye Delo*, 1938, no. 7, pp. 16–24 (in Russian).

[42]Streltsov, V.V. On the effect of low barometric pressure upon the human body. *Voyenno-Sanitarskoye Delo*, 1933, no. 5, pp. 11–17 (in Russian).

[43]Rubissow, G.J., and Mackay, R.S. Ultrasonic imaging of in vivo bubbles in decompression sickness. *Ultrasonics,* 1971, vol. 9, no.10, pp. 225–234.

[44]Hornberger, W. Decompression sickness. In: USAF Surgeon General. *German Aviation Medicine in World War II*, Washington, D.C., U.S. Government Printing Office, 1950, vol. 1, pp. 354–394.

[45]Marbarger, J.; Kadet, W.; and Hausen, J. The occurrence of decompression sickness following denitrogenation at ground level and altitude. *Journal of Aviation Medicine,* 1957, vol. 28, no. 2, p. 127.

[46]Nims, L.F. Environmental factors affecting decompression sickness. Part 1. A physical theory of decompression sickness. In: Fulton, J.F., Ed. *Decompression Sickness*. Philadelphia, Saunders, 1951, pp. 192–222.

[47]Brooks, C. Loss of cabin pressure in Canadian Air Force ejection seat aircraft. 1962–1982. *Aviation, Space, and Environmental Medicine*, 1984, vol. 55, pp. 1154–1163.

[48]Rayman, R.B., and MacNaughton, G.B. Decompression sickness: USAF experience 1970–80. *Aviation, Space,*

and Environmental Medicine, 1983, vol. 54, no. 3, pp. 258–260.

[49]Wirjosemito, S.A.; Touhey, J.E.; and Workman, W.T. Type II altitude decompression (altitude decompression sickness): U.S. Air Force experience with 133 cases. *Aviation, Space, and Environmental Medicine*, 1989, vol. 60, pp. 256–62.

[50]Gray, J.S. Constitutional factors affecting susceptibility to decompression sickness. In: Fulton, J.F., Ed. *Decompression Sickness*. Philadelphia, Saunders, 1951, pp. 182–191.

[51]Belgov, I.M.; Vyadro, M.D.; Gorbov, F.D.; and Panfilov, A.S. Decompression disorders in flight personnel. *Voyenno-Meditsinskiy Zhurnal*, 1954, no. 11, pp. 38–42 (in Russian).

[52]Haymaker, W., and Johnston, A.D. Pathology of decompression sickness. *Military Medicine*, 1955, vol. 117, pp. 285–306.

[53]Chryssanthou C.; Palaia, T.; Goldstein G.; and Stenger, R. Increase in blood-brain barrier permeability by altitude decompression. *Aviation, Space, and Environmental Medicine*, 1987, vol. 58, no. 11, pp. 1082–1086.

[54]Ferris, E.G., and Engel, G.L. The clinical nature of high altitude decompression sickness. In: Fulton, J.F., Ed. *Decompression Sickness*. Philadelphia, Saunders, 1951.

[55]Rozenblyum, D.Ye. Nature of altitude sickness (Reports 1 and 2). *Byulleten Eksperimentalnoy Biologii i Meditsiny*, 1943, vol. 16, no.1, pp. 2–4 (in Russian).

[56]Gorodinskiy, S.M.; Kartsev, A.N.; Kuznets, Ye.I.; and Levinskiy, S.V. On the possibility of extended human exposure to a modified atmosphere in an enclosed environment. In: *Proceedings of the Seventh Lecture Series on the Development of The Scientific Legacy of K.E. Tsiolkovskiy*. Moscow, Izdatelstvo Instituta Istorii Yestestvoznaniya i Tekhniki, 1973, pp. 28–35 (in Russian).

[57]Behnke, A.R. Decompression sickness incident to deep sea diving and high altitude ascent. *Medicine*, 1945, vol. 24, pp. 381–402.

[58]Arthur, D.C., and Margulies, R.A. The pathophysiology, presentation, and triage of altitude-related decompression sickness associated with hypobaric chamber operation. *Aviation, Space, and Environmental Medicine*, 1982, vol. 53, no. 5, pp. 489–497.

[59]Zagryadskiy, V.P.; Sidorov, O.Yu.; and Sulimo-Samuylo, Z.K. The effect of a modified gas atmosphere on the origin and course of decompression disorders. In: *Problems of Space Medicine, Conference Proceedings*. Moscow, Nauka, 1966, pp. 175–176 (in Russian).

[60]Beard, S.E.; Allen, T.H.; McIver, R.G.; and Bancroft, R.W. Comparison of helium and nitrogen in production of bends in simulated orbital flights. *Aerospace Medicine*, 1967, vol. 38, no. 4, pp. 331–337.

[61]Roth, E.M. Gas physiology in space operations. *New England Journal of Medicine*, 1966, vol. 275:, no.1, pp. 144–154, no. 2, pp. 196–203, no. 3, pp. 255–263.

[62]Dean, R.B. The formation of bubbles. *Journal of Applied Physiology*, 1944, vol. 15, pp. 446–451.

[63]Fulton, J.F. The origin of bubbles in tissues. In: Fulton, J.F., Ed. *Decompression Sickness*. Philadelphia, Saunders, 1951.

[64]Gazenko, O.G.; Gippenreiter, Ye.B.; and Malkin, V.B. Altitude decompression sickness and methods of its prophylaxis and therapy (a review). *Kosmicheskaya Biologiya i Aviakosmicheskaya Meditsina,* 1989, vol. 23, no.3, pp. 17–22 (in Russian).

[65]Balke, B. Rate of gaseous nitrogen elimination during rest and work in relation to the occurrence of decompression sickness at high altitude. USAF SAM Project No. 21-1201-0014, Report No. 6, Brooks AFB, Texas, USAF School of Aviation Medicine, 1954.

[66]Apollonov, A.P.; and Shik, L.L. Denitrogenation at an altitude of 8,000 m. *Arkhivy Biologicheskikh Nauk*, 1941, vol. 64, no. 1, p. 2 (in Russian).

[67]Ardashnikova, L.I. The role of respiration and circulation changes during hypo- and hypercapnia in nitrogen washout from the body. In: *On the Regulation of Respiration, Circulation and Gas Exchange*. Moscow, Medgiz, 1948, pp. 103–104 (in Russian).

[68]Behnke, A.R. The application of measurements of nitrogen elimination to the problem of decompression divers. *U.S. Naval Medicine Bulletin*, 1937, vol. 35, pp. 219–240.

[69]Jones, H.B. Gas exchange and blood-tissue perfusion factors in various body tissues. In: Fulton, J.F., Ed. *Decompression Sickness*. Philadelphia, Saunders, 1951, pp. 278–321.

[70]Yakobson, M.I. *Caisson Disease*. Moscow, Medgiz, 1950 (in Russian).

[71]Bondaryov, E.V.; Genin, A.M.; Gurvich, G.I.; Draguzya, M.D.; Yegorov, V.A.; Yeleshin, Yu.N.; Yelinskiy, M.P.; Krykalova, O.K.; Parfenova, E.N.; and Rastsvetayev, V.V. Use of a two-component artificial atmosphere in manned space vehicles. *Kosmicheskaya Biologiya i Meditsina*, 1969, vol. 3, no. 2, pp. 17–25 (in Russian).

[72]Genin, A.M.; Gurvich, G.I.; Kuznetsov, A.G.; Chernyakov, I.N.; Bondaryov, E.V.; Polischuk, I.P.; and Draguzya, M.D. Altitude decompression disorders in man exposed to a rarefied atmosphere and different denitrogenation regimens. In: *Proceedings of Fifth Lecture Series on the Development of the Scientific Legacy and Concepts of K.E. Tsiolkovskiy*. Moscow, Izdatelstvo Instituta Istorii Yestestvoznaniya i Tekhniki, 1970, pp. 65–67 (in Russian).

[73]Bonura, M.S., and Nelson, W.G. Engineering criteria for spacecraft cabin atmosphere selection. NASA-CR-891, Washington, D.C., NASA, 1967.

[74]Genin, A.M., and Malkin, V.B. Artificial atmosphere. *Nauchnaya Mysl* (Bulletin of the Academy of Pedagogical Sciences), 1968, no. 7, pp. 38–51 (in Russian).

[75]Kuznetsov, A.G. The phenomena of boiling and vaporization in the body at high altitudes. *Izvestiya Akademii Nauk SSSR*, 1957, no. 3, pp. 293–305 (in Russian).

[76]Boyle, R. New pneumatical experiments about respiration. *Philosophical Transactions*, London, 1670, vol. 5, pp. 2011–2058.

[77]Parfenova, O.I., and Streltsov, V.V. The effect of low barometric pressures in the course of ontogenetic develop-

ment. In: *Proceedings of the Central Aviation Medicine Laboratory*. Moscow, 1938, vol. 5, pp. 127–131 (in Russian).

[78]Burch, B.N.; Kemph, I.P.; Vail, E.G.; and Hitchcock, F.A. Some effects of explosive decompression and subsequent exposure to 30 mm Hg upon the hearts of dogs. *Journal of Aviation Medicine*, 1952, vol. 23, no. 2, pp. 159–167.

[79]Marlowe, B.L. Altitude hypoxia. *Flying Safety*, 1986, vol. 42, no. 6, pp. 16–21.

[80]Ernsting, J. Mild hypoxia and the use of oxygen in flight. *Aviation, Space, and Environmental Medicine*, 1984, vol. 55, pp. 407–410.

[81]Kovalenko, Ye.A., and Chernyakov, I.N. *Tissue Oxygen in Response to Extreme Flight Factors. Problems of Space Biology, Volume 21*. Moscow, Nauka, 1972 (in Russian).

[82]Lubbers, D.W., and Kessler, M. Oxygen supply and rate of tissue respiration. In: Lubbers, D.W., et al., Eds. *Oxygen Transport in Blood and Tissues*. Stuttgart, Thieme, 1968, p. 90.

[83]Sechenov, I.M. The theory of the composition of air in the lungs. In: *Selected Works*. Moscow, Izdatelstvo Vsesoyuznogo Instituta Eksperimentalnoy Meditsiny imeni A.M. Gorkogo, 1935 (in Russian)

[84]West, J.B. Hypoxic man: Lessons from extreme altitude. *Aviation, Space, and Environmental Medicine*, 1984, vol. 55, pp.1058–1062.

[85]Opiz, E. Uber akute Hypoxie *Ergebnisse der Physiologie*, 1941, vol. 44, p. 315 (in German).

[86]Bert, P. *La Pression Barometrique*. Paris, G. Masson, 1878 (in French).

[87]Bonvallet, M.; Hugelin, A.; and Dell, P. The milieu interieur and automatic activity of the mesencephalic reticular cells. *Journal de Physiologie*, Paris, 1956, vol. 48, pp. 403–406 (in French).

[88]Dell, P., and Bonvallet, M. Direct and reflex control of the activity of the ascending activating reticular system of the brain stem by oxygen and carbon dioxide in blood. *Comptes Rendus de la Société de Biologie*, 1954, vol. 148, nos. 9–10, pp. 855–859 (in French).

[89]Asyamolova, N.M. The use of electroencephalography in various hypoxic tests. Dissertation for the degree of Candidate in Medical Sciences, Moscow, 1969 (in Russian).

[90]Kovalenko, Ye.A. Changes in oxygen tension in tissues during hypoxia. Abstract of a dissertation for the degree of Doctor of Medical Sciences, Moscow, 1966 (in Russian).

[91]Ernsting, J. Respiration and anoxia. The effects of anoxia on the central nervous system; the metabolic effects of anoxia. In: Gillies, J.A., Ed. *A Textbook of Aviation Physiology*. Oxford, Pergamon Press, 1965, pp. 215–302.

[92]Strughold, H. Reserve time following interruption of oxygen breathing at high altitudes. *Luftfahrtmed.*, 1938, vol. 3, pp. 55–63; 1940, vol. 5, pp. 66–75 (Reports 1–2, in German).

[93]Prast, L.W., and Noell, W.K. Indication of earlier stages of human hypoxia by electroencephalometric means. *Aviation Medicine*, 1948, vol. 19, no. 6, pp. 426–434.

[94]Davis, P.A.; Davis, H.; and Thompson, W. Progressive changes in the human electroencephalogram under low oxygen tension. *American Journal of Physiology*, 1938, vol. 123, no. 1, pp. 51–52.

[95]Gibbs, F.A.; Williams, D.; and Gibbs, E.L. Modification of the cortical sequence by changes in CO_2 blood sugar and O_2. *Journal of Neurophysiology*, 1940, vol. 3, no. 1, pp. 49–58.

[96]Noell, W.K. The human EEG during anoxia. In: USAF Surgeon General. *German Aviation Medicine in World War II*. Washington, D.C., U.S. Government Printing Office, 1950, vol. 1, pp. 301–302.

[97]Malkin, V.B. Fundamentals of automatic diagnosis of the hypoxic state. In: *Oxygen Deficit*. Kiev, Izdatelstvo Akademii Nauk, Ukrainskoy SSR, 1963, pp. 563–571 (in Russian).

[98]Skrypin, V.A. Physiological limits and time to unconsciousness of the pilot in response to oxygen shutoff or sudden pressure drop at high altitudes. Abstract of dissertation for the degree of Candidate in Medical Sciences, Moscow, 1956, p. 272 (in Russian).

[99]Kornmuller, A.E.; Palme, F.; and Strughold, H. Recording brain action currents as a method of studying altitude sickness. *Klin.-Wochenschr.*, 1942, vol. 21, p. 55 (in German).

[100]Malkin, V.B., and Gippenreiter, Ye.B. *Acute and Chronic Hypoxia. Problems of Space Biology, Volume 35*. Moscow, Nauka, 1977 (in Russian).

[101]Sirotinin, N.N. Results of studying hypoxia. *Patologicheskaya Fiziologiya i Experimentalnaya Therapiya*, 1957, vol. 5, pp. 13–20 (in Russian).

[102]Barbashova, Z.I. *Acclimation to Hypoxia and its Physiological Mechanisms*. Moscow-Leningrad, Izdatelstvo Akademii Nauk SSSR, 1960 (in Russian).

[103]Meyerson, F.Z.; Maizelis, M.Ya.; and Malkin, V.B. On the role of synthesis of nucleic acids and proteins in adaptation to altitude hypoxia. *Izvestiya Akademii Nauk SSSR, Seriya Biologicheskaya*, 1969, no. 6, pp. 819–831 (in Russian).

[104]West, J.B., and Lahiri. S. *High Altitude and Man*. Washington, D.C., American Physiological Society, 1984.

[105]Zharov, S.G.; Ilyin, Ye.A.; Kovalenko, Ye.A.; Kalinichenko, I.R.; Karpova, L.I.; Mikerova, N.S.; Osipova, M.M.; and Simonov, Ye.Ye. Study of prolonged human exposure to an atmosphere with a high CO_2 content. In: Parin, V.V., Ed. *Aviation and Space Medicine*. Moscow, Akademiya Nauka SSSR, 1964, pp 155–158 (in Russian).

[106]Malkin, V.B.; Belkin, V.Sh.; Kayumov, L.Yu.; and Landukhova, N.F. *Methods of Increasing Resistance to Altitude Hypoxia*. Dushanbe, Donish, 1989 (in Russian).

[107]Malkin, V.B., and Gazenko, O.G. On the optimization of an artificial atmosphere with an irreversible decrease of PO_2. *Doklady Akademii Nauk SSSR*, 1969, vol. 184, no. 4, pp. 995–998 (in Russian).

[108]Vasilyev, P.V.; Malkin, V.B.; Volozhin, A.I.; Kotovskaya, A.R.; Krasnykh, I.G.; Loginova, Ye.V.; Orlova, T.A.; Potkin, V.Ye.; Roschina, N.A.; Tikhonov, M.A.; and Uglova, N.N. Experimental data about the effect of the hypodynamic syndrome. In: *Fifth Lecture Series on the De-*

velopment of the Scientific Legacy and Concepts of K.E. Tsiolkovskiy. Moscow, Izdatelstvo Instituta Istorii Yestestvoznaniya i Tekhniki, 1970, pp. 51–59 (in Russian).

[109]Sergeyev, A.A. *Essays on the History of Aviation Medicine*. Moscow, Leningrad, Akademiya Nauk SSSR, 1962 (in Russian).

[110]Bruner, H., and Klein, K.E. Hypoxia as stressor. *Aerospace Medicine,* 1960, vol. 32, pp. 1009–1018.

[111]Gershenovich, Z.S. Molecular mechanisms of action of increased oxygen pressure. The effect of increased oxygen pressure on the body. In: *Effects of Elevated Oxygen Pressure on the Organism. All-Union Inter-VUZ Conference Materials*, Dec. 1968, Rostov, Izdatelstvo Rostovskogo Universiteta, 1969, pp. 16–18 (in Russian).

[112]Zhironkin, A.G. *Oxygen. Physiological and Toxic Effects*. Leningrad, Nauka, 1972 (in Russian).

[113]Kaplan, Ye.Ya. Regulation of biooxidation processes as a method of increasing resistance to hypo- and hyperoxia. Dissertation for degree of Doctor of Medical Sciences, Moscow, 1972 (in Russian).

[114]Forward, S.A.; Landowne, M.; Follansbee, J.N.; Hansen, J.E. Effect of acetazolamide on acute high altitude sickness. *New England Journal of Medicine*, 1968, vol. 279, no. 16, pp. 839–845.

[115]Hamilton, R.W.; Doebler, G.F.; and Schreiner, H.R. Biological evaluation of various spacecraft atmospheres. *Space Life Sciences*, 1970, vol. 2, no. 3, pp. 307–334.

[116]Lambertsen, C.S. Oxygen toxicity. In: *Fundamentals of Hyperbaric Medicine*. Washington, D.C., National Research Council, Committee on Hyperbaric Oxygenation, NRC Pub. No. 1298, 1965, pp. 21–32.

[117]Jamieson, D.; Chance, B.; Cadenas, E.; and Boveris, A. The relation of free radical production to hyperoxia. *American Review of Physiology*, 1968, vol. 48, pp. 703–719.

[118]Gille, J.P.; Wortelboer, H.M.; and Joenie, H. Effect of normobaric hyperoxia on antioxidant defenses of HeLa and EHO cells. *Free Radical Biology and Medicine*, 1988, vol. 4, pp. 85–91.

[119]Freman, B.A.; Mason, R.J.; Williams, M.C.; and Crapo, J.D. Antioxidant enzyme activity in alveolar type II cells after exposure of rats to hyperoxia. *Experimental Lung Research*, 1986, pp. 203–222.

[120]Wood, C.D., and Perkins, G.F. Factors influencing hypertension and pulmonary edema produced by hyperbaric O_2. *Aerospace Medicine*, 1970, vol. 41, pp. 869–872.

[121]Genin, A.M.; Tikhonov, M.A.; Malkin, V.B.; Glazkova, V.A.; Grishin, Ye.P.; Drozdova, N.T.; Loginova, Ye.V.; Lushina, L.A.; Roshchina, N.A.; and Solovyov, V.I. Physiological criteria of early toxic manifestations of normobaric hyperoxia. *Izvestiya Akademiya Nauk SSSR*, 1973, no. 3, pp. 378–390 (in Russian).

[122]Romanova, L.K. Specific features of the ultrastructural organization of the surfactant system of the lung in the norm and under the action of pathogenic factors. *Vestnika AMN SSSR*, 1983, no. 11, pp. 44–53 (in Russian).

[123]Malkin, V.B.; Gramenitskiy, P.M.; Loginova, Ye.V.; Romanova, L.K.; Roshchina, N.A.; and Yurova, K.S. A rational regimen of hypoxia training and the limit of oxygen toxicity. In: *K.E. Tsiolkovskiy and Progress in Science and Engineering,* Moscow, Nauka, 1982, pp. 96–101 (in Russian).

[124]Kotovskiy, Ye.F., and Shimkevich, L.L. *Functional Morphology During Extreme Exposures. Problems of Space Biology, Volume 15*, Moscow, Nauka, 1971 (in Russian).

[125]Kistler, G.S.; Caldwell, P.R.; and Weibel, E.R. Development of fine structural damage to alveolar and capillary lining. *Journal of Cell Biology*, 1967, vol. 32, pp. 605–628.

[126]Balakhovskiy, I.S.; Mansurov, A.R.; Yazdovskiy, V.I. The effect of pure oxygen breathing on the lungs and heart of white rats. *Byulleten Eksperimentalnoy Biologii i Meditsina*, 1962, vol. 53, no. 2, pp. 43–47 (in Russian).

[127]Brooksby, G.A.; Dennis, R.L.; and Staley, R.W. Effects of continuous exposure of rats to 100% oxygen at 450 mm Hg for 64 days. *Aerospace Medicine*, 1966, vol. 37, no. 3, pp. 243–246.

[128]Roth, E.M., Ed. Compendium of human responses to the aerospace environment. Volumes I, II, III, and IV, NASA-CR-1205. Washington, D.C., NASA, 1968.

[129]DuBois, A.B.; Turaids, T.; Mammen, R.E.; and Nobrega, F.T. Pulmonary atelectasis in subjects breathing oxygen at sea level or at simulated altitude. *Journal of Applied Physiology*, vol. 21, pp. 828–836.

[130]Genin, A.M.; Zharov, S.G.; Kaplan, Ye.Ya.; Ogleznev, V.V.; and Solovyov, V.I. Investigation of long-term effect of a reduced pressure oxygen atmosphere on animals and man. In: *Transactions of 18th Congress of the International Astronautical Federation*. Belgrade, 1967, vol. 17, pp. 25–30 (in Russian).

[131]Kann, H.E.; Mendel, C.E.; Smith, W.; and Horton, B. Oxygen toxicity and vitamin E. *Aerospace Medicine*, 1964, vol. 35, no. 9, pp. 840–844.

[132]Kaplan, H.P. Hematologic effects of increased oxygen tensions. In: *Proceedings of the 2nd Annual Conference on Atmosphere Contamination in Confined Spaces*. AMRL-TR-66-120, Wright-Patterson AFB, Ohio, Medical Research Laboratories, 1966, pp. 200–222 ,

[133]Guan, Jiangin. Oxygen toxicity and lung damage. In: *Proceedings of the International Congress on Hypoxia and Pulmonary Pathophysiology*, Chongqing China, Oct. 10–12, 1990, p. 81.

[134]Fischer, C.L.; Johnson, P.C.; and Berry, C.A. Red blood cell mass and plasma volume changes in manned space flight. *Journal of the American Medical Association*, 1967, vol. 200, pp. 579–583.

[135]Kaplanskiy, A.S.; Durnova, G.N.; Kalinichenko, I.R.; Portugalov, V.V.; and Agadzhanyan, N.A. Phagocytic activity and parameters of carbohydrate metabolism of neutrophils in men exposed to increased oxygen concentrations. *Kosmicheskaya Biologiya i Meditsina*, 1969, vol. 3, no. 2, p. 65 (in Russian).

[136]Portugalov, V.V.; Durnova, G.N.; Kaplanskiy, A.S.; and Babchinskiy, F.V. Histological study of internal organs of mice exposed for 20 days to an atmosphere with an increased

oxygen concentration. *Kosmicheskaya Biologiya i Meditsina*, 1969, vol. 3, no. 5, pp. 35–39 (in Russian).

[137]Helvey, W.M. Effects of prolonged exposure to pure oxygen on human performance. RAC-393-1, ARD-807–701 (Final report), Farmingdale, N.Y., Republic Aviation Corporation, 1962.

[138]Morgan, T.E.; Ulvedal, F.; Cutler, R.G.; and Welch, B.E. Effects on man of prolonged exposure to oxygen at a total pressure of 190 mm Hg. *Aerospace Medicine*, 1963, vol. 34, pp. 588–592.

[139]Welch, B.E.; Morgan, T.E.; and Clamann, H.G., Jr. Time concentration effects in relation to oxygen toxicity in man. *Federal Proceedings*, 1963, vol. 22, pp. 1053–1065.

[140]Messier, A.A., and Fisher, H.W. Sensitivity of cultured mammalian cells to oxidative stress adaptation to repeated exposures of hyperbaric oxygen. *Undersea Biomedical Research*, 1990, vol. 17, no. 46, pp. 305–322.

[141]Bean, J.W. Tris buffer CO_2 and sympathoadrenal system in reaction to O_2 at high pressure. *American Journal of Physiology*, 1961, vol. 201, no. 4, pp. 737–739.

[142]Babchinskiy, F.V. Study of potential adaptation of the body to hyperoxia. In: *Materials from the Effect of Increased Oxygen Pressure on the Body. All-Union Inter-VUZ Conference*. Dec. 1968, Rostov, Izdatelstvo Rostovskogo Universiteta, 1969, pp. 4–5 (in Russian).

[143]Breslav, I.S. *Perception of the Breathing Environment and Gas Preferences of Man and Animals*. Leningrad, Nauka, 1970, pp. 4–5 (in Russian).

[144]Marshak, M.Ye. *Physiological Significance of Carbon Dioxide*. Moscow, Meditsina, 1969 (in Russian).

[145]Schaefer, K.E. Gaseous requirements in manned space flights. In: Schaefer, K.E., Ed. *Bioastronautics*. New York-London, Macmillan, 1964, pp. 76–110.

[146]Malkiman, I.I.; Polyakov,V.N.; and Stepanov, V.K. The effect of breathing gas mixtures containing 3–9% CO_2 on the human body. *Kosmicheskaya Biologiya i Meditsina*, 1971, vol. 5, no. 5, pp. 23–29 (in Russian).

[147]Levinskiy, S.V., and Malkiman, I.I. The formation of the functional state of respiration and thermal control systems when working in an atmosphere with an increased CO_2 content. *Fiziologiya Cheloveka*, 1990, vol. 16, no.1, pp. 133–141 (in Russian).

[148]Schaefer, K.E. A concept of triple tolerance limits based on chronic carbon dioxide toxicity studies. *Aerospace Medicine*, 1961, vol. 32, pp. 197–204.

[149]Albitskiy, P.M. On the reverse or after effects of carbon dioxide and on the biological significance of CO_2 occurring in the body. *Izvestiya Voyenno-Meditsinskoy Akademii*, St. Petersburg, 1911, vol. 22, pp. 117–141, 227–251, 351–386, 601–635 (in Russian).

[150]Schaefer, K.E.; Nichols, G.; and Carey, C.R.; Jr. Acid-base balance and blood and urine electrolytes of man during acclimatization to CO_2. *Journal of Applied Physiology*, 1964, vol. 19, no. 1, pp. 48–58.

[151]Mendeleyev, D.I. Air flight from the city of Klin during a solar eclipse, 1887. In: *Collected Works*. Moscow-Leningrad, Izdatelstvo Akademii Nauk SSSR, 1946, vol. 7, pp. 471–549 (in Russian).

[152]Tsiolkovskiy, K.E. Exploration of outer space by jet rockets. In: *Selected Works*. Moscow, Izdatelstvo Akademii Nauk SSSR, 1954 (in Russian).

[153]Gazenko, O.G., and Genin, A.M. Introduction. In: Gazenko, O.G., and Genin, A.M, Eds. *Man in Space and Undersea*. Moscow, Voyenizdat, 1967, pp. 5–14 (in Russian).

[154]Genin, A.M. Principles of formation of space cabin atmospheres. In: Sisakyan, N.M., and Yazdovskiy, V.I., Eds. *Problems of Space Biology, Volume 3*. Moscow, Nauka, 1964, pp. 59–65. (in Russian).

[155]Ivanov, D.I.; Malkin, V.B.; Chernyakov, I.N.; Popkov, V.L.; Popova, Ye.O.; Flekkel, A.B.; Arutyunov, G.A.; Terentyev, V.G.; Buyanov, P.V.; Vorobyov, N.A.; and Sturua, G.G. The effect of prolonged exposure of man to a low barometric pressure and relative isolation. In: Chernigovskiy, V.N., Ed. *Work Performance. Issues of Habitability and Biotechnology. Problems of Space Biology, Volume 7*. Moscow, Nauka, pp. 269–280 (in Russian).

[156]Kuznetsov, A.G.; Agadzhanyan, N.A.; Bizin, Yu.P.; Yezepchuk, N.I.; Kalinichenko, I.R.; Karpova, L.I.; Neumyvakin, I.P.; and Osipova, M.M. Respiratory and cardiovascular changes during extended exposure to low barometric pressure. In: Parin, V.V., Ed. *Aviation and Space Medicine*. Moscow, Akademiya Nauka SSSR, 1964, pp. 318–321 (in Russian).

[157]Spasskiy, V.A. *Physiological and Hygienic Support of Manned Flights in the Stratosphere*. Moscow, Medgiz, 1940 (in Russian).

[158]Boriskin, V.V.; Oblapenko, P.V.; Rolnik, V.V.; and Savin, B.M. The potential for development of animals in a helium-oxygen atmosphere. *Doklady Akademii Nauk SSSR*, 1962, vol. 143, no. 2, pp, 475–478 (in Russian).

[159]MacHattie, and Rahn, H. Survival of mice in the absence of inert gas. *Proceedings of the Society of Experimental Medicine and Biology*, 1960, vol. 104, pp. 772–775.

[160]Wright R.A.; Kreglow, E.S.; and Weiss, H.S. Effects of changing environmental factors on embryonic development in a helium-oxygen atmosphere. *Aerospace Medicine*, 1966, vol. 37, no. 3, p. 309.

[161]Dianov, A.G. On the possibility of substituting helium for nitrogen and the efficacy of using a helium-oxygen atmosphere for space suit ventilation. *Kosmicheskiye Issledovaniya*, 1964, vol. 2, no. 3, pp. 498–503 (in Russian).

[162]Dianov, A.G., and Kuznetsov, A.G. On the possibility of substituting helium for nitrogen in space cabins. In: Parin, V.V., Ed. *Aviation and Space Medicine*. Moscow, Akademiya Nauka SSSR, 1964, pp. 162–165 (in Russian).

[163]Adams, J.D.; Conkle, J.P.; and Mabson, W.E. The study of man during a 56-day exposure to an oxygen-helium atmosphere at 258 mm Hg total pressure. II, Major and minor atmospheric components *Aerospace Medicine*, 1966, vol. 37, no. 6, pp. 555–558.

[164]Bartek, M.J.; Ulvedal, F.; and Brown, H.E. Study of man during a 56-day exposure to an oxygen-helium atmo-

sphere at 258 mm Hg total pressure. IV, Selected blood enzyme response. *Aerospace Medicine*, 1966, vol. 37, no. 6, pp. 563–566.

[165]Cordaro, J.T.; Sellers, W.M.; Ball, R.J.; and Schmidt, I.P. Study of man during a 56-day exposure to an oxygen-helium atmosphere at 258 mm Hg total pressure. X, Enteric microbial flora. *Aerospace Medicine*, 1966, vol. 37, no. 6, pp. 594–596.

[166]Epperson, W.L.; Quigley, D.G.; Robertson, W.G.; Welch, B.E.; and Behar, V.S. Observations on man in an oxygen-helium environment at 380 mm Hg total pressure. III, Heat exchange. *Aerospace Medicine,* 1966, vol. 37, no. 5, pp. 457–462.

[167]Dianov, A.G. The physiological effect of nitrogen replacement with helium in an atmosphere with decreased oxygen and increased carbon dioxide. In: Chernigovskiy, V.N., Ed. *Work Performance. Issues of Habitability and Biotechnology. Problems of Space Biology, Vol. 7*. Moscow, Nauka, pp. 220–232 (in Russian).

[168]Kulik, A.M. Breathing helium-oxygen when gas exchange in the lungs is impaired. *Byulleten Eksperimentalnoy Biologii i Meditsiny*, 1960, vol. 49, no. 5, pp. 32–35 (in Russian).

[169]Zeft, H.J.; Ulvedal, F.; Shaw, E.G.; Welch, B.E.; Behar, V.S.; and Quigley, D.G. Observations on man in an oxygen-helium environment at 380 mm Hg total pressure. 1. Clinical. *Aerospace Medicine*, 1966, vol. 37, no. 5, pp. 449–453.

[170]Kuznetsov, V. S. Specific features of speech in a modified atmosphere. In: Chernigovskiy, V.N., Ed. *Work Performance. Issues of Habitability and Biotechnology. Problems of Space Biology, Vol. 7*. Moscow, Nauka, pp. 232–237 (in Russian).

[171]Heidelbaugh, N.D.; Vanderveen, J.E.; Kicka, M.V.; and O'Hara, I. Study of man during a 56-day exposure to an oxygen-helium atmosphere at 258 mm Hg total pressure. VIII, Observations of feeding bite size foods. *Aerospace Medicine*, 1966, vol. 37, no. 6, pp. 583–590.

[172]Morgan, T.E.; Ulvedal, F.F.; and Welch, B.E. Observation in the SAM two-man space-cabin simulator. II, Biomedical aspects. *Aerospace Medicine*, 1961, vol. 32, no. 6, p. 591.

[173]Lamb, L.E. Hypoxia—an anti-deconditioning factor for manned space flight. *Aerospace Medicine*, 1965, vol. 36, no. 2, pp. 97–100.

[174]Genin, A.M.; Shepelev, Ye.Ye.; Malkin, V.B.; Voskresenskiy, A.D.; Krasnykh, I.G.; Loginova, Ye.V.; Maksimov, D.G.; Fomin, A.M.; and Khalturin, V.S. On the potential use of an artificial atmosphere with nonstationary gas composition in an enclosed cabin. *Kosmicheskaya Biologiya i. Meditsina,* vol. 3, no. 3, pp. 119–129 (in Russian).

[175]Genin, A.M., and Shepelev, Ye.Ye. Some problems and principles of the formation of a habitable environment based on matter turnover. In: *Proceedings, XV International Astronautical Congress,* NASA-TT-F-9131, Warsaw, Sept. 7–12, 1964, Washington, D.C., NASA, 1964, pp. 17–23.

[176]Lynch, T.N.; Jensen, R.L.; Stevens, P.M.; Johnson, R. L.; and Lamb, L.E. Metabolic effects of prolonged bed rest: Their modification by simulated altitude. *Aerospace Medicine*, 1967, vol. 38, no. 1, pp. 10–20.

[177]Stevens, P.M.; Miller, P.B.; Lynch, T.N.; Gilbert, C.A.; Johnson, R. I.; and Lamb, L.E. Effects of lower body negative pressure on physiological changes due to four weeks of hypoxic bed rest. *Aerospace Medicine*, 1966, vol. 37, no. 5, pp. 466–474.

[178]Luft, U.C., and Bancroft, R.W. Transthoracic pressure in man during rapid decompresssion. SAM TR-56-62, Brooks AFB, Texas, USAF School of Aviation Medicine, 1956, vol. II, p. 60.

Chapter 2

Toxicology of Airborne Gaseous and Particulate Contaminants in Space Habitats

John T. James and Martin E. Coleman

I. The Challenge of Space-Flight Toxicology

The goal of space-flight toxicology is to protect crewmembers from the adverse effects on health, comfort, and performance that could result from chemical exposures during all aspects of space exploration. This includes not only missions in low Earth orbit but also missions to the Moon and planets and periods of time when outposts and bases are inhabited on these bodies. Achieving this goal requires detailed knowledge of potentially hazardous chemicals in space habitats, recognition of the unique constraints of space exploration, familiarity with the physiological and biochemical changes experienced by crewmembers, and a thorough understanding of how to apply the principles of toxicological and analytical chemistry to reduce risks to crew health. The scope of the present chapter is limited to toxicological issues related to inhalation exposures to gaseous and particulate contaminants (not including microbes, which are covered in Chapter 4 of this volume).

Sources of potentially hazardous atmospheric contaminants must be considered from a normal perspective and from the contingency perspective. For periods of normal operation, the toxicologist is concerned primarily with the accumulation of contaminants that could cause adverse health effects as a result of prolonged exposures. For contingency situations, the toxicologist must consider the acute effects of either an accidental large release of specific chemicals or the formation of toxic mixtures that could result from the thermodegradation of materials. Decrements in crew performance are the primary concern during contingency chemical releases.

Space habitats place strict constraints on the strategies developed to protect crewmembers from contaminants. Instrumentation to monitor contaminants must comply with limits on weight, size, and power consumption. Escape and medical treatment options are considerably fewer than on Earth and may entail additional risks. Microgravity environments do not permit settling of large particles, and combustion behavior is significantly altered in the absence of convection. High radiation levels may change airborne chemicals to more toxic species in space habitats beyond low Earth orbit. Each of these unique factors must be considered before effective strategies are developed to protect the crew from airborne contaminants.

Space-flight crews undergo a number of physiological and biochemical changes that could affect their susceptibility to chemical exposure. Changes that are of particular concern to the toxicologist include effects on the cardiovascular and central nervous systems, hematological changes, changes in tissue enzymes, and immunological changes. The data bases in these disciplines are rapidly improving; however, because of our limited experience with space flight, the magnitudes and mechanisms of these changes are not always well established. The toxicologist must compare mechanisms of toxicity with mechanisms that cause changes in microgravity to estimate crew susceptibility to chemicals.

Basic principles of toxicology and analytical chemistry must be used to build a framework for protecting crew health. If possible, spacecraft maximum allowable concentrations (SMACs) must be based on data obtained from high-quality studies using appropriate species and routes of administration. The results of mechanistic toxicological studies must also be utilized, if available, to develop a logical rationale for setting SMACs. Unfortunately, toxicological data bases often contain seriously flawed data or are incomplete. Analytical monitoring must provide sensitive, specific, and timely results on many potential contaminants within the weight, size, and power constraints of a spacecraft. It is simply impossible to obtain sensitivity, specificity, and real-time responses without giving up the ability to measure a broad range of compounds. Monitoring strategies must be based on careful consideration of the relative risks of chemical contamination to crew health.

II. Definitions and Concepts

A. Definition of Toxicology and Application of Toxicological Principles

Traditionally, toxicology has been defined as the study of poisons, with the caveat that dose makes the poison. Modern toxicology has expanded and refined this basic concept through careful scientific investigation; however, an important part of toxicology still remains an art form. The "cre-

The authors gratefully acknowledge the support of Dr. V.P. Savina of the Institute of Biomedical Problems, who provided information on toxic contaminants on Soviet space stations.

ative" side of toxicology continues to be essential because toxicologists are often asked to communicate recommendations to nontoxicologists, based on incomplete information. The toxicologist's conclusions must be conveyed with the appropriate degree of confidence; however, genuine uncertainties inherent in the recommendations must be skillfully communicated to avoid irrational reaction to the information. This is often difficult to do, with the result that whole industries have formed from overreactions to perceived problems. An example of public overreaction is the response to the potential carcinogenicity of asbestos fibers, which has resulted in expensive regulatory policies that are of questionable benefit to public health.[1]

The modern science of toxicology involves descriptive, regulatory, and mechanistic toxicology. Descriptive toxicology involves characterizating the response of a test system (usually an animal) to chemical exposure. The description may include clinical signs, mortality data, behavioral changes, physiological changes, pathological and clinical laboratory findings, and specialized endpoints. Regulatory toxicology involves the systematic application of descriptive data to achieve a specific degree of health protection (or risk) in human populations. For example, the acceptable risk of an adverse health effect may be one in a million for the general population, whereas for selected high-risk occupations the acceptable risk may be one in a thousand. Estimating the hazard presented by chemical exposure, even in a well-defined situation, may be difficult because of limitations in the descriptive data base. Mechanistic toxicology involves scientific studies designed to improve understanding of the results of descriptive studies. Regulatory toxicologists are beginning to use the results of mechanistic toxicology studies to better predict the human health hazards. For example, one may want to understand why formaldehyde causes neoplasia in the nasal cavities of rodents more easily than in man.[2] Answers to such questions will enable regulatory toxicologists to judge the relevance of descriptive findings to the prediction of human health hazards. Understanding mechanisms of toxicity may involve biochemistry, molecular biology, and pharmacokinetic modeling. Space-flight toxicology represents a specialized application of descriptive, regulatory, and mechanistic toxicology to protect the health of space crews during missions.

Descriptive toxicology utilizes a number of basic concepts that have been developed during decades of toxicity testing. The cumulative knowledge relating to these basic concepts is embodied in the regulatory guidelines that place constraints on how descriptive studies are performed. Species selection, routes of administration, dose levels, lengths of exposure, and toxic endpoints are basic to any descriptive study. Variations of more than a hundredfold in the susceptibility of different sexes, species, strains, and even substrains are well documented in the literature.[3–5] Ideally, the choice of species should be made on the basis of similarity to man; however, the mechanistic data are seldom complete enough to clearly indicate the best choice of species. In the absence of data to the contrary, regulatory guidelines, cost limitations, and historical experience typically lead to selection of a rodent species.[6] The route of administration of a test chemical should be identical to the expected route of human exposure. Generally, human beings are exposed by the oral, dermal, or inhalation route. Data from other routes of administration may be useful under some conditions; however, considerable uncertainty will be introduced when predicting human exposure hazards from data obtained by a route that is different from the human route. Dosages are generally selected to elicit a clear toxic response (highest dose), an intermediate toxic response, and a no-observed-adverse-effect level (NOAEL). Carcinogenesis bioassays have generally used the maximum tolerated dose; however, this approach has been criticized as irrelevant to human exposures, which tend to be much lower.[7] Most long-term exposure protocols specify intermittent exposures designed to mimic the pattern of industrial worker exposures. For space-flight applications, exposures will be continuous, so data from intermittent exposures must be extrapolated to continuous exposures. The choice of toxicological endpoints to measure during a study will have a profound effect on the value of the results. One must ask whether endpoints observed in animal models predict similar effects in human beings. For example, the renal effects induced in male rats by hydrocarbons cannot be taken to predict the same effect in human beings, because mechanistic studies have shown that interaction of hydrocarbons with a protein unique to male rats causes the injury.[8] Endpoints are particularly important when considering a NOAEL. A NOAEL is only meaningful when a battery of endpoints has been used to detect chemical injury. On the other hand, adaptive responses to chemical exposure must be distinguished from toxic responses.

Given a reasonably complete descriptive toxicology data base for a single chemical, a regulatory toxicologist can set safe human exposures by extrapolation from animal data. For noncarcinogens, the first step is to determine the NOAEL in animals for endpoints relevant to human beings. Depending on the type and quality of the data and the population potentially exposed, a safety factor of 10 to 1000 is applied to the NOAEL to set a permissible exposure level. For demonstrated mammalian carcinogens, a model is fit to the animal data at high concentrations to predict the risk of cancer at much lower human exposures. The choice of suitable low-dose extrapolation models has been the subject of much scientific research and controversy.

B. Constraints of Space Flight

Space flight imposes a set of unique constraints on the process of ensuring that cabin atmospheres are safe to breathe for extended periods. Clean air is the most urgent requirement of spacecraft crews. The cabin environment must contain the requisite amount of oxygen and be sufficiently free of chemical contaminants to pose no threat to crew health. During missions, crews are exposed continuously to whatever chemical contaminants are present in the air. This is in marked contrast to the vast majority of Earth-based workers, who are exposed only intermittently to workplace contaminants. In the early days of space flight, clean air was provided from high-pressure tanks as part of totally "open loop" systems. As the length of missions has increased, the methods of providing oxygen (O_2) and removing contaminants, including carbon dioxide (CO_2), have become more sophisticated. The ultimate goal is to achieve nearly "closed loop" operation so that very long missions can be undertaken without prohibitive resupply requirements. As systems become more closed, the opportunity for accumulating unremoved minor contaminants is increased. The toxic effects that can be tolerated in Earth-based workers or the general population are usually greater than those for astronauts. This is because 1) astronauts may be called upon to perform more sophisticated tasks than most Earth-based workers, and 2) the rescue and treatment options for astronauts are severely limited compared to the options on Earth.

C. Effects of Space Flight on Susceptibility

The process used to set safe contaminant levels must provide for the possibility that astronauts will be more susceptible to toxic chemicals because of mission-related stresses, microgravity-induced physiological adjustments, and biochemical changes. Data on these changes come from both animal exposures to space flight and human experience in space. On flights lasting only a few days, the most obvious clinical effect is space motion sickness. Typically, this problem develops during the first 6 h of flight and may last 3 to 4 days. The symptoms include sensitivity to motion and head movements, headache, nausea, and vomiting.[9] Additional physiological changes include cephalad fluid shifts, postural changes, cardiopulmonary adjustments, bone loss, and muscular atrophy.[10–12] Biochemical effects include reduction in plasma volume, loss of red cell mass, decreases in the number and function of T-lymphocytes, hormonal changes, and a decrease in enzyme activity.[13] Some of these effects (e.g., fluid shifts) seem to be self-limited, whereas other effects appear to increase in severity with the length of the mission (e.g., bone density loss). As research continues, it is hoped that countermeasures will at least minimize the extent of the physiological and biochemical effects. At present, it is not possible to predict in any quantitative way how space flight affects susceptibility to chemical exposures.

D. Chemical Release Contingencies

The constraints of space flight demand a well-reasoned, preventive strategy and a high degree of preparedness to deal with plausible contingencies. In the Space Shuttle Program, hazards from payload and utility chemicals are based on toxicity and amount at risk for release into the internal atmosphere; chemicals are categorized as nonhazards, critical hazards, or catastrophic hazards. Nonhazardous chemicals are flown with one or zero levels of containment, critical hazards

with two levels, and catastrophic hazards with three levels of containment.[14] An extensive flammability certification program limits the risk of combustion products in spacecraft environments.[15] These strategies have proven to be effective ways of controlling accidental chemical releases into the cabin atmosphere. Although chemical releases have occurred, their frequency has declined as preventive measures improve. On the space station, a thorough air monitoring system with associated decontamination capability is being planned to deal with contingency releases.[16] On the space station, the most likely sources of accidental chemical releases are synthetic material combustion, release from a utility chemical system, release from a payload experiment, and release from stored chemical wastes. It is also possible that highly toxic propellants (such as hydrazine), which are present outside the spacecraft, could enter the cabin through the airlocks following extravehicular activity (EVA).

E. Monitoring of Contaminant Concentrations

Any discussion of airborne chemical contamination would be incomplete without a consideration of how contaminant levels will be monitored. Monitoring strategies should be targeted to the highest risk chemicals and must provide detection at the appropriate concentration and in the appropriate time frame to protect crew health. The current Shuttle program provides for archival air sampling with later ground-based analysis for contaminant concentrations. There is no flight hardware currently capable of quantitating toxic gases on orbit; however, a prototype combustion products analyzer has been flown as part of a program to develop a capability to detect potentially toxic combustion products. In addition, an effort is underway to develop real-time particle detectors suitable for space flight.[17] Since the U.S. space station will be inhabited for decades and experiments will involve large quantities of potentially hazardous chemicals, a comprehensive monitoring strategy has been devised. Its goal is to limit any accidental chemical release to no more than one structural element by rapid detection of the release and quick isolation of the affected area. This is a difficult goal to achieve because of power, weight, and volume constraints, as well as technological limitations on chemical monitoring hardware. The long-term goal of the program is to ensure that no chemical contaminant accumulates to concentrations that could be harmful to crew health.

F. Environments Analogous to Space Habitats

Space habitats are not without Earth-based analogs; however, no single analog provides an adequate model to predict chemically induced health effects. The tight building with its sealed windows and recirculated air is similar in some ways to sealed spacecraft. The "tight" or "sick" building syndrome experienced on Earth illustrates the type of health effects that could occur as a result of stays in the closed cabin of a spacecraft.[18] For example, there is evidence that inhalation of relatively low concentrations of mixtures of volatile organic compounds similar to those found in tight buildings can have adverse effects on memory.[19] Submarine air quality has long been a concern to the U.S. Navy, and, in many ways, the concerns parallel those for spacecraft.[20] Submarine crews are exposed continuously to chemical contaminants and also experience stresses related to being in a confined space. However, submarine crews do not undergo microgravity-induced changes and have more complete medical treatment available and better escape options.

III. Toxicological Incidents During Past Space Missions and Ground Simulations

A. Severe Illness in Test Subjects During Manned Environmental Systems Assessment (MESA) Project (1963)

The NASA-sponsored MESA system was designed to evaluate the effectiveness of a regenerative air, water, and biological life support system in maintaining the health and well-being of five men living in a closed-loop environment for 30 days.[21,22] The test chamber atmospheric decontamination system included charcoal and silica gel adsorption beds to remove organic contaminants, lithium hydroxide (LiOH) to remove metabolic CO_2, sodium superoxide (Na_2O_2) to remove CO_2 and generate O_2, and a Hopcalite high-temperature catalytic oxidizer to completely oxidize CO_2, hydrogen, and organic compounds. During this study, the Na_2O_2 began to react with aluminum components of its container and to produce H_2. To remove the H_2 more rapidly, air flow through the Hopcalite was increased, resulting in a lowered Hopcalite temperature. This caused incomplete oxidation of many organic compounds.[21,22]

After less than 48 h, the test subjects complained of a sweet-sour and highly irritating odor. After 3 days, they experienced nausea and vomiting, sore gums, headaches, and painful jaws; the project was terminated on the fourth day. Most of the symptoms persisted for several days, after which the test subjects fully recovered.[21,22]

Analyses of desorbed contaminants from the charcoal revealed 23 volatile organic compounds, including two unusual compounds, dichloroacetylene (DCA) and monochloroacety-lene (MCA). Trichloroethylene (TCE) levels were especially high; TCE had been used as a cleaning solvent before the test. A literature review by the project scientists revealed that TCE is partially degraded to MCA and DCA by alkaline materials and some catalytic oxidizers. DCA is known to be highly toxic with toxic effects resembling those experienced by the chamber test subjects. Considering its structural similarity to DCA, MCA is probably also highly toxic. The TCE was apparently degraded to DCA and MCA by the LiOH, $Na2O_2$, and the Hopcalite catalytic oxidizer (operating at a substandard temperature).[21,22] The MESA experiment was repeated after complete removal of the residual TCE and installation of larger charcoal beds and a modified Na_2O_2 unit. It then proceeded for 30 days without difficulty.[22]

B. Apollo Fire Resulting in Lethal Concentrations of Combustion Products (1967)

The sudden death of three astronauts in the Apollo 204 fire during a ground simulation test shocked the nation and resulted in the grounding of the Apollo spacecraft for more than 3 years. Alleged flame-resistant materials became flammable in the Apollo spacecraft because of the use of 100 percent oxygen at a pressure of 260 mm Hg (5 psia),[23] which exceeded the oxygen partial pressure of the Earth's atmosphere (150 mm Hg, 2.9 psia). Since a postmortem examination of the three crewmembers revealed very high carboxyhemoglobin levels, CO_2 intoxication was listed as the cause of their deaths.[23] Other thermodegradation products of polymeric wire insulation, such as hydrogen cyanide, along with heat and smoke, were believed to be contributory to the crewmembers' deaths.[23,24]

After the Apollo fire in 1967, NASA implemented even more stringent flammability requirements for flight articles. Most electrical wire insulation in the habitable areas of the Shuttle is made of either Teflon® or Kapton®, two highly heat- and flame-resistant materials. Largely to reduce the flammability hazard, the usual composition of the Shuttle atmosphere is about the same as that of normal air (79 percent N_2 and 21 percent O_2).

C. Nitrogen Tetroxide and Monomethylhydrazine Exposure After Descent Following the Apollo-Soyuz Mission (1975)

During descent of the Apollo command module after the successful Apollo-Soyuz mission, the crew failed to activate the Earth Landing System (ELS) and to disarm the Reaction Control System (RCS) on time.[25,26] Therefore, they had to deploy the drogue parachute and forward heat shield manually after entering the Earth's atmosphere. This resulted in severe pitching and swaying of the command module, causing the RCS to fire its roll thrusters for 30 s in an attempt to stabilize the spacecraft. The roll thrusters released unreacted nitrogen tetroxide (N_2O_4) and monomethyl hydrazine (MMH) for 7 s, and then N_2O_4 alone for 23 s. Simultaneously, the cabin pressure relief (air intake) valve opened automatically to equalize the pressure inside the command module (260 mm Hg) with that of the Earth's atmosphere. Since the roll thrusters were located only about 0.6 m from the pressure relief valve, the cabin was immediately flooded with unignited MMH and nitrogen dioxide (NO_2). About 30 s later, the crew deployed the ELS with the main parachutes, which stabilized the spacecraft and caused the release of toxic gases from the roll thrusters to cease. The crewmembers experienced considerable eye and respiratory irritation, coughing, and nausea; and one crewmember lost consciousness. However, the others managed to go through the landing checklist and to bring down the Apollo spacecraft safely. After splashdown in the Pacific Ocean, the crew donned their oxygen masks, preventing further inhalation exposure. The unconscious crewmember quickly regained consciousness when an oxygen mask was held to his face.[25,26] Abnormal pulmonary function and radiographic findings were reported in all crewmembers.[27] After a 2-week stay in a Honolulu hospital, the crew fully recovered and made extensive tours of the United States and the Soviet Union.

This type of event is very unlikely to occur in the Shuttle, since no vents are open during ascent and descent. Even if a noxious gas should enter the Shuttle cabin during ascent or descent, all crewmembers would be protected, because they wear pressurized launch-entry suits and breathe oxygen from a central reservoir during this time. The Shuttle hatch is not opened for about 15 to 20 min after the Shuttle comes to a standstill upon landing as a further protection against toxic gas exposures.

D. Eye and Respiratory Irritation Caused by Lithium Hydroxide Dust (1981–1988)

After at least six Shuttle missions, crewmembers reported dust in the vicinity of the LiOH canisters during changeouts. The LiOH dust often caused minor eye irritation and coughing (personal communications of crewmembers after their respective missions). The two 5-lb LiOH cartridges used to remove metabolic CO_2 from the cabin atmosphere are alternately changed out at 6- to 12-h intervals, depending on the crew size.[28] The crewmembers admitted that they could have avoided this irritation by shutting off the cabin fan air flow through the LiOH cartridges or by donning filter masks and goggles before the changeout. However, they did not think that the irritation was severe enough to justify this additional effort. Preflight procedures implemented in 1989 and 1990 to reduce the release of LiOH dust included using a screen and shaker apparatus to remove smaller particles before packing the LiOH, vacuuming repacked LiOH cartridges at the Kennedy Space Center (KSC), and then vacuuming the LiOH again after checking for air resistance at KSC [personal communication from John Whalen, former subsystem manager for LiOH/charcoal (LiOH/C) air scrubbers, NASA Johnson Space Center (JSC) Crew and Thermal Systems Division, December 12, 1990]. Apparently because of these procedures, irritation from LiOH dust seldom has been mentioned by the flight crews after the STS-28 mission.

E. Escape of Payload Chemicals During Shuttle Missions

For Shuttle cabin middeck payload chemicals with significant toxicity potential, NASA normally requires double or triple containment (or other equivalent safeguards), depending on the magnitude of the potential toxicity. In one instance in which single containment was allowed for a nonvolatile buffer of low toxicity, a sizable amount of the buffer escaped. After the water evaporated, a residual particle lodged

Table 1 Production rate of human metabolites

Contaminant	Metabolic production rate[29] (mg/day/man)
Acetaldehyde	0.08
Acetone	0.13
Ammonia	250
n-Butyl alcohol	1.3
Carbon monoxide	33
Caprylic acid	9.2
Ethyl alcohol	4
Ethyl mercaptan	0.8
Hydrogen	50
Hydrogen sulfide	0.08
Indole	25
Methyl alcohol	1.4
Methane	600
Methyl mercaptan	0.8
Propyl mercaptan	0.8
Pyruvic acid	210
Skatole	25
Valeraldehyde	0.8
Valeric acid	0.8
Carbon dioxide	1,180,000 (maximal)[30] 990,000 (nominal) 910,000 (minimal)

in the eye of a crewmember, causing severe pain for several hours (personal communications of crewmembers after mission). In another instance, crewmembers reported that a nontoxic buffer escaped as a fine mist from a very small reservoir, causing mild, transient eye irritation. Since these incidents, more stringent containment safeguard requirements for payload chemicals have been implemented, making future occurrences less likely.

IV. Sources Of Environmental Contamination

A. Continuous Sources

1. Crew Metabolism

Crew metabolism is typically the major source of atmospheric contamination. The normal rates of metabolic generation of a variety of gases (determined in ground studies) are given in Table 1.[29,30] Of the compounds listed in this table, ammonia, the sulfur compounds, the alcohols, indole, skatole, methane, and hydrogen are produced primarily by micro-organisms in the intestines and to a much lesser extent by micro-organisms on the skin. Acetone, the aldehydes, and the organic acids are produced in the body primarily by metabolic processes. At the nominal CO_2 production rate of 990 grams/person/day (see Table 1) without a CO_2 scrubber system, a crew of five in the Shuttle cabin would generate an atmospheric concentration of about 4.1 percent of CO_2 in 1 day. This would necessitate a mission abort. Carbon monoxide (CO) is generated by human metabolism in much lesser

Mass Concentration Data:
STS-32 and Indoor Environments

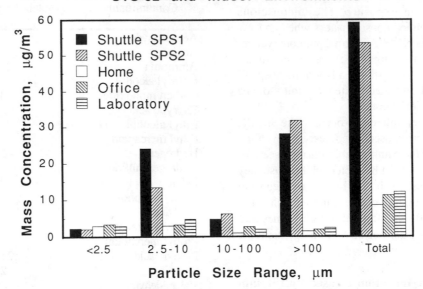

Fig. 1 Particle mass concentration data from STS-32 compared to concentration data from indoor environments. [Reprinted with permission 1991, Society of Automotive Engineers, Inc.]

amounts; but, without removal from the atmosphere, it could cause toxicity problems during long-term missions.

There is evidence that generation of some metabolic products may be significantly increased during space flight. Recently, breath samples from eight cosmonauts collected during space flight were analyzed. Results indicated that levels of the metabolic products ethane and ethylene (assayed together) increased more than sevenfold; acetaldehyde and methanol increased about threefold; acetaldehyde and n-butane doubled; and acetone increased significantly during 3–8 months of space flight, as compared to basal ground levels in the same persons.[31]

2. Offgassing

Practically all nonmetallic materials continuously release (offgas) trace amounts of gases, both from a gradual breakdown of these materials and from the escape of gases trapped in their matrices. In the closed-loop environment of a spacecraft, offgassed products could possibly accumulate to toxic levels. A wide variety of offgassed products, predominantly low-to-medium-weight organic chemicals, have been found during offgas testing but usually at rather low levels. Practically all candidate flight articles or component materials are subjected to offgas testing as a requisite for flight certification. Offgas testing and toxicological evaluation procedures are given in Section V.B.1, Offgas Testing of Flight Articles.

3. Use of Utility Chemicals

Utility chemicals, such as cleansers and adhesives, also contribute to the Shuttle's atmospheric contamination load. For example, each of the wet wipes used by crewmembers to clean their hands contains about 0.5 grams of ethyl alcohol (Dr. Fred Dawn, crew equipment manager, personal communication, April 1987 and February 1990). Isopropyl alcohol swabs are commonly used to disinfect the skin prior to venipunctures and for cleaning electronic equipment during Shuttle missions (Dr. Fred Dawn, personal communication, April 1987 and February 1990). During the STS-2 mission, unusually high atmospheric levels (but below the SMAC) of toluene[32] resulted from repeated gluing of Velcro® to the orbiter cabin walls (Paul Ledoux, manager, Materials and Processing Group, McDonnell Douglas, NASA JSC engineering support contractor, personal communication, July 1985).

4. Particulates

Free-floating particulates are commonly seen during every Shuttle mission. The number and size distribution of particulates from a typical Shuttle mission, as compared to those in a normal indoor Earth environment, are given in Fig 1.[17] The high concentration of large particulates in the spacecraft atmosphere is because, in a microgravity environment, they remain suspended in the air rather than falling to the floor. Spacecraft particulates include flakes of paint, flakes of skin, lint, dust, and food crumbs. Inertia may cause large particulates to remain suspended in the air for many hours before moving to an air filter.

Recent hardware and procedural changes, such as using a 40- to 70-μm mesh cabin air filter (Air Revitalization System air filter) in place of a 280- to 300-μm mesh filter and extensive preflight cleaning of the Orbiter cabin interior at KSC, have reduced the concentrations of particulates during recent Shuttle missions. (John E. Whalen, subsystem manager for cabin air fan and cabin air filter, NASA JSC Crew and Thermal Systems Division, seminar presentation, July 23, 1987.)

B. Contingency Sources

1. Qualitative Risk Analysis Applied to Management of Accidental Chemical Releases

Potential sources of a contingent chemical release must be identified in order to develop monitoring and decontamination strategies. Once potential sources of contamination have been identified, they should be evaluated in terms of the probability of a chemical release occurring and the severity of the hazard posed. Resources should be applied to the management of chemical sources that have a relatively high probability of releasing a toxic chemical and the potential to cause a severe toxicity hazard.

2. Thermodegradation of Synthetic Materials

After the Apollo fire in 1967, NASA enacted stringent flammability and thermodegradation resistance requirements for all materials used in pressurized spacecraft modules . As a result, only a few minor thermodegradation events have occurred, and these were the result of wiring shorts[33,34] or overheated circuits.[35] However, thermodegradation of synthetic materials, such as those used to insulate wiring on spacecraft, continues to cause some concern because of the highly toxic nature of the combustion products. For example, the present wiring insulation on the Space Shuttle and that planned for space station consist largely of polytetrafluoroethylene and polyimide. These insulating materials have considerable resistance to combustion; however, polyimide has some tendency to arc track; and, because it is in contact with other insulators, toxic gases such as hydrogen cyanide, hydrogen fluoride (HF), and CO could be produced.[36–38] It has also been shown that the particulate fraction from combustion of perfluoropolymers is highly toxic under some conditions.[39] Because of widespread use of automatic fire extinguishing systems, it can be concluded that the risk of a moderate-sized combustion incident is fairly small but the severity of the outcome is high.

3. Payload Chemicals

Experience with the Shuttle has indicated that material from payload experiments periodically escapes containment and causes minor, transient, adverse effects on the crew. It is expected that space station payloads containing chemicals will be more massive and involve a wider variety of chemicals than Shuttle payloads. Experiments on permanently orbiting stations are also of longer duration than those on reusable vehicles. Space station payloads will require on-orbit installation and checkout, periodic sample loading and equipment maintenance, and in-rack payload waste storage.[40] For long-lived space vehicles or space outposts in which many experiments are performed, the risk of a payload chemical release appears to be moderate. The consequences of the release of a payload chemical do not appear to be as severe as those resulting from a moderate-sized fire. Obviously, chemicals with high potential for toxicity will be better contained than those that are less toxic. It can be concluded that the risk of rapid, accidental release of chemicals from payloads is moderate, and the severity of the resultant hazard is moderate.

4. Fire Extinguishants

Because of a moderate fire or an accidental release, fire extinguishant materials may be dispersed into the internal atmosphere of the cabin. The Shuttle employs Halon® 1301 (bromotrifluoromethane) as the fire extinguishant. The material has very low toxicity, as evidenced by controlled human exposures for 24 h at 1 percent, showing that only minor changes were detected in a few performance and clinical parameters.[41] One percent is the Halon® concentration that would result from the discharge of all three hand-held extinguishers aboard the Shuttle. Halon® is difficult to remove from spacecraft atmospheres; it remains in the air for many days after accidental release. The toxic decomposition products of Halon® 1301 include HF, hydrogen bromide (HBr) and trace quantities of carbonyl fluoride (COF_2) and carbonyl bromide ($COBr_2$); however, if the extinguishant is applied rapidly when a fire is small, these products do not pose a serious toxic hazard.[42] The level for safe continuous exposure to Halon® for 90 days has been set at 100 parts per million (ppm) by the National Research Council.[43] Even though small concentrations of bromotrifluoromethane are occasionally detected in cabin atmospheres, there have been no instances of large releases into the Shuttle cabin. An alternative fire extinguishant is CO_2, which has been proposed for space station. CO_2 is not as effective as Halon®; however, it is readily removed from air by filters containing basic materials and is somewhat less toxic. Based on Shuttle experience, it appears that the risk of fire extinguishant release is fairly low and the consequences of any releases would be no more than moderate.

5. External Chemicals

Chemicals outside a spacecraft may accidentally contaminate the internal environment after EVA. Typically, the chemicals of concern are highly toxic propellants, such as a hydrazine or NO_2. During the Space Shuttle Program, there has been no evidence that EVA chemicals are a problem for internal environments, even though a "strong odor" was noted in the airlock after an EVA on one mission. For activities involving assembly of large structures in space (e.g., space station), there will be an increased risk of EVA-caused contamination simply because of the number of EVAs. Although propellant chemicals are often very toxic, they tend to be reactive and easily removed from the internal atmosphere. Therefore, if they did enter the cabin in the small quantities possible from EVAs, the toxic hazard would be only moderate. It can be concluded that the probability of chemical contamination from EVAs is small and the potential hazard moderate.

6. Utility Chemicals

The sudden release of fluid-systems chemicals or utility chemicals is another potential source of concern. Such chemicals are selected with toxicity in mind and are generally well contained. An example is dichlorofluoromethane (Freon® 21), which is doubly contained in the cabin heat exchanger but has the potential to be hazardous if it escapes in moderate quantities.[44] There have been no significant accidental releases of utility or fluid-systems chemicals during Shuttle missions. Even though these chemicals are of moderate toxicity, they tend to be used in large quantities; therefore, the severity of release into the internal environment would be moderate. Just as for fire extinguishants and EVA chemicals, the probability of release of utility and fluid-system chemicals is low.

V. Predicting, Measuring, and Removing Airborne Chemical Contaminants

A. Chemical Load Models for Spacecraft

The design of spacecraft air revitalization systems depends on a reasonably accurate prediction of the chemical load that will be placed into the air and on the air quality standards that must be met to protect crew health. There is considerable uncertainty in predicting airborne chemical loads; however, progressively improved models have been formulated to develop predictions. In the late 1960s, an early load model including more than 150 chemicals for spacecraft air was developed based on a variety of information sources.[45] The information included offgassing test data, contaminants detected in ground-based testing of human beings in closed environments, contaminants from known experiments, and contaminants detected on charcoal adsorption beds of Gemini and Mercury space flights. The model was developed in support of an isotope-heated catalytic oxidizer system. A later version of this model reduced the nonbiological loading by a factor of 10 because offgassing is highest early in a mission and falls off rapidly late in the mission.[29] The model was again updated in 1976, using measured payload contaminant generation rates in preparation for Spacelab experiments aboard the Space Shuttle.[46] With each model, a number of assumptions were necessary to estimate contaminant levels from data compiled from many sources.

The space station contaminant load model began with data from experimental offgassing of the fully configured Spacelab. Spacelabs 1 and 3 were offgassed to obtain two lists of trace contaminants, and the higher of the two measured values for each contaminant was incorporated into the space station model by a weight proportioning factor of 7.9.[47] Additional information was incorporated into the model based on predicted leakage rates from space station subsystems, potential introduction of propellant contaminants through EVAs, and release of indole, a normal human metabolite present in bodily wastes.[47] While efforts to predict contaminant levels are essential,[48] it is equally important to recognize that the predictions provided by contaminant models are, at best, within an order of magnitude of reality. A significant confounding factor may be the reactions that occur among the chemicals present in the air.[49] Additional in situ measurements of labile contaminants and grab samples (e.g., samples trapped in an evacuated bottle) have been recommended as an approach to validating models of contaminant loading and their reactions.[49]

B. Preflight Assessment of Contaminants

1. Offgas Testing of Flight Articles

Since offgassing is a major source of atmospheric contamination (see Section II, Sources of Environmental Contamination), NASA requires that all candidate flight articles to be flown in a spacecraft living environment (or the component materials in these articles) be offgas tested as a requisite for flight certification. The offgas test serves as a screen for articles or materials that might release toxic amounts of offgassed products into the Shuttle atmosphere.

In the standard offgas test procedure, an article or component material sample is placed in a sealed chamber at 49 °C (120 °F) for 72 h. Air samples taken from the chamber are then analyzed for offgassed products by gas chromatography/mass spectrometry.[50] If offgas test results for all of the component materials in an article are available, a summation of offgassed products released from these materials, prorated to the amount used in the article, may be used instead of an offgas test of the article itself. The toxicologist evaluates the results of an offgas test in light of the concentration of offgassed chemicals compared to their SMACs and the potential additive toxicity factor (T-value) of all offgassed products (see Section III.E, Exposure to Mixtures of Compounds). If a candidate flight article releases unacceptable amounts of offgassed products, the article must either be conditioned to reduce offgassing and then retested or eliminated from further consideration for flight.

2. Offgas Test of Flight Configured Orbiter Cabin and Spacelab

A 6-h offgas test is performed on the flight-configured crew cabins of all new and extensively refurbished spacecraft, of spacecraft that have not flown for more than 2 years, and for all habitable Spacelabs. This test serves as a final check to determine if the sum of offgassed products from all components of the cabin interior and the entire cargo (including payloads, housekeeping equipment, and communication equipment) is likely to reach a toxic level during the mission.

The test is usually performed in the KSC Orbiter Processing Facility, about 4 to 6 weeks before launch. After the hatch is closed, five pairs of air samples are collected through a vent line into evacuated stainless steel cylinders over a period of 6 h. The air samples are then returned to the NASA JSC Toxicology Laboratory for analysis[50] and subsequent toxicological evaluation. Detailed procedures for collecting and handling air samples during this test are given in Test 12 in NASA document NHB 8060.1.[15]

C. In-Flight Assessment of Airborne Contaminants

1. Particulate Contaminants

Before STS-32, which flew in early 1990, there had never been real-time analysis of airborne particles during a U.S. space flight. Understanding of particulate contamination had come from postflight microscopic examination and chemical analysis of materials trapped on large-mesh filters during the mission. Two types of particle samplers were flown aboard STS-32.[17] Shuttle particle samplers (Fig. 2) collected airborne particles in four size ranges as follows: 0–2.5 μm, 2.5–10 μm, 10–100 μm, and >100 μm. A second system, the Shuttle particle monitor (Fig. 3), took real-time counts of particles using a photometer and a data logger. The mass concentrations of particle fractions collected by the Shuttle particle sampler were determined gravimetrically after the instrument was returned to Earth. Preliminary data indicate that the atmospheric concentrations of particles in the three largest size categories were well above typical values found in Earth environments (previously shown in Fig. 1). This was not unexpected, since large particles do not settle in a microgravity environment. The increased concentrations seen in the 2.5–10 μm range would be of toxicological concern, since they are within the respirable range.[51] However, the concentrations found were well below the maximum level of 200 μg/m^3 recommended for space flights more than 1 week in length.[52] Chemical characterization of the particles obtained during STS-32 is underway, and additional flights of the instruments are planned on STS-40.

2. Gaseous Contaminants

Prior to 1990, the only gaseous contaminants quantitated analytically during space missions were hydrazines and the major constituents O_2 and CO_2. Beginning with the STS-41 mission, a combustion products analyzer (Fig. 4) with electrochemical sensors for four toxic combustion gases was flown.[53] The sensors were targeted to HCl, HCN, HF, and CO. The combustion products analyzer was flown as a test instrument for the purpose of developing flight hardware to give quantitative information on these four gases in the event of thermodegradation of synthetic material in the cabin. Baseline readings were taken during the missions, and analyses of bottle samples collected during the missions revealed that the CO sensor was responding to the accumulation of

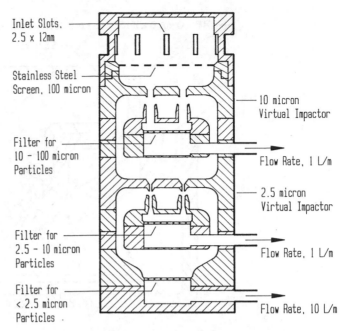

Fig. 2 Cross section of the Shuttle particle sampler, which separates particles into the size range of >100 μm, 10-100 μm, 2.5-10 μm, and <2.5 μm. [Reprinted with permission 1991, Society of Automotive Engineers, Inc.]

hydrogen in the cabin air. The accumulation of hydrogen had been unexpected, and the CO sensor was redesigned to reduce hydrogen cross-sensitivity. At this writing, the instrument is undergoing further development and testing so that a thoroughly tested flight unit will be available for real-time monitoring in the event of a combustion incident.

Flying a real-time analytical monitor for potentially toxic gases marks the beginning of a new era in U.S. spacecraft air monitoring. Previous measurements depended on samples trapped in evacuated bottles or adsorbent materials and analyzed in Earth-based laboratories after the mission. If human beings are to continue permanent occupation of space, then the air within space habitats must be monitored independently of Earth-based laboratories. Some monitoring must be in real time in order to detect potentially hazardous gases in time to protect crew health. For example, a goal for air monitoring in space station is to contain hazardous contaminants to the element in which they originate. This can be accomplished only with instruments having rapid response times to targeted compounds or rapid responses to groups of compounds. Examples of instruments planned for the man-tended phase of space station are compound-specific analyzers and a total hydrocarbon analyzer. The compound-specific analyzer will respond rapidly to a small group of toxic gasses with specific sensors, whereas the total hydrocarbon analyzer will respond quickly to a wide range of nonmethane hydrocarbons and halocarbons. To determine the level of toxic hazard, the total hydro-

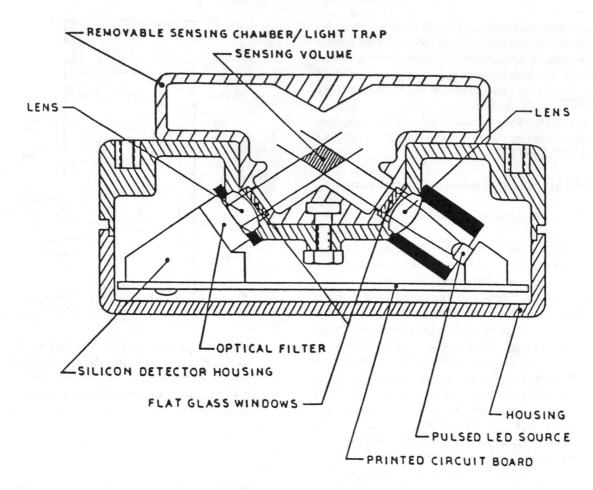

REMOVABLE SENSING CHAMBER/LIGHT TRAP
SENSING VOLUME
LENS
LENS
OPTICAL FILTER
SILICON DETECTOR HOUSING
FLAT GLASS WINDOWS
HOUSING
PULSED LED SOURCE
PRINTED CIRCUIT BOARD

Fig. 3 Shuttle particle monitor capable of real-time detection of airborne particles.

carbon analyzer will be backed up by a volatile organic analyzer capable of identifying compounds detected by the total hydrocarbon analyzer. The organic analyzer will also be used to identify and quantitate airborne organics on a periodic basis by desorption of those organics from an organic sampler, which can be placed in various locations throughout the station.

D. Retrospective Measurement of In-Flight Atmospheric Contaminant Levels

Atmospheric contaminant levels during Shuttle flights are monitored retrospectively through the collection of in-flight air samples for postmission analysis. Usually, one 0.3-liter air sample is collected into an evacuated stainless steel cylinder immediately before flight and another is collected near the end of the mission or at any time that air contamination is suspected.[54] At least four cylinder samples are routinely collected from the Spacelab during Spacelab missions.[55] During some Shuttle missions, the cabin atmosphere is sampled continuously for 24 h with a Tenax® resin column in the solid sorbent air sampler (Fig. 5).[56] The Tenax® resin traps the volatile organic contaminants, which are thermally desorbed from the Tenax® during the subsequent ground-based analy-

sis. A fresh Tenax® column is selected after 24 h of continuous air sampling. Since relatively large air volumes are sampled by this method (3.25 liters of air in 24 h through each Tenax® tube), many contaminants may be detected and quantitated in the parts per billion range. On the other hand, many low molecular weight compounds, such as methane and CO_2, are not retained by Tenax®; so they are not identified by this sampling method. Analytical results of air cylinder samples collected from the Shuttle cabin during the STS-26, STS-27, STS-28, and STS-33 missions[57–60] are shown in Table 2. As of this writing (May 1991), no contaminant has ever exceeded its SMAC in any air sample collected during a Shuttle mission. This demonstrates the high effectiveness of the contamination control measures and Air Revitalization Systems (ARSs) for the Shuttle and Spacelab (see Section V.D.1, Toxic Contaminant Removal Capabilities in the Space Shuttle).

In many respects, the measurement of airborne contaminants in the permanently manned Russian Mir has paralleled the approach used in the reusable Shuttle. Typically, contaminant samples are obtained in several locations (exercise trainer, toilet, and workstations) by drawing 0.5 liters of air through a Tenax® tube. The filter material is returned to Earth for desorption of contaminants and identification by gas chro-

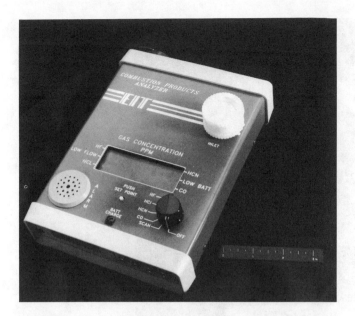

Fig. 4 Combustion products analyzer being developed to measure carbon monoxide, hydrogen cyanide, hydrogen fluoride, and hydrogen chloride in the event of a combustion contingency in the Shuttle.

matography. The major contaminants during the visits of prime crews 3 and 4 were similar, typified by the following averages obtained during the visit of prime crew 3: acetone, 1.1 mg/m^3; acetaldehyde, 1.0 mg/m^3; ethanol, 7.6 mg/m^3; ethyl acetate, 0.6 mg/m^3; and methyl ethyl ketone, 0.8 mg/m^3. These contaminants tended to increase when cargo vehicles were unloaded or when cosmonauts used the exercise machine.

Contaminant levels during the visit of prime crew 5 were somewhat higher than those seen during the visits of prime crews 3 and 4. The major contaminants and their ranges of concentration were as follows: acetone, 0.9 to 1.4 mg/m^3; acetaldehyde, 0.8 to 3.7 mg/m^3; ethanol, 30.6 to 107.3 mg/m^3; ethyl acetate, 0.3 to 1.8 mg/m^3; and methyl ethyl ketone, 0.6 to 12.4 mg/m^3. It is important to note that the maximal values were found for no more than 4 h per day, based on the results of a diurnal study of contaminant concentrations. The study of airborne contaminants was expanded during the visit of prime crew 6. The usual contaminant samples were obtained three times per day during certain periods, and ammonia and CO$_2$ were detected using indicator tubes. After docking with the "T" module, the sample taken immediately after opening the hatch proved to contain the contaminants listed above, as well as isopropanol, isobutanol, and heptane.

1. Toxic Contaminant Removal Capabilities in the Space Shuttle

The Shuttle ARS includes a variety of particulate and vapor filters, and other types of contaminant collection devices designed to function during both normal operations and contingency situations (Fig. 6). If properly used, the various ARS systems may make it possible to decontaminate the Shuttle cabin atmosphere after a small-to-moderate-scale toxicological accident. Specific data regarding each ARS component are given in Table 3.[28,30,61–69]

The LiOH in the LiOH/C cartridges is designed specifically to remove CO$_2$. During Shuttle missions, the LiOH/C cartridges must be changed at intervals of 5.5–24 h depending on crew size.[28] A maximum of 32 reserve units is initially available. In a combustion contingency in which toxic acid gases are produced, the alkaline LiOH would efficiently remove those gases from the air.

Three types of charcoal are used in various ARS air filter configurations. Untreated activated charcoal, which lines the radial inlet of the LiOH/C cartridges, efficiently removes most odorous and toxic chemicals. It is particularly effective against compounds that are reactive and not highly volatile;[61] it is not effective against certain gases such as CO, hydrogen, and ammonia (NH$_3$). The amount of charcoal in each LiOH/C cartridge (86–115 grams) would be sufficient to remove only a rather small amount of a well-adsorbed volatile chemical. The ambient temperature catalytic oxidizer (ATCO) includes both activated charcoal and platinum-treated charcoal (Pt/C). The activated charcoal protects the platinum from reactive compounds that would poison its catalytic properties.[62] The Pt/C catalyzes the oxidation of CO and H$_2$ to CO$_2$ and H$_2$O, respectively. The CO$_2$ and H$_2$O are then removed by other systems. The ATCO has a very low airflow rate (1.7 m^3/h), which limits its value for removing CO in a combustion contingency. On recent Shuttle flights, the ATCO has been supplemented (for contingency use) with a reserve ATCO unit consisting of an LiOH/C cartridge containing about 2300 grams of Pt/C, which could be inserted in the place of one of the regular LiOH/C cartridges. Each LiOH/C cartridge filters a much greater air volume per hour (46 m^3/h) than does the ATCO (2.5 m^3/h).[28] The third type of charcoal air filter is the proprietary acid-treated charcoal in the waste collector system odor/bacteria filter, which is designed to remove ammonia and other odorous nitrogenous compounds, such as indole and skatole. This acid charcoal has also been shown to effectively remove many nonalkaline gases, such as phenol and hydrogen sulfide.[67] Considering the large amount of charcoal in this unit (2.27 kg) and the fact that there is also an identical reserve unit in the waste management compartment, this charcoal may be very useful in the event of release and vaporization of a rather large amount of a well-adsorbed volatile chemicals. The Spacelab tunnel air scrubber contains all three types of charcoal; however, its effectiveness is limited by a relatively low airflow (2.5 m^3/h).

Toxic and nuisance particles are routinely filtered from the cabin atmosphere by 40- to 70-μm mesh filters preceding the cabin fan and many of the flight deck avionics instrument panels, which need filtered air for cooling. The odor/bacteria filter in the waste collection system contains a 0.45-μm bacteria filter. The movement of particulates to the cabin filters is somewhat limited by inertia, which is proportional to the size of these particulates. Therefore, the orbiter vacuum

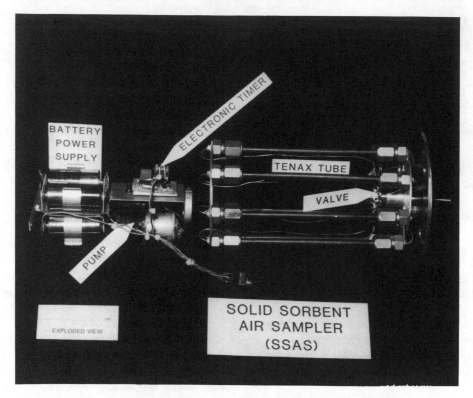

Fig. 5 Solid sorbent air sampler used on many Shuttle missions to trap airborne gaseous contaminants for later ground-based analysis.

Table 2   Contaminants found in the air cylinder samples collected during typical STS missions

	Concentrations(mg/m^3) during STS missions			
Compound	STS-26	STS-27	STS-28	STS-33
2-methyl-2-propanol	0.86			
2-propanol			0.15	0.32
2-propanone		0.56		
1,1,1-trichloro-1,2,2-trifluoroethane	0.04			
1,1,1-trichloroethane	0.06	0.06		
1,1,2-trichloro-1,2,2-trifluoroethane		0.38		1.62
Acetaldehyde		0.25	0.13	
C$_4$-alkane(1)			0.07	
C$_4$-alkane(2)			0.06	
Chloromethane			0.004	
Dichloromethane	0.46	0.33	0.17	0.29
Ethanol	6.4	3.6	0.4	6.1
Ethoxyethyl acetate	0.67			
Hexamethylcyclotrisiloxane	0.2			0.07
Methane			78.5	25.0
Octamethylcyclotetrasiloxane	1.22			0.18
Propanone	0.87		0.35	0.65
Toluene	0.02	0.01		

cleaner may be very useful after the escape of toxic particulates, since it could be brought into the immediate vicinity of the escape. It is routinely used to remove particles and lint from the cabin filters. The condensing heat exchanger, even though it does not use filters, is effective in removing most water-soluble gaseous contaminants (e.g., alcohols and ammonia). Relatively insoluble contaminants (e.g., toluene and benzene) are moderately well removed by the heat exchanger.[64] Depending on the ambient temperature and thermostat setting, from 30–100 percent of the cabin air flow

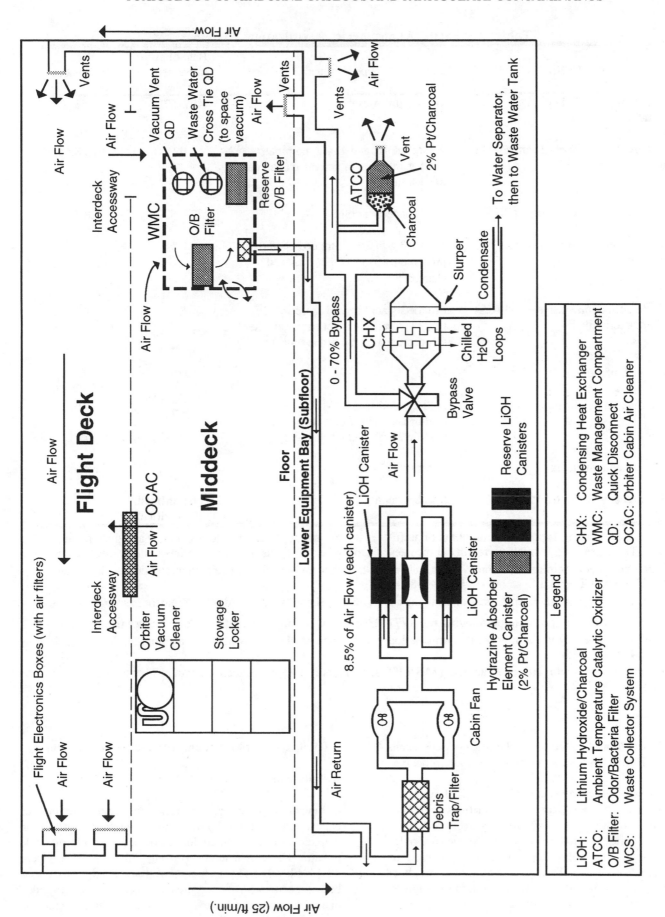

Fig. 6 Atmospheric decontamination system in the Shuttle cabin. Major areas indicated are the waste management system, ambient temperature catalytic oxidizer (ATCO), and the condensing heat exchanger (CHX).

Legend

LiOH:	Lithium Hydroxide/Charcoal	CHX:	Condensing Heat Exchanger
ATCO:	Ambient Temperature Catalytic Oxidizer	WMC:	Waste Management Compartment
O/B Filter:	Odor/Bacteria Filter	QD:	Quick Disconnect
WCS:	Waste Collector System	OCAC:	Orbiter Cabin Air Cleaner

Table 3 Shuttle Atmospheric Revitilzation Systems[a]

Device	Type air filter[a]	Rate of air movement (m^3/hr)[a]	References
Cabin fan (preceded by orbiter cabin air filter)	40—70 μm mesh[b]	497–578	63
LiOH/C air scrubber (2 canisters in line, 32 reserve canisters)	2.3 kg LiOH[c] and 114 g, nominal,[c] or 85 g, minimal of activated charcoal in each canister	92	61,28,65
Condensing heat exchanger (CHX)	Cold condensor coils	232–529	28,66
Ambient temperature catalytic oxidizer (ATCO)	327+ 2.3 g of 2% Pt-treated charcoal, preceded by 511+57 g of activated charcoal[d]	1.7	62,28
Waste collection subsystem (WCS) odor/bacteria filter	Proprietary acid-treated charcoal (2.27 kg/unit) 0.45-μm bacterial filter (1 operational and 1 reserve unit)	65	67
Spacelab tunnel fan	None	210	30
Spacelab tunnel air scrubber	2.38 kg of charcoal 1.81 kg of acid-treated charcoal 0.31 kg 2% Pt-treated charcoal	2.5	30
Orbiter vacuum cleaner	Filter paper	60	68,69
Contingency vacuum hoses[e]	Space vacuum	1.3 (1st orifice)[f] 0.77 (2nd orifice)[f]	

[a] In most instances, approximate amounts of air filter materials and approximate rates of airflow are given in this table. There are always small variations in the rates of airflow and amounts of filter materials in the respective units.

[b] ARS air filters: seminar by John Whalen, subsystem manager for the cabin fan, air filter, and debris trap system, JSC Crew and Thermal Systems Division, 1987.

[c] CO_2 adsorber cartridge: specification drawing no. SV75510, Hamilton Standards Co., Windsor Lock, Conn.

[d] ATCO cartridge: Specification drawing no. SV774230, Rev. C, Hamilton Standards Co., Windsor Lock, Conn.

[e] Three contingency vacuum hoses that may be connected to one another are available in the Shuttle; they are 3, 3, and 2.4 m in length.

[f] Communication with Hubert Brasseau, NASA JSC Life Support Systems Branch, Crew and Thermal Systems Division, Dec. 12, 1990.

(about 500 m^3/h) is directed across the cold condenser coils,[28] so this unit may remove some types of contaminants very rapidly.

The three contingency vacuum hoses (which may be connected to either of two space vacuum orifices or to one another) have a relatively low aspiration rate (0.8 or 1.3 m^3 air/h). However, they would be effective in the removal of localized gaseous or particulate contaminants, such as the gases and smoke from a fire. The hoses would also be ideal for removing volatile liquids that would otherwise vaporize if collected on the cabin air filters.

III. Spacecraft Maximum Allowable Concentrations

A. Rationale for Setting SMACs

Several regulatory agencies and private organizations set exposure levels for airborne chemicals to which workers or the general population could be exposed with minimal risk of harm. There are a number of compelling reasons why permissible levels set by such organizations cannot be used as a basis for setting SMACs. A great number of exposure guidelines come from the American Conference of Governmental

Industrial Hygienists, which sets threshold limit values at levels to "which it is believed that nearly all workers may be repeatedly exposed day after day without adverse effect." They specifically state that threshold limit values are not intended for use "in estimating the toxic potential of continuous, uninterrupted exposures or other extended work periods."[70] The Occupational Safety and Health Administration sets permissible exposure limits for regulation of industrial exposures based, in part, on recommended exposure levels published by the National Institute for Occupational Safety and Health and the threshold limit values.[71] None of these standards is suitable for the continuous exposures that people in space habitats will experience. A few pollutant exposure levels (National Ambient Air Quality Standards) have been set by the Environmental Protection Agency, but these values are targeted at a broad population, including persons with heart and respiratory diseases, which is very different from the relatively healthy astronaut population.

To some extent, the problem of continuous exposures has been considered by the Board on Toxicology and Environmental Health Hazards of the National Research Council. In a series of publications, they have set Emergency Exposure Guidance Levels and Short-term Public Emergency Guidance Levels.[72] However, these apply to continuous exposures only up to 24 h and are available only on a limited number of compounds. To provide guidance to the U.S. Navy on submarine operations, approximately fifty 90-day continuous exposure guidance levels have been set by the National Research Council.[20] These limits are probably the closest to being applicable to spacecraft air standards; however, they are not directly applicable to space habitats for several reasons. First, the scope of these values is limited to the extent that no values have been set for many compounds of interest to NASA. The toxic endpoints (performance decrements) acceptable to the U.S. Navy may be significantly different from those acceptable to NASA, particularly in view of the limited escape options available to astronauts compared to escape options from submarines. People living in space habitats will be subjected to varying degrees of gravity deprivation, with concomitant physiological and biochemical changes that may induce increased susceptibility to toxicants. Potentially increased susceptibility must be considered when SMACs are set.

B. History of SMACs

Since the mid-1960s, the National Research Council Committee on Toxicology has been closely involved in the process of setting SMACs. In 1968, they recommended 90-day limits on 23 chemicals, 1000-day limits on 11 contaminants, and 60-min limits on 5 contaminants.[73] Following NASA's request, the Committee on Toxicology set SMACs in 1972 on 52 compounds for exposure times varying from 10 min to 6 months.[74] These limits were provisional and subject to change as more data became available. A few years later, NASA expanded the list of compounds to 190 and set values

for 7 and 30 days; the list was later modified to exclude the 30-day SMACs.[15] The limitation to all these values is that no documentation was developed to support the levels set. This is a major shortcoming and makes it nearly impossible to defend the existing values or to review them in light of new data. In 1988, NASA again asked the Committee on Toxicology to become involved in the SMAC process by providing guidelines that NASA toxicologists could use to set SMACs.[75] Table 4 presents scientifically based SMACs established at JSC. This table is being used by NASA in the design of future life support systems but still requires official approval.

C. Goals of the SMAC Program

1. Specific Goals

The goal of the SMAC Program is to provide a basis, in terms of maximum acceptable contaminant levels, that will ensure protection of crew health at risk levels acceptable to NASA.[44] Implementation of this goal involves the use of SMACs to interpret data from the offgassing of flight materials. The SMACs are also used to set requirements for the sensitivity of monitoring instruments and for the effectiveness of air revitalization systems in keeping potentially hazardous chemicals at acceptable levels. Finally, when the quantity of a payload chemical at risk for accidental release is known, SMACs may be used to determine if the payload requires single, double, or triple containment.

2. Noncarcinogens

For noncarcinogens to which a crew may be exposed for 7, 30, or 180 days, the goal is to set SMACs to ensure that no adverse health effects will result from the exposure. These exposure intervals were chosen to correspond with mission lengths for the Shuttle, Extended Duration Orbiter, and space station, respectively. For emergency or short-term exposures, the 1- and 24-h SMACs are set to permit reversible effects as long as those effects do not impair astronaut performance. For example, mild eye irritation would be acceptable; however, loss of visual acuity would be unacceptable.

3. Carcinogens

For individual carcinogens, the goal is to keep the crewmember's risk from exposure below a lifetime incidence of 1 in 10,000 for each mission. While this would never be an acceptable risk for a large, diverse population, it seems conservative in light of the acceptable risk of carcinogenesis from radiation exposure in space. The risk presently accepted for radiation is "a career limit 3-percent risk of cancer mortality for space activities for both sexes and all ages."[76] It should be emphasized that the chemical risk is indexed to occurrence of cancer, whereas the radiation risk is indexed to death as a result of cancer. It is anticipated that no more than five

Table 4 Current Spacecraft Maximum Allowable Concentrations Established at NASA JSC [NASA JSC internal document dated April 13, 1993]

Chemical (CAS #)		Potential Exposure Period					Year Set or Reviewed	Remarks
		1 hr	24 hr	7 d	30 d	180 d		
Acetaldehyde (75-07-0)	ppm:	10 Irr	6 Irr	2 Irr	2 Irr	2 Irr	1992	Carcinogen
	(mg/m3):	(20)	(10)	(4)	(4)	(4)		
Acrolein (107-02-08)	ppm:	0.075 Irr	0.035 Irr	0.015 Irr	0.015 Irr	0.015 Irr	1992	Ceiling values
	(mg/m3):	(0.2)	(0.08)	(0.03)	(0.03)	(0.03)		
Ammonia (7664-41-7)	ppm:	30 Irr	20 Irr	10 Irr	10 Irr	10 Irr	1991	Ceiling values
	(mg/m3):	(20)	(14)	(7)	(7)	(7)		
1,3- Butadiene (106-99-0)	ppm:	2 SGt	2 SGt	0.3 SGt	0.15 SGt	0.06 Crc	1992	Carcinogen
	(mg/m3):	(4)	(4)	(0.7)	(0.3)	(0.13)		
Carbon dioxide (124-38-9)	ppm:	13000 CNS	13000 CNS	7000 Hv	7000 Hv	7000 Hv	1992	
	(mg/m3):	(23000)	(23000)	(13000)	(13000)	(13000)		
Carbon monoxide (630-08-0)	ppm:	55 CNS Hrt	20 CNS Hrt	10 CNS Hrt	10 CNS Hrt	10 CNS Hrt	1991	Carboxyhemoglobin target
	(mg/m3):	(60)	(20)	(10)	(10)	(10)		
Dichloroacetylene (7572-29-4)	ppm:	0.6 CNS Kdy Lvr	0.04 CNS Kdy Lvr	0.03 CNS Kdy	0.025 CNS Kdy	0.015 CNS Kdy	1992	
	(mg/m3):	(2.4)	(0.16)	(0.12)	(0.10)	(0.06)		
1,2- Dichloroethane (107-06-2)	ppm:	0.4 GI	0.4 GI	0.4 GI	0.4 GI	0.2 Crc	1992	Carcinogen
	(mg/m3):	(2)	(2)	(2)	(2)	(1)		
2 - Ethoxyethanol (110-80-5)	ppm:	10 RBC	10 RBC	0.8 RBC	0.5 RBC	0.07 RBC	1992	
	(mg/m3):	(40)	(40)	(3)	(2)	(0.3)		
Formaldehyde (50-00-0)	ppm:	0.4 Irr	0.1 Irr	0.04 Irr	0.04 Irr	0.04 Irr	1991	Ceiling values, Carcinogen
	(mg/m3):	(0.5)	(0.12)	(0.05)	(0.05)	(0.05)		

CNS - Central Nervous System　　Hda - Headache　　Kdy - Kidney Injury　　Odr - Odor　　　　　　SGt - Sperm Genotoxicity
Crc - Carcinogen　　　　　　　　Hrt - Heart　　　　Lvr - Liver　　　　　　RBC - Red Blood Cell　Tes - Testis
Dth - Death　　　　　　　　　　Hv - Hyperventilation　Nau - Nausea　　　Rsp - Respiratory System Injury　Vis - Visual Disturbances
GI - Gastrointestinal　　　　　　Irr - Irritant　　　Nsl - Nasal Injury　　SM - Sperm Morphology　Xpl - Explosive

(Table 4 continued on next page)

Table 4 (continued) Current Spacecraft Maximum Allowable Concentrations Established at NASA JSC [NASA JSC internal document dated April 13, 1993]

Chemical (CAS #)		Potential Exposure Period					Year Set or Reviewed	Remarks
		1 hr	24 hr	7 d	30 d	180 d		
Freon 113 (76-13-1)	ppm:	50 Hrt	50 Hrt	50 Hrt	50 Hrt	50 Hrt	1991	
	(mg/m3):	(400)	(400)	(400)	(400)	(400)		
Hydrazine (302-01-2)	ppm:	4 Dth	0.3 Lvr	0.04 Lvr	0.02 Lvr	0.004 Lvr	1992	Carcinogen
	(mg/m3):	(5)	(0.4)	(0.05)	(0.03)	(0.005)		
Hydrogen (1333-74-0)	ppm:	4100 Xpl	4100 Xpl	4100 Xpl	4100 Xpl	4100 Xpl	1990	Ceiling values are 10% of the Lower Explosive Limit
	(mg/m3):	(340)	(340)	(340)	(340)	(340)		
Indole (120-72-9)	ppm:	1.0 Nau	0.3 Nau	0.05 Nau RBC	0.05 Dth RBC	0.05 Dth RBC	1992	Normal turnover of indole used to establish a lower bound of 0.05 ppm.
	(mg/m3):	(5)	(1.5)	(0.25)	(0.25)	(0.25)		
Mercury (7439-97-6)	ppm:	0.01 CNS	0.002 CNS	0.001 CNS	0.001 CNS	0.001 CNS	1992	
	(mg/m3):	(0.1) Rsp	(0.02) Rsp	(0.01) Kdy	(0.01) Kdy	(0.01) Kdy		
Methane (74-82-8)	ppm:	5300 Xpl	5300 Xpl	5300 Xpl	5300 Xpl	5300 Xpl	1990	Ceiling values are 10% of the Lower Explosive Limit
	(mg/m3):	(3800)	(3800)	(3800)	(3800)	(3800)		
Methanol (67-56-1)	ppm:	30 Vis	10 Hda	7 Hda	7 Hda	7 Hda	1992	
	(mg/m3):	(40)	(13) Vis	(9) Vis	(9) Vis	(9) Vis		
Methyl Ethyl Ketone (78-93-3)	ppm:	50 Irr	50 Irr	10 Irr	10 Irr	10 Irr	1992	Ceiling values
	(mg/m3):	(150)	(150)	(30)	(30)	(30)		
Methyl hydrazine (60-34-4)	ppm:	0.002 Nsl	0.002 Nsl	0.002 Nsl	0.002 Nsl	0.002 Lvr Nsl RBC	1991	Carcinogen
	(mg/m3):	(0.004)	(0.004)	(0.004)	(0.004)	(0.004)		
Methylene chloride (75-09-2)	ppm:	100 CNS	35 CNS	15 Hrt	5 Lvr	3 Lvr	1992	CO formation, Carcinogen
	(mg/m3):	(350) Hrt	(120) Hrt	(50)	(20)	(10)		

CNS - Central Nervous System	Hda - Headache	Kdy - Kidney Injury	Odr - Odor	SGt - Sperm Genotoxicity
Crc - Carcinogen	Hrt - Heart	Lvr - Liver	RBC - Red Blood Cell	Tes - Testis
Dth - Death	Hv - Hyperventilation	Nau - Nausea	Rsp - Respiratory System Injury	Vis - Visual Disturbances
GI - Gastrointestinal	Irr - Irritant	Nsl - Nasal Injury	SM - Sperm Morphology	Xpl - Explosive

(Table 4 continued on next page)

Table 4 (continued) Current Spacecraft Maximum Allowable Concentrations Established at NASA JSC [NASA JSC internal document dated April 13, 1993]

Chemical (CAS #)		Potential Exposure Period					Year Set or Reviewed	Remarks
		1 hr	24 hr	7 d	30 d	180 d		
Nitromethane (75-52-5)	ppm: (mg/m3):	25 RBC (65)	15 RBC (40)	7 RBC (18)	7 RBC (18)	5 RBC (13)	1992	
Octamethyltrisiloxane (107-51-7)	ppm: (mg/m3):	400 Dth (4000)	200 Dth (2000) Lvr Kdy	100 Lvr (1000) Kdy	20 Lvr (200) Kdy	4 Lvr (40) Kdy	1992	Based on structure activity relationships
2-Propanol (67-63-0)	ppm: (mg/m3):	400 CNS (1000) Irr	100 CNS (240) Irr Lvr	60 CNS (150) Irr Lvr	60 CNS (150) Irr	60 CNS (150) Irr	1992	
Toluene (108-88-3)	ppm: (mg/m3):	16 CNS (60)	16 CNS (60)	16 CNS (60) Irr	16 CNS (60) Irr	16 CNS (60) Irr	1992	
Trichloroethylene (79-01-6)	ppm: (mg/m3):	50 CNS (270)	11 CNS (60)	9 Kdy (50) Lvr	4 Kdy (20) Lvr	2 Crc (10) Kdy Lvr	1992	See dichloroacetylene if alkali scrubber is present. Possible carcinogen.
Trimethylsilanol (1066-40-6)	ppm: (mg/m3):	150 CNS (600)	20 CNS (70)	10 CNS (40)	10 CNS (40)	10 CNS (40)	1991	
Vinyl chloride (75-01-4)	ppm: (mg/m3):	130 Irr (330) Hda CNS Lvr	30 CNS (75) Lvr	1 Tes (3) Lvr	1 Tes (3) Lvr	1 Tes (3) Lvr	1992	Carcinogen
Xylene (1330207 (mixed))	ppm: (mg/m3):	100 Irr (430) CNS	100 Irr (430) CNS	50 Irr (220)	50 Irr (220)	50 Irr (220)	1992	Applies to each individual xylene isomer and mixtures of xylene isomers.

CNS - Central Nervous System	Hda - Headache	Odr - Odor	SGt - Sperm Genotoxicity
Crc - Carcinogen	Hrt - Heart	RBC - Red Blood Cell	Tes - Testis
Dth - Death	Hv - Hyperventilation	Rsp - Respiratory System Injury	Vis- Visual Disturbances
GI - Gastrointestinal	Irr - Irritant	SM - Sperm Morphology	Xpl - Explosive
	Kdy - Kidney Injury		
	Lvr - Liver		
	Nau - Nausea		
	Nsl - Nasal Injury		

missions would be flown by an individual astronaut, so the maximum lifetime risk of cancer resulting from exposure to a chemical carcinogen is 1 in 2000.

D. Methods Used to Set SMACs for Individual Compounds

1. Literature Review

The initial step in setting a SMAC is to review the chemical and toxicological literature. From printouts of abstracts, the investigator must identify those studies that appear to have the most suitable data. First priority is given to controlled human inhalation exposures. For some compounds, these data are available for short-term exposures but almost never for long-term exposures. Epidemiological data may be useful in estimating potential hazards from long-term human exposure. Second priority is given to inhalation studies involving nonhuman primates, particularly if they have been exposed continuously and suitable toxicological endpoints have been examined. Third priority is given to inhalation studies involving other mammalian species, such as rodents, which are the most likely to be well studied. Last priority is given to studies done by routes of administration other than inhalation; it is very difficult to judge inhalation toxicity from data obtained by other routes of administration. The original publication for each important study must be obtained and evaluated for quality and suitability of the results.

2. Quality of Key Studies

Unfortunately, the toxicological literature contains many flawed or incomplete studies; therefore, each potentially important study must be carefully evaluated to ensure that the reported results are of acceptable quality.[77] A partial checklist for evaluating studies is provided below.

1) Were suitable controls used, and were the exposures and observations free of significant bias? Were there sufficient numbers of experimental subjects?

2) Was the test chemical sufficiently pure? Was it quantitated in the gaseous state by an accurate analytical method, and was it disseminated in a way that led to uniform distribution and good recovery in the inhalation chamber? If the recovery was low, could the cause of the low recovery be explained?

3) Were well-defined and appropriate endpoints examined, and were the group comparisons made with suitable statistical methods?

Studies that are found to be of acceptable quality are compared for consistency. If the results of one study differ markedly from those of other studies, then the investigator should attempt to explain the discrepancy. This review process should result in identification of target organs for the toxicological action of the compound. The target organs and mechanisms of toxicity may vary with exposure times over the range of times considered (1 h to 180 days).

3. Determination of the Most Sensitive Endpoint (Toxic Effect)

For each potential exposure time the data should suggest a number of toxicological endpoints. Each endpoint must be analyzed to determine which is predicted to be the most sensitive in human beings. For example, hydrazine, a common propellant used by NASA, induces a number of toxicological effects, including the following: mucosal irritation, nephrotoxicity, hepatotoxicity, carcinogenesis, and death.[78,79] The effects reported depend on the species exposed and the duration of exposure.[80]

Carcinogenic risks are calculated using the linearized multistage model with the number of stages set to three (worst case) and minimum age of exposure set at 30 years.[75] The SMAC document for methylene chloride provides an example of how pharmacokinetic data may be used to predict human toxicity from rodent data.[81,82] Similarly, the SMAC document for formaldehyde illustrates the use of tissue macromolecular binding levels to predict, from rodent date, the human risk of nasal cancer.[2,83] When available, mechanistic data such as these impart much more precision to the process of setting SMACs than relying only on descriptive data and safety factors.

4. Safety Factors

When the descriptive data base is limited and no mechanistic studies are available, a conservative approach to setting SMACs must be taken. In the absence of adequate data, safety factors must be considered for the following extrapolations:

From	To	Value
Observed adverse effect	No adverse effect level	3-100
Nonhuman exposures	Human exposures	1-100
Short exposures	Long exposures	X time
Intermittent exposures	Continuous exposures	1-3
Gravity-based subjects	Microgravity-conditioned subjects	1-10

The magnitude of the safety factors may vary from 1 to 100 depending on the quality of the data and the severity of the toxic effect. Extrapolation of results of short-term exposures to predict effects of long-term exposures is often done in proportion to the exposure times involved (X time); that is, the product of the concentration times the exposure duration (ct) gives a constant toxic effect.[84] This approach tends to be conservative when extrapolating from short-term to long-term exposures; however, it should not be used in the opposite direction, since the resultant short-term values may not be safe. In any case, the "constant ct" approach should be used only as a last resort, since its accuracy has seldom been demonstrated for exposure times differing by more than a factor of 10. The SMAC support document must detail the magnitude of each safety factor rather than provide a "blanket" safety factor. This forces the toxicologist to examine the degree of uncertainty associated with each factor and, from that analysis, identify data gaps. Documenting specific safety factors also makes revision of the SMAC easier when new data become available.

E. Exposures to Mixtures of Compounds

1. Normal and Contingency Mixtures

The normal space habitat is filled with air containing a complex mixture of many contaminants at relatively low concentrations. Under laboratory conditions, it has been shown that subtle performance decrements can occur in healthy individuals as a result of exposure to a low-concentration mixture of volatile organic compounds known to be indoor air pollutants.[19] In a thermodegradation contingency, the air may contain relatively high levels of toxic gases and particles; the combined effects of combustion products have been the subject of several investigations.[85] Unfortunately, the mixture of pyrolysis products from synthetic materials may vary greatly depending on the conditions in which the materials are burned; the resultant toxicological variations approach three orders of magnitude in some cases.[86] Real-time measurements of the toxic pyrolysis products and knowledge of how they interact toxicologically are the best methods for dealing with such a contingency in space habitats. For normal operations where trace contaminants accumulate and toxic effects may be subtle, a summation by target organ has been used to predict the toxicity of mixtures.

2. Summation Method for Mixtures of Chemicals

Following a method used previously,[70,89,90] the toxicity (T-value) of a defined mixture is estimated by adding the ratios of each measured concentration (C_i) to the appropriate SMAC for every compound in the mixture that has the same target organ and mechanism of action.

$$T = C_1/\text{SMAC}_1 + C_2/\text{SMAC}_2 + \cdots C_n/\text{SMAC}_n$$

For example, noncarcinogenic respiratory irritants and pulmonary carcinogens would not be in the same group, even though the target organ is the same. If this summation exceeds unity for any group, then the SMAC has been exceeded for that group. This approach does not apply to compounds known to have synergistic or potentiating effects; however, it is unusual that this information would be known for contaminants at relatively low concentrations. An example is described below for a mixture of three compounds with SMACs of 5, 10, and 50 ppm and measured concentrations of 2, 1, and 15 ppm, respectively. The T summation value is

$$T = 2/5 + 1/10 + 15/50 = 0.8$$

For this mixture of three compounds, the SMAC is not exceeded.

3. Establishment of Group SMACs

More than 650 different compounds without a SMAC have been detected during offgas tests of candidate flight articles since 1974; many were found only on rare occasions. Some of these compounds, such as the C_6 aliphatic hydrocarbons, were not completely identified. Many candidate payload chemicals that were reviewed also did not have a SMAC. All of these offgassed and payload chemicals required a toxicological evaluation, based largely on a comparison between their projected orbiter cabin concentrations and their SMACs. Developing a SMAC for each of these chemicals within the short time available before an upcoming mission would severely tax the manpower and financial resources of the JSC Toxicology Group. Therefore, that group has developed group SMACs for several narrowly defined classes of structurally related chemical compounds. Chemicals that are unusually toxic (as compared with other members of their chemical class), carcinogens, chemicals that already have an individual SMAC, and chemicals with functional groups other than the ones specified in the chemical class description are exempted from the respective group SMACs.

The general procedure for establishing a group SMAC for a specific chemical class is as follows:

1) Summarize the available toxicological data on at least seven prototype compounds, including test concentrations or dosages, animal species, and quantitative estimates of toxic effects. Toxicity data from compounds that already have a SMAC may be used, but not data from other exempt compounds.

2) Establish several potential group SMACs using different toxicological endpoints, such as mortality, behavioral effects, hepatotoxicity, etc.

3) Make adjustments from each data point to be used on the basis of possible differences between the animal species and humans, extrapolation from toxic levels to no-effect levels, etc.

4) Take the lowest adjusted value derived by these procedures as the tentative group SMAC. If adjusted values for one compound are out of line with the others, this compound may be placed on the exempt compound list.

Examples of chemical classes for which tentative group SMACs have been assigned are saturated aliphatic hydrocarbons (C and H only), unsaturated aliphatic hydrocarbons (C and H only), and saturated aliphatic ketones ($>C_2$).

VII. Toxicological Challenges for Future Space Habitats

A. Extended Duration Orbiter

The length of missions flown by the Space Shuttle will be extended to at least 16 days in the near future. In order to avoid the requirement to carry many LiOH canisters for removal of CO_2, the present LiOH system is being replaced with a regenerable, solid-amine sorbent bed. Even though this system will be well tested prior to launch, there is some risk that unexpected contaminants may be produced on the bed and enter the Shuttle's internal environment. Since low concentrations of organic compounds can affect performance in subtle ways, it will be important to know on orbit if new contaminants have entered the environment. To accomplish this objective, a volatile organic analyzer and detector is under development. It will use gas chromatography/ion mobility spectrometry to separate and quantitate trace contaminants. This technology offers many advantages over alternatives, such as gas chromatography/mass spectrometry, which are heavier, consume more power, and require frequent maintenance.

B. Space Station

Monitoring hardware developed as part of the Space Shuttle and Extended Duration Orbiter programs will serve as a basis for developing instruments for use on space station. The space station will include small-scale industrial operations that involve relatively large quantities of chemicals. The processes will be operated over extended periods of time, and changeouts by the crew will be necessary. In addition, chemical wastes will be stored in the experimental units until they can be returned to Earth. Clearly, on-orbit monitoring of potentially hazardous chemicals will be required to protect crew health and well-being. The present strategy to achieve this goal includes first-alert monitors for contingencies and more complete instruments to separate and quantitate potential chemical contaminants. A particularly challenging problem is the monitoring of metal aerosols with sufficient speed to give a warning to the crew that materials have escaped from one of the many experiments involving metal alloys. Except for contingency instruments, space station instruments must be more sensitive than those used on Shuttle missions. This is because astronauts will be staying up to 180 days on the space station, and 180-day SMACs will generally be lower than those for 7-day Shuttle missions.

C. Lunar and Martian Outposts

Extended stays on the Moon or Mars present special concerns to the toxicologist. It is expected that the ARS will be radically transformed by the advent of such bases. For example, the air in such habitats may be partially purified by plants grown within the habitat.[87] The air-quality concerns that pertained to shorter manned missions will be magnified by the longer duration stays in space, the reduced access to medical treatment and escape options, and larger-scale operations (e.g., mining). There will be increased opportunities for materials to enter the internal environment from sources external to the outpost. For example, a major area for investigation is the toxicity of martian dust, which will certainly enter the internal environment as a result of human activi-

ties outside a martian habitat. Evidence from Viking missions shows that martian soil releases oxygen upon addition of water, oxidizes organic nutrients, and fixes CO_2.[88] To some extent, it will be possible to estimate the potential toxicity of martian soil by further chemical analyses done on future Mars landers. However, conclusive toxicological data will require that carefully sampled martian soil be returned to Earth and subjected to thorough in vivo toxicological testing. A tier approach should be used for experimental testing on Earth. The descriptive phase of the study should begin with exposures of lower species and end with long-term human exposures that simulate potential exposures on Mars. In vitro toxicology studies and mechanistic studies would be valuable complements to the descriptive studies in mammals.

References

[1]Abelson, P.H. The asbestos removal fiasco (Editorial). *Science*, 1990, vol. 247, pp. 1017.

[2]Heck, H.d'A.; Casanova, M.; and Starr, T.B. Formaldehyde toxicity—new understanding. *Critical Review of Toxicology*, 1990, vol. 20, pp. 397–426.

[3]Gibson, J.E., and Bus, J.S. Current perspectives on gasoline (light hydrocarbon) induced male rat nephropathy. In: Maltoni, C., and Selikoff, I.J., Eds. *Living in a Chemical World*. New York, New York Academy of Sciences, 1988, pp. 481–485.

[4]Hottendorf, G.H. Species differences in toxic lesions. In: Roloff, M.V., Ed. *Human Risk Assessment*. London, Taylor & Francis, 1987, pp. 87–95.

[5]Pohjanvirta, R., and Tuomisto, J. Letter to the editor. *Toxicology and Applied Pharmacology,* 1990, vol. 105, pp. 508–509.

[6]Gross, S.B. Issues of regulatory requirements for inhalation toxicology testing. In: Salem, H., Ed. *Inhalation Toxicology*. New York, Marcel Dekker, Inc., 1987, pp. 361–383.

[7]Abelson, P.H. Incorporation of new science into risk assessment (Editorial). *Science,* 1990, vol. 250, p. 1497.

[8]Swenberg, J.A.; Short, B.; Borghoff, S.; Strasser, J.; and Charbonneau, M. The comparative pathobiology of α_{2U} globulin nephropathy. *Toxicology and Applied Pharmacology*, 1989, vol. 97, pp. 35–46.

[9]Homick, J.L., and Vanderploeg, J.M. The neurovestibular system. In: Nicogossian, A.E.; Huntoon, C.L.; and Pool, S.L., Eds. *Space Physiology and Medicine*. Philadelphia, Lea & Febiger, 1989, pp. 154–166.

[10]Bungo, M.W. The cardiopulmonary system. In: Nicogossian, A.E.; Huntoon, C.L.; and Pool, S.L., Eds. *Space Physiology and Medicine*. Philadelphia, Lea & Febiger, 1989, pp. 179–201.

[11]Schneider, V.S.; Leblanc, A.; and Rambaut, P.C. Bone and mineral metabolism. In: Nicogossian, A.E.; Huntoon, C.L.; and Pool, S.L., Eds. *Space Physiology and Medicine*. Philadelphia, Lea & Febiger, 1989, pp. 214–221.

[12]Nicogossian, A.E. Overall physiological response to space flight. In: Nicogossian, A.E.; Huntoon, C.L.; and Pool,

S.L., Eds. *Space Physiology and Medicine*. Philadelphia, Lea & Febiger, 1989, pp. 139–153.

[13]Huntoon, C.L.; Johnson, P.C.; and Cintron, N.M. Hematology, immunology, endocrinology, and biochemistry. In: Nicogossian, A.E.; Huntoon, C.L.; and Pool, S.L., Eds. *Space Physiology and Medicine*. Philadelphia, Lea & Febiger, 1989, pp. 222–239.

[14]National Aeronautics and Space Administration. Space Transportation Operations: Safety policy and requirements for payloads using the space transportation system (STS). NSTS 1700.7B, NASA, 1989.

[15]National Aeronautics and Space Administration. Flammability, odor, and offgassing requirements and test procedures for materials in environments that support combustion. NHB 8060.1B, Houston, NASA Johnson Space Center, 1981.

[16]National Aeronautics and Space Administration. Space Station *Freedom* hazardous contamination study. Operations Integration Office, Houston, NASA Johnson Space Center, Dec. 1990.

[17]National Aeronautics and Space Administration. Airborne particle measurement in the Space Shuttle. NASA, 1989.

[18]Limero, T.F.; Taylor, R.D.; Pierson, D.L.; and James, J.T. Space Station *Freedom* viewed as a "tight building." Paper SAE 901382, presented at the 20th International Conference on Environmental Systems, Williamsburg, VA, 1990.

[19]Molhave, L.; Bach, B.; and Pedersen, O.F. Human reactions to low concentrations of volatile organic compounds. *Environment International,* 1986, vol. 12, pp. 167–175.

[20]National Research Council, Committee on Toxicology. *Submarine Air Quality*. Washington D.C., National Academy of Sciences, 1988.

[21]Saunders, R.A. A new hazard in closed environmental atmospheres. *Archives of Environmental Health,* 1967, vol.14, pp. 380–384.

[22]Saunders, R.A. A dangerous closed atmosphere toxicant, its source and identity. In: *Proceedings of the 2nd Annual Conference on Atmospheric Contamination in Confined Spaces*, May 1966.

[23]United States Senate. Apollo Accident: Hearing Before the Committee on Aeronautical and Space Science, First Session of 90th Congress, Feb. 7, 1967.

[24]Report of Panel 11 Medical Analysis Panel, Appendix 10–11 to final report of Apollo 204 Review Board, 1967, pp. D11–D27.

[25]Ezell, E.C., and Ezell, L.N. *The Partnership: A history of the Apollo-Soyuz Test Project.* NASA SP-4209, Washington, D.C., NASA Hq., 1978.

[26]National Aeronautics and Space Administration. Apollo-Soyuz mission evaluation report. JSC-10607, Houston, NASA Johnson Space Center, 1975, pp. 14.4–14.11.

[27]De Journette, R.L. Rocket propellant inhalation in the Apollo-Soyuz astronauts. *Radiology,* 1977, vol. 125, pp. 21–24.

[28]National Aeronautics and Space Administration. Shuttle operational data book. Shuttle systems performance and con-

straints data. JSC-08934, Houston, NASA Johnson Space Center, 988, Rev. E., vol. 1, pp. 4.6.1.10–4.6.1.17.

[29]Olcott, T.M. *Development of a sorber trace contaminant control system including pre-and post-sorber for a catalytic oxidizer.* NASA CR-20276, Washington, D.C., NASA Hq., 1972.

[30]European Space Agency. Spacelab payload accommodation handbook. SLP-2104-3, European Space Agency, 1985, Appendix C, pp. 3-229, 4-155.

[31]Savina, V.P.; Mikos, K.N.; and Ryzhkova, V.E. Space flight effects on volatile metabolites in exhaled breath of cosmonauts. *Kosmicheskaya Biologiya i Aviakosmicheskaya Meditsina,* 1988, vol. 22., pp. 47–50 (in Russian).

[32]Rippstein, W.J. Shuttle toxicology. STS-2 medical report, NASA TM 58245, Houston, NASA Johnson Space Center, 1982.

[33]Coleman, M.E. STS-6 Summary report for DTO 0602, Spacecraft cabin atmospheric analysis. Memorandum SD482-215, Houston, NASA Johnson Space Center, 1982.

[34]Coleman, M.E. Thermodegradation products of an STS-28 power cable. Memorandum SD489-275, Houston, NASA Johnson Space Center, 1989.

[35]James, J.T. Toxicological Analysis of STS-35 Atmosphere. Memorandum SD491-027, Houston, NASA Johnson Space Center, 1991.

[36]Purser, D.A. Toxicity assessment of combustion products. In: Di Nenno, P.J., et al., Eds. *The SFPE Handbook of Fire Protection Engineering*. Quincy, Mass., National Fire Protection Association, 1988, Sec. 1, pp. 200–245.

[37]Williams, S.J.; Baker, B.B.; and Lee, K.P. Formation of acute pulmonary toxicants following thermal degradation of perfluorinated polymers: Evidence for a critical atmospheric reaction. *Fundamentals of Chemical Toxicology,* 1987, vol. 25, pp. 177–185.

[38]National Research Council, Board on Environmental Studies and Toxicology, Commission on Life Sciences. *Reviews of Combustion- and Pyrolysis-Product Toxicology of Ten Plastics*. Washington, D.C., National Academy Press, 1987.

[39]Warheit, D.B.; Seidel, W.C.; Carakotas, M.C.; and Hartsky, M.A. Attenuation of perfluoropolymer fume pulmonary toxicity: effect of filters, combustion method and aerosol age. *Experimental and Molecular Pathology,* 1990, vol. 52, pp. 309–329.

[40]Lunar & Planetary Institute. Space Station *Freedom* science facility assessment. Houston, NASA, 1990.

[41]National Aeronautics and Space Administration. Halon 1301 human inhalation study. JSC 23845, Houston, Johnson Space Center, Aug. 1989.

[42]Grant, C. Halon design calculations. In: Di Nenno, P.J., et. al., Eds. *The SFPE handbook of fire protection engineering*, Quincy, Mass., Society of Fire Protection Engineers, 1988, Sec. 3., pp. 59–87.

[43]Board on Toxicology and Environmental Health Hazards, Commission on Life Sciences, National Research Council. *Emergency and Continuous Exposure Limits for Selected*

Airborne Contaminants: Volume 3 Bromotrifluoromethane. Washington, D.C., National Academy Press, 1984.

[44]National Aeronautics and Space Administration. Spacecraft maximum allowable concentrations for airborne contaminants. JSC 20584, Houston, NASA Johnson Space Center, 1990.

[45]Olcott, T.M. Study and preliminary design of an isotope-heated catalytic oxidizer system. NASA CR-66346, Washington, D.C., NASA Hq., 1967.

[46]Jagow, R.B. Development of a computer program for space contaminant control analysis. LMSC-D550710, Sunnyvale, Calif., Lockheed Missiles & Space Co., 1977.

[47]Leban, M.I., and Wagner, P.A. Space Station trace contaminant control. In: Proceedings *of 19th Intersociety Conference on Environmental Systems,* Paper SAE 891513, San Diego, Calif., 1989.

[48]Wydeven, T., and Golub, M.A. Generation rates and chemical compositions of waste streams in a typical crewed space habitat. NASA TM-102799, Washington, D.C., NASA Hq., 1990.

[49]Brewer, D.A., and Hall, J.B. A simulation model for the analysis of Space Station gas-phase trace contaminants. *Acta Astronautica,* 1987, vol. 15, pp. 527–543.

[50]National Aeronautics and Space Administration. Standard procedure for nonmetallic offgas analysis by gas chromatography mass spectrometry data systems. In: *Toxicology Laboratory Procedures Manual,* JSC 23611, Houston, NASA Johnson Space Center, 1988.

[51]Svartengren, M.; Falk, R.; Linnman, L.; Philipson, K.; and Kramer, P. Deposition of large particles in human lung. *Experimental Lung Research,* 1987, vol. 12, pp. 75–88.

[52]National Aeronautics and Space Administration. Airborne particulate matter in spacecraft. NASA Conference Publication 2499, Houston, NASA Johnson Space Center, 1988.

[53]Limero, T.; James, J.; Cromer, R.; and Beck, S. A combustion products analyzer for contingency use during thermodegradation events on spacecraft. In: Proceedings *of 21st Intersociety Conference on Environmental Systems,* Paper no. 91000, San Francisco, 1991.

[54]National Aeronautics and Space Administration. Detailed Test Objective (DTO) 0616, JSC 17462, Houston, NASA Johnson Space Center, 1982.

[55]National Aeronautics and Space Administration. Change Configuration Board Directive, Spacelab 4495. Huntsville, Ala., Marshall Space Flight Center, 1985.

[56]National Aeronautics and Space Administration. Detailed Test Objective (DTO) 0623, JSC 17625, Rev. F, Houston, NASA Johnson Space Center, 1984.

[57]Coleman, M.E. Postflight report for STS-26 atmospheric analysis. Memorandum SD488-387, Houston, NASA Johnson Space Center, 1988.

[58]Coleman, M.E. Postflight report for STS-27 atmospheric analysis. Memorandum SD488-042, Houston, NASA Johnson Space Center, 1988.

[59]Coleman, M.E. Postflight report for STS-28 atmospheric analysis. Memorandum SD489-316, Houston, NASA Johnson Space Center, 1989.

[60]James, J.T. Toxicological analysis of STS-33 atmosphere. Memorandum SD489-432, Houston, NASA Johnson Space Center, 1989.

[61]Barneby & Sutcliff Corporation, Activated Carbon Division. Relative holding capacity of Type AC Carbon for various contaminant vapors, a descriptive brochure. P.O. Box 2526, Columbus, Ohio, Barneby & Sutcliff Corporation, undated, pp. 3–5.

[62]Hamilton Standard Co. Catalytic charcoal specifications. Specification no. SVHS 8741, Rev. A, Windsor Lock, Conn., undated, pp. 3–4.

[63]Hamilton Standard Co. Cabin Fan and Debris Trap Assembly. Specification no. SVHS 6401, Windsor Lock, Conn., undated.

[64]Ray, C.C., and Stanley, J.B. Spacelab baseline ECS contaminant removal program. NASA TM 78135, Huntsville, Ala., NASA Marshall Space Flight Center, 1977, pp. 28–29.

[65]CO_2 adsorber element intermediate and depot maintenance requirements. Specification no. 61V006.000.

[66]National Aeronautics and Space Administration. Environmental systems console handbook. JSC-19935, Houston, NASA Johnson Space Center, 1985, Rev. A, Sec. 6, pp. 26–37.

[67]General Electric Company. Waste Collection Subsystem (WCS): Certification of requirements by analysis. Rockwell specification MC 282-00669C, Valley Forge Space Center, Philadelphia, General Electric Company, 1983, pp. 13–17.

[68]Mission Operations Directorate, Systems Division. Inflight maintenance tool catalog. Houston, NASA Johnson Space Center, 1990, pp. 6–10.

[69]Moon L.J. Orbiter Vacuum Cleaner evaluation test report. Houston, NASA Johnson Space Center, 1979, p. 4.

[70]American Conference on Governmental Industrial Hygienists. Threshold limit values and biological exposure indices for 1990–1991. Cincinnati, Ohio, American Conference on Governmental Industrial Hygienists, 1990.

[71]Air contaminants—permissible exposure limits. U.S. Code of Federal Regulations, Title 29, Part 1910.1000, Washington, D.C., 1989.

[72]National Research Council, Committee on Toxicology. Emergency and continuous exposure limits for selected airborne contaminants. Washington, D.C., National Academy of Sciences, 1984–1988, vols. 1–8.

[73]National Research Council, Committee on Toxicology. Atmospheric contamination in spacecraft. Washington, D.C., National Academy of Sciences, 1968.

[74]National Research Council, Committee on Toxicology. Atmospheric contaminants in spacecraft. Washington, D.C., National Academy of Sciences, 1972.

[75]National Research Council, Committee on Toxicology. Guidelines for developing spacecraft maximum allowable concentrations (SMACs) for space station contaminants. Washington, D.C., National Academy Press, 1991.

[76]National Research Council, National Council on Radiation Protection and Measurements. Guidance on radiation

received in space activities. Report no. 98, Washington, D.C., National Academy Press, 1989.

[77]Task Force of Past Presidents of the Society of Toxicology. Animal data in hazard evaluation: Paths and pitfalls. *Fundamentals of Applied Toxicology,* 1982, vol. 2, pp. 101–107.

[78]Weatherby, J.H., and Yard, A.S. Observations on the subacute toxicity of hydrazine. *A.M.A. Archives of Industrial Health*, 1955, vol. 11, pp. 413–419.

[79]Vernot, E.H.; MacEwan , J.D.; and Bruner, R.H., et al. Long-term inhalation toxicity of hydrazine. *Fundamentals of Applied Toxicology,* 1985, vol. 5, pp. 1050–1064.

[80]Garcia, H. Hydrazine SMAC document. Houston, NASA Johnson Space Center, 1991.

[81]Wong, K.L. Methylene Chloride SMAC document. Houston, NASA Johnson Space Center, 1991.

[82]Anderson, M.E.; Clewell, H.J.; Gargas, M.L.; Smith, F.A.; and Reitz, R.H. Physiologically based pharmacokinetics and the risk assessment process for methylene chloride. *Toxicology and Applied Pharmacology,* 1987, vol. 87, pp. 185–205.

[83]Wong, K.L. Formaldehyde SMAC document. Houston, NASA Johnson Space Center, 1991.

[84]Haber, F. *Funfvortage Ausden Jahren.* Springer-Verlag, Berlin, 1924, pp. 1920–1923 (in German).

[85]Levin, B.C.; Paabo, M.; Gurman, J.L.; and Harris, S.E. Effects of exposure to single or multiple combinations of the predominant toxic gases and low oxygen atmospheres produced in fires. *Fundamentals of Applied Toxicology,* 1987, vol. 9, pp. 236–250.

[86]Williams, S.J.; Baker, B.B.; and Lee, K.P. Formation of acute pulmonary toxicants following thermal degradation of perfluorinated polymers: Evidence for a critical atmospheric reaction. *Fundamentals of Chemical Toxicology,* 1987, vol. 25, pp. 177–185.

[87]Oberg, J.E., and Gardens, A.R. *Pioneering Space.* New York, Mcgraw-Hill, 1986, Chapter 8.

[88]Arvidson, R.E.; Gooding, J.L.; and Moore, H.J. The Martian surface as imaged, sampled, and analyzed by the Viking landers. *Review of Geophysics*, 1989, vol. 27, pp. 39–60.

[89]Lazarev, A.G. *Principles of Industrial Toxicology.* Moscow, Medgiz, 1938, p. 53 (in Russian).

[90]Averyanov, A.G. On evaluating the atmosphere in work environments for the presence of certain harmful components. *Gigiyena i Sanitariya*, 1957, vol. 8, pp. 64–67 (in Russian).

Chapter 3

Heat Balance in Space Operations and Explorations

James M. Waligora

I. Introduction

A. Importance of Thermoregulation

On April 11, 1970, Apollo 13 was launched on what was to be the third visit to the surface of the Moon. When the mission was 55 h 53 min in flight, one of the oxygen tanks in the service module supplying oxygen to the command module exploded. The story of the subsequent 87 h—as the spacecraft continued to the Moon, circled it, and successfully returned to Earth—is one of survival under extremely difficult conditions. One threat to survival was the thermal environment in the spacecraft. After the command module was powered down and the lunar module was configured for minimum power, the temperatures of both spacecraft modules fell rapidly, stabilizing at approximately 3 °C in the command module and 11 °C in the lunar module. The crew donned spare constant-wear garments but remained very cold, to the extent that they had difficulty sleeping. The lunar module was powered up about 2 h before reentry to provide some warmth; this left about 3 h of spare battery power at the time of successful reentry.[1]

On May 14, 1973, the unmanned Skylab spacecraft was launched atop a Saturn 5 launch vehicle. During the second minute of the flight, there were indications of meteoroid shield deployment and separation of a solar array wing beam fairing. All other systems were normal, and the vehicle was successfully placed into orbit. After the spacecraft systems were deployed, it was determined that the solar array wing had not been properly deployed. In addition, temperature readings in the workshop showed that the meteoroid shield was not affecting the temperature as intended. The workshop temperatures stabilized as high as 58 °C.

The first mission to Skylab was scheduled for May 15 but was delayed 10 days to allow the development of means and procedures for repairing the damage. One of these means was a solar shade to be deployed from inside the Skylab through the scientific airlock. One activity conducted in that 10-day period was analysis and empirical testing of crew tolerance to the workshop environment. It was determined that the crew could work in the environment for about 2 h, after which time they would have to move to the cool command module, with about equal periods of time in each environment.[2] The first mission to visit the Skylab was launched on May 25, 1973. During the first day, the nature and extent of the damage was confirmed. On the second day, the crew entered the workshop and successfully deployed the Skylab parasol after about 4 h, moving at intervals from the cool command module to the workshop environment. In the next few days, the parasol lowered the Skylab temperature to the comfort level.[3]

It has been suggested that spacecraft temperature environments might be remarkable because of their blandness and monotony, since the temperature is controlled at the will of the crew by the cabin environmental control system (ECS). The contingencies just described are evidence that this is not always the case. Moreover, the need to minimize weight and power in ECSs has led physiologists and engineers to interact to ensure a balance between the needs of humans for heat and the need to minimize weight and power.

The existence of humans on Earth is a specific case of heat balance in space. Earth's temperature is a function of the planet's position in space and the balance between radiant heat input from the Sun and radiant heat loss to space. Temperatures are further defined by the characteristics of the atmosphere, the varying albedo of the surface of the Earth, the rotation of the Earth, and the axis of the planet's rotation relative to the plane of orbit. Humans are homeothermic animals, which utilize regulatory mechanisms to maintain a relatively constant core temperature.

Because humans evolved in tropical regions, where the average temperature was from 22–28 °C,[4] their evolutionary heritage is the same as that of a tropical animal. However, by means of a strong physiological control system and, much more important, by means of behavioral control of the microenvironment, humans can now exist in any locale on the Earth and can bring a habitable environment (including an acceptable thermal environment) into space.

The 37 °C human body temperature control point is 10–15 °C above the typical ambient temperature. This temperature gradient is such that a balance can be reached between heat production in the body and heat loss to the environment. A body temperature fixed within a narrow range provides many benefits for the organism: chemical reactions in the body can proceed at an optimum rate at a given temperature, and activity can be variable and not tied to body temperature.

Animals (including humans) with temperature control prosper and enjoy significant advantages over animals whose body temperatures track the temperature of the environment. However, the temperature range in which all terrestrial animals can survive is narrow, -2–46 °C for the vertebrates, while potential temperatures in space range from -273–5750 °C temperature at the surface of the Sun, on up through the millions of degrees Celsius postulated during supernova events.[5] Although this chapter relates to regulation of temperature flux to retain heat balance, the temperature range within which we must work is determined by our position in space.

B. Challenges of the Space Environment

While much of the influence of the spacecraft environment on heat balance relates to the spacecraft's position relative to the Sun, a number of other factors are important as well. Among these are the loss of the moderating factors of the Earth itself on the organism's temperature balance at the planet's surface: the tilt of the Earth; one's geographical location, rotation, and albedo; and the influence of the atmosphere. Some of these factors are replicated to some extent by the characteristics of spacecraft; e.g., rate of rotation around the Earth, rate of rotation around its own axis, and the surface reflectivity or emissivity. In addition, a number of potential variations in the spacecraft atmosphere influence heat balance. There is no atmosphere in space. The atmosphere provided in the spacecraft must be created by the designers of its ECS. In the brief history of space travel, a number of different combinations of pressures and atmospheric compositions have been implemented and many more have been considered. Atmospheric pressure has ranged from the 34.5 kPa (1 kPa = 0.145 psi) cabin pressures used in the U.S. Mercury, Gemini, Apollo, and Skylab Programs, to the 69.1 kPa pressure of the Apollo-Soyuz docking module, to the pre-extra-vehicular-activity (EVA) 70.3 kPa pressure option on the U.S. Space Shuttle Orbiter, to the normal Earth pressure of 101 kPa or slightly higher, which is the nominal pressure for the Shuttle and for all Soviet (Russian) space vehicles to date. Other pressures have been considered or at least investigated and discussed in both the U.S. and Soviet programs.[6]

In the similarly isolated environment of submarines, pressures in excess of 101 kPa have been considered to provide normoxic atmosphere at a reduced percentage of oxygen concentration, thereby reducing the fire hazard related to flammable materials.[7] Gas composition has varied from 100 percent oxygen in the Mercury, Gemini, and Apollo Programs to essentially normoxic in all of the other vehicles with nitrogen as the diluent gas. Other diluent gases have been considered in both U.S. and Soviet programs. Considerations of gas composition and pressure are treated in depth in Chapter 1 of this volume, but their impact on heat balance through changes in convection and evaporation must also be considered in this chapter.

The microgravity environment in Earth orbit and in unpowered transit can affect heat exchange in a number of ways—some demonstrable and some speculative. Microgravity virtually eliminates the free convection that provides a base level of convection on the Earth's surface. Microgravity affects the behavior of sweat on the surface of the skin and potentially influences the wet area available for evaporation and the ability to maintain elevated sweat rates over a period of time. Microgravity may also influence heat production or metabolic rate in ways ranging from a simple difference in the amount of physical work done in an average day to a more basic change in sustaining metabolism. Changes in heat production would, of course, directly affect heat balance and could possibly affect the status of the thermoregulatory control system. This control system utilizes several physiological systems in the body; thus, any changes in these systems initiated by microgravity could have a secondary effect on thermoregulation. All of the considerations we have mentioned thus far in relation to the spacecraft environment also apply to space-suit environments, with the additional considerations of high work rates and special cooling systems.

C. Record of Performance to Date

Given all of these considerations, there have been remarkably few problems in maintaining heat balance in manned space operations. The problems encountered have typically been associated with failure of a nominal system and have been successfully controlled with backup systems. The relative freedom from problems is the result of appropriate attention to the comfort requirements, tolerance requirements, and special problems associated with the spacecraft and spacesuit environment. In dealing with these requirements and considerations, models of thermoregulation and heat balance have been increasingly useful and productive of good design solutions that have maintained heat balance and crew safety.

D. Challenges for the Future

We are still at the beginning of the age of human space travel and exploration, and a number of challenges remain that relate to maintaining human heat balance. To a certain extent, we have avoided potential problems by designing effective and forgiving temperature control systems in our spacecraft and pressure suits. There has been little investigation into the effects of space flight, and microgravity in particular, on heat balance and thermoregulation; thus, further, more detailed investigations are needed to maintain our good record with respect to heat balance in space. As manned space programs (particularly those associated with interplanetary travel) progress to longer stays in space,we will encounter more challenging problems of heat balance. Our experience in space to date has been in a region, in Earth orbit, and even on the Moon, with a fairly constant mean solar heat flux. As we expand exploration to other planets, we will encounter greater challenges in maintaining the crewmembers' heat balance and body temperature.

II. Characteristics of Maintaining Heat Balance in Humans

A. Heat Production

A prime consideration in heat balance is the rate of heat production. For convenience, this can be divided into the basal metabolic rate (that energy production required to maintain the organism when all activity has been at a minimum for some time) and the active metabolic rate (everything above the basal rate, including maximum anaerobic work). The basal metabolic rate for an astronaut of typical size and age would be about 80 W. To avoid the residual effects of exercise, the basal metabolic rate is measured in the postabsorptive state, while lying down, after sleep, or after a long period of rest. A less restrictive resting metabolic rate is about 105 W. The peak metabolic rate can be very high indeed; during the 10 s of a 100-yd dash, it is about 8500 W. The maximum metabolic rate that can be sustained varies with time. A maximum effort of several minutes' duration is limited by the maximum rate of aerobic metabolism or the maximum oxygen consumption. In a well-trained individual, 100 percent of maximal oxygen uptake can be maintained during 10 min, 95 percent during 30 min, 85 percent during 60 min, and 80 percent during 120 min.[8] These combinations of maximum output and time are for activities involving large muscle groups (such as running) for which the individual is well trained. Individuals involved in actual productive work over long periods of time are able to work at diverse useful tasks at only a fraction of those rates. In general, work rates of 50 percent maximum oxygen consumption are considered very heavy and are seldom sustained for longer than 10–20 min. Average metabolic rates over a 24-h period measured in military men engaged in a range of duties vary from 10–20 percent of maximum oxygen consumption.[9]

The thermal mass of the body acts to damp the short-term, very high metabolic rates that are interspersed with longer periods of lower rates. To raise the temperature of the body 1 °C requires about 70 W, or two-thirds of the resting metabolic rate, over a 1-h period. In any model of thermoregulation in the body, it is critical to depict the passive generation, accumulation, and transfer of heat in the body accurately. Figure 1 depicts the output of a model of thermoregulation in a body with the regulatory system inactivated. It demonstrates effectively how the intermittent nature of most work activity can interact with the thermal mass of the body to minimize the need for thermoregulatory control.

B. Heat Exchange Pathways

To maintain the body's heat balance, the level of heat produced must be balanced with the heat flow from the body to achieve an average body temperature (as moderated by the thermal mass of the body) that is within acceptable limits for both comfort and tolerance. The avenues for heat loss or gain to the surrounding environment are convection, radiation,

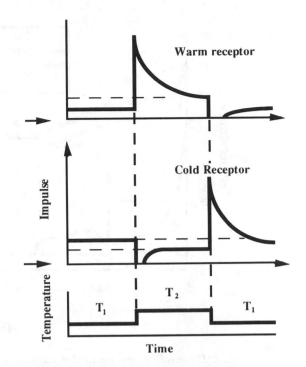

Fig. 1 Output of a model of thermoregulation in man during intermittent exercise in a 10 °C environment when the controller parameters are set to zero (from Stolwijk, Ref. 64).

conduction, and evaporation. As a result of the multiple pathways for heat exchange from the body, a large number of environmental factors can affect heat balance. A change in any of these factors can affect heat balance and, thus, body temperature.

Convection is the transfer of thermal energy from one surface to another through an intervening fluid in motion. To calculate the rate of convective heat exchange between a human and an air environment, we must know the skin temperature, characteristic dimensions of the body (shape and size), air temperature, pressure, velocity of air across the body, and gravity.

Radiation is the transfer of thermal energy from one surface to another without dependence on an intervening medium. Radiation depends only on the temperatures and natures of the two surfaces. Thermal energy can be transmitted by radiation throughout the electromagnetic spectrum. To calculate the rate of radiant heat exchange between a human and the environment, we must know skin temperature, effective surface area, reflectivity of the skin, mean radiant temperature, emissivity of the environment, and temperature of radiant sources.

Conduction is the flow of heat from one surface to another through an intervening medium without the physical transfer of material. Conduction can occur in solids, gases, and liquids. To calculate the rate of conductive heat exchange between a human and the environment, we must know the skin temperature, contact area, thickness of the conductor,

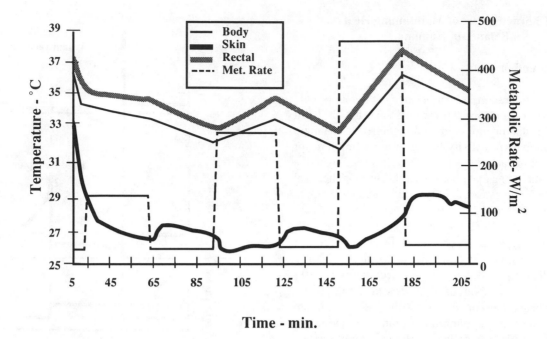

Fig. 2 Dynamic response of the warm and cold skin receptors. A temperature increase from
T_1 **to** T_2 **causes a rapid rise in warm receptor discharge, returning to a new resting level.**
Conversely, the cold receptor is temporarily inhibited. When the temperature reverts from
T_1 **to** T_2**, the pattern of discharge is reversed. (Reprinted with permission from Ref. 13).**

temperature of the conducting medium, and specific thermal conductivity of the medium.

Evaporative heat exchange occurs when a change of state of an intervening medium transfers thermal energy from one surface to another. The skin and respiratory tract are two major body sites in which evaporative heat exchange occurs. To calculate evaporative heat exchange between a human and the environment, we must know the wet area percentage, air temperature, air velocity over the body surface, relative humidity, skin temperature, and characteristic dimensions of the body.

C. Control Mechanisms

Humans generate heat by metabolism at the cellular level throughout the body. Multiple pathways for heat exchange with the environment are available. The second element in maintaining heat balance is temperature control, or control of heat loss from the body. Temperature control is ubiquitous in the animal kingdom and is characteristic of both homeothermic and poikilothermic animals. One of the most basic responses that can be demonstrated in any organism with motility is avoidance of temperature extremes. But a human is a homeotherm with physiological temperature control and, as with all animals possessing physiological temperature control, has the advantages and disadvantages of a relatively fixed body temperature. Advantages include optimum temperature for chemical reactions within the body, greater freedom from the restrictions of environmental temperature, and greater freedom to vary levels of metabolism

independently of environmental temperature. Disadvantages include a higher requirement for food and reduced tolerance for extremes of body temperature.

Physiological temperature regulation differentiates poikilothermic and homeothermic animals. Both types of animal display behavioral regulation. Physiological temperature regulation allows humans to maintain a central body temperature of 37 ± 0.5 °C. At this temperature the body is capable of high energy exchange rates and the most rapid transmission of information. The physiological thermoregulatory system is typical of controlled systems in that it requires sensors to be able to quantitate the controlled variable (in this case, temperature or heat quantity or heat flux), an integration and regulation site or mechanism, and effector systems to alter the avenues of heat loss.

The concept of specific thermal receptors in the skin and elsewhere was first referred to in the work of sensory physiologists in the 19th century. In 1840 Muller spoke of specific thermoreceptors, and in 1882 Blix identified localized sensory spots on the skin that produced thermal sensation.[10] Thermoreceptors are nerve endings excited only or preferentially by temperature stimuli. There are specific receptors for warmth and cold, and they behave in a complementary fashion. Warm receptors respond with an overshoot of discharge on sudden warming and are transiently inhibited on cooling. Cold receptors respond with an overshoot of discharge on sudden cooling and are transiently inhibited by heating (see Fig. 2).

The characteristics of temperature receptors are that they have a static discharge at constant temperature, they respond dynamically to temperature change with either a positive temperature coefficient (warm receptors) or a negative coefficient (cold receptors), they are not excited by mechanical stimuli, and they respond well within the temperature ranges bordered by pain sensation. There are wide variations in the density of sensors in the skin and in the distribution of the hot and cold sensors between species, in different individuals, and on different areas of the body.

The first central temperature receptors identified were those in the hypothalamus. They were identified in experiments in which the temperature of the hypothalamus was independently modified from that of the rest of the body. Hypothalamic central temperature sensors, or receptors, are still thought to be the most significant central temperature sensors; however, other areas of the central nervous system (including the thalamus, midbrain, and spinal cord) have been identified as being thermally sensitive.[11,12] In some animals, the heating or cooling of the abdomen elicits a thermoregulatory response suggesting thermosensitivity of tissue in this area.[13] There is also some evidence of and speculation about thermosensitivity in the walls of blood vessels and in muscle.[14]

The integration of thermal inputs and the regulatory control of body temperature reside primarily in the hypothalamus. As early as 1885, it was demonstrated that temperature control could be largely eliminated by lesions of the brain.[15] The specific site was identified in 1922 to be the hypothalamus.[16] With the identification of the hypothalamus as a site of both thermosensitivity and temperature control, as well as identification of specific sites in the hypothalamus for sensing and/or integration of hot and cold sensing, elegant theories of temperature control were proposed. These theories depended primarily on temperature sensing internal to the hypothalamus for most thermoregulation, with neuronal input from skin sensors only for cold inputs below some critical skin temperature.[15] In the last few years, numerous studies have revealed a much more complicated control system with a great deal of redundancy, multiple pathways, multiple sensors, possible secondary sites with some regulatory capacity, neuronal and neurohumoral pathways, and local and spinal cord reflex inhibition of efferent signals. The controlled temperature would appear to be one of several proposed combinations of central and peripheral temperature.[10,11,14,16,17] Despite the additional complexity of current views, the general scheme remains one of thermal perception based on peripheral and central sensors with thermoregulatory control in the hypothalamus incorporating sensors in the hypothalamus and possibly other central sites modified by peripheral sensors.

Given the temperature-sensing systems and the integration and regulation system, the third component of the physiological thermoregulation system encompasses the effector mechanisms that alter heat loss and retention in the body. These mechanisms include sweating, which provides evaporative cooling on the skin surface; shivering, which greatly increases heat production in the body by involuntary muscular contraction; and vasomotor control, which can increase or decrease temperature gradients from the core to the skin by increasing or decreasing skin blood flow above or below the value at thermoneutrality.

Sweating is a very powerful means of increasing heat loss; the change of state that occurs during the evaporation of sweat releases 2.45 kJ/g (0.585 kcal/g). The sweat that is important in thermoregulation is excreted by the eccrine sweat glands. These glands are distributed over the entire skin surface, with the density of distribution in various areas differing in various individuals and groups of individuals. The total number of sweat glands is about $3–4 \times 10^6$, and their mass is about 100 grams.[13] The sweat glands filter blood plasma to excrete a dilute solution on the skin surface for evaporation. Excreted sweat is always hypotonic and is most dilute when sweat rates are low. As sweat rates approach maximum values, the composition of the sweat becomes less hypotonic and may approach the ionic content of plasma. Very high rates of sweat production are possible, as high as 2–3 liters/h for short periods of time and 1 liter/h for several hours.[18] Sweat rates may be maintained in the face of some level of dehydration but will begin to fail as dehydration reaches 9–10 percent.[18] High sweat rates can be maintained in dry environments if water intake can be maintained. This is very difficult, however, because intake must be very frequent and drinking the required amount may be subjectively unpleasant. A lack of appropriate water intake (called voluntary dehydration) can also be a problem in chronic heat exposure.[19] Sweat rates can be maintained at high levels for many hours in a dry environment where skin wetness is low. In hot, humid environments that result in a high level of skin wetness, the sweat rate is progressively reduced after the second hour of sweating. This reduction is characterized by reductions in the number of active sweat glands and in the sweat output per gland. This phenomenon of sweat reduction is called hidromeiosis.[20,21] Hidromeiosis is most likely caused by physical obstruction of the sweat gland by swelling of the stratum corneum at the surface of the sweat duct, as stripping of a layer of stratum corneum will restore high sweat rates.[22]

Shivering is repeated muscle contraction in response to cold stimulation, which, at moderate levels, has some subjective component and may be temporarily under voluntary control. As the cold stimulus increases in intensity, shivering becomes more dramatic. Few individuals have experienced violent shivering. In violent shivering, the contractions cause involuntary flexing and jerking of the limbs, produce a great deal of heat, and cause extreme fatigue. Peak levels of energy production in shivering are as high as five times the basal rate. The level that can be sustained for several hours is lower, probably two to three times the basal rate.[4] The rate of shivering depends on the thermoregulatory state but can be modified by temperature distribution and rate of skin temperature change. Maximum shivering rates occur when an unclothed individual is exposed to rapid cooling. Fatal hypothermia may occur in slow cooling of clothed individuals with relatively minor shivering.

Vasomotor control is the control of the effective conductance of the body. The skin temperature of an individual at rest and in a thermally neutral state, comfortable and without thermal stress, will vary over the body surface from about 34 °C on the trunk and face to about 30 °C on the hands and feet. In this state, there is considerably more blood flow to the hands and feet than is required to support metabolism; and, in fact, there is extensive shunting of blood in the hands and feet, resulting in a partial extension of core temperature into the large, deep blood vessels in the extremities. In the thermally neutral state, the extremities are heated by a shunted blood flow in excess of the metabolic needs of the extremities. In this same state, the smooth muscles in the arterioles of the skin and the arterial venous shunts are partially constricted by stimulation of sympathetic innervation, resulting in a level of muscle tone in these smooth muscles. When the body is heated above thermoneutrality, the muscle tone is reduced or inhibited, resulting in vasodilation; i.e., an increase in blood flow and blood volume in the peripheral vessels. When the body is cooled below thermoneutrality, the muscle tone is increased, resulting in vasoconstriction; i.e., a fall in skin blood flow and in skin temperature. The reduction of excess blood flow through the arterial venous shunts or anastomoses also reduces blood flow through the limbs, which results in progressive distal to proximal cooling of the limbs and further reduces skin temperature in the extremities. The extent of vasomotor control varies over the surface of the body. The range of blood flows is greatest in the hands and feet and least in the skin of the face and trunk. As a result, the range of local conduction in the hands can be as much as 10–1, while the range in the face is 1.5–1.[23]

The end result of vasomotor control is a wide variability of the gradient between skin temperature and core temperature. Vasoconstriction maximizes the temperature difference between the skin and core temperatures and conserves heat in the core of the body. Vasodilation minimizes the temperature difference between the skin and core temperatures and increases heat loss.

When humans are subjected to hot or cold exposure involving thermal stress over a period of several days or a week, changes occur in the thermoregulatory system that increase its efficiency and effectiveness. Characteristics of heat acclimatization include sweat rate increases at a given body temperature, reduced sweat thresholds, increased skin blood flow at a given body temperature, and reduced threshold of vasodilation.[23–26] All of these responses result in an increase in the flow of heat from core to skin at a given environmental temperature. Exercise in even a neutral environment greatly increases metabolic heat production in the body, increases body temperature, stimulates the thermoregulatory system, and results in vasodilation and sweating. Changes in thermoregulatory responses are similar after thermal stress without exercise, exercise in a moderate environment, and exercise in a hot environment. The greatest changes occur when exercise and heat stress are combined.

Acclimation to cold is more difficult to demonstrate in humans. In some species of mammals, repeated cold exposure increases the nonshivering thermogenesis related to brown fat deposits. Brown fat and nonshivering thermogenesis are either not present or present to an insignificant extent in humans. Some patterns of response to cold change with time in humans exposed to cold without clothing. They show a reduced shivering and a greater fall in core temperature. There is also evidence of increased fat deposition and insulation on cold exposure.[4,15] What is clear is that prolonged cold exposure is not common in humans, even in cold environments. It is avoided by behavioral thermoregulation.

Behavioral thermoregulation includes all voluntary actions that humans may take to control heat balance, from changing postural position to decrease or increase effective surface area and heat loss to the environment to designing an ECS for a spacecraft. The basis for all behavioral thermoregulation is the avoidance of pain or discomfort, and this avoidance relates to the perception of the thermal environment. The aforementioned temperature sensors in the skin have a function in physiological thermoregulation. They also influence behavioral regulation. Strong sensations of heat and cold are unpleasant and, in themselves, stimulate behavior to reduce them. Such sensations are more pronounced in response to changes in temperature, facilitating an avoidance response.

The effector responses of the thermoregulating system also generate sensations of discomfort. Vasoconstriction results in lower skin temperature in the extremities and accentuates the perception of cold from these areas. Shivering is uncomfortable at any level and becomes increasingly disagreeable and painful as it increases in intensity. Sweating, except in a very dry environment, creates a condition of skin wetness. The percentage of skin wetness is correlated with discomfort (at least at rest).[27] When combined with heat exposure, exercise can lead to an unpleasant feeling of exhaustion that is not present at equivalent work rates in a cold environment. All of these unpleasant sensations accompany a lack of heat balance and stimulate behavior to alter the heat balance.

One of the most basic behavioral responses seen in simple mobile life forms, as well as in humans, is the avoidance of and movement away from a thermally disagreeable environment and the selection of or movement toward a comfortable one. Body position can influence the effective surface areas for convection and radiation; i.e., we stretch out when we are warm and curl up when we are cool. Although humans evolved as tropical animals, clothing allowed them to live in temperate and polar climates. In temperate climates, there has been a progressive trend to reduce insulation values of typical indoor clothing as the reliability, availability, effectiveness, and ease of control of central heating systems have become common. Indoor clothing outfits have been reduced from a 1.5 clo outfit suitable for a 15–17 °C temperature to a 0.6 clo outfit suitable for a 24 °C temperature. [Clo is a unit of insulation or resistance to heat flow and is defined as 0.18 °C/(kcal/m^2/h).] On the other hand, the thermoneutral point for a nude human is 30 °C.

The ultimate behavioral thermoregulation is the control of the environment by the use of modern heating and cooling technologies to provide any desired temperature environment with appropriate gas and wall temperature for the desired activity level and clothing assembly. Even with available power and technology to heat and cool an environment, knowledge of the characteristics of heat transfer and the physiological and behavioral needs of humans is essential to designing and providing a comfortable, thermally controlled environment.

III. Variables Imposed by the Space Environment

A. External Space Environment

The near-space environment refers to the environment encountered in Earth orbit and translunar flight. It can be characterized as having approximately the same solar flux or insolation as the Earth, or exposure to some intermittent portion of that flux interspersed with or complemented by radiant heat flux from the Earth or Moon. In this environment, particle density is so low that the average velocity of these particles or their temperature has no significance as far as the thermal balance of a spacecraft or space suit is concerned. Generally speaking, it is possible to achieve thermal balance in a spacecraft or space suit with a fixed energy production by coating the external surface with material of the appropriate emissivity and reflectivity. A useful characteristic of this environment is that it facilitates controlled sublimation of water from the spacecraft that can serve as a heat sink for an ECS to handle variations in energy production in the spacecraft or space suit.

In interplanetary space, solar flux is a function of distance from the Sun. The solar flux, planetary albedo, and atmosphere combine to produce maximum temperatures rnaging from 342 °C on Mercury to -217 °C on Neptune. Manned spacecraft would need means to vary reflectivity and emissivity to venture closer to the Sun. At distances farther from the Sun, some means of collecting and concentrating solar flux would have to be utilized.

B. Characteristics of the Space Habitat Environment

The characteristics of the external space environment that have been enumerated provide many difficult and challenging tasks to the designers and engineers responsible for environmental control in space habitats and pressure suits, but the external space environment is not the one to which crewmembers are directly exposed. The external space environments that we have described are uniform only in that human life cannot exist in them without intervention and modification. It is the controlled environment of spacecraft, space habitats, and pressure suits with which we are concerned when we speak of the human thermal environment in space. The challenges of this environment depend on the decisions and tradeoffs that are made in the design of these controlled

environments. These challenges are nonetheless real and deserving of our attention, consideration, and investigation.

In stable orbital space habitats and in the unpowered transit phase of interplanetary flight, crewmembers will experience microgravity unless specific measures are taken to generate a simulated gravity force. Microgravity will or may have a number of effects (some well known and some speculative) on heat balance. These effects can be because of physical factors, a combination of physical factors affecting physiological response, or a physiological response to microgravity directly or indirectly affecting heat exchange.

A physical change in heat transfer in microgravity is the lack of free or natural convection. Free convection is the movement of air in a volume caused by the differential effect of gravity on dense cool gas and less dense warm gas when there are surfaces and objects of different temperatures in the volume. In any volume there may be a greater or lesser number of objects with surfaces hotter or cooler than the mean temperature. In a volume that is losing heat to an external environment, the walls will be cool and a heating system will offset heat loss by presenting a hot surface in the environment or infusing heated gas. The opposite condition will occur in a volume gaining heat from an external environment. An environment containing electrical, electronic, and mechanical systems will generate heat (or in some cases act as a heat sink) and present a different surface temperature to the environment. Even if humans were not present in such a volume, there would be currents of air and a measurable air velocity caused by free convection. When a human is present in this volume, the body presents a higher temperature surface at the skin or clothing interface with the environment. In addition to the currents of gas motion in the volume caused by other sources, free convection creates an upward moving stream of gas over the surface of the body. A number of authors have speculated on the impact of a lack of free convection on heat transfer in spacecraft.[28,29] As the velocity of any forced convection increases, it at some point masks and overwhelms the effect of free convection caused by temperatures of surfaces commonly encountered in a volume. For that reason, it is a convention in heat balance studies involving humans, particularly in partitional calorimetry, to assume that forced convection predominates above a certain velocity [4.6–9.2 m/min (15–30 ft/min)] and that free convection predominates and provides a stable minimum of about 4.6 m/min (15 ft/min) below that level. With these considerations in mind, physiologists responsible for environmental spacecraft requirements in both the U.S. and U.S.S.R. programs have specified minimum levels of forced air motion to minimize the effect of the lack of free or natural convection.[6] Despite minimum forced convection levels, it is difficult to fully predict the effect of a loss of free convection. Free or natural convection provides a dependable minimum air motion. Forced convection is subject to shadowing (a directionality with high velocity on one side of the body and very low velocity on the other) and creates the potential for "dead" areas in the habitable volume with very low velocities and a resultant lack of convective heat transfer. Czechoslovakian, Soviet, and Polish investigators[30,31] used an instrument complex that included an electrically heated and controlled Kata thermometer in combination with a bank of six skin temperatures to investigate the effect of microgravity on convective heat loss. A basic Kata thermometer measures turbulent air motion as a function of the time required for a heated thermometer with a specific geometry to cool from one temperature to another. The Electrical Dynamic Katathermometer is a Kata thermometer that measures the energy necessary to maintain the thermometer at 37 °C—an approximation of body temperature. The instrument was used on the biosatellite Cosmos 936 and in the orbital complexes Soyuz 28/Salyut 6 and Soyuz 30/ Salyut 6. Measurements were made at rest and during exercise on a bicycle ergometer. The Kata thermometer proved to be reliable for assessing the effect of convection and evaluating differences in convection in flight and on the ground. There was a tendency in the in-flight measurements for temperatures to be lower and gas velocities to be higher. Where in-flight instrument readings were similar to laboratory readings associated with comfort at a given work rate, the in-flight crewmembers were also comfortable. However, distribution of skin temperatures was not the same: trunk temperatures were higher and extremity temperatures were lower in space. The authors expressed the intent to use these measurements to design fans, determine fan location, and design clothing.[30,31]

The lack of gravity also affects the behavior of sweat excreted as a thermoregulatory control mechanism in a hot environment. In a 1-g environment, sweat is normally excreted from the sweat glands and either evaporates or accumulates in the area of the sweat gland. If sweat accumulates, it will be visible first as tiny droplets, then as droplets in a sheen of wetness, and finally as larger droplets leading to running sweat. The maximum evaporation rate is limited in part by the percentage of skin wetness (maximum skin wetness is about 76 percent).[32] The skin is kept from being 100-percent wet by hydrophobic secretions and films on the skin and by the fact that sweat running off the body limits accumulation. Optimal maximum cooling should occur when sweat evaporates from a very thin accumulation of sweat covering the whole body.

Skylab astronauts noticed that in conditions of prolonged exercise sweat could accumulate in sheets on the skin. The crewmembers did not consider this a particular problem, but they did speculate on towel-based absorbent systems that might be used to collect or remove the sweat.[33] The Skylab environment did not have high air velocities available from the distributed ECS, but portable fans were available that could provide gas velocities in excess of 305 m/min (100 ft/min) over the body. (The portable fans took some time to set up.) Sweat sheeting was not reported when the portable fans were in use. The effect of sweat sheeting is not intuitively obvious. It may allow a higher percentage of skin wetness and increase the surface area available for evaporation, thereby increasing cooling. However, sheets of sweat with a significant thickness would remove the surface of evaporation from the skin, impose an intervening sweat layer, and thereby decrease cooling. The sweat rates that result in sweat sheeting in microgravity are conditions that result in sweat running off the body in 1-g. A high percentage of skin wetness in either of these conditions will result in extreme discomfort and possible limitation of sweat rates by hidromeiosis. Sweat sheeting has occurred under conditions of significant thermal stress that would not commonly be experienced, except for the extensive periods of high exercise that are being implemented, or considered as countermeasures against deleterious effects of microgravity. All of these difficulties and sweat sheeting can be eliminated by maximizing environmental conditions that encourage evaporation, principally by reducing humidity and increasing the gas velocity with fans.

Microgravity might also affect heat balance if it changed the level of heat production of the crewmembers. There is a widely held misconception that microgravity imposes a hypokinetic existence on crewmembers. Some of the first measurements of crewmembers in spacecraft simulators[9] and in the very cramped early spacecraft that did not allow crew movement[34] contributed to this misconception (as do bed rest and water or dry immersion simulations of microgravity). Measurements of crewmember metabolism in long-duration exposures, where they are free to move about and have a busy schedule of activities, reveal that their metabolic rates in flight are not reduced from the rates recorded in their busy preflight schedules.[35,36] The average metabolism that is measured is determined primarily by crewmember activity. However, it is possible that microgravity may affect the basal or resting metabolism because of a reduction of tone in the postural muscles or some other mechanism. Basal metabolism has not been measured in flight.

It is possible that microgravity might affect heat balance in space by altering physiological control. This could be a direct effect of thermoregulatory sensors, integration and regulatory centers, or effector mechanisms; or it could be indirect—imposed by changes in the neurological, cardiovascular, pulmonary, or hormonal systems that incidentally influence temperature regulation. No in-flight investigations have been specifically directed at thermoregulation, and no specific operational problems or incidents indicative of a change in crewmembers' heat balance have occurred. There have been some changes in body temperature and circadian rhythms[37,38] in animals. In general, these animals have been hypokinetic during their exposure to microgravity.

Hypokinesia itself seems to affect thermoregulatory systems. In bed rest studies involving a 200–300 kcal/day reduction in heat production,[39] a reduction in skin temperature, a greater variation in deep body temperature oscillation, and reduced thermal sensitivity were reported. A recent review on the effects of bed rest on energy and thermoregulation[40] reported that the stability of the basal metabolic rate during bed rest is unclear. Some investigators reported decreases of 2–22 percent, but others found no change. Exercise was performed during bed rest in some of the studies in both categories. The nonstandard conditions may have contributed to the mixed results.

A change in peak VO_2 was a more consistent result of bed rest. Where there were no remedial procedures, the decrement in peak VO_2 was a linear function of the duration of bed rest. Exercise minimized the decrement in peak VO_2, but only in investigations with high levels of exercise designed to maintain exercise capacity was the pre-bed-rest VO_2 maximum approached.[40] Similar disparate results are reported on the effect of bed rest on thermoregulation. Some investigators have found a reduction in basal temperature after bed rest, and others have not. Several different investigators have reported increased levels of core temperature during exercise after bed rest, which suggests impaired thermoregulation, although the details of this impairment have not been consistent from one study to another.[40]

Partial gravity or a force field of less than 1-g would be encountered on the lunar and Martian surfaces and could be encountered in a spacecraft being rotated to generate simulated gravity. A partial or reduced gravity field would have free convection but with reduced strength. Similarly, it could be hypothesized that any effect that microgravity might have on thermoregulation would be modified or reduced by a partial gravity force field.

Gravitational field is not the only factor in a spacecraft environment that can influence heat balance. Several different atmospheres have been used in flight—from the 34.5 kPa, 100-percent-oxygen Mercury spacecraft to the Earth's normal 101 kPa, 20-percent-oxygen/80-percent-nitrogen atmosphere on U.S. and Soviet spacecraft. Both pressure and gas composition influence heat balance. A reduced pressure gaseous environment has a lower density. Convection is a direct function of density; therefore, heat loss by convection is directly related to the atmospheric pressure. Reduced pressure increases the rate of evaporation. The rate of evaporation is primarily related to the difference in water vapor pressure between the liquid surface and the gaseous environment. However, the total pressure does affect evaporation by influencing the boundary layer. The physical basis for the increased rate of evaporation at lower pressures has been empirically demonstrated by several investigators.[41,42] The upper comfort band calculated for the Skylab environment (5.0 psi, 70 percent oxygen/30 percent nitrogen) was about 1 °C lower than that of an Earth-normal environment.[43] The thermal characteristics of the diluent gas selected for the environment could also influence heat balance.[44] To date, all spacecraft have used either 100 percent oxygen or a mixture of oxygen and nitrogen; however, other diluents such as argon, neon, and helium could be used. Helium would have the greatest impact on heat balance by significantly increasing convective heat transfer and resulting in a higher temperature comfort range.

The design, volume, and thermal mass of the habitat or spacecraft also will influence heat balance. Very small and light spacecraft, such as the Mercury and Gemini, are likely to have greater variations in wall temperature from location to location and as a function of time and position of the space-

Table 1 EVA Comparison

Spacecraft	Hours	Metabolic rate
Apollo	159	271 W[46]
Skylab	84	267 W[47]
Space Shuttle	137	228 W

craft. They are less likely to have a stable, uniform temperature; and they rely on a good range of compensatory gas heating or cooling to offset wall temperature variations.

In larger spacecraft and habitats, the thermal mass of the vehicle results in a more stable environmental temperature. The quantity, location, and cooling provisions allocated to electrical, electronic, and mechanical systems, which consume power and generate heat, increase in importance. Ideally, systems generating significant amounts of heat would be cooled locally rather than allowed to radiate heat directly or through a wall surface into the habitat volume. As thermal mass and uniformity of an environment increase, thermostatic control becomes easier and more desirable.

The possible impact of microgravity on heat balance through an effect on heat production has been discussed. However, the activity level of crewmembers in spacecraft and space suits definitely has a major effect on heat balance. Metabolic rates in flight are discussed in detail in Chapter 8 of this volume. It can be briefly stated here that in small spacecraft that restrict activity, metabolic rates are low.[45] In larger spacecraft and habitats, crewmembers have been very active, with busy schedules, and have had metabolic rates as high as on the ground.[46,47] Both the United States and the Soviet Union have encouraged high levels of in-flight aerobic exercise on the order of 60–80 percent of maximum consumption as a countermeasure. This level of activity results in elevated body temperature, strong vasodilation, and heavy sweat rates, which significantly challenge the thermoregulatory system. To support these work rates, the ECS must provide an environment with relatively low humidity and substantial capability to increase the gas stream velocity. The metabolic rates encountered in flight will depend to a predominant extent on activity levels, which are controlled by the crewmembers and their work schedules. If the current approach of using exercise as a countermeasure to microgravity-induced adaptive changes is effective and worthwhile, it is unlikely that long periods of inactivity will be planned. It is more likely that low activity will be avoided even if operational tasks on long missions do not always require activity. However, there will always be situations beyond the planners' control, such as illness or injury, that will require low activity.

EVA requires an elevated level of activity (see Table 1).

Peak metabolic rates were as high as 585 W for periods of 30 min on U.S. EVAs.[48] Metabolic rates during Soviet EVAs have been reported as 180–550 W.[49]

IV. Comfort and Tolerance Requirements, Approaches, and Experience

A. Comfort Zones

"Thermal comfort is that condition of mind which expresses satisfaction with the thermal environment" (American Society of Heating, Refrigerating and Air Conditioning Engineers Standard 55-66). A large number of environmental and physiological factors affect heat balance. The same factors combine to produce comfort or discomfort. Research on thermal comfort has been directed at identifying combinations of thermal factors that result in thermal comfort in a population or in the largest possible percentage of a given group of people. The approach has been to empirically expose many people to combinations of air temperature, wall temperature, humidity, air motion, clothing insulation, and activity level. Some of the early trials used to develop the original effective temperature scales determined equivalency by assessing comparative comfort levels immediately after moving from one controlled environment to another. These trials consistently overestimated the deleterious effect on comfort of increasing humidity in a steady-state environment. The currently accepted approach is to expose subjects to a controlled environment long enough to achieve steady-state conditions and assess comfort by means of a subjective scale.[51] Using these and other subjects and the same techniques developed at the Institute for Environmental Health at Kansas State University,[50,51] Fanger conducted tests in which he combined the empirical relationship of skin temperature and sweat rate with biophysical calculations of heat loss to arrive at an equation to calculate optimum comfort.[52]

B. Comfort Design Approaches

The specifications for the Mercury, Gemini, and Apollo spacecraft called for a temperature range of 65–75 °F with a relative humidity of 30–70 percent during all operational conditions of spacecraft heat exchange with the outside and during all operational power levels. In the early design of Skylab (when the program was called the Apollo Applications Program), the plan was to outfit an empty fuel tank in flight. The initial analysis indicated significant wall temperature cycling and variations in air and wall temperatures.[53] Although the final Skylab vehicle was fully outfitted on launch and more thermally stable, these differential temperatures were a consideration in the development of comfort criteria using empirical data and a computer model of heat exchange and thermoregulation in humans.[43] This model was used to generate comfort boxes for various combinations of air temperature, wall temperature, air motion, and metabolic rate.

Water vapor pressure was controlled above 1.0 kPa and less than 95 percent saturated. In this humidity range within the comfort box temperature, humidity does not significantly affect comfort. Touch temperatures were nominally maintained between 12.8 and 40.5 °C, and surfaces warmer than 45 °C were carefully restricted and identified.[43,53,54] Minimum air motion of 4.6 m/min was required at all times, well above the bulk flow rate of the Skylab ECS. To achieve this minimum flow rate, flow restrictions were designed into diffusers, which acted as air pumps and generated additional turbulent flow in the habitable area.

In the Space Shuttle Program and in the current design of the Space Station, the comfort design approach is to provide thermostatic temperature selection between 18.3 and 26.7 °C with a selectability of 1 °C. Humidity is restricted within a range of 0.8–1.9 kPa and air motion of 6.2–12.4 m/min. Air motion up to 25 m/min will be provided for use with the exercise countermeasure devices.

Clothing variation has not been an integral part of the U.S. thermal comfort requirements prior to Space Station. On the station, however, clothing variations will be used to achieve heat balance and comfort in degraded performance modes and in safe haven modes.

C. Temperature Tolerance Limits

In the Mercury and Gemini Programs, temperature and humidity limits were adopted and modified from aviation limits.[55] For the Apollo Program, these limits were not adequate, so heat storage limits were adopted from Blockley and others[56–58] and combined with the model of heat exchange and thermoregulation previously mentioned.[43] The model incorporated both shirtsleeve and pressure suit options and could be used to assess the rate of storage and accumulated heat storage in either mode. A conservative limit of 75 kcal heat storage was adopted; this is approximately 75 percent of the tolerance threshold and is considered a level of assured performance.[56] The heat storage limits and model were used extensively in the Apollo and subsequent programs as a design tool, and resulted in sizing emergency systems and defining the limits of normal and emergency capabilities.

V. Heat Balance in Pressure Suits

A. Suit Characteristics

EVA pressure suits share all of the requirements of spacecraft and other space habitats regarding the maintenance of heat balance in crewmembers. Detailed descriptions of pressure suits and associated life support systems are presented in Chapter 14 of this volume. Briefly stated, the suit must maintain a heat balance in the crewmember through a wide range of internal heat production rates. It must control heat flow in and out of the pressurized volume of the suit to acceptable levels and deal with the heat exchange with the external environment in the overall heat balance of the person in the suit. It must maintain acceptable surface temperatures on the inside of the suit to avoid local discomfort, to ensure crew comfort during nominal operations, and to keep the body temperature within tolerable limits during peak transient conditions and contingency conditions.

The EVA pressure suits minimize heat exchange with the external environment by means of effective insulation outside the pressure retention layers. Much of the surface of the suit is covered with insulation composed of reflective layers separated by mesh, all at a vacuum. This insulation limits heat flow in or out of the suit to a maximum of ±75 kcal/h when exposed to the hottest or coldest external environments. The EVA suits and life support system for the Space Shuttle have been designed to support crew metabolic rates of 116–464 W for steady-state operations and rates as high as 580 W for 30-min periods. The Russian Federation's pressure suits have similar performance capabilities and are designed to handle metabolic rates as high as 250–400 W with short peaks to 600 W.[49]

It has been the practice to cool pressure suits used in aircraft with gas ventilation, and this has been adequate for the low metabolic rates encountered in aircraft cabins. When higher metabolic rates (as may be encountered during EVA) are considered, the limits of gas cooling become a problem.[59] When work rates exceed about twice the rates while resting, the major portion of heat removal must be by evaporation, specifically evaporation of sweat.[60]

Since the thermoregulatory system acts as a proportional controller, the core temperature must rise to produce sweat. The limited air motion possible in a pressure suit results in evaporation from a skin surface with a substantial percentage of skin wetness. Under these conditions (elevated core temperature and wet skin), crewmembers are uncomfortable; hidromeiosis and dehydration will limit exposure. Current U.S. and Russian EVA pressure suits use liquid-cooled garments that can handle maximum operational work rates with a minimum of thermal stress. For the Apollo Program, the United States developed a liquid-cooled garment based on a British design to provide cooling in aircraft cockpits with high environmental heat loads.[61,62] Current liquid-cooled garments worn by astronauts and cosmonauts have similar design characteristics and can handle peak EVA work rates with only minimal sweating. Although a number of designs for automatic control of liquid-cooled garments have been developed and demonstrated,[63] manual temperature control has proved to be simple, effective, and acceptable to the crewmembers.

B. Crewperson Characteristics

EVA pressure suits support crewmembers' capability for useful work outside the spacecraft. This work requires good hand mobility. For that reason, insulation is minimized in the area of the hand. There has been some experience of overcooling the hands when dealing with cold surfaces, but this has almost always been associated with low metabolic rates and heat leakage from the suit in a cold environment resulting in a general overcooling in the suit. Design requirements for future suits would allow metabolic rates as low as 73 W and maximum heat leaks without a negative heat balance on the crewmember. Positive heat storage approaching tolerance levels has not been a problem with an active liquid-cooled garment. Contingency gas cooling is limited in cooling capability: it will support metabolic rates of 204–234 W for a few hours or higher metabolic rates for very limited durations when using acceptable heat storage.

VI. Modeling of Heat Exchange and Thermoregulation and Its Application

Space is a hostile environment, and survival requires human intervention in designing ECSs for habitats and pressure suits. Since physiological thermoregulation is an important and complex variable, the engineers responsible for designing ECSs rely on environmental physiologists to specify human thermal requirements and to define physiological thermoregulation and acceptable comfort and tolerance values. Engineers and physiologists need to communicate in detail about the components of heat balance of crewmembers in the space environment; they need to jointly consider the complex heat exchange equations. Many of the values relating to humans in these equations are not constants but, rather, are variables that for any state of thermal exchange depend on the status of physiological thermoregulation. At the same time, tolerance of these thermal conditions depends not only on the status of the temperature at heat balance but also on the capability of the body to maintain the heat balance.

What was needed was a set of equations that would describe the heat balance between the space environment and the space habitat or suit, the heat balance between the habitat or suit and crewmember, and the human thermoregulatory responses to specific environments. This is, in fact, a description of a model, and simple working models of thermoregulation and heat balance had been used for years. The computer, however, has allowed the development of more complicated models, interactive solutions of equations as a function of time, and interaction of physiological thermoregulation with the environment as a function of time. The multiple variables, avenues of heat exchange, and multiple physiological systems of the thermoregulatory system make it particularly suitable for computer modeling. The first computer model of a physiological system to be used in the space program was a model of thermoregulation in humans developed by Stolwijk at the John B. Pierce Foundation Laboratory under NASA sponsorship.[63,64] The model was first structured for an analog computer, then reconfigured for a digital computer. The thermoregulatory model was then combined with models of heat transfer in spacecraft cabins and pressure suits by NASA contractors.[65]

The Stolwijk model consisted of a controlled system of six compartments with four layers in each; a central blood compartment was common to the six compartments. Characteristic dimensions, heat transfer coefficients, blood flow rates, metabolism, and specific heats of each segment and each layer allowed the calculation of heat flow in the passive model. The control system consisted of sensing mechanisms, an integrator controller, and effector systems. The model used receptors in the skin layer of each segment in the core segment of the head. The controller consisted of control equations for sweating vasodilation, vasoconstriction, and shivering. Each control equation had a term consisting of the product of a control coefficient and a central temperature signal; a term consisting of the product of a control coefficient and an integrated skin temperature signal; and a term consisting of the product of a control coefficient, a central temperature signal, and a skin temperature signal. The effector systems were described by equations defining shivering as a function of the control signal producing increased metabolism, increased or decreased blood flow to the skin, and sweat on the skin surface.

One of the first practical uses of the model was for analyzing comfort in spacecraft environments. Earlier in this chapter, it was stated that comfort is subjective and empirically determined; but the thermal model allowed extrapolation of comfort determinations under specific thermal conditions. The assumption was that thermal stimuli generating equal levels of thermal sensation and increased or decreased body temperatures would be perceived as equally comfortable. The changes in body temperature associated with the limits of comfort are small and within the ranges of circadian variations of the set points. The changes in heat storage in this instance are theoretical changes in the steady-state model, not actual measurable changes in body temperature. The thermal comfort criteria allowed extrapolation of the resting comfort conditions of Nevins[66] and the exercise comfort condition of McNall[50] to any metabolic rate in that range and any combination of environmental conditions, including changes in pressure and gas composition.[43]

The model was also used to assess thermal tolerance in spacecraft and space suits. In this case, thermal tolerance was defined in terms of heat storage; and the heat storage criteria for the model were a more direct application than the comfort criteria. Heat storage is an acceptable correlate of tolerance, and the heat storage prediction of the model can be expected to relate to actual heat storage.[56] Heat storage limits have been important determining factors in the design of contingency life support systems and just as important in the evaluation of their operational capacity. For example, heat storage limits define, in part, the flow rate provided by the contingency gas supply in the extravehicular mobility unit (EMU). They also define the metabolic rates that can be safely supported by this system under worst-case conditions. Similarly, heat storage was a consideration in defining EVA traverse limits on the lunar surface to ensure that heat storage limits would not be exceeded if contingency systems were utilized. In the 25 years since a thermal model was first used in the space program, there has been a tremendous expansion in the number, type, and purposes served by thermal models. The Stolwijk model remains the basis for many of those models.[67–69] Models are used for a number of purposes, including the prediction of tolerance and performance,[70,71] the evaluation of hyperthermic medical treatments,[72] and as an iterative tool in investigations of thermoregulation.[73,74] It is the latter use of the model that may be of particular value

in investigating the impact of microgravity on thermoregulation.

VII. Monitoring and Temperature Control in Spacecraft

The complexity of any thermal environment, particularly that of a spacecraft, mandates the use of multiple temperature sensors and of sensors that respond in a representative way to the thermal environment. Care must be taken to avoid placing sensors where temperatures will not be representative of a significant portion of the environment. A reliable technique is to use multiple temperature sensors and to choose their locations on the basis of spacecraft modeling, spacecraft heat exchange with the external environment, spacecraft or habitat heat sources, and the ECS.[54,75]

Spacecraft temperature control systems rely on a passive balance between the spacecraft and the external environment. The balance can be modified by the emissivity and reflectivity characteristics of the external surface of the spacecraft, as well as by heating or cooling the interior to deal with the variation of temperature because of cyclic power requirements and to vary crew activity and metabolic rate.

The Skylab system used external panels of varying emissivity combined with insulation to maintain much of the heat balance with passive systems. Since some of the greatest variations in heat generation in the spacecraft relate to heat produced by equipment, a major consideration in spacecraft design is gas cooling or cold plate cooling of these equipment items. Most ECSs have relied on gas temperature control for the fine control of the temperature in the crew compartment, with the crew able to increase or decrease gas temperature or thermostatic control.

VIII. Future Challenges

It has been more than 30 years since the first pioneering space flights of Yuri Gagarin and others in the Soviet Union and the United States. In the Soviet program, cosmonauts remained in space for 1 year. In all of this time, no operational difficulties have indicated a degradation of thermoregulation. At the same time, no in-flight studies have addressed thermoregulation, although some bed-rest studies have suggested a potential effect on thermoregulation. Certainly the physical environment is modified in microgravity, and any effect on the cardiovascular system and respiratory system, or any changes influencing metabolism at rest or during exercise, would have a collateral effect on thermoregulation. A careful long-term assessment of thermoregulation in microgravity will certainly be important to future missions, particularly long-duration space station exposures that may be conducted in verification of and preparation for interplanetary flight.

Interplanetary travel will require long exposure to both space and microgravity or, if necessary, to a simulated gravity field. Either environment will provide special challenges to crew heat balance. Interplanetary travel will mean that the spacecraft habitat will be moving in a changing external heat flux environment and that all systems to support the crew will have to compensate for the full range of the external environments. Decisions in the design of the environment for such a mission may well lead to the consideration of an alternate atmosphere at a lower pressure or with a different gas composition, with all of the heat balance considerations this would entail. Finally, a mission of this duration would require the consideration of long-term contingency situations and definition of long-term tolerance to an unfavorable heat balance environment.

One of the long-term goals of the U.S. Space Program is to establish an outpost on the Moon and possibly Mars. An extended return visit or a permanent outpost on the lunar surface will have to address the fact that the average temperature of the lunar environment is colder than that on Earth because of the lack of a heat-trapping atmosphere. EVA will be an important lunar surface activity, but consumable considerations may not allow the use of sublimators in the EMU for cooling the pressure suit. Both of these considerations will be of even greater significance on a Martian surface mission. At a greater distance from the Earth and with a less dense atmosphere, Mars has an average temperature that is much cooler than on the Earth or the Moon. The most important need for EVA heat control will be not so much a mechanism to allow heat loss (that will be easy enough) but a heat buffer that will allow variation from the 175 W heat loss rate measured as an average on lunar EVA missions, without unacceptable positive or negative heat storage.

Whatever the nature of our future activities in space, maintenance of heat balance will be one of the essential and difficult considerations in maintaining the health and well-being of our astronauts and cosmonauts.

References

[1]National Aeronautics and Space Administration. Mission operations report, Apollo 13. MSC-02680, Manned Spacecraft Center, Houston, NASA, 1970.

[2]Waligora, J.M. Medical position on temperature requirements for entry into the OWS (Hot Workshop Test Report). Johnson Space Center, Houston, NASA internal report, 1973.

[3]National Aeronautics and Space Administration. Skylab Mission Report, First Visit, August 1973. JSC-08414, Johnson Space Center, Houston, NASA, 1973.

[4]Burton, A.C., and Edholm, O.G. Man in a Cold Environment. London, Edward Arnold Ltd., 1955, pp. 16–20.

[5]Swan, H. Thermoregulation and Bioenergetics. New York, American Elsevier, 1974, p. 2.

[6]Waligora, J.M.; Horrigan, D.J.; and Nicogossian, A.E. The physiology of spacecraft and space suit atmospheric selection. In: Proceedings of the Eighth International Academy of Astronautics, Man in Space Symposium, IAA-T-114, Tashkent, U.S.S.R., September 29–October 3, 1989.

[7]Eckenhoff, R.G.; Osborne, S.F.; Parker, J.W.; and Bondi, K.R. Direct ascent from shallow air saturation exposures. Undersea Biomedical Research, 1986, vol. 13, no. 3, pp. 305–316.

[8]Astrand, P.O., and Rodahl, K. Textbook of Work Physiology. St. Louis, McGraw-Hill, 1970, p. 304.

[9]Webb, P. Work heat and oxygen cost. In: Parker, J.F., and West, V.R., Eds. Bioastronautics Data Book. Second Edition, NASA SP-3006. Washington, D.C., NASA, 1973, Chapter 18, p. 853.

[10]Hensel, H. Thermoreception and Temperature Regulation. In: Monographs of the Physiological Society. Number 38, New York, Academic Press, 1981.

[11]Gordon, C.J., and Heath, J.E. Integration and central processing in temperature regulation. Annual Review of Physiology, 1986, vol. 48, pp. 595–612.

[12]Tahuer, R. Thermosensitivity of the spinal cord. In: Hardy, J.D.; Gagge, A.P.; and Stolwijk, J.A.J., Eds. Physiological and Behavioral Temperature Regulation. Springfield, Ill., Thomas, 1970, pp. 472–492.

[13]Houdas, Y., and Ring, E.F.J. Human Body Temperature, Its Measurement and Regulation. New York, Plenum Press, 1982.

[14]Simon, E.; Pierau, F.K.; and Taylor, D.C.M. Central and peripheral thermal control of effectors in homeothermic temperature regulation. Physiological Review, April 1986, vol. 66, no. 2, pp. 235–299.

[15]Bensinger, T.H., and Kitzinger, C. The human thermostat. In: Herzfeld, C.M., Ed. Temperature, Its Measurement and Control in Science and Industry. New York, Reinhold, 1963, vol. 3, pp. 637–665.

[16]Bligh, J. Temperature Regulation in Mammals and Other Vertebrates. New York, American Elsevier, 1973, p. 8.

[17]Houdas, Y., and Guieu, J.D. The human thermoregulatory system: Regulated system or servo system? NASA TTF-16256, 1975.

[18]Herrington, L.P. The range of physiological response to climatic heat and cold. In: Newburg, L.H., Ed. Physiology of Heat Regulation and Science of Clothing. Philadelphia, W.B. Saunders, 1949, pp. 262–277.

[19]Greenleaf, J.E., and Sargent, F. Voluntary dehydration in man. Journal of Applied Physiology, 1965, vol. 20, no. 4, pp. 719–724.

[20]Sargent, F. II. Depression of sweating in man. In: Montagna, W.; Ellis, R.A.; and Silver, A.F., Eds. Advances in Biology of Skin. New York, Pergamon Press, 1962, vol. III.

[21]Brown, W.K.; Sargent, F. II; and Waligora, J.W. Skin wettness and eccrine sweat gland function in development of hidromeiosis. Journal of Laboratory and Clinical Medicine, 1962, vol. 60, p. 863.

[22]Brown, W.K. Studies on the mechanism of the progressive depression of sweating in man (hidromeiosis). Ph.D. Thesis, Physiology, University of Illinois, 1964.

[23]Stolwijk, J.A.J. A study of heat exchange between man and his environment in Project Apollo. Final Report, NAS9-4522, Johnson Space Center, Houston, NASA, 1967.

[24]Taylor, N.A.S. Eccrine sweat glands adaptations to

physical training and heat acclimation. *Sports Medicine*, 1986, vol. 3, pp. 387–397.

[25]Libert, J.P.; Amoros, C.; Di Nisi, J.; Muzet, A.; Fukuda, H.; and Ehrhart. Thermoregulatory adjustments during continuous heat exposure. *European Journal of Applied Physiology*, 1988, vol. 57, pp. 499–506.

[26]Brengelmann, G.L. Circulatory adjustments to exercise and heat stress. *Annual Review of Physiology*, 1983, vol. 45, pp, 191–212.

[27]Gagge, A.P.; Stolwijk, J.A.J.; and Nishi, Y. The prediction of thermal comfort when thermal equilibrium is maintained by sweating. *ASHRAE Transactions*, 1969, vol. 75, pp. 108–125.

[28]Novak, L. Heat exchange between the organism and environment under conditions of weightlessness, methodical approach. In: *Life Sciences and Space Research XIV, Proceedings of the Open Meeting of the Working Group on Space Biology*, May 29–June 7, 1975. Berlin, Akademic-Verlog, 1976, pp. 330–333.

[29]Kuznetz, L.H. Analysis of the effects of free stream gas velocity upon astronaut thermal comfort. NASA TM-79823, Johnson Space Center, Houston, NASA, 1968.

[30]Novak, L.; Genin, A.M.; and Kozlowski, S. Skin temperature and thermal comfort in weightlessness. *The Physiologist*, 1980, vol. 23, Supplement.

[31]Baranski, S.; Bloszczynyski, R.; Hermaszewski, M.; Kubiozkowa, J.; Piorko, A.; Saganiak, R.; Sarol, Z.; Skibniewski, F.; Stendera, J.; and Walachnowski, W. Investigation of cooling properties of the gaseous medium of a space station. *Postepy Astronautyki*, 1979, vol. 12, no. 4, pp. 81–84.

[32]Berglund, L.G., and Gonzalez, R.R. Evaporation of sweat from sedentary man in humid environments. *Journal of Applied Physiology. Respiratory, Environmental and Exercise Physiology, 1977*, vol. 43, no. 5, pp. 767–772.

[33]Pogue, W.R.; Carr, G.P.; and Gibson, E.G. Skylab 1/4 medical debriefing. JSC-08811, Johnson Space Center, Houston, NASA, 1974, p. 160.

[34]Michel, E.L. Summary of flight metabolic data, Mercury 8–Apollo 11 (DB6-72). Johnson Space Center, Houston, NASA internal report, 1969.

[35]Rambaut, P.C.; Leach, C.S.; and Leonard, J.J. Observations in energy balance in man during space flight. *American Journal of Physiology,* 1977, vol. 233, no. 5, pp. R208–R212.

[36]Bogomolov, U. V.; Popova, I.A.; Yegorov, A.D.; and Kozlovskaya, I.B. The results of medical research during the 326-day flight of the second principle expedition on the orbital complex "Mir." In: Gazenko, O.G., Ed. P*roceedings of Second U.S./U.S.S.R. JWG Conference on Space Biology and Medicine*, 1988.

[37]Jauchem, J.R. Environmental stressors during space flight: Potential effects on body temperature. Mini Review, *Comparative Biochemical Physiology*, 1988, vol. 91A, no. 3, pp. 425–427.

[38]Klimovitskiy, V.Ya.; Alpatov, A.M.; Sulzman, F.M.; Fuller, C.A.; and Moore-Ede, M.C. In-flight simian circadian rhythms and temperature homeostasis aboard Cosmos-1514 biosatellite. *Kosmicheskaya Biologiya i Aviakosmicheskya Meditsina,* 1981, vol. 21, no. 5, pp. 14–18 (in Russian).

[39]Panferova, N. Ye. Heat regulation under prolonged limitation of muscular activity. *Fiziologiya Cheloveka*, 1978, vol. 4, no. 5, pp. 835–839 (in Russian).

[40]Greenleaf, I.E. Energy and thermal regulation during bed rest and space flight, Brief Review. *Journal of Applied Physiology,* 1989, vol. 67, no. 2, pp. 507–516.

[41]Chernyakov, I.N.; Maksimov, I.V.; and Azhevskiy, P.Ya. Evaporation under low atmospheric pressure conditions. *Kosmicheskaya Biologiya i Meditsina*, 1968, vol. 2, no. 3, pp. 81–86, (in Russian).

[42]Hale, F.C.; Westland, R.A.; and Taylor, G.L. The influence of barometric pressure and vapor pressure on insensible weight loss in nude resting man. WADC TR-57-9, Wright-Patterson AFB, Ohio, Wright Air Development Center, USAF, 1957, pp. 57–59.

[43]Waligora, J.M. Thermal comfort and tolerance design criteria. BRO DB-57-67, Rev. B, Johnson Space Center, Houston, NASA internal report, 1970.

[44]Hamilton, R.W., Jr.; Doebbler, G.F.; and Shreiner, H.R. Biological evaluation of various spacecraft cabin atmospheres. *Space Life Sciences,* 1970, vol. 2, pp. 307–334.

[45]Verostko, C.E. *LiOH Analysis Data for STS-1 through STS-8.* Report EC11883, Johnson Space Center, Houston, NASA internal report, 1983.

[46]Waligora, J.M., and Horrigan, D.J. Metabolism and heat dissipation during Apollo EVA periods. In: Johnston, R.S.; Dietlein, L.S.; and Berry, C.A., Eds. *Biomedical Results of Apollo,* SP-368, Washington D.C., NASA, 1975, pp. 115–128.

[47]Waligora, J.M., and Horrigan, D.J. Metabolic cost of extravehicular activities. In: Johnston, R.S., and Dietlein, L.S., Eds. *Biomedical Results from Skylab*, SP-337, Washington D.C., NASA, 1977, pp. 395–399.

[48]Horrigan, D.J., and Waligora, J.M. Overview of crew member energy expenditure during shuttle flight 61-B ease/access task performance. In: *Proceedings of a Conference held at NASA Langley Research Center*, Hampton Va., NASA Conference Publication 2490, 1986.

[49]Abramov, I.P., and Severin, G.I. *Pressure Suits and Systems for Working in Open Space.* Moscow, Mashinostroyeniye, 1984 (in Russian), Translation 1987, FTD-ID(RS)T-1313-86; Foreign Technology Division, Wright Patterson AFB, Ohio, USAF, p. 27.

[50]McNall, P.E.; Jax, I.; Rohles, F.H.; Nevins, R.G.; and Springer, W. Thermal comfort (thermally neutral) conditions for three levels of activity. *ASHRAE Transactions,*1967, p. 73.

[51]Koch, W.; Jennings, B.H.; and Humphreys, U. Environmental study II—Sensation responses to temperature and humidity under still air conditions in the comfort range. *ASHRAE Transactions*, 1960, p. 66.

[52]Fanger, P.O. *Thermal Comfort: Analysis and Applica-*

tions in Environmental Engineering. Copenhagen, Danish Technical Press, 1970.

[53]Cody, J.C. *Environmental Control of Apollo Applications Program Orbital Assembly*. Society of Automotive Engineers, Paper 690622, 1969.

[54]Hopson, G.D. Skylab life support and habitability system requirements and implementation. In: *Proceedings of the 22nd International Astronautical Congress*, 1971.

[55]Taylor, G.L. Thermal requirements for aircraft cabins. Army Air Force Headquarters, Air Technical Service Command Engineering Division Report, 1945.

[56]Blockley, W.V.; McCutchan, J.W.; and Taylor, C.L. Prediction of human tolerance for heat in aircraft: A design guide. WADC Technical Report 53-346, Wright Patterson AFB, Ohio, Wright Air Development Center, USAF, 1954.

[57]Blockley, W.V., and Roth, H.P. Limits of endurance for heat stress arising from work while totally insulated. NASA CR-108419, Washington, D.C., NASA, 1970.

[58]Dasler, A. Heat stress and strain in men wearing impermeable clothing. Ph. D. Thesis, Michigan State University, 1966.

[59]Genin, A.M., and Golovkin, L.G. *The problem of prolonged autonomous human existence in a space suit*. Translation of Paper Presented at the 17th International Astronautical Congress, Madrid, Oct. 9–15, 1966. NASA TT F-10.

[60]Waligora, J.M., and Michael E.L. Application of conductive cooling for working men in a thermally isolated environment. *Aerospace Medicine,* May 1968, vol. 39, no. 5.

[61]Burton, D.R., and Collier, L. The development of water-conditioned suits. Royal Aircraft Establishment Technical Note No. Mech. Eng. 400, 1964.

[62]Nunneley, S.A. Water cooled garments: A review. *Space Life Sciences,* 1970, vol. 2. pp. 335–360.

[63]Stolwijk, J.A.J., and Hardy, J.D. Temperature regulation in man: A theoretical study. *Pflugers Archives,* 1966, vol. 291, pp. 129–162.

[64]Stolwijk, J.A.J. A mathematical model of physiological temperature regulation in man. NASA CR-1855, Washington, D.C., NASA, 1970.

[65]Morgan, L.W.; Collett, G.; and Cook, D. W. Transient metabolic simulation program. Computer program documentation, Manned Spacecraft Center, Houston, NASA, 1969.

[66]Nevins, R.G.; Rohles, F.H.; Springer, W.; and Feyerherm, A.M. A temperature-humidity chart for thermal comfort of seated persons. *ASHRAE Journal,* 1966, p. 55.

[67]Werner, J. Thermoregulatory models. *Scandinavian Journal of Work and Environmental Health,* 1989, vol. 15, Suppl. 1, p. 34–46.

[68]Halsom, R.A., and Parsons, K.C. A comparison of models for predicting human response to hot and cold environments. *Ergonomics,* 1987, vol. 30, no. 11, pp. 1599–1614.

[69]Werner, J. Do black-box models of thermoregulation still have any research value? Contributions of system-theoretical models to the analysis of thermoregulation. *The Yale Journal of Biology and Medicine,* 1986, vol. 59, pp. 335–348.

[70]Halsom, R.A., and Parsons, K.C. Quantifying the effects of clothing for models of human response to the thermal environment. *Ergonomics*, 1988, vol. 31, no. 12, pp. 1787–1806.

[71]Shapiro, Y., Moran, D., and Epstein, Y. Adjustment and validation of the mathematical prediction model for sweat rate, heart rate, and body temperature under outdoor conditions. AD-A222 599, Fort Detrick, Frederick, Md., U.S. Army Medical Research and Development Command, 1989.

[72]Charny, C.K.; Hagman, M.J.; and Levin, R.L. A whole body thermal model of man during hyperthermia. *IEEB Transactions on Biomedical Engineering*, 1987, vol. BME-34, no. 5, pp. 375–387.

[73]Song, W.J.; Weinbaum, S.; and Jiji, L.M. A theoretical model for peripheral tissue heat transfer using the bioheat equation of Weinbaum and Jiji. *Journal of Biomechanical Engineering,* 1987, vol. 109, no. 1, pp. 72–78.

[74]Werner, J.; Buse, M.; and Foegen, A. Lumped versus distributed thermoregulatory control: Results from a three-dimensional dynamic model. *Biological Cybernetics*, 1989, vol. 32, no.1, pp. 63–73.

[75]Waligora, J.M.; Sauer, R.I..; and Bredt, J.H. Spacecraft life support systems. In: Nicogossian, A.E.; Huntoon, C.L.; and Pool, S.L., Eds. *Space Physiology and Medicine*. Second edition. Philadelphia, Lea & Febiger, 1989, pp. 104–120.

Chapter 4

Microbiological Contamination

Duane L. Pierson, Michael R. McGinnis, and Aleksandr N. Viktorov

Micro-organisms are ubiquitous in spacecraft environments, as they are on Earth. Microbes are amazingly adaptive to a wide range of environmental extremes in temperature, pressure, and desiccation. The vast majority of microbial species are harmless to humans, and many have proven remarkably beneficial. Their capability to degrade complex organic materials into simple substances is essential in maintaining the natural balance on Earth. This property may make them useful in the bioremediation of waste materials (e.g., human wastes) on planetary outposts. As space exploration continues, microbes will be increasingly involved in food production and air and water purification. Unfortunately, however, microbial biodeterioration also may degrade materials responsible for maintaining environmental safety, such as airlock seals.

Relatively few microbial species cause infectious diseases in humans. However, the crowded, closed environment of the spacecraft may predispose crewmembers to the problems associated with the "tight building syndrome" on Earth.[1] An example is allergic reactions induced by fungal propagules and mycelium, which produce discomfort and decrease productivity.

Microbes will colonize an ecological niche that contains sufficient moisture and nutrients. Even though space vehicles, space stations, and planetary bases are closed environmental systems, microbial development and its associated problems will be dynamic. The initial resident microbial population will change over time as crews are exchanged and experiments involving plants, micro-organisms, and animals are conducted. As the environments evolve, each crewmember will be at risk for infections caused by the changing microbe populations.[2–4] Many opportunistic infections observed in spacecraft environments have been caused by crewmembers' normal flora. Experiences from the U.S.S.R. (currently Russian) and American space programs have demonstrated clearly that morbidity resulting from opportunistic infections can reduce crew health and productivity.[5] Greater knowledge of the effects of microgravity on microbial function is critical to understanding the potential for opportunistic infections and potential biodeterioration of materials.

Unquestionably, air, water, and interior surfaces in spacecraft will become contaminated. Environmental monitoring systems, acceptability limits, and appropriate countermeasures to protect the health of the crews, as well as the integrity of their space habitats, must be formulated and tested.[5,6] Monitoring systems must incorporate flexibility in their designs to take advantage of technological advances over time. Microbial standards will change as new information on health effects becomes available. Finally, the microbial populations themselves will change through human habitation, periodic crew exchange, docking of resupply vehicles, biological experiments, and the presence of experimental plants and animals. Many micro-organisms will find niches in the interior of the space habitat regardless of preventive measures, because no environmental control system will be able to remove all micro-organisms. Furthermore, it is expected that environmental selection for changes in microbial metabolic activities will affect microbial virulence and sensitivity to disinfectants and antibiotics.

This chapter presents the sources of microbial contaminants and the principal means of infectious disease transmission in the closed environment of a spacecraft. Onboard capabilities for monitoring micro-organisms in the environment and decontamination procedures are also described. Tentative plans for the microbiology subsystem of the U.S. Space Station are discussed. Finally, some thoughts are presented on future directions for the field of microbiology in space exploration.

I. Infectious Diseases in Spacecraft

Infectious diseases remain an important concern associated with space flight.[5–8] The morbidity and potential mortality associated with infectious diseases in space are exacerbated by the limited diagnostic capabilities and few countermeasures available to crewmembers during flight. In addition, the relatively small closed environment, crowded conditions, and lack of appropriate isolation facilities in the space habitat greatly increase the potential for transmission of disease-causing microbes among crewmembers.

Infections result from agents that are both endogenous and exogenous to the host. Endogenous infections result from changes in the relationship between the host and its commen-

Christine Wogan provided invaluable help in the preparation of this paper.

sal microflora. This relationship represents a delicate balance, and factors upsetting this balance may predispose individuals to infection from their own flora. The commensal flora normally protect the host from microbial pathogens through several mechanisms, including competition for nutrients, production of bactericides, and stimulation of the immune system in preparation for invading pathogens.[9] Illnesses caused by the indigenous microbiota follow changes in either the host's resistance, the host's flora, or both. Exogenous infections, on the other hand, occur following the transmission of an infectious agent from an exogenous source to a susceptible host. Infectious agents are transmitted primarily via four routes: contact, common vehicle, air, and vector. Understanding the routes of transmission allows interruption of the chain of events that leads to infection and may provide a form of "countermeasure" in the closed spacecraft environment.

Contact between an infectious source and a host can be direct or indirect. Direct contact implies physical contact between the host and the source. Indirect contact refers to the passive transfer of micro-organisms from the source to the host, usually by means of an inanimate object. In common vehicle transmission, an infectious agent is transmitted to multiple hosts via a single inanimate vehicle, such as food, water, or airborne particles. Infectious agents can be aerosolized (see "Modes of Transmission") and reach potential hosts via airborne transmission. Potential pathogens may also be transferred via a vector (e.g., an insect); this route, although deserving of consideration in the preflight period, is unlikely to play a role in disease transmission during space flight.

Clearly, the host-microbe relationship will determine the probability of the onset of infectious diseases in spacecraft or in planetary habitats. The effects of the stresses associated with space habitation (reduced gravity, radiation, physiological changes, isolation, and others) on the host-microbe relationship are unknown. Although much work remains to be done in the study of this area, evidence suggests that the human immune response is attenuated somewhat during space flight.[10–13] Blunting of the delayed-type hypersensitivity response after as few as 3 to 5 days in flight was reported by Taylor and Janney.[14] Changes in the immune response have been observed in the cell-mediated component of the immune system; however, significant changes in the humoral immune response have yet to be demonstrated. The microbial agent is the other important aspect of the host-microbe relationship. The effects of space flight on microbial structure and function leading to changes in pathenogenicity have not been demonstrated conclusively.[6,15,16] Some bacteria, such as *Escherichia coli* and *Staphylococcus aureus*, have exhibited decreased susceptibility to selected antibiotics in space flight. Moatti et al.[17] demonstrated similar findings during the German Spacelab D-1 mission. These in vitro findings, if consistent in vivo, may affect in-flight antibiotic dosages for infections. Probable changes in drug pharmacodynamics resulting from in-flight fluid shifts and other physiological changes

will exacerbate the problems associated with determining antibiotic dosages.

The environment also plays an important role in the chain of infection by affecting the infectious agent, the route of transmission, and the host. Environmental factors of interest in the space-flight environment include temperature, moisture, radiation, air pressure, ventilation, and the presence of chemicals and toxins. Environmental factors may promote or limit the infection process from or prevent it from progressing to clinically apparent disease.

To understand the role of the many stresses associated with space flight on the increased risk of infectious disease, we must first understand the changes in the host-microbe relationship. Specifically, space-flight-induced clinically relevant effects on the human immune response and the pathogenic potential of micro-organisms must be determined and evaluated.

That infectious diseases can have serious effects on crew health and performance during space missions has been recognized from the inception of the U.S. space program. The highest incidence of infectious diseases before and during flight was reported in the early Apollo missions, before the crews were routinely isolated from potential sources of infection before missions. During this period, 57 percent of the Apollo crewmembers reported illnesses during the 21-day period before. These illnesses included upper respiratory infections, gastroenteritis, urinary tract infections, and various skin infections.[18] The Apollo 9 mission was delayed because an astronaut had an upper respiratory illness.[18] After Apollo 13, the Flight Crew Health Stabilization Program was formulated and implemented, dramatically reducing the occurrence of infectious diseases. Infectious diseases reported during Skylab missions were restricted primarily to gingivitis and skin infections such as dermatitis, sty formation, and boils.[19] Few infectious diseases have been reported during the Space Shuttle Program, attesting to the effectiveness of the present Health Stabilization Program for the relatively brief missions. However, the launch of U.S. Space Shuttle mission STS-36 was delayed because of a crewmember's upper respiratory infection.

II. Sources of Micro-Organisms

Micro-organisms are plentiful in the spacecraft environment; moreover, they are capable of surviving in quite hostile conditions. During the Apollo 16 mission to the Moon, the survival rate of spores of *Bacillus subtilis* and *B. thuringiensis* placed outside the command module and exposed to solar ultraviolet radiation and the space vacuum was no different than that observed using ground-based controls.[7] The ribonucleic acid (RNA) and deoxyribonucleic acid (DNA) viruses can survive conditions duplicating those in space.[20] Micro-organisms have survived in the artificial Mars apparatus used to reproduce various extreme environmental conditions.[21] Soviet scientists have identified 94 species of micro-organism onboard their space stations (see Table 1).

Table 1 Micro-organisms isolated on Soviet spacecraft

Bacteria	No. of species	Fungi	No. of species
Acinetobacter	1	Alternaria alternata	
Achromobacter		Aspergillus	11 *
Aeromonas	1	Candida albicans	
Alcaligenes	1	Cladosporium	2
Arizona		Fusarium	2
Bacillus	9 *	Mucor	1
Citrobacter	1	Oidiodendion cerealis	
Corynebacterium	7 *	Penicillium	13 *
Enterobacter	4 *	Rhizopus arrhizus	
Escherichia	1 *	Rhodotorula	
Flavobacterium		Stemphylium botryosum	
Klebsiella	4 *		
Micrococcus			
Moraxella	2		
Neisseria	5		
Proteus	3		
Pseudomonas	5		
Staphylococcus	3 *		
Streptococcus	6		
Streptomyces			

*Always present.

The crew is the primary source of micro-organisms in the closed environment of space habitats. Microbes are shed continuously from the skin, the respiratory tract, the gastrointestinal tract, and the genito-urinary tract. For example, approximately 10^{10} skin particles are shed per person per day and each particle contains an average of 4 viable bacteria. Thus, 1 person can shed 40 billion bacteria from the skin alone in 1 day.[22] The respiratory tract is another common source of micro-organisms. Sneezing, coughing, singing, and talking all produce aerosols, which provide an effective means of spreading micro-organisms in crowded, closed conditions.

Crews will harbor a broad spectrum of bacteria, fungi, and, to a lesser extent, viruses. Organisms such as S. aureus, S. epidermis, Klebsiella, Bacteroides, Proteus, Pseudomonas, Flavobacterium, Serratia, Mima, Moraxella, Corynebacterium, Neisseria, Enterobacter, Haemophilus, Streptococcus, Micrococcus, Mycoplasma, Escherichia, and Candida are expected.[5] Of these microbes, the major bacteria dispersed and surviving in the spacecraft environment will probably be Staphylococcus, Micrococcus, Streptococcus, and a few others. During the Apollo 14 lunar exploration, and during Skylabs 2 and 4, the numbers of aerobic microbes, such as S. aureus, increased, although the numbers of anaerobic bacteria decreased. In general, during the Apollo mission series, the absolute numbers of micro-organisms increased, while the diversity and number of anaerobes decreased. The number of fungal isolates decreased, as was the case during the Skylab missions. Different fungi were identified during different missions. The implementation of a preflight quarantine period was undoubtedly an important factor in the smaller numbers of both aerobic and anaerobic bacteria found during later missions.[23]

Not surprisingly, micro-organisms were exchanged among the Apollo crewmembers. Bacterial exchange among crewmembers was demonstrated by bacteriophage typing of S. aureus isolated from nares. A high carrier rate for Mycoplasma was also documented.[5] Staphylococci were also reportedly exchanged among crews on the Soviet space station Salyut 6.[24] Microbial exchange among crewmembers has many implications.[7] The population dynamics of each individual's flora and the interactions between that flora and a host whose immune response may become compromised, establish one dimension for potential autoinfection. The transfer or exchange of the normal flora of one host to another host also has serious implications. Microbiological results from the Apollo, Skylab, and Apollo-Soyuz Test Project have been reported previously.[19,25–27] During the Skylab missions, gross microbial contamination by normal flora microbes, intercrew transfer of known pathogens, minor in-flight infections, and microbial simplification of anaerobes were all documented.[19]

Although humans are the chief contributors to the microbial populations aboard spacecraft, other sources exist as well. During the assembly and testing associated with developing planetary quarantine requirements, it was reported that about 25 percent of the micro-organisms found with the Viking lander capsules, orbiters, and shrouds were soil bacteria. The remaining 75 percent were considered indigenous human flora.[28] Some of these microbes survived even the terminal heat treatment of the Viking spacecraft.[28] The location and type of environment in which spacecraft are assembled and tested has a profound effect on which micro-organisms will appear on the vehicles. The Explorer 33 spacecraft showed a microbial burden of 2.6×10^5 micro-organisms at launch.[29] Similarly, at the assembly and testing phases for Apollo 10 and 11, the command module was contaminated by 2.7×10^4 micro-organisms per square foot.[29] Approximately 95 percent of the micro-organisms recovered in both cases were indigenous human flora.[30] In addition, each time supplies and materials are brought to an existing spacecraft or planetary base, new organisms may be introduced. During the Skylab missions, small numbers of various fungi were detected, except in the third mission, in which the spacecraft was widely contaminated by species of Aspergillus and Penicillium. The sources of the fungi were traced to the liquid-cooling garment for the space suits.[31]

Other sources of micro-organisms in the space-flight environment are experimental animals and plants. Bacteria can be exchanged easily among experimental animals and their

Table 2 Some bacterial and viral zoonoses that can be transmitted to humans

Disease	Etiological agent	Host	Method of infection
Herpes B viral encephalitis	*Herpesvirus simiae*	Old World monkeys	Bites, contact with infected material
Leptospirosis	*Leptospira interrogans*	Mice, rats	Contact with contaminated food and water
Listeriosis	*Listeria monocytogenes*	Mice, rats	Unknown
Lymphocytic choriomeningitis	Arbovirus	Mice, rats, monkeys	Inhalation or ingestion of contaminated materials
Melioidosis	*Pseudomonas pseudomallei*	Mice, rats	Arthropod vectors, contaminated food and water
Pasteurellosis	*Pasteurella multocida*	Mice, rats	Animal bites
Rat bite fever	*Spirillum minus, Streptobacillus moniliformis*	Mice, rats	Bites
Salmonellosis	*Salmonella* sp.	Mice, rats	Direct contact, contaminated food

Adapted from Youmans, G. P. Zoonoses. In: Youmans, G. P.; Paterson, P. Y.; and Sommers, H. M., Eds. *The Biologic and Clinical Basis of Infectious Diseases*. Philadelphia, London, Toronto; W. B. Saunders, 1980. Reprinted with permission.

human caretakers, particularly in enclosed environments.[32] Zoonoses, or infectious diseases transmitted from animals to humans, range from inconsequential to lethal. *Herpes virus simiae* is frequently carried by Old World monkeys, such as the rhesus monkey. *H. simiae* causes a relatively benign, self-limited infection of the oral mucosa in the rhesus monkey, not unlike a *Herpes simplex* Type I infection in humans. In humans, however, *H. simiae* can lead to fatal encephalitis.[33] Zoonotic agents can be transmitted by a variety of means, including direct contact with the animal or its excreta, contamination of foodstuffs, animal bites, and insect vectors (e.g., mosquitos). Infectious aerosols have been demonstrated to transmit disease among animals; thus, airborne transmission must be considered in human infections. Because many zoonoses are restricted to one or a few animal species, different species pose different infectious threats. Examples of some bacterial and viral zoonoses in species of interest to NASA are shown in Table 2. On Earth, various opportunistic pathogens often are first identified through instances of animal infections.

Rats and squirrel monkeys are at present the only mammals that have flown on manned U.S. spacecraft. An upcoming joint France-U.S. project will use rhesus monkeys. Safeguards taken to protect the space crewmembers from animal-borne infectious agents are described in further detail later in this chapter.

As for experimental plants, most plant diseases are caused by fungi, viruses, and insects; bacterial infections are rare. Plant viruses are highly host specific and the insects and bacteria pathogenic to plants are not major causes of disease in humans. This is not the case, however, with fungi, which account for the majority of plant diseases. Fungi have been incriminated frequently in the etiology of superficial, subcutaneous, and mucocutaneous infections in humans.[34] Members of the genera *Alternaria* and *Fusarium* are the examples in this context. Cases of systemic or deep-seated infections in immune-compromised individuals have been attributed occasionally to these as well as other genera of plant pathogenic fungi.[34] Since long-duration space missions may compromise astronauts' immunity, the possibility of human infection from plant pathogenic fungi deserves to be taken seriously.

III. Modes of Transmission—Aerosols

Transmission of micro-organisms in space is most likely to take place via direct and indirect contact among crewmembers and common vehicles such as contaminated food, water, and air. Because particles of all sizes remain suspended in microgravity, microbial aerosolization presents a unique challenge to the health of the flight crews. Aerosols are liquid or solid particles suspended in air, which can then be inhaled. Bioaerosols are aerosols of micro-organisms or microbial products. Production of a microbial aerosol requires a reservoir, which can be a human, an animal, or an environmental niche; amplification, which occurs during favorable growth of the micro-organism in its host or environmental source; and dissemination or aerosolization through mechanisms such as coughing or sneezing. Several micro-organisms are capable of causing respiratory infections upon inha-

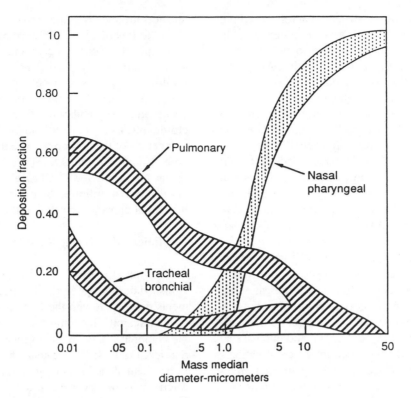

Fig. 1 Deposition of particles of different sizes in the human respiratory tract.

lation by a susceptible host. Both solid and aqueous airborne particulates can harbor microbes; therefore, both are important in the airborne transmission of disease.

The size and surface area of the particulates comprising aerosols are extremely important in determining their clinical effect. The diameter of individual aerosol particles can range from less than 0.1 μm to greater than 100 μm. As an example, a 2-μm droplet of water is large enough to contain a single cell of *Legionella pneumophila*;[35] larger particles may contain greater numbers of organisms. In general, aerosol particles up to 1 μm in size present the greatest hazard because of the likelihood of their being deposited in the lower respiratory tract[36] (see Fig. 1), where they may remain, become locally established, and eventually produce pathology.[37]

In 1-g, particles larger than 1 μm cannot remain long in suspension; for example, a 40-μm particle settles to the floor in about 60 s. Therefore, fewer potentially infective airborne particles are available for dispersion, and those particles that are inhaled often cannot efficiently negotiate beyond the upper respiratory passageways. In microgravity, however, even large or dense particles, which can accommodate many micro-organisms, will remain suspended in the spacecraft atmosphere and may penetrate more deeply into the respiratory system. Dense particles, with their greater mass and inertia, can also cause physical damage as they impact the walls of the respiratory system, even in the upper portion of the respiratory tract.

Relative humidity can also affect the size and disposition of bioaerosols. As atmospheric humidity decreases, the size of aqueous particles decreases because of fluid evaporation.

On the other hand, air is humidified to approximately 95 percent relative humidity by the body upon inhalation.[37] If hygroscopic viral aerosols are inhaled, their size increases through hydration: a 1.5-μm viral-aerosol particle can increase to nearly 4 μm through the addition of moisture from the respiratory tract.[38] Droplet nuclei are classic infectious units; in tuberculosis, the droplet nuclei are less than 5 μm in size. If their matrix contains proteinaceous materials, these materials can help retain the water associated with the droplet nuclei, thereby increasing the possibility of microbial survival.

The relative humidity of the atmosphere can also affect bioaerosols in other ways. The stability of some viruses in aerosols is governed by the presence or absence of lipids in the virion, the air temperature, and the relative humidity of the atmosphere.[39] Some lipid-enveloped RNA viruses (e.g., influenza and measles) are relatively stable in dry atmospheres (<40 percent relative humidity), whereas lipid-free viruses (e.g., enterovirus and rhinovirus) prefer higher moisture content (>60 percent relative humidity). Deposition of viruses in the lower regions of the respiratory tract is not necessary to initiate disease. Unlike bacteria, respiratory viruses, such as influenza, often cause infections when deposited in the upper respiratory tract.

It is clear that some bacteria, such as *Pseudomonas aeruginosa* and *Serratia marcescens*, can be spread as components of aerosols. A related question of great import in microgravity is whether bacteria can reproduce in aerosols. Experiments using *S. marcescens* have demonstrated that bacteria can grow, be metabolically active, and divide in aqueous particles and that these processes are enhanced when the particles are greater than 5 μm in size.[38] Anaerobic bacteria, however, may not behave like their aerobic counterparts in aerosols. Anaerobic bacteria tend to produce nonvolatile products, which may accumulate as potential toxins. Anaerobic bacteria also require slightly reduced molecules as an energy substrate for metabolism and subsequent growth.

Disease transmission by aerosols in microgravity will also be influenced by inertial impaction, Brownian motion, and air circulation patterns.[40] In the space-flight environment, particles are not deposited on surfaces by natural sedimentation; an enormous number of particles of differing sizes remain suspended in the air. These larger particles may carry larger numbers of micro-organisms, which, in turn, might survive longer with greater amounts of substrate. Because the deposition of aerosols in the respiratory tract is normally influenced by particle size and density as well as the involved site in the respiratory tract, the lack of sedimentation in microgravity may result in deposition at different sites and changes in retention relative to a gravity environment. Aerosols can also participate in other modes of infection, including contamination of eyes, skin, equipment, and internal surfaces of the space habitat. Direct contact among crewmembers who have touched contaminated surfaces or inhaled infectious droplets further increases the probability of transmitting infectious agents among the crew.

IV. Microbial Acceptability Limits and Monitoring Strategies

Given that achieving and maintaining spacecraft sterility is neither a realistic nor a desirable goal, appropriate microbial limits must be set to protect the health of space crews and the physical integrity of the environment. Although Soviet scientists did collect some information on micro-organisms present in the spacecraft environment (Table 1), most data in both U.S. and Soviet (currently Russian) space programs have been restricted to preflight-to-postflight comparative measurements. Few data are available concerning the interactions of micro-organisms with their substrates or their human hosts in the space environment, although Zaloguyev, Konstantinova, and others[24,41–43] have observed that microfloral status tends to change in cyclical rather than linear fashion during flight, probably in response to selection pressures from the environment. The changes microbes undergo in response to environmental selection, in turn, affect their interactions with that environment. A further complication in predicting microbial acceptability limits from a health standpoint is the possibility that human immune function is altered in microgravity.[10–14] Finally, implementing and verifying acceptability limits during flight will require the use of monitoring strategies appropriate to the space-flight environment. Onboard diagnostic and monitoring equipment—and its associated procedures—must conform to the physical and operational limitations imposed by space flight. These limitations include requirements for low power, weight, and volume; simplicity of operation; high reliability and low main-

tenance; limited crew time and expertise; and, of course, the ability to function in the absence of gravity.

Despite these difficulties, some microbial limits have been set as experience has been gained from space flight and from Earth-based studies of closed environments. The following paragraphs present a brief history of microbial surveillance efforts and acceptability limits for numbers and types of micro-organisms in the U.S. and Soviet space programs. Further details of the philosophy underlying the selection of microbial limits for the U.S. Space Station can be found in a recent NASA review.[44] Clinical monitoring strategies are discussed first, followed by plans for monitoring the microbial populations in the spacecraft environment.

A. Clinical Monitoring Strategies

The first U.S. space crew microbiology program was established during the Apollo Program in response to requirements developed with the Interagency Committee on Back Contamination. This committee included representatives from the National Academy of Sciences, the U.S. Public Health Service, the U.S. Department of Agriculture, and the U.S. Department of the Interior. The committee recommended characterizing each crewmember's microflora in detail, in part to identify contaminants of terrestrial origin that might appear in lunar soil samples and, also, to provide a tool for clinical screening. Thus, microbial pathogens could be detected before flight, aiding in the diagnosis and treatment of ill crewmembers; and changes in microfloral population dynamics resulting from space flight could be observed.[25] The reasoning behind this study is still valid today, although most assessments are made only before and after flight.

Under the Apollo Program, specimens were collected from each crewmember three times before launch (30 days, 14 days, and immediately before flight) and once immediately after flight. Urine and fecal samples were collected, as well as swab specimens from the nose, throat, and skin. In addition, the immune status of each crewmember was determined serologically for mumps, rubella, and rubeola. Antibody titers were also determined for Influenza A and B, echovirus, adenovirus, *Herpes simplex* 1, parainfluenza, cytomegalovirus, respiratory syncytial virus, and *Mycoplasma pneumoniae*. Microbiological surveillance during the Skylab Program was similar to that described for the Apollo Program. Additional sample collections were added at 45 days before flight and at approximately 2 and 10 days after flight.

As part of the Health Stabilization Program, U.S. Space Shuttle crewmembers are screened for the presence of bacteria, fungi, and parasites during examinations for Astronaut Corps selection, in the course of recertification examinations, and before and after missions. Standards and procedures for selection and recertification examinations are described elsewhere.[45] Mission-related clinical evaluations begin 3 months before flight, when the crew's immune status to selected viral agents is reviewed. Specimens are next collected for bacterial, fungal, parasitic, and viral culture 10 days before flight.

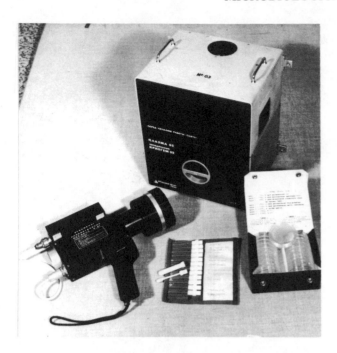

Fig. 2 Microbiological monitoring equipment used on Mir; includes thermostat, air sampler, test-tube rack for smears, and nutrient media.

Although viral results generally are not available until after the flight because of culture time requirements, these data are used for diagnostic and epidemiological purposes. Microbial sampling is repeated 1 to 2 days before launch and again after landing to evaluate any change in the microbial flora and to detect cross-contamination among crewmembers. Clinical monitoring in both the U.S. Space Shuttle Program and the Russian space program includes a period of isolating crewmembers before flights and limiting their contacts with other people, all of whom undergo medical examinations to identify potentially infectious agents.

As part of the "Plan for Sanitation, Hygiene, and Epidemic Prevention in Spacecraft," Russian cosmonauts also undergo microbiological and immunological testing with the goal of characterizing each individual's microflora and identifying occult infectious states. The latter are defined as the presence of pathogenic micro-organisms (e.g., Group A streptococci), or "dysbacteriosis" of the intestinal microflora. In cases where such deviations are identified, the cosmonaut undergoes a course of prophylaxis, including bifidobacterin or lactobacterin preparations, immunoprophylaxis, and other means of correcting the microflora. The effectiveness of these actions is verified through re-examination, and the results are used to determine whether that person is allowed to fly.[3,46]

During Salyut and Mir missions, signs of increase in staphylococci and gram-negative bacteria were observed in cosmonaut nasal, oral, and throat cultures in association with crew exchange.[24,42,47,48] As new crews were exposed, they became carriers of *S. aureus*; some developed clinical symptoms of disease, and some remained asymptomatic. Other microfloral changes noted during flight included colonization

of mucous membranes in the nose, mouth, throat, and occasionally the skin by species of *Proteus, Klebsiella, Enterobacter, Citrobacter,* and *E. coli.*

Lizko[43] compared characteristics of cosmonauts' intestinal microflora during preflight training to those after space flights varying in duration. Minor aberrations tended to be present before flight (e.g., decreased numbers of bifidobacteria and lactobacilli), although the statistical significance of these aberrations is unclear. The state of the intestinal microflora after flight tended to depend upon the degree of dysbiosis observed before flight. In general, lactobacilli and bifidobacteria levels were decreased, and levels of opportunistic enterobacteria such as proteidae, clostridia, and enterococci were found to have increased.

B. Environmental Monitoring Strategies

Space-flight crews must also be protected from exogenous agents of infection during their missions. Maintaining the microbial safety of the space environment, including its air, water, food, and internal surfaces, is just as critical to ensuring in-flight health, safety, and performance as is maintaining the clinical safety of the crew. Moreover, maintaining limits on environmental contamination is also useful in preventing the mechanical or material failures associated with biodeterioration. *Pseudomonas aeruginosa*, for example, is an opportunistic pathogen that can grow on the polymers used in hermetically sealed chambers[49,50] and on 2-methylstyrene;[51] pseudomonads were isolated from Soviet space stations (see Table 1).

Despite deliberate attempts to minimize microbial contamination of spacecraft components by assembling them in highly filtered "clean rooms," with airlock chambers used as sterile passageways to these rooms, and testing and disinfecting during the vehicle preparation process, micro-organisms were found to be present during both U.S. and Soviet space missions. Observations of Salyut 7 over several years revealed a periodic, cyclical pattern to fungal colonization of the station; the 13 micromycete species isolated during occupation by the first prime crew decreased to 4 with the second crew and increased again to 8 with the third. Because of concern over the structural stability of space station materials under conditions of fungal colonization, a bank of strains isolated from Salyut and Mir were established with regular checks of the air and structural materials onboard Mir using the equipment pictured in Fig. 2.

The following sections review microbiological findings; identify microbial limits established for air, internal surfaces, water, food, and experimental animals; and outline monitoring strategies planned for the U.S. Space Station.

C. Air

Acceptability limits have been set for the air quality in the U.S. Space Shuttle, but assessments of success in achieving these limits are generally restricted to measurements taken

Table 3 Bacteria and fungi isolated from orbiter air

Bacteria	Fungi
Acinetobacter calcoaceticus*	Acremonium sp.
Corynebacterium sp.	Alternaria sp.*
Flavobacterium	Curvularia sp.
Staphylococcus sp.*	Nigrospora sp.
Staphylococcus aureus	Pithomyces sp.
Bacillus species*	Aspergillus fumigatus
Enterobacter agglomerans	Aspergillus sp.*
Micrococcus sp.*	Cladosporium sp.
Streptococcus sp.	Bipolaris sp.
	Penicillium sp
	Rhodotorula sp.

*Frequently isolates.

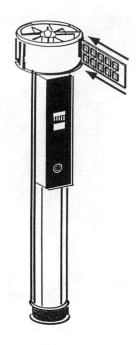

Fig. 3 A prototype air sampler being tested for in-flight use. A known volume of air is drawn into the device by rotating vanes (top), where it impacts an agar strip (arrows).

before and after flight. Air samples are collected from the Space Shuttle crew compartment approximately 25 days before launch to verify the effectiveness of cleanup procedures. Samples are collected again within 1 day of launch to obtain preflight baseline levels, and a third time at landing to assess microbial buildup during flight. The air in the crew quarters at Johnson Space Center and Kennedy Space Center is also monitored and the microbial content evaluated before these areas are occupied by the crewmembers. Typical organisms detected during Space Shuttle flights are shown in Table 3.

At present, air samples are collected in the U.S. space program using a centrifugal air sampler. The Russian program uses an air sampler consisting of a manual pump with a reflux valve and a set of removable cassettes containing a fibrous capron filter soaked with preservative. Air samples will be collected on the U.S. Space Station, using portable, battery-powered devices that collect airborne particles onto an agar medium attached to a plastic strip. After sample collection, the strip is incubated for an appropriate interval and microbial colonies are enumerated and their morphology recorded. If the test sample reveals potentially harmful airborne micro-organisms, isolation and identification procedures are then performed. Figure 3 depicts an air-sampling device that has been used successfully on U.S. Space Shuttle flights and will be modified for use aboard Space Station.

The density and type of fungal propagules present in the Space Station's internal atmosphere will also be monitored using another device that eliminates the need for culturing filamentous fungi, thus reducing the risk of fungal-propagule contamination. Air contaminants will be collected on a sterile 0.45-μm membrane filter during filtration of a known volume of air. The filter is then treated with reagents, stained, and examined under a microscope. The underlying principles, concepts, and functional approach of this portable device are described elsewhere.[52]

NASA has established an acceptability limit for airborne micro-organisms on Space Station of 1000 colony-forming units (CFUs) per cubic meter.[53] This level, which includes both bacteria and fungi, is typical in U.S. office buildings.[1] Like Mir, Space Station's air revitalization system includes strategically placed air filters and is designed to avoid stagnant areas and cross-contamination. Its air filters are expected to achieve the 1000-CFU limit by removing particulate matter larger than 0.3 μm. Standards for unacceptable organisms, that is, those that must not be present on Space Station, are under consideration,[44] with the classification system of the National Institutes of Health, Centers for Disease Control, being used as a model.

D. Internal Surfaces

Swab samples of Space Shuttle interior surfaces are collected with the preflight and postflight air samples. Approximately 20 sites throughout the Shuttle's flight deck, middeck, and Spacelab are swabbed with duplicate calcium alginate swabs, which are then stored in tubes containing phosphate buffers for later analysis. Surfaces showing visible contamination, or contamination exceeding 100 CFUs per 25 cm^2 are disinfected before launch. Disinfectants are provided onboard in the event of visible growth on surfaces. On Russian stations, cosmonauts use a device consisting of a cotton swab attached to a capillary tube containing a preservative, all of which are housed in a test tube with a screw cap. This device was used to collect samples from the crew's skin and mucous membranes, as well as to take smears from the interior of the spacecraft. Cosmonaut samples are typically returned to Earth for analysis within 6 days of their collection.

The crew of Salyut 6 described a "white film" on parts of the interior, including the rubber straps of the exercise machine. This film was found to consist of micromycetes belonging to the genera *Aspergillus, Penicillium,* and *Fusarium.*[24] On Salyut 7, visible growth on the hull, joints, and cables in the work module was found to contain *Penicillium* (mostly *P. chrysogenum*), *Aspergillus, Cladosporum, Mucor,* and actinomycetes. In the Soyuz transport vehicle that was docked with Mir for 6 months, the viewing window was nearly obscured with fungi, as well as spore-forming bacteria, such as *Bacillus polymixa.* In some of these instances, the contaminated materials have shown physical changes and structural damage.[49,50,54] Future plans to protect the spacecraft interior include selection of structural materials that are resistant to degradation, efforts to make surfaces water-repellant, and efforts to incorporate antiadhesive, antibacterial, and antifungal properties in construction materials wherever possible. Plans for the U.S. Space Station at present include collecting swab samples as needed. Routine sampling of internal surfaces is not anticipated, although a means of collecting and analyzing samples will be onboard in the event of visible growth.

E. Water

The Space Shuttle's onboard potable water supply is maintained and monitored at the launch site; microbial isolates are identified and characterized before and after flight; and samples are analyzed for chemical and microbial content, including the presence and numbers of anaerobic, aerobic, and coliform bacteria and yeasts and molds.

The U.S. Environmental Protection Agency has established a limit of 1 CFU of coliform bacteria per 100 mL for public potable water supplies.[55] The present microbial acceptability limit for the Space Shuttle potable water system is 1 CFU of any bacteria per 100 mL of water. This stringent microbial limit has also been set for the potable water system aboard Space Station. This low number was derived under the assumption that no onboard capability for identifying bacterial contaminants will exist; further details on current and planned water sampling and analysis procedures can be found elsewhere in this volume.

F. Food

Crewmembers can become ill from food contaminated with toxic chemicals or pathogenic micro-organisms. In addition, the management of leftover food and cleanliness of the dining areas are as important in controlling pathogens as is aseptic packaging of microbiologically safe foods. In the U.S. Space Shuttle Program, random food-lot samples are evaluated microbiologically before flight. Random samples of nonthermostabilized food to be consumed on U.S. spacecraft

may not exceed 10,000 aerobic bacteria per gram;[56] in addition, these foods must not contain pathogens such as *Clostridium botulinum, Salmonella* sp., *Shigella* sp., *S. aureus,* or *Bacillus cereus.* Frozen foods planned for use aboard Space Station will require similar testing. It should be noted, however, that aerosolized food particles can supply a rich source of nutrients for microbial growth. Controlling this nutrient source will depend upon housekeeping procedures and the efficiency of air filtering devices onboard space vehicles.

G. Animals

The two major means of protecting the crewmembers from zoonotic agents are careful microbiological screening of all animals to be used in the space environment and isolating the animals from the crewmembers through the use of specially designed containment facilities and judicious animal husbandry practices. Animals to be flown on U.S. missions must be certified before flight as free of specified pathogens (see Table 4).

Rats were first flown on a U.S. Space Shuttle during the STS-8 mission. In addition to meeting microbiological standards, the animals were contained within an animal enclosure module (AEM, Fig. 4), a self-contained cage designed to fit on the orbiter middeck so that neither servicing nor direct contact was required during flight. Food was provided to the animals as prepackaged nutrient bars and potatoes served as a water source. Air from the crew compartment was drawn by two fans into a plenum that directed it through a filter at the rear of the unit. The air was pulled across the cage and exited at the front of the AEM through electrostatic filter material and charcoal to the crew compartment. Animal waste was entrained by the air flow and moved from the front to the back of the AEM into an absorbent material serving as a prefilter to the electrostatic air filter. This unit successfully contained odors and micro-organisms, in addition to maintaining its rodent inhabitants.

A more elaborate animal containment system, the research animal holding facility (RAHF), was designed at the NASA Ames Research Center to accommodate both rats and squirrel monkeys (Fig. 5). The RAHF was first flown on STS-51B [the U.S. Spacelab Life Sciences (SLS) 3 mission] with 32 rats contained in one section and 2 squirrel monkeys in the other. Although the SLS-3 animals generated many important biochemical and physiological findings, the RAHF did not contain food particles and waste products as well as expected, and some contamination of the Spacelab and orbiter resulted. After SLS-3, several features of the RAHF were redesigned, notably the addition of an auxiliary fan that minimized the probability of the cage contents escaping, even when the RAHF was being serviced or animals were being removed from the facility. After rigorous ground-based testing, the improved RAHF was flown on the SLS-1 mission (STS-40). Both this RAHF and a general-purpose workstation (a modified Class II cabinet) successfully contained particulate matter. Although the animal containment facilities planned for

Table 4   Exclusion criteria for animals to be used during flight

Rats

Bacteria	Viruses
Streptobacillus moniliformis	Lymphocytic choriomeningitis virus
Spirillum minus	Rat parvoviruses
Streptococcus pneumoniae	Rat coronavirus
Streptococcus pyogenes	Sialodacryadenitis virus
Bacillus piliformis	Sendai virus
Corynebacterium kutscheri	
Salmonella sp.	**Fungi**
Pasteurella pneumotropica	All dermatophytes
Leptospira sp.	
Campylobacter sp.	

Squirrel Monkeys

Bacteria	Fungi
Shigella sp.	All dermatophytes
Salmonella sp.	
Streptococcus pneumoniae	**Endoparasites**
Mycobacterium tuberculosis	*Trichomonas*
Pasteurella multocida	Acanthocephalans
Campylobacter sp.	*Strongyloides*
Leptospira sp.	*Entamoeba histolytica*
Streptococcus pyogenes	Hemoprotozoa
Viruses	
Lymphocytic choriomeningitis virus	
Herpes tamarinus	
Herpesvirus saimiri	

Rhesus monkeys

Bacteria	Viruses
Mycobacterium tuberculosis	*Herpesvirus simiae*
Shigella sp.	Yaba
Salmonella sp.	Yaba-like viruses
Pasteurella multocida	(OrTeCu, BEMP, Tanapox)
Yersinia pseudotuberculosis	Monkey pox
Yersinia enterocolitica	Measles (Rubeola)
Streptococcus pyogenes	Lymphocytic choriomeningitis virus
Campylobacter sp.	Rabies
Leptospira sp.	SAIDS (SRV-1, SRV-2)
HIV	
STLV III	
Parasites	**Fungi**
Hymenolepis nana	All dermatophytes
Entamoeba histolytica	
Giardia intestinalis	
Giardia lamblia	
Balantidium coli	
Trichomonas hominis	
Ascaris sp.	
Strongyloides sp.	
Acanthocephalans	

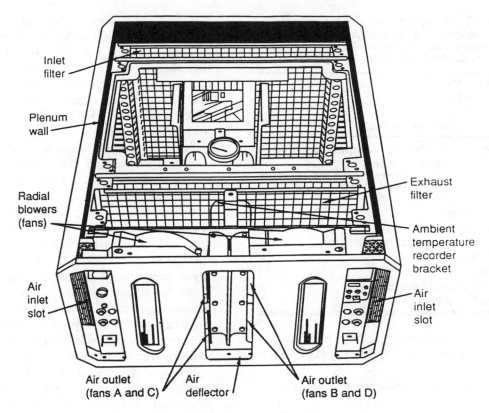

Inlet filter

Plenum wall

Radial blowers (fans)

Air inlet slot

Exhaust filter

Ambient temperature recorder bracket

Air inlet slot

Air outlet (fans A and C)

Air deflector

Air outlet (fans B and D)

Fig. 4 The U.S. animal enclosure module.

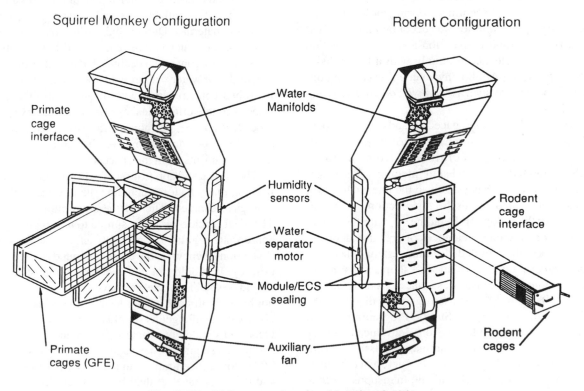

Squirrel Monkey Configuration

Rodent Configuration

Primate cage interface

Water Manifolds

Humidity sensors

Water separator motor

Module/ECS sealing

Primate cages (GFE)

Auxiliary fan

Rodent cage interface

Rodent cages

Fig. 5 The U.S. research animal holding facility.

Table 5   Techniques for near-real-time microbial monitoring

Direct detection of micro-organisms
Direct microscopy
Stains
Dyes
Fluorescent antibodies

Detection of microbial components and metabolites
Gas chromatography (GC)
GC/mass spectrometry
Pyrolysis
Raman spectrometry
Infrared/ultraviolet spectrometry
Photometry
Fluorometry
Polymerase chain reactions
Nucleic acid probes

Space Station have not been finalized, the level of bioisolation is expected to be similar to that exhibited by the RAHF.

H. Disinfection and Decontamination Procedures

Control of contamination during space flight has been of concern to NASA and the Soviet programs since the first manned missions. During the Gemini missions, crewmembers cleansed themselves with *Phisohex*, a topical disinfectant, before flight to reduce skin shedding in the spacecraft interior.[57] This practice was discontinued during the Apollo missions, and the spacecraft interior was decontaminated only if problems arose. The food preparation and waste collection areas, however, were cleaned routinely with a liquid disinfectant. Predictably, the Apollo environment was often contaminated with organisms such as *Staphylococcus aureus* and *Aspergillus fumigatus*.[25]

Gross contamination of both spacecraft and crew was documented during Skylab 3.[19] *Staphylococcus aureus* was isolated throughout the spacecraft and from all three crewmembers, and led to several skin infections. The possibility that *S. aureus* could have survived the interim between Skylab 3 and 4 prompted successful disinfection of the interior surfaces with the iodophor, Betadine™, with the arrival of the Skylab 4 crew. Other incidences of contamination associated with Skylab included the inadvertent release of *Serratia marcescens* into the orbital workshop compartment, after which this micro-organism was isolated from the air and crewmembers. Betadine™ was used again for disinfection.

With the advent of the Space Shuttle Program, the reuse of space vehicles for multiple missions introduced another set of concerns. Not only was contamination possible during missions, but there was also potential for microbial carryover and contamination during refurbishment. In response to concerns about this issue, maintenance of clean rooms for vehicular assembly, regular use of iodine and other disinfec-

tants, and routine sampling have all been instituted to maintain a clean living and work environment. Despite these precautions, numerous potential pathogens have been isolated from flight hardware and the cabin atmosphere. The waste management area is disinfected during Shuttle flights with a mixture of denatured ethanol (10 percent), Lysol™ liquid (5 percent), Palmolive™ soap (1.5 percent), and distilled water (83 percent). Routine cleaning is performed with disposable wet wipes containing benzalkonium chloride.

Water systems, particularly those supplying potable water, present special disinfection problems. A further discussion of water systems of the U.S. space program is presented elsewhere in this volume. Iodine is used to disinfect water aboard the U.S. Space Shuttle; it has also been proposed as a water and surface disinfectant for Space Station. The disadvantages of iodine include its corrosiveness and its propensity to stain surfaces. The use of iodine in the Shuttle water system has already demonstrated the propagation of iodine-resistant bacteria;[58,59] these resistant forms could eventually prove catastrophic to a space station's life support system. Moreover, the toxicological effects of iodine and its organic complexes are not understood completely.

Living in space, whether on spacecraft or on planetary bases, requires an environmental control system that provides safe air and water for crew consumption. Although sterility is not a realistic goal, microbial contamination must not be allowed to reach unsafe levels. Careful selection of structural materials to be used in spacecraft is a first step. Russian engineers have attempted to solve this problem by searching for ways to make surfaces water-repellant and seeking methods of incorporating antiadhesive and biocidal properties in construction materials. During flight, filtration of the air, purification of the water before reuse, good housekeeping practices, and environmental designs that do not allow accumulation of dirt or water will probably be effective in maintaining microbial contamination within safe limits. The possibility of occasional spills or leakage of biological materials (e.g., food, feces, urine, or vomitus), however, requires the capability for decontamination; i.e., the removal of pathogenic micro-organisms from the spacecraft.

The choice and application of a disinfectant or biocide depend on many factors, including the physical, chemical and biological characteristics of the environment to be treated. The ideal biocide would be simple to use, registered with an appropriate regulatory agency (such as the Environmental Protection Agency), and well documented as to its safety and efficacy. It should not cause deterioration of materials. It should be soluble, stable, and have "wetting action." It should not have significant human health effects (i.e., it should be nontoxic, nonallergenic, should not cause cancer or birth defects, and should not irritate skin or mucous membranes). In addition, it should not have a noxious odor; it should act rapidly at low concentrations in the presence of organic debris; and it should have residual biocidal activity. Unfortunately, no biocide exists that meets all these criteria.[60]

The closed nature of the spacecraft environment dictates

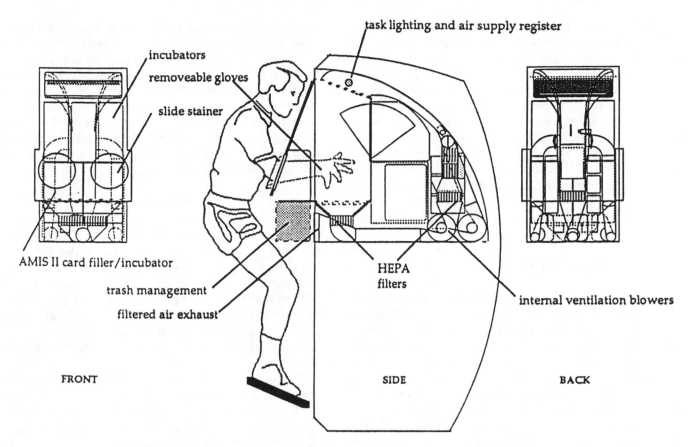

Fig. 6 An artist's conception of the bioisolation facility planned for Space Station.

that chemical germicides be used only in situations where physical methods (heat and ultraviolet light) are impractical and when microbiological hazards outweigh toxicological concerns. A nontoxic detergent, such as hydrogen peroxide, could be used for prophylactic treatment, routine disinfection, and microbial control. In addition, a more potent disinfectant should be available to counteract microbial spills from biological experiments, food, or biological wastes; glutaraldehyde is an example of such an agent. Biological control measures, such as the use of secondary microbial metabolites or antibiotics, may also hold promise for long-term space habitation.

VI. Microbiology Facilities for the U.S. Space Station

The Space Station microbiology subsystem is being designed to detect, collect, identify, and archive micro-organisms isolated from the crew and environment (air, water, and surfaces). In conjunction with the Health Maintenance Facility (HMF), the microbiology subsystem also identifies micro-organisms from clinical specimens and provides information on their antibiotic sensitivity.[52] All sample processing, culturing, and maintenance will take place in bioisolation facilities to reduce the possibility of cross-contamination between crew and biological specimens.

A microbiology safety cabinet will serve as the principal bioisolation facility. The exposure of crewmembers to con-

taminants will be minimized by the inward flow of cabin air, high-efficiency filtration, vertical laminar air flow, and an access compartment fitted with ultraviolet lights for decontamination. This device will meet Class II requirements for biological containment cabinets, as defined by the National Sanitation Foundation.[61] All microbiological equipment will be located close to the cabinet; some devices, such as the slide-staining apparatus, incubators, and the automated microbial system, will be operated within the bioisolation work space (Fig. 6).

Clinical and environmental isolates will be identified using an automated system being designed in collaboration with BioMérieux Vitek Systems, Inc. This device, which is being tested on the U.S. Space Shuttle, consists of a filler module and a reader/incubator module that are capable of identifying a wide array of bacteria and yeasts from environmental and clinical sources, as well as determining their susceptibility to antimicrobial agents. A detailed description of this device has been presented elsewhere.[62]

A specialized slide staining apparatus has also been designed for use in microgravity.[63] This self-contained, compact manual unit requires no spacecraft power and uses a minimal amount of reagents and stains. This device may be used to test micro-organisms, as well as blood smears, sputum, and other clinical specimens.

A combined bright field-phase contrast-fluorescent microscope will be used to examine stained slides, microbial filters, wet mounts, and other specimens. Video and 35-mm images can be downlinked by telemetry to investigators at the NASA Johnson Space Center for consultation. Similar systems are already in use at other specialized facilities.[64,65] Once the specimen has been prepared for microscopic examination by the crew, image telemetry and image analysis by the ground-based microbiology laboratory can expedite the analysis of a wide variety of samples and organisms. A system capable of archiving microbiological samples and specimens collected from the Space Station's air, water, food, surfaces, and clinical sources will be provided onboard. It is expected that some analyses will require the extensive analytical capabilities of sophisticated microbiological facilities on Earth.

VII. Conclusion

Meeting the challenges of future space exploration (including Space Station missions, a lunar base, and Mars exploration) will require increased knowledge of the interactions of micro-organisms with their human hosts. The effects of the space environment on microbial properties, such as virulence, antibiotic susceptibility, genetic stability, and population dynamics, are not well understood. Perhaps equally important is the need to determine the effect of space flight on the human immune system. Clinically significant decrements in the immune system during long stays in space could prove catastrophic to space crews and to the success of their missions.

In addition to being etiological agents of infectious diseases, micro-organisms are important sources of biodegradation. This property may prove detrimental to the integrity of the spacecraft or a Mars or lunar outpost. For example, microbial degradation of materials in airlock seals or extravehicular space suits may seriously compromise the safety of the pressurized closed environment.

Ensuring habitability of the space environment over long periods of time will require sophisticated monitoring equipment and technologies. Technologies must be developed to rapidly and reliably detect important contaminants such as *Legionella*. Rapid detection is essential to allow immediate containment and disinfection. In addition to environmental monitoring, diagnostic capabilities that detect and identify clinically important pathogens directly from clinical specimens are essential. All monitoring equipment and diagnostic technologies must meet the obvious requirements, such as minimal weight, volume, and power consumption; but equipment for long-duration missions must be vastly improved in the areas of reliability and maintainability. In addition, intense competition for crew time during flight dictates that equipment be automated whenever possible.

Although micro-organisms may pose obstacles to long stays in space because of their ability to cause illnesses and biodegrade foodstuffs and critical materials, the microbial world may prove invaluable in other ways. For example, the management of trash and biological waste products is an immense logistical problem for long stays in space and one in which microbes may play a key role in bioremediation. Microbes may also play key roles in processes associated with regenerative life support systems, food production, water purification, and removal of airborne chemical contaminants. Given the ubiquity of micro-organisms, space exploration will ultimately benefit from an understanding of the host-microbe relationship in space, which allows us to exploit microbial functions to our advantage while minimizing their potential detriment to human health.

References

[1]Burge, S.; Hedge, A.; and Wilson, S. Sick building syndrome: A study of 4373 office workers. *Annual Review of Occupational Hygiene*, 1987, vol. 31, no. 4A, pp. 493–504.

[2]Zaloguyev, S.N.; Viktorov, A.N.; and Startseva, N.D. Sanitary microbiological and epidemiological aspects of habitability. In: Chernigovskiy, V.N., Ed. *Sanitary-Hygienic and Physiological Aspects of Manned Spacecraft.Problems in Space Biology. Volume 42.* Moscow, Nauka, 1980, pp. 80–140 (in Russian).

[3]Shilov, V. M., and Lizko, N.N. The microecology of the intestine under extreme conditions. In: Chernigovskiy, V.N., Ed. *Sanitary-Hygienic and Physiological Aspects of Manned Spacecraft.Problems in Space Biology. Volume 42.* Moscow, Nauka, 1980, pp. 140–170 (in Russian).

[4]Zaloguyev, S.N.; Viktorov, A.N.; Gorshkov, V.P.; Norkina, T.Yu.; and Shinkareva, M.M. Prophylaxis of staphylococcal infections in humans during space flight. *Kosmicheskaya Biologiya i Aviakosmicheskaya Meditsina,* 1981, no. 5, pp. 27–29 (in Russian).

[5]Berry, C.A. View of human problems to be addressed for long-duration space flights. *Aerospace Medicine*, 1973, vol. 44, pp. 1136–1146.

[6]Rodgers, E. The ecology of micro-organisms in a small closed system: potential benefits for Space Station. NASA TM 86563, Huntsville, Ala., NASA Marshall Space Flight Center, 1986.

[7]Taylor, G.R. Cell anomalies associated with spaceflight conditions. *Advanced Experimental Medicine and Biology*, 1976, vol. 225, pp. 259–271.

[8]Zaloguyev, S.N.; Utkina, T.G.; and Sinkareva, M.M. The microflora of the human integument during prolonged confinement. *Life Science Space Research*, 1971, vol. 9, pp. 55–59.

[9]Stiehm, E.R.; Sztein, M.B.; and Steeg, P.S., et al. Deficient antigen expression on human cord blood monocytes. Reversal with lymphokines. *Clinical Immunology and Immunopathology*, 1984, vol. 30, pp. 430–436.

[10]Taylor, G.R.; Neale, L.S.; and Dardano, J.R. Immunological analyses of U.S. Space Shuttle crew members. *Aviation, Space, and Environmental Medicine*, 1986, vol. 57, pp. 213–217.

[11]Meehan, R.T. Human mononuclear cell in vitro activation in microgravity and post-spaceflight. *Advances in Ex-*

perimental Medicine, 1987, vol. 225, pp. 273–286.

[12]Konstantinova, I.V. Problems of space biology. The immune system under extreme conditions. *Space Immunology*, 1988, Washington, D.C., NASA Hq., 1990 (translated from Russian).

[13]Manie, S.; Konstaninova, I.; Breittmayer, J.P.; Ferrua, B.; and Schaffar, L. Effects of long-duration spaceflight on human T-lymphocyte and monocyte activity. *Aviation, Space and Environmental Medicine,* 1991, vol. 62, 12, pp. 1153–1158.

[14]Taylor, G.R., and Janney R.P. *In vivo* testing confirms a blunting of the human cell-mediated immune metabolism during space flight. *Journal of Leukocyte Biology*, 1992, vol. 51, no. 2, pp. 129–132.

[15]Dickson, K.J. Summary of biological space flight experiments with cells. *American Society for Gravitational and Space Biology (ASGSB) Bulletin*, 1991, vol. 4, no. 2, pp. 151–260.

[16]Cioletti, L.A.; Pierson, D.L.; and Mishra, S.K. Microbial growth and physiology in space: a review. Paper presented at the 21st International Conference on Environmental Systems, San Francisco, July 1991. *Society for Automotive Engineers Technical Paper Series,* no. 911512, Warrendale, Pa., 1991.

[17]Moatti, N.; Lapchine, L.; Gasset, G.; Richoilley, G.; Templier, J.; and Tixador, R. Preliminary results of the "Antiobio" experiment. *Naturwissenschaften,* 1986, vol. 73, pp. 413–414.

[18]Hawkins, W.R., and Ziegleschmid, J.F. Clinical aspects of crew health. In: Johnston, R.S.; Dietlein, L.F.; and Berry, C.A., Eds. *Biomedical results of Apollo.* NASA SP-368, Washington, D.C., NASA Hq., 1975, pp. 43–81.

[19]Taylor, G.R.; Graves, R.C.; Brockett, R.M.; Ferguson, J.K.; and Mieszkuc, B.J. Skylab environmental and crew microbiology studies. In: Johnston, R.S., and Dietlein, L.F., Eds. *Biomedical Results from Skylab.* NASA SP-377, Washington, D.C., NASA Hq., 1977, pp. 53–63.

[20]Hotchin, J.; Baker, F.D.; and Benson, L. Survival of RNA and DNA viruses in space on the Gemini XII satellite. *Life Sciences Space Research*, 1969, vol. 7, pp. 67–68.

[21]Imshenetsky, A.A.; Murzakov, B.G.; Yevdokimova, M.D.; and Dokofeyeva, I.K. The survival of bacteria studied in the artificial Mars apparatus. *Mikrobiologiya,* 1984, vol. 53, pp. 731–737 (in Russian).

[22]Mims, C.A. *The Pathogenesis of Infectious Disease.* Third Edition, New York, Academic Press, 1987, pp 8–47.

[23]Carmichael, C., and Taylor, G.R. Evaluation of crew skin flora under conditions of a full quarantine lunar-exploration mission. *British Journal of Dermatology*, 1977, vol. 97, pp. 187–196.

[24]Zaloguyev, S.N.; Viktorov, A.N.; Shilov, V.M.; Gorshkov, V.P.; Zarubina, K.V.; Shinkareva, M.M.; and Norkina, T.Yu. Results of mirobiological studies performed during the use of the Salyut-6 space station. *Kosmicheskaya Biologiya i Aviakosmicheskaya Meditsina,* 1985, no. 3, pp. 64–66 (in Russian).

[25]Ferguson, J.K.; Taylor, G.R.; and Mieszkov, B.J. Microbiological investigations. In: Johnston, R.S.; Dietlein, L.F.; and Berry, C.A., Eds. *Biomedical Results of Apollo.* NASA SP-368, Washington, D.C., NASA Hq., 1975, pp. 83–103.

[26]Taylor, G.R. Recovery of medically important microorganisms from Apollo astronauts. *Aerospace Medicine,* 1972, vol. 4, pp. 824–828.

[27]Taylor, G.R. Medical microbiological analysis of U.S. crewmembers. In: Nicogossian, A.E., Ed. *The Apollo-Soyuz Test Project Medical Report.* NASA SP-411, Washington, D.C., NASA Hq., 1977, pp. 69–85.

[28]Puleo, J.R.; Fields. N.D.; Bergstrom, S.L.; Oxborrow, G.S.; Stabekis, P.D.; and Koukol, R.C. Microbiological profiles of the Viking spacecraft. *Applied Environmental Microbiology*, 1977, vol. 33, pp. 379–384.

[29]Powers, E.M. Microbiological burden on the surfaces of Explorer XXXIII spacecraft. *Applied Microbiology*, 1967, vol. 15, pp. 1045–1048.

[30]Puleo, J.R.; Oxborrow, G.S.; Fields, N.D.; and Hall, H.E. Quantitative and qualitative microbiological profiles of the Apollo 10 and 11 spacecraft. *Applied Microbiology*, 1970, vol. 20, pp. 384–389.

[31]Brockett, R.M.; Ferguson, J.K.; and Henney, M.R. Prevalence of fungi during Skylab missions. *Applied Environmental Microbiology*, 1978, vol. 36, pp. 243–246.

[32]Kniazev, V.M.; Korolkov, V.I.; Viktorov, A.N.; Pozharskiy, G.O.; and Petrova, L.N. Sanitary and microbiologic aspects of the concurrent residence of man and animals in hermetic quarters. *Kosmicheskaya Biologiya i Aviakosmicheskaya Meditsina,* 1986, vol. 20, pp. 80–82 (in Russian).

[33]Drew, W.L., and Rawls, W.E. Herpes simplex viruses. In: Lennette, E.H., Ed. *Manual of Clinical Microbiology.* Washington, D.C., American Society for Microbiology, 1985, pp. 705–710.

[34]Ajello, L. Hyalohyphomycosis and phaeohyphomycosis: Two global disease entities of public health importance. *European Journal of Epidemiology*, 1986, vol. 2, pp. 243–251.

[35]Baron, P.A., and Willeke, K. Respirable droplets from whirlpools: Measurements of size distribution and estimation of disease potential. *Environmental Research*, 1986, vol. 39, pp. 8–18.

[36]Steere, N.V. *Handbook of Laboratory Safety.* Cleveland, Ohio, CRC Press, 1967.

[37]Knight, V.; Couch, R.B.; and Landahl, H.D. Effect of lack of gravity on airborne infection during space flight. *Journal of the American Medical Association,* 1970, vol. 214, pp. 513–518.

[38]Dimmik, R.L.; Chatigny, M.A.; Wolochow, H.; and Stroat, P.E. Evidence for propagation of aerobic bacteria in particles suspended in gaseous atmospheres. In: *Life Sciences and Space Research XV: Proceedings of the Open Meeting of the Working Group on Space Biology*. Philadelphia, Pa., June 8–19, 1976. Oxford-New York, Pergamon Press, 1977, pp. 41–45.

[39]Stephenson, E.H.; Larson E.W.; and Dominik, J.W. Ef-

fect of environmental factors on aerosol-induced lassa virus infection. *Journal of Medical Virology*, 1984, vol. 19, pp. 295–303.

[40]Fox, L. The ecology of micro-organisms in a closed environment. *Life Sciences Space Research*, 1971, vol. 9, pp. 69–74.

[41]Konstantinova, I.V., and Antropov, Ye.N. Immunological reactivity in inhabitation of space environments. In: Chernigovskiy, V.N., Ed. *Sanitary-Hygienic and Physiological Aspects of Manned Spacecraft. Problems in Space Biology. Volume 42.* Moscow, Nauka, 1980, pp. 191–213 (in Russian).

[42]Tashpulatov, R.Yu., and Guseva, Ye.V. Study of the microbial flora and immunity of the crew of Salyut-3. *Kosmicheskaya Biologiya i Aviakosmicheskaya Meditsina,* 1979, no. 2, pp. 40–43 (in Russian).

[43]Lizko, N.N. Dysbacteriosis of extreme states. *Antibiotiki i Meditsinskaya Biotekhnologiya,* 1987, vol. 3, pp. 184–186, 1987 (in Russian).

[44]Pierson D.L.; McGinnis M.R.; Mishra S.K.; and Wogan, C.F., Eds. *Microbiology of Space Station Freedom.* NASA Conference Publication 3108, Washington, D.C., NASA Hq., 1991.

[45]National Aeronautics and Space Administration, Medical Operations Branch. NASA astronaut medical standards, selection and annual medical certification. JSC-24834, Houston, NASA Johnson Space Center, 1991.

[46]Zaloguyev, S.N.; Viktorov, A.N.; and Prokhovor, V.Ya., et al. An experimental approach to the rationale for one of the multimethod prophylactic treatments for cosmonauts. *Kosmicheskaya Biologiya i Aviakosmicheskaya Meditsina,* 1983, no. 2, pp. 83–86 (in Russian).

[47]Zaloguyev, S.N.; Savina, V.P.; and Mukamediyeva, L.N., et al. Sanitary and hygienic characteristics of the living environment of the Salyut-7 station. *Kosmicheskaya Biologiya i Aviakosmicheskaya Meditsina,* 1984, no. 2, pp. 40–43 (in Russian).

[48]Zaloguyev, S.N.; Shilov, V.M.; and Viktorov, A.N. Cosmonaut health status: Microflora status. In: Gazenko, O.G., Ed. *Results of Medical Research Performed on the Orbital Scientific Complex Salyut-6-Soyuz.* Moscow, Nauka, 1985, pp. 80–86 (in Russian).

[49]Novikora, N.D.; Orlova, M.I.; and D'yachenko, M.B. Investigation of reproductive capacity of microflora on polymer materials used in hermetically sealed cabins. *Kosmicheskaya Biologiya i Aviakosmicheskaya Meditsina,* 1986, vol. 20, pp. 71–73.

[50]Novikova, N.D., and Saloguyev, S.N. Formation of volatile substances in the process of destruction of polymers by *Pseudomonas aeruginosa. Kosmicheskaya Biologiya i Aviakosmicheskaya Meditsina,* 1985, no. 4, pp. 74–76 (in Russian).

[51]Dzhusupora, D.B.; Baskunov, B.P.; Goloblera, L.A.; Aliyera, R.M.; and Ilyaletdirov, A.N. Specifics of oxidation of Alpha methylstrene by bacteria of the genus *Pseudomonas. Mikrobiologiya,* 1985, vol. 54, pp. 136–140 (in Russian).

[52]Cioletti, L.A.; Mishra, S.K.; Richard, E.; Taylor, R.; and Pierson, D.L. Microbiology facilities aboard Space Station Freedom (SSF). *Society of Automotive Engineering (SAE) Technical Paper Series,* no. 901262, 20th Intersociety Conference on Environmental Systems, 1990.

[53]National Aeronautics and Space Administration. Space Station program definition and requirements. SSP 30000, Section 3: Space Station requirements (Revision J), Reston, Va., NASA Langley Research Center, Space Station Freedom Program Office, 1990.

[54]Nefyodov, Yu.G.; Novikova, N.D.; and Surovezhin, I.N. Products of microbiological damage to polymer materials as a factor of potential pollution of the atmosphere of pressurized environments by toxic substances. *Kosmicheskaya Biologiya i Aviakosmicheskaya Meditsina,* 1988, no. 3, pp. 67–71 (in Russian).

[55]U.S. Environmental Protection Agency. National Interim Primary Drinking Water Regulations. EPA Publication no. 570/9-76-003, Washington, D.C., EPA, 1976.

[56]National Aeronautics and Space Administration. General specifications—microbiological specification and testing procedure for foods that are not thermostabilized. JSC SD-T-0251H, Houston, NASA Johnson Space Center, Aug. 1987.

[57]Wheeler, H.O. Effects of space flight upon indigenous microflora and Gemini crewmembers. *Bacteriological Proceedings,* 1967, pp. 1–16.

[58]McFeters, G.A., and Pyle, B.H. Consequences of bacterial resistance to disinfection by iodine in potable water. *Society of Automotive Engineering Technical Paper Series,* no. 871498, 17th Intersociety Conference on Environmental Systems, 1987.

[59]Pyle, B.H., and McFeters, G.A. Iodine sensitivity of bacteria isolated from iodinated water systems. *Canadian Journal of Microbiology,* 1989, vol. 35, pp. 520–523.

[60]Burge, H.A. Biocides. In: *Guidelines for the Assessment of Bioaerosols in the Indoor Environment.* Cincinnati, Ohio, American Conference of Governmental Industrial Hygienists, 1989.

[61]National Sanitation Foundation, Standard no. 49 for Class II (Laminar Flow) Biohazard Cabinetry. Ann Arbor, Mich., National Sanitation Foundation, 1987.

[62]Brown, H.D.; Scarlett, J.B.; Skweres, J.A.; Fortune, R.L.; Staples, J.L.; and Pierson, D.L. Microbial identification systems for Space Station Freedom. *Society of Automotive Engineering Technical Paper Series,* no. 891540, 19th Intersociety Conference on Environmental Systems, 1989.

[63]Molina, T.C.; Brown, H.D.; Irbe, R.M.; and Pierson, D.L. Gram-staining apparatus for space station applications. *Applied Environmental Microbiology,* 1990, vol. 56, pp. 601–606.

[64]Mishra, S.K.; Brown, H.D.; Taylor, R. D.; and Pierson, D.L. Telemycology: A novel approach to monitoring envi-

ronmental microbial load in Space Station Freedom. *Society of Automotive Engineering Technical Paper Series*, no. 891542, 19th Intersociety Conference on Environmental Systems, 1989.

[65]Weinstein, R.S.; Bloom, K.J.; and Rozek, S. Telepathology and the networking of pathology diagnostic services. *Archives of Pathology and Laboratory Medicine*, 1987, vol. 111, pp. 646–652.

Chapter 5

Noise, Vibration, and Illumination

Charles D. Wheelwright, Robert C. Lengel Jr., and Anton S. Koros

It is essential that the spacecraft environment be safe and habitable. Therefore, upper limits for vibration and noise and minimum levels of illumination must be established so that crewmembers can accomplish their tasks in a timely and efficient manner. This chapter presents recommendations and suggestions that will aid in designing, developing, and verifying a suitable living environment for flight. Such an environment would ensure crew safety and comfort and allow crewmembers to perform their visual tasks.

I. Adverse Effects of Airborne Noise

Human reaction to exposure to airborne noise is a complex subject. Typically, low-level energy exposure is adapted to over time in a phenomenon referred to as habituation. However, humans never completely adapt to noise, and so it is crucial that the effects of noise be understood and addressed in the design of manned spacecraft. Noise exposure effects can be divided roughly into physiological and performance effects. Figure 1 presents the noise level at which adverse effects are likely.

A. Physiological Effects

A principal physiological effect of noise is temporary threshold shift (TTS), a transient increase in a person's threshold for sound. The occurrence and severity of such hearing loss depend upon the duration of exposure, the physical characteristics of the sound (intensity, frequency, narrow or wide bandwidth), and the nature of the exposure (continuous or intermittent). TTS varies among individuals but generally occurs when the overall noise level exceeds 75 decibels A-weighted [dB(A)]. The likelihood of TTS increases as the noise level and duration of exposure increase (up to a median of 6 h, when it reaches a plateau); if the sound is limited to very few frequencies (especially between 2000 and 6000 Hz); and if the noise is continuous.

Permanent hearing loss, or noise-induced permanent threshold shift (NIPTS), can result from exposure to an intense impulse of noise or from repeated (or extreme) TTS. Permanent hearing loss can arise in two very different ways: when an intense impulse of noise causes structural damage to the inner ear and/or eardrum, or when long-term exposure to moderate noise leads to hearing loss due to degeneration of the hair cells along the basilar membrane. This area has been the subject of much research and concern on the part of the space community, since permanent hearing loss is avoidable and directly related to spacecraft habitability. Low-frequency NIPTS is more serious because it raises a person's hearing threshold in the human speech spectrum.[1]

In addition to hearing loss, noise is responsible for several other physiological effects:

1) The onset of a loud noise will cause a startle reflex. This is characterized by dilation of the pupils, vasoconstriction in the peripheral regions, changes in the heart rate, and longer and slower breathing movements. These responses are short-lived.[2]

2) Long-term noise exposure has been related to abnormal heart rhythms.[3]

3) Changes in blood chemistry have been noted, including increases in the concentration of corticosteroids and alterations in the glucose level.[3]

4) Electrolytic imbalances of magnesium, potassium, sodium, and calcium occur in the presence of noise.[3]

5) High-intensity noise causes the stapedius and tensor tympani muscles to contract, stiffening the middle ear ossicular chain (approximately 10 ms after onset of the noise).[3]

6) Highintensity noise is related to alterations in the nerve cells that perceive sound and influence the functional and psychological state of the central nervous system.[4]

Although some research indicates that many adverse effects, such as hypertension and abnormal heart rhythms, usually do not occur until levels reach 95 dB(A), continued exposure to noise at lower levels has been linked to gastrointestinal ulcers.

B. Performance Effects

Human performance is critical during space flight because of time limitations and the severe consequences of error. Thus, the adverse effects of noise on performance have been the subject of much scrutiny. Typically, these effects are divided into the categories of interference with communication, annoyance, and sleep effects.

Interference with communication has received considerable attention because it can severely compromise crewmem-

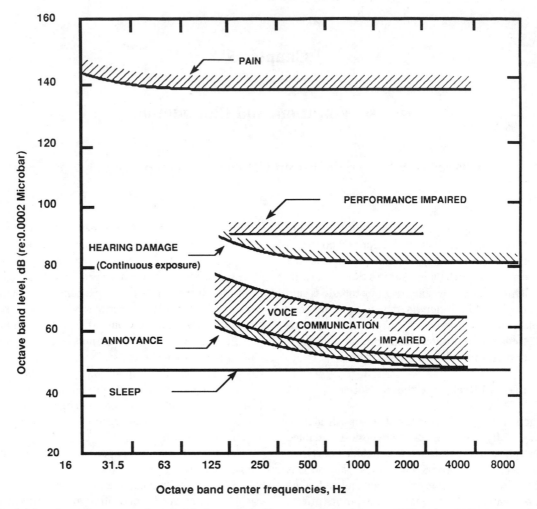

Fig. 1 Physical and performance thresholds for noise effects. (Adapted from: Willshire, K.F. Human response to vibroacoustic environments of space vehicles. TM86316, Langley, VA, NASA Langley Research Center, p. 20)

ber efficiency and increase the possibility of human error. Speech can be rendered completely inaudible in the presence of extreme levels of noise.

Voice communication occurs in the bandwidth of 200-6000 Hz; and, in the normal communicating voice, volume is approximately 55-80 dB(A). Speech intelligibility deteriorates progressively as ambient noise levels exceed 50 dB(A) in the bandwidth of human speech. More details are presented in Table 1. Noise affects communication more severely if living areas are highly reverberant, as speech becomes blurred. Extremely short reverberation periods should also be avoided, since the amplitude of the spoken word decays rapidly, precluding propagation across the room in extreme cases.

Annoyance refers to the "unwantedness" of a particular sound. Although level of annoyance is affected by the intensity of the source, it is highly dependent on the attitude of the individual toward the source. Noise that is intermittent, pure in tone, or perceived to be beyond the individual's control will more likely be considered annoying. Noise is especially annoying when it interferes with low-level conversation.

Interference with sleep during space flight has been a concern, both in the past and today. High levels of noise delay

the onset of rest and can awaken individuals or shift them to a shallower sleep. Sleep does not seem to be disturbed until levels of 65 dB(A) are reached. However, if the source is transient, sleep disturbance may occur at 50 dB(A).[5] Research also suggests that women are more easily disturbed than men, and the elderly more than the young.

Exposure to infrasonic noise (below 16 Hz) has also been shown to produce adverse effects. Persons subjected to low-frequency noise have experienced insomnia, a feeling of increased pressure in the head, headaches, a feeling of vibration of the body, and thought disruption.[6] The combined effects of noise and infrasound suggest that the infrasonic energy induces drowsiness.[7]

Effects on task performance have also been noted. Noise causes a narrowing of attention and can have both beneficial and adverse effects. The following activities are most compromised by noise[8]:

1) Those that have to be conducted over long intervals, especially if the noise is continuous.

2) Those that involve steady posture and uninterrupted vision, which are affected by sudden bursts of noise.

3) Those that require an effort to initiate, especially if the

Table 1 Speech interference level (SIL) criteria for voice communications (Adapted from: National Aeronautics and Space Administration. Man-Systems Integration Standards, Volume I, Rev. A. NASA-STD-3000, Houston, NASA Johnson Space Center, 1989, pp. 5–60)

Speech interference level (dB)	Person to person communication
30 - 40	Communication in normal voice satisfactory
40 - 50	Communication satisfactory in normal voice 1 to 2 m (3 to 6 ft), and raised voice 2 to 4 m (6 to 12 ft)
50 - 60	Communication satisfactory in normal voice 30 to 60 cm (1 to 2 ft), raised voice 1 to 2 m (3 to 6 ft)
60 - 70	Communication with raised voice satisfactory 30 to 60 cm (1 to 2 ft) slightly difficult 1 to 2 m (3 to 6 ft). Ear plugs and/or ear muffs can be worn with possible adverse effects on communication.
70 - 80	Communication slightly difficult with raised voice 30 to 60 cm (1 to 2 ft), slightly difficult with shouting 1 to 2 m (3 to 6 ft). Ear plugs and/or ear muffs may aid communication.
80 - 85	Communication slightly difficult with shouting 30 to 60 cm (1 to 2 ft). Ear plugs and/or ear muffs may aid communication.
Overall speech level (dB) minus SIL (dB)	**Communications via earphones or loudspeaker.**
+ 10 dB or greater	Communication satisfactory over range of SIL 30 to maximum SIL permitted by exposure time.
+ 5 dB	Communication slightly difficult. About 90 percent of sentences are correctly heard over range of SIL 30 to maximum SIL permitted by exposure time.
0 dB to - 10 dB	Special vocabularies (i.e., radio-telephone voice procedures) required. Communication difficult to completely unsatisfactory over range of SIL 30 to maximum SIL permitted by exposure time.

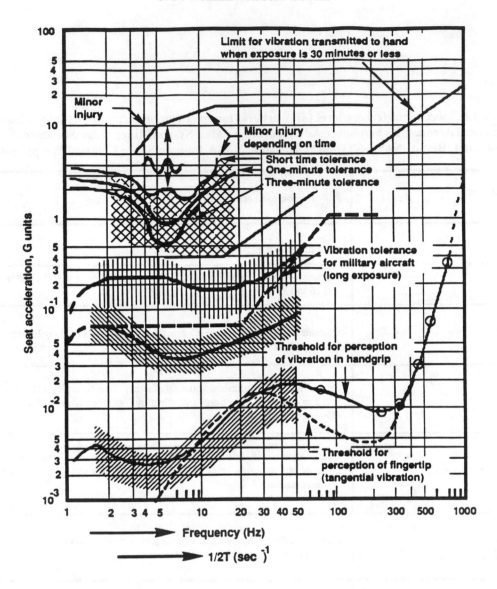

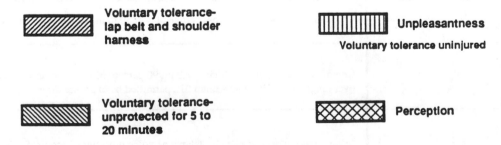

Fig. 2 Short-term vibration tolerance limits. (Adapted from: Broch, T. Mechanical Vibration and Shock Measurements. Marlboro, Mass., Bruel & Kjaer Instruments, Inc., 1980)

noise appears to be beyond the person's control.

4) Those that demand comprehension of meaning rather than rote learning.

5) Those that demand some flexibility of response, such as a response to a sudden change in circumstances.

II. Adverse Effects of Vibration

As with exposure to acoustical energy, the human body reacts to exposure to vibration energy. Limits to human vibration perception and comfort are detailed in Fig. 2.

Table 2   Body-part vibration resonant frequency region (1-g bias) [Ref. International Standards Organization (ISO).   Guide for the Evaluation of Human Exposure to Whole Body Vibration. ISO 2631-1978 (E), Geneva, Switzerland, 1978]

Body Component	Resonant Frequency (Hz)
Whole body, standing erect	6 & 11-12
Whole body, standing relaxed	4-5
Whole body (transverse)	2
Whole body (sitting)	5-6
Head	20-30
Head, sitting	2-8
Eyeball	40-60
Eardrum	1000
Head/shoulder, standing	5 & 12
Head/shoulder, seated	4-5
Shoulder/head, transverse rib	2-3
Main torso	3-5
Shoulder, standing	4-6
Shoulder, seated	4
Limb motion	3-4
Hand	1-3
Hand	30-40
Thorax	3.5
Chest wall	60
Anterior chest	7-11
Spinal column	8
Thoraco-abdominal viscera (semi-supine)	7-8
Abdominal mass	4-8
Abdominal wall	5-8
Abdominal viscera	3-3.5
Pelvic area, semi-supine	8
Hip, standing	4
Hip, sitting	2-8
Foot, seated man	>10

A. Physiological Effects

Human exposure to vibration is typically classified as belonging to one of two broad categories—whole-body vibration or hand-arm vibration. The former occurs in people exposed to vibration while standing, seated, or prone. The latter occurs during operation of a hand-held device that produces significant vibrational energy. An introduction to the biomechanical characteristics of the human body is necessary prior to discussing specific effects attributed to either type of vibration exposure.

Body cavity dimensions and musculoskeletal structure provide the basis for the biomechanical response observed in the human body. Cavity resonances and structural modes define the natural frequencies determined with test subjects. Table 2 provides a summary of these findings. When the body is subjected to vibrational energy at the natural frequency of a particular body, the component response is enhanced. Symptoms produced by exposure to vibrational energy at a particular frequency are described in Table 3. These symptoms are brought about by exposure to fairly high levels of vibrational energy. Clinical disorders that result from long-term exposure to lower levels of vibrational energy have also been identified. Although the research on the combined effects of vibration with linear acceleration is limited, it appears that an acceleration bias can change some body resonances as well as lower vibration tolerance limits.

Early investigations of the human body's exposure to vibration focused on subjects exposed to high vibration levels—aircraft pilots, operators of heavy work vehicles, and hand-tool operators.[9] This pioneering work discovered that whole-body vibration exposure can cause permanent damage to various body components or affect the nervous system. Hand-arm vibration from hand-held tools has been found to produce Raynaud's Syndrome ("white finger disease") in exposed workers.

Table 3 Sensitive vibration frequencies for discomfort symptoms. (Ref. Rasmussen, G. Human Body Vibration Exposure and Its Measurement. Technical Review, Marlboro, Mass., Bruel & Kjaer Instruments, Inc., 1982)

Symptom	Frequency (Hz)
Motion sickness	0.1 - 0.63
Abdominal pains	3 - 10
Chest pain	3 - 9
General discomfort	1 - 50
Complaints	4 - 8
Musculoskeletal discomfort	3 - 8
Head symptoms	13 - 20
Lower jaw symptoms	6 - 8
Influence on speech	13 - 20
"Lump in throat"	12 - 16
Urge to urinate	10 - 18
Influence on breathing	4 - 8
Muscle contractions	4 - 9
Testicular pain	10
Dyspnea	1 - 4

Raynaud's Syndrome appears to be most common in workers exposed to high hand-vibration levels, which result in lower finger blood pressure than normally found in a healthy population.[10] The onset of this disorder may be abated by higher ambient working temperatures; fewer cases have been noted in warmer climates.[11] Typically, high levels of hand-arm vibration result in a higher required gripping force (relative to no vibration) applied by the affected subject.[12] A supplementary effect, fatigue, is thus induced.

Long-term whole-body vibration can affect the circulatory, urological, and musculoskeletal systems and cause central nervous system disturbances, including fatigue, insomnia, headache, and "shakiness."[9] Short-term exposure causes a decrease in aortic and cerebral blood flow rate[13] and an increase in stomach motility.[14] Neurosensory disorders in the peripheral extremities (hand, arm, leg, foot) may be caused by long-term exposure.[15] Ischemic lumbago, a condition affecting the lower spinal region, has been attributed to long-term whole-body vibration.[9]

B. Performance Effects

Performance degradation from exposure to lower level whole-body vibration is caused primarily by the movement of visual cues relative to the body's reference plane. This effect is embodied in the inability to read text or displays and monitors.[16] Lower level hand-arm vibration exposure produces annoyance during fine motor skill tasks that require highly focused concentration. Observed effects include the inability to perform high-accuracy tactile tasks and increases in task completion times. A summary of vibration frequencies affecting various human performance tasks is presented in Table 4.

Compounding effects on human reaction to vibration exposure are related to the characteristics of the vibrational energy. Inclusion of shock or impulse energy in the vibration spectrum causes significantly greater irritation in exposed subjects.

C. Effects of Simultaneous Exposure to Noise and Vibration

Few studies have attempted to define the effects of simultaneous exposure to noise and vibration. Generally, simultaneous exposure produces greater irritation in subjects than does exposure to noise or vibration alone. Thus, a reduced threshold is expected in the case of simultaneous exposure.

Effects of simultaneous noise and vibration exposure are illustrated in a study of ride comfort ratings.[17] Figure 3 shows the test subject's comfort rating as a function of vibration and noise level. The high noise curve represents actual helicopter noise as a function of vibration level. Significant reduction of vibration alone did not meaningfully improve perceived ride quality. In the presence of ambient background noise, reducing acceleration yielded improvements in perceived ride quality. These results (as well as the moderate noise level curve) suggest that the vibration and noise fields interact to create a complex environment that the evaluator judges *in toto*, not independently.

III. Airborne Noise and Structureborne Vibration in Space Flight

Acoustical energy during space flight is highest during lift-off. Here, the high-level jet noise is reflected from the ground and coupled to the exterior skin of the spacecraft. Structureborne propagation and re-radiation into the crew compartment produce the high levels measured. As the vehicle lifts

Table 4 Sensitive vibration frequencies affecting human performance (Adapted from: National Aeronautics and Space Administration. Man-Systems Integration Standards, Volume I, Rev. A. NASA-STD-3000,Houston, TX., NASA Johnson Space Center, 1989, pp. 5–61)

Activity	Frequency range (Hz)
Equilibrium	30 - 300
Tactile sense	30 - 300
Speech	1 - 20
Head movement	6 - 8
Reading (texts)	1 - 50
Tracking	1 - 30
Reading errors (instruments)	5.6 - 11.2
Manual tracking	3 - 8
Depth perception	25 - 40, 60 - 40
Hand grasping handle	200 - 240
Visual task	9 - 50

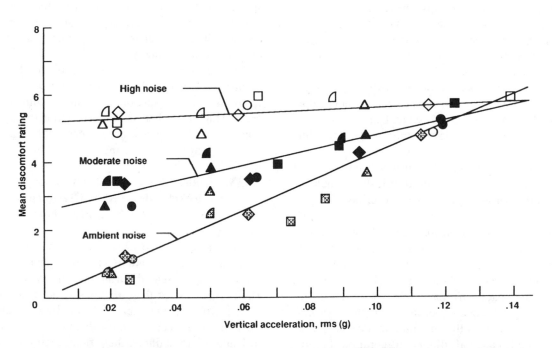

Fig. 3 Mean discomfort response to high, moderate, and ambient noise in the presence of vibration. (Reprinted from: Leatherwood, J.D.; Clevenson, S.A.; and Hollenbrough, D.D. Evaluation of ride quality prediction methods for helicopter interior noise and vibration environment. TP-2261, NASA, 1984, p. 40)

higher into the air, acoustical energy impinging on the exterior surface is decreased by the spreading loss of jet noise from the vehicle to and from the ground. Also, jet noise amplitude decreases as forward velocity increases. Increasing spacecraft velocity produces higher aerodynamic flow, and boundary layer turbulence becomes an ever-increasing noise source until the point of maximum dynamic pressure. Aero-

dynamic noise decreases progressively from this point on, becoming insignificant approximately 2 min after lift-off.

In orbit or during transorbital flight, spacecraft noise is generated solely from internal equipment. Primary sources of acoustical energy are the Environmental Control and Life Support System (ECLSS) and avionics cooling fans and pumps. These sources are predominantly continuous, with

Note: **Descent sound pressure level (SPL) of approximately 110 and 103 dB measured at drogue and main parachute deployment, respectively**

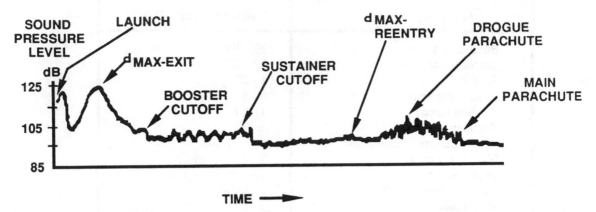

Fig. 4 Internal Mercury capsule broad bandwidth, acoustic noise level, time history for Big Joe launch. (Reprinted from: National Aeronautics and Space Administration. Vibroacoustic noise source data— literature survey results. JSC-24148, Houston, NASA Johnson Space Center, 1990, p. H-4)

little variation during operation. Additional noise during these portions of the flight regime is generated by systems that operate intermittently, including pumps, fans, and valves for the personal hygiene station and waste control system. Fluid pressure regulation and flow systems also contribute noise at various times during flight. Reaction Control System thruster firings can also produce significant intermittent noise.

Atmosphere re-entry noise is dominated by boundary layer turbulence. The energy level is similar to that generated during maximum dynamic pressure of ascent. Duration of maximum levels, however, can be significantly longer than during ascent.

Figure 4 provides an example of acoustical levels observed during the flight of the Mercury capsule/Big Joe launch vehicle. The variation of acoustical levels described above is observed.

Significant levels of vibration are observed during the lift-off and ascent phases. Low-frequency vibration is most prominent when the spacecraft shudders during ignition and lift-off. Vibrational energy characteristics change as fuel is burned (decreasing spacecraft mass), and spacecraft geometry changes during staging and booster separation. This effect is caused by changes in the structural mode characteristics inherent in each spacecraft flight configuration. Significant vibration levels from the aerodynamic response of the spacecraft are observed at maximum dynamic pressure during ascent. Guidance corrections can produce low frequency transverse oscillations during various flight conditions.

As is the case with acoustics, spacecraft vibration is generated solely from internal equipment once on orbit or during transorbital flight. Thus, the ambient vibration levels to which the crewmember may be exposed are significantly lower during these phases. Whole-body vibration is transmitted only when the crewmember is restrained. Otherwise, the crewmember's ability to float freely about the compartment

without contacting the vibrating structure greatly reduces vibration exposure levels. Under this condition, crewmembers spend little time in direct contact with the spacecraft structure. Vibration is transmitted through hand-arm and foot-leg contact with the structure as crewmembers attempt to secure themselves within the cabin.

Re-entry vibration levels are significant, but not as high as during the launch phase. The magnitude and frequency of the oscillations depend on entry angle, with steeper angles causing higher oscillations. The oscillation frequency is maximum at the re-entry deceleration peak. Vibration amplitudes decrease progressively during deceleration.

IV. Airborne Noise and Structureborne Vibration Effects Observed by Crewmembers During NASA Missions

Vibroacoustic energy observed during space flight varies in character and level as a function of flight regime. The highest levels are observed during launch, ascent, and re-entry. High levels during these regimes suggest the potential for crew performance problems initiated by noise and vibration phenomena. Indeed, the most dramatic problems have historically occurred during these flight regimes.

Mercury crewmembers noted a severe vertical vibration approximately 110-120 s into flight. The phenomenon was named "Pogo" after the child's toy that produces a similar effect. The source of the vibration was an 11-Hz oscillation initiated by the first-stage booster fuel pump, which was coupled to a longitudinal structural mode. The result was vibration levels recorded at 0.5-6.0 g in an acceleration bias of 3.1-4.4 g. The oscillation blurred crewmembers' vision during this phase of the ascent.

High acoustic energy during launch caused Apollo crewmembers to note difficulty with capsule/ground control

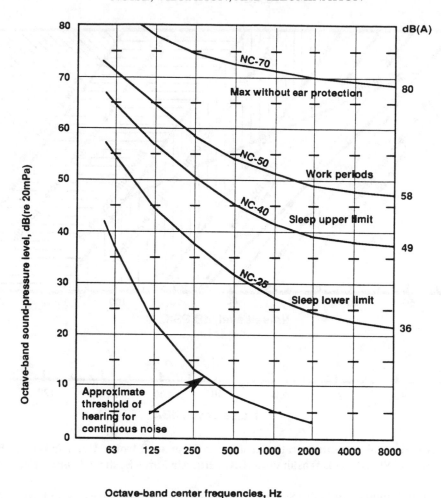

Fig. 5 Indoor noise criteria (NC) curves. (Reprinted from: National Aeronautics and Space Administration. Man-Systems Integration Standards, Volume IV, Rev. A. NASA-STD-3000, Houston, NASA Johnson Space Center, 1981, pp. 5–12)

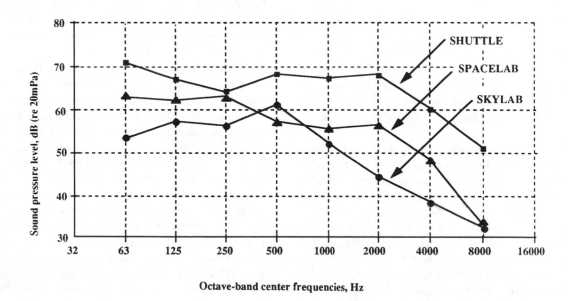

Fig. 6 Comparison of the internal noise levels measured during flight for Skylab, Space Shuttle, and Spacelab.

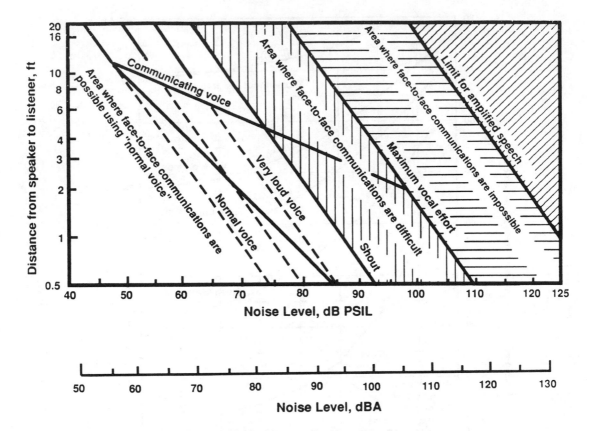

Fig. 7 PSIL and effective voice communication distance. (Reprinted from: U.S. Air Force. Human Factors Engineering. AFSC DH 1-3, Washington, D.C., Hq. Air Force Systems Command, 1972, p. 2)

communication during this initial flight regime. The Saturn 5 booster produced significantly higher internal noise levels than any other spacecraft to date. Experiments determined that maximum noise attenuation was provided by the helmet and head set. Reverberation room tests showed that the increase in headset amplifier gain during launch could offer a solution.

Apollo crewmembers also noted high levels of cabin noise during the translunar coast. Noise was controlled in flight by securing the offending equipment for brief intervals. Ground tests of individual capsule equipment identified the electrical system inverter, space suit compressor, cabin fans, and glycol pump as primary noise sources. These components, both individually and in aggregate, exceeded the acoustic design goal of 80 dB.[18]

On Skylab, problems associated with noise were primarily speech intelligibility and crewmember annoyance. Skylab was one of the quietest spacecraft built, primarily because of low atmospheric pressure (5 psia) and large internal volume, which provided significant gaps between equipment. However, habitability assessments by the crew indicated some sleep disturbance as well as communication problems. The latter were attributed to the low atmospheric pressure and long reverberation time in the volume. Crewmembers often had to shout to be understood at long distances. The longest duration mission provided the most noise complaints. Preflight and postflight audiograms determined that these crewmembers

suffered TTS despite the low ambient noise levels measured on orbit.[19]

Shuttle noise levels are due mainly to the ECLSS fans and avionics cooling fans. Levels measured with all systems operational are in excess of the NC-55 contour (see Fig. 5). Raised voices are often required for crewmembers to be heard between decks. Although no direct complaints of annoyance have been recorded, nearly 75 percent of those responding to recent Shuttle crewmember surveys recommended lower noise levels for the orbiter.

Vibration exposure problems have not been described by most Shuttle crewmembers. However, crewmembers noted annoyance from ambient vibrations while operating the Shuttle's Remote Manipulator System during recovery of the Long-Duration Exposure Facility. This experience is corroborated by a finding at the Jet Propulsion Laboratory (JPL) that defined adverse affects of vibration relative to control force feedback for remote manipulators.[20]

Overall sound pressure levels measured during a ground simulation of an Apollo mission were in excess of 80 dB. Skylab, Shuttle, and Spacelab spectral levels are compared in Fig. 6. The Skylab levels are an average of measurements taken throughout the internal volume and have been corrected from 1/3 to 1 atm to allow direct comparison. Shuttle levels were measured at the middeck location. Spacelab levels are an average of measurements throughout the internal volume but do not include measurements made at either end of the

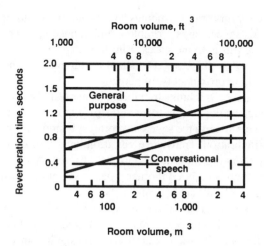

Fig. 8 Preferred reverberation time. (Adapted from: National Aeronautics and Space Administration. Man-Systems Integration Standards, Volume I, Rev. A. NASA-STD-3000, Houston, NASA Johnson Space Center, 1989, pp. 5–53)

access tunnel. The Skylab, Shuttle, and Spacelab spectrums can be converted to 64, 76, and 68 dB overall sound levels, respectively.

V. Recommended Vibroacoustic Limits for Manned Spacecraft

A crucial goal for designing manned spacecraft is to ensure crew safety, comfort, and productivity. The environment must be conducive to the exceptional performance demanded in space. The requirements are addressed in detail below.

A. Acoustic Design Goals

Acoustically, the spacecraft should be designed to prevent hearing loss, minimize speech disruption and annoyance, and ensure a comfortable acoustic environment. Acoustic limits are presented in terms of hearing conservation, voice communications, and annoyance.

1. Hearing Conservation

Hearing conservation measures are critical during the launch and re-entry phases, because noise levels during these times typically reach the 110 overall sound pressure level (OASPL) inside the spacecraft. Hearing conservation techniques are also required during several on-orbit conditions. NASA has developed a hearing conservation program, which specifies noise levels at which hearing protection is required. Crewmembers are required to wear hearing protection when
- Constant sound levels reach or exceed 85 dB(A)
- Total noise exposure over 24 h exceeds 80 dB(A)
- Sound levels exceed 115 dB(A) for 2 min over 24 h
- Sound levels exceed 120 dB(A) in any octave band or 135 dB OASPL

- Narrow-band components, pure tones, or beat frequencies are within 10 dB of the octave band that contains the component
- Impulse noise exceeds 140 dB peak sound pressure
- Infrasonic (1-16 Hz) sound pressure levels exceed 120 dB over a 24-h period
- Ultrasonic (greater than 20 kHz) sound pressure levels exceed 110 dB, 115 dB, or 115 dB at 25 kHz, 31.5 kHz, or 40 kHz (one-third octave band), respectively

It should be noted that it is impractical to provide hearing protection in the infrasonic hearing range.

2. Voice Communication

Successful task performance frequently relies on oral communication. Therefore, good speech intelligibility is crucial. Intelligibility has been defined as the percentage of speech units (words, phrases, or sentences) correctly recognized by a listener. Minimal intelligibility levels of 75 percent are satisfactory for face-to-face communication.

Direct (face-to-face) communication is evaluated using the Preferred Speech Interference Level (PSIL) index. Figure 7 presents the PSIL relationship relative to effective communication distances. In addition to distance between the speaker and listener, other important variables that should be considered are reverberation time, background noise level, voice level, ambient air pressure and gaseous composition of the atmosphere. Preferred reverberation time (in the speech communication frequencies) is a function of room characteristic, as depicted in Fig. 8.

Indirect communication lacks the visual cues that enhance voice communication, and a more conservative measure is used to evaluate intelligibility. An Articulation Index (AI) of 0.7-1.0 defines very good to excellent communications capability and is recommended.

Hearing protectors may affect verbal communication differently, depending on the sound pressure level. With continuous noise levels of 85 dB(A) or more, hearing protection may increase the intelligibility of speech; however, a reduction may be noted when levels fall below 80 dB(A). An additional concern is raised by findings that suggest that speakers wearing hearing protectors typically lower their voice by 3-4 dB.[8]

3. Annoyance

Annoyance refers to the discomfort or irritation caused by a noise source. Specific guidelines have been proposed to minimize the impact of annoying sounds. If noise levels are high enough to cause annoyance, it is likely that communication will be hampered and sleep delayed.

In work areas the NC-50 contour has been recommended as the maximum noise level. Levels that correspond to this contour are considered quiet, and no extra vocal effort is required to communicate over 0.9-3 m (3-10 ft). However, if tones are present, their level should be 10 dB lower than the

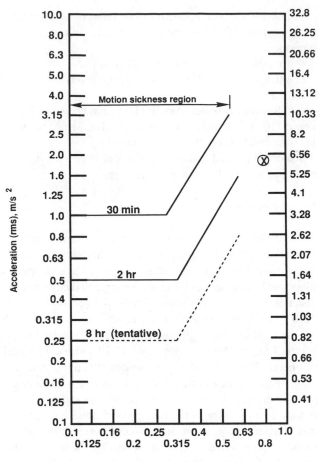

Fig. 9 Longitudinal (z-axis) acceleration limits (0.1–0.63 Hz) and severe discomfort boundaries. (Reprinted from: National Aeronautics and Space Administration. Man-Systems Integration Standards, Volume IV, Rev. A. NASA-STD-3000, Houston, NASA Johnson Space Center, 1991, pp. 5–18)

corresponding octave band level.

Research suggests that the sleep disturbance threshold is about 65 dB(A), except for transient noises when 50 dB(A) causes a 50 percent probability of sleep disturbance.[5] It is recommended that sleeping area noise levels be maintained between the NC-25 and NC-40 contours. Pure narrow bandwidth energy should be avoided in sleeping areas.

B. Vibration Design Goals

The effects of vibration on human performance should be considered when designing manned spacecraft. NASA has specified vibration limits as a function of expected human response between 0.1 and 80 Hz. Frequencies between 0.1 and 80 Hz are termed "low frequency" and dealt with independently of higher frequencies.

Vibrational energy between 0.1 and 0.63 Hz produces symptoms of motion sickness. Pallor and dizziness should be

expected for mild cases, whereas nausea and/or vomiting occurs during severe cases. Complete functional disability may be expected in extreme cases. Limiting exposure to levels below 1.4 m/s/s (0.1-0.315 Hz) should limit the incidence of vomiting to approximately 10 percent.

Figure 9 specifies limits for vibration energy in the 0.1-0.63 Hz frequency domain as a function of exposure duration. These levels specify the severe discomfort boundary for longitudinal vibration. Transverse vibration level limits are derived by reducing these levels 30 percent. Another 25-percent reduction is required if other types of vibration (particularly pitch and roll) are present.

Specified limits for vibration exposure (1-80 Hz) are defined as a function of exposure time and expected human response. Response to z-axis vibration differs significantly from x- and y-axis vibration, so limits are defined accordingly.

Vibration design goals are typically defined by the following three criteria:

1) *Fatigue-decreased proficiency boundary* defines the level that, if exceeded, will likely lead to degraded performance because of crewmember fatigue. Figures 10 and 11 define acceptable limits relative to exposure time and excitation frequency for the x- and y-axis, and the z-axis, respectively.

2) *Exposure limit* defines the maximum level to which crewmembers should be exposed during the mission. The limit is reduced by 10 percent during launch to accommodate the effect of linear acceleration bias. To determine the maximum exposure limits for the x- and y-axis, and the z-axis, multiply the acceleration values presented in Figs. 10 and 11 by 2.

3) *Reduced comfort boundary*. Activities such as eating, reading, and writing are vulnerable if this boundary is exceeded. The recommended limits can be calculated by dividing the acceleration values in Figs. 10 and 11 by 3.15.

VI. Vibroacoustic Control Techniques

Vibroacoustic control engineering is the use of engineering design to minimize the source of noise energy (either vibrational or acoustical), its coupling to or transmission through a structural system, and subsequent radiation into a compartment. Control of acoustical energy is, therefore, integrally dependent on the control of vibrational energy. Minimization of vibrational and/or acoustical radiation of a source, its transmission path, or radiation mechanism are the primary methods of vibroacoustic control. A secondary, and traditionally less desirable, method is control of vibroacoustic energy at the receiver—in this case, the crewmember.

The approach defined above may be further modified for the case of vibroacoustic energy control onboard spacecraft. Weight and volume constraints make it necessary to apply primary noise control to the source rather than to its propagation path or radiation mechanism. Modifying structures to change stiffness, resonance, damping, and structural coupling may increase weight and volume. Similarly, modifying ducts and interior spaces through the addition of silencers, enclo-

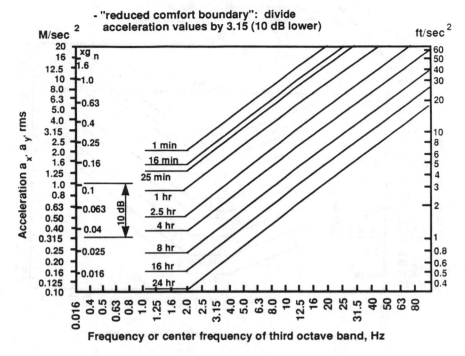

Fig. 10 Transverse (x-axis) and lateral (y-axis) acceleration limits "fatigue-decreased proficiency boundary." (Reprinted from: U.S. Department of Defense. Human Engineering Design Criteria for Military Systems, Equipment, and Facilities. MIL-STD-1472C, Huntsville, AL p. 175)

sures, barriers, and absorptive material incurs the same penalties. The best solution is obvious: specify equipment that meets vibroacoustic criteria.

Initial vibroacoustic design of a spacecraft would begin with development of a noise budget for the various systems and components to be installed. An analysis of budgeted levels relative to available equipment operating levels would identify possible noise source problems. Once identified, noise sources may be classified as vibration, impact, friction, and fluid-flow turbulence sources. The equipment could be evaluated in the laboratory and modified according to the methodologies listed in Fig. 12. Some solutions are more applicable to spacecraft than others.

Vibrating sources are the dominant sources of continuous noise and deserve additional attention. Vibrational energy sources may be classified as structural, torsional, or bending; flexural or bending plate-mode; translational or axial rigid-body; intermittent; or random/miscellaneous. Typical sources of these types of vibrational energy are summarized in Table 5. Suggested vibration control methods for these sources are presented in Table 6.

Controlling vibrational energy along its transmission path is the recommended secondary method of vibroacoustic control onboard spacecraft. Table 7 identifies traditional methods for controlling various types of vibration. The applicability of these methods is defined by the constraints implied

by the spacecraft under consideration.

The tertiary method of vibroacoustic control is application of a control methodology at the crewmember. Acoustical energy control is typically achieved through hearing protection in the form of helmet/headset or ear plugs/muffs. Protecting the crewmember from residual vibrational energy requires attention to body posture and support. Severe vibration in the x-, y-, or z-axis, especially under high-acceleration bias loads, is best withstood in the semisupine position. Seated position loads result in high z-axis loads, whereas the standing position results in high x-, y-axis vibration. Support for crewmembers should be designed so that resonant frequencies are at one-half the lowest vibration frequency of significance. Vibration protection could be provided through:

- Contoured seats
- Contoured and adjustable couches
- Elastic seat cushions
- Suspension seats
- Body restraints
- Rigid or semirigid body enclosures
- Head restraints
- Vibration absorbent hand/foot pads

The highly dynamic lift-off, ascent, and re-entry phases typically demand application of receiver control methodologies. Designing the spacecraft to control these high vibroacoustic loads would, of course, be impractical, since

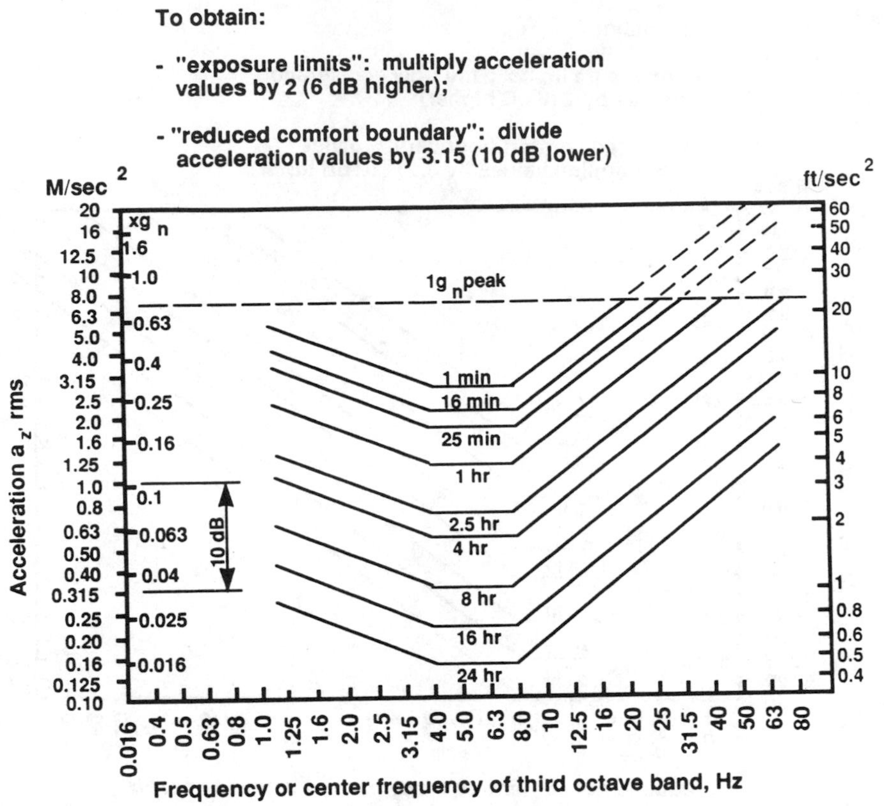

To obtain:
- "exposure limits": multiply acceleration values by 2 (6 dB higher);
- "reduced comfort boundary": divide acceleration values by 3.15 (10 dB lower)
M/sec 2
ft/sec 2
xg n
1g n peak
Acceleration a z, rms
20
16
12.5
10
8.0
6.3
5.0
4.0
3.15
2.5
2.0
1.6
1.25
1.0
0.8
0.63
0.50
0.40
0.315
0.25
0.20
0.16
0.125
0.10
1.6
1.0
0.63
0.4
0.25
0.16
0.1
0.063
0.04
0.025
0.016
10 dB
1 min
16 min
25 min
1 hr
2.5 hr
4 hr
8 hr
16 hr
24 hr
60
50
40
30
20
10
8
6
5
4
3
2
1
0.8
0.6
0.5
0.4
0.016
0.4
0.5
0.63
0.8
1.0
1.25
1.6
2.0
2.5
3.15
4.0
5.0
6.3
8.0
10
12.5
16
20
25
31.5
40
50
63
80
Frequency or center frequency of third octave band, Hz

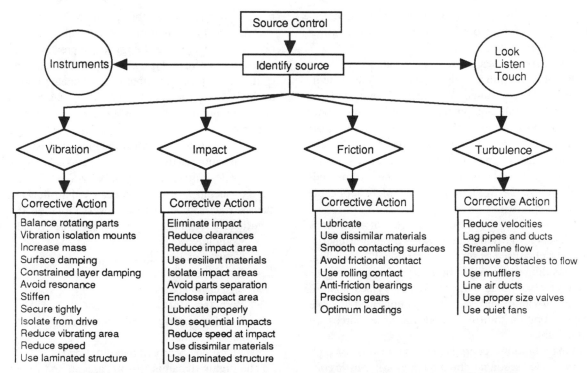

Fig. 11 Longitudinal (z-axis) acceleration limit "fatigue-decreased proficiency boundary." (Reprinted from: U.S. Department of Defense. Human Engineering Design Criteria for Military Systems, Equipment, and Facilities. MIL-STD-1472C, Huntsville, AL, p. 175)

Source Control
Identify source
Instruments
Look
Listen
Touch
Vibration
Impact
Friction
Turbulence
Corrective Action
Balance rotating parts
Vibration isolation mounts
Increase mass
Surface damping
Constrained layer damping
Avoid resonance
Stiffen
Secure tightly
Isolate from drive
Reduce vibrating area
Reduce speed
Use laminated structure
Corrective Action
Eliminate impact
Reduce clearances
Reduce impact area
Use resilient materials
Isolate impact areas
Avoid parts separation
Enclose impact area
Lubricate properly
Use sequential impacts
Reduce speed at impact
Use dissimilar materials
Use laminated structure
Corrective Action
Lubricate
Use dissimilar materials
Smooth contacting surfaces
Avoid frictional contact
Use rolling contact
Anti-friction bearings
Precision gears
Optimum loadings
Corrective Action
Reduce velocities
Lag pipes and ducts
Streamline flow
Remove obstacles to flow
Use mufflers
Line air ducts
Use proper size valves
Use quiet fans

Fig. 12 Typical noise source corrective actions. (Reprinted from: National Aeronautics and Space Administration. Man-Systems Integration Standards, Volume I, Rev. A. NASA-STD-3000, Houston, NASA Johnson Space Center, 1989, pp. 5–56)

Table 5 Sources of vibration.
(Adapted from: National Aeronautics and Space Administration. *Man-Systems Integration Standards* Volume I, Rev. A (NASA-STD-3000). Johnson Space Center, Houston, TX., NASA, 1989, pages 5-75.)

Torsional vibration

    Reciprocating devices
        Valves
        Compressors
        Pumps
        Engines
    Rotating devices
        Electric motors
        Fans
        Turbines
        Gears
        Turntables

Translational, axial, or rigid-body vibration

    Reciprocating devices
        Engines
        Compressors
        Shakers
    Motors
    Devices on vibration mounts

Bending vibration

    Shafts in motors
    Springs
    Belts
    Pipes

Intermittent vibration

    Impacts on floor
    Impacts on walls
    Impacts on the hull
    Typewriters
    Stepping motors
    Relays

Flexural and plate-mode vibration

    Hulls and decks
    Turbine blades
    Gears
    Floors
    Walls

Random and miscellaneous vibration

    Rocket combustion
    Aerodynamic turbulence
    Gas and fluid flow
        interacting in pipes and
        ducts

required performance design objectives, such as maximum payload accommodation, would be adversely affected. A simple example provides perspective.

The acoustical levels observed inside the Shuttle crew compartment during launch and on orbit are presented in Fig. 13. The launch load levels are severe enough to cause hearing damage and interfere with communications. Vibroacoustic control methods suggest controlling the source, path, and/or receiver in order to provide acceptable levels within the compartment.

Reducing the acoustical level by controlling the source, i.e., the rocket motors, would decrease the thrust capability, resulting in a lower payload limit—an unacceptable design alternative. Controlling the energy transmission path through structural modifications would most likely add weight, and, again, decrease the payload limit. Control of the acoustical

Table 6 Vibration control methods at the source (Reprinted from: National Aeronautics and Space Administration. Man-Systems Integration Standards, Volume I, Rev. A. NASA-STD-3000, Houston, NASA Johnson Space Center, 1989, page 5–76)

<u>Gas or fluid flow vibrations</u>

    Reduce flow rate
    Use less pressure
    Use quieter valve
    Modify impeller
    Smooth pipe or duct
    Lagging of pipe or duct
    Use flow turning vanes at bends

<u>Gear vibrations</u>

    Use proper lubrication
    Reduce speed
    Balance gear
    Replace worn/damaged gears
    Use higher quality gears
    Use different material gear

<u>Rotor vibrations</u>

    Balance rotor/coupling
    Modify force or speed
    Alter rotor bearings
    Add damping
    Reduce mass of moving elements

<u>Bearing vibrations</u>

    Lubricate properly
    Adjust bearing alignment
     or mounting
    Reduce speed
    Replace worn or damaged
    bearings
    Different bearing type

<u>Magnetic vibration</u>

    Use quieter motor, choke,
     or transformer
    Isolate or enclose
    Relocate

<u>Belt/chain vibration</u>

    Adjust tension
    Adjust alignment
    Lubricate properly
    Reduce speed
    Change material or type

<u>Pump noise</u>

    Reduce speed
    Reduce pressure
    Alter pressure cycle
    Isolate

<u>Combustion noise</u>

    Correctly adjust burner
    Use lower pressure
     barrier

<u>Impact vibration</u>

    Avoid it
    Cushion it
    Apply damping

energy at the crewmember is the only feasible alternative. A NASA helmet equipped with communication-type ear muffs provides 5-42 dB attenuation from 63-8000 Hz, reducing launch noise at the crewmember's ears to approximately 93 dB(A).

The short duration of high-intensity noise at launch makes this solution acceptable relative to hearing conservation requirements. Degradation of speech communication is overcome by utilizing higher gain in the headset during these high-noise periods. Further, hearing protection is not required on orbit, since airborne noise levels during this flight regime are much lower and acceptable relative to hearing protection

Table 7   Control of path vibration.
(Reprinted from: National Aeronautics and Space Administration.
***Man-Systems Integration Standards* Volume I, Rev. A (NASA-STD-3000).**
Johnson Space Center, Houston, TX., NASA, 1989, pp. 5-76.)

<u>Vibrating wall, floor and frames</u>

    Reduce area
    Add mass
    Change stiffness
    Detune resonances
    Add dampening material

<u>Source/receiver location</u>

    Position source or receiver at vibration nodes
    Change position of source or receiver or both
    Increase distance between source and receiver

<u>Gas or fluid flow vibrations</u>

    Use resilient pipe/duct connectors
    Use resilient pipe hangers and supports

<u>Equipment mount vibrations</u>

    Isolate sections with soft mounts
    Fasten external parts at vibration nodes
    Detune-avoid resonant buildup

and speech communication criteria. Hence, noise control at the crewmember is an acceptable solution for this particular problem.

VII. Spacecraft Vibroacoustic Measurements

The unknown characteristics of space flight during the early days of manned missions provided an impetus for the acquisition of information about and the analysis of vibroacoustic energy aboard spacecraft. Accelerometers and microphones were installed throughout the craft to measure structural vibration and airborne noise levels. Data were telemetered in real-time to mission control for recording and were analyzed postflight.

The high levels measured during lift-off, ascent, and reentry were immediately evident. Human factors analyses defined performance degradation during these flight conditions, so little emphasis was placed on determining ambient vibroacoustic levels during the relatively quiescent on-orbit flight regime. Measurements of on-orbit vibroacoustic energy did not become a concern until longer duration missions—specifically, Skylab.

The Skylab Program was the first in which significant noise control measures were integrated into the spacecraft during design. Noise control treatments were included in design of the cabin ventilation system.[21] An on-orbit measurement program used a portable sound level meter. Readings were taken throughout the internal volume. Triaxial force functions, generated by a variety of crew activities, were also measured.[22] A force plate was installed on the cabin walls to measure crew push-off and landing forces.

On-orbit vibroacoustic measurements continued with the Shuttle and Spacelab programs. Portable sound level meters have provided the acoustical measurements to date. Ambient vibration level measurements produced by crew activity and onboard systems have been obtained using either resident accelerometers or temporarily installed transducer systems. Signal processing and analysis of vibration data are typically performed at mission control from either the telemetered or recorded data.

A permanent VibroAcoustic Monitoring System (VAMS) concept has been developed for Space Station.[18] The system, through a distributed transducer/signal processing system, would be capable of continuously measuring the ambient vibroacoustic environment at significant locations throughout the Space Station. VAMS would autonomously qualify the data relative to NASA Standard 3000 requirements. Should a hazardous vibroacoustic environment be detected, the re-

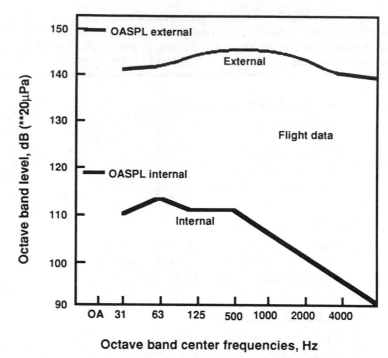

Fig. 13 Space Shuttle orbiter-crew module noise survey launch phase. (Reprinted from: National Aeronautics and Space Administration. Man-Systems Integration Standards, Volume I, Rev. A. NASA-STD-3000, Houston, NASA Johnson Space Center, 1989, pp. 5–40)

sults of that analysis would be transmitted to the crew and mission control over the Space Station Data Management System (DMS). A caution and warning hierarchy would alert the crew, prompting appropriate corrective action. Design constraints have precluded incorporation of VAMS into Space Station; however, the concept is valid for utilization on other platforms.

VIII. General Illumination

The lighting system for spacecraft presents unique problems. The hardware must be designed to withstand the extreme environment of the spacecraft and function for the duration of the mission. Therefore, reliability and redundancy are of major importance in providing good continuous illumination to the crewmembers throughout the mission. The lighting specification for a spacecraft requires a high level of quality and reliability to ensure excellent readability of the displays and controls and also to ensure that the lighting conditions are appropriate for adequate monitoring of subsystem performance.

The primary source of light during any space mission will be artificial illumination. Therefore, the lighting levels specified should achieve the most pleasing living and working environment, with the proper correlation between illumination and visual acuity, decoration, wall and ceiling reflection, source dispersion, and power and weight requirements.

The lighting subsystem should provide interior and exterior lighting to allow the crewmembers to locate, operate, and read all displays, controls, and nomenclature. The interior lighting should provide sufficient illumination for visual access to all interior compartment surfaces, storage for retrieval of all flight and personnel crew equipment and articles, and for location and orientation of the crewmembers within the crew quarters and other specialized compartments. The exterior lighting should provide orientation to allow crewmembers to conduct acquisition, tracking, docking, and extravehicular activity (EVA). The total lighting systems should provide illumination levels great enough to allow the crew visual access to the following areas and functions:

Interior: General interior
                 Personal hygiene area
                 Health maintenance area
                 Crew quarters
                 Wardroom/galley
                 Workstations
                 Display and control panels
                 Hatches, ladders and emergency exit
                 Equipment storage areas

Exterior: Acquisition and tracking
                 Docking interface and docking aids
                 Orientation
                 EVA traverse routes and EVA worksite

IX. Interior Illumination

The design of spacecraft lighting should produce a controllable lighting system adequate for providing a visual en-

Table 8 Area illumination and suggested source lamps.

A) <u>Controls and displays</u>

Electroluminescent
Transluminescent
Incandescent fiber optics
Incandescent projection
Light emitting diode
Liquid crystals

B) <u>Night light</u>

Electroluminescent
Chem-light
Incandescent
Light emitting diode
Phosphorus diode

C) <u>Crew quarters</u>

Fluorescent
Incandescent (lamp)
Projection lighting

D) <u>Work areas</u>

Fluorescent
Incandescent
Projection
Low pressure plasma

E) <u>General areas</u>

Fluorescent fixed/auxiliary
Incandescent fixed/auxiliary
Low pressure plasma

F) <u>Exterior</u>

High pressure plasma
Low pressure plasma
Incandescent

G) <u>CRT - graphic displays</u>

Ambient dedicated flood lighting

vironment that will permit crewmembers to operate all flight systems with an acceptable visual performance for prolonged periods of time. In designing the lighting subsystem for a multiactivity spacecraft, the ambient illumination from one activity center may either interfere with or benefit the activities in an adjacent center. Therefore, activities that require illumination will benefit from the "spillover" of ambient illumination while some areas, such as photographic and sleep areas, will need to have this ambient "spillover" occluded. The architecture layout, therefore, should recognize these areas and place the luminaire to take advantage of "spillover" and to maximize scatter. Some suggested lamp sources and their specified areas of use are shown in Table 8.

White light is preferred for the work and living areas. White light imparts a more natural appearance to objects and people. It also improves visual color acuity when color coding of controls and displays are used. The light intensity should be sufficient to allow crewmembers to perform their visual tasks efficiently. Therefore, supplemental task lighting should be provided when required; the lighting system should be dimmable to allow crewmembers to optimize their luminance environment. In the past, in areas where dark adaptation is required, red lighting has been the standard. However, under red lighting, color codes may not be as effective; the crewmember's color acuity is jeopardized. Also, older persons do not see fine instrument indices as well under red light. The same effect or benefit can be accomplished by providing dimming mechanisms on all task lighting systems and providing integral display lighting that can be dimmed.

X. Illumination Criteria

In general, lighting provides two functions for the individual: illumination for the visual scene and a photobiological function that results in direct and indirect physiological and biochemical responses. The result of the direct response of the photobiological function is a sensitive photochemical response of the skin. The indirect result stimulates the neural systems responsible for control of human circadian rhythms.

Research on artificial lighting systems has demonstrated that there can be beneficial effects for the individual when the indoor artificial illumination matches the natural environment.[23] Recent studies have shown that various sleep and mood disorders can be corrected by exposure to bright light. Czeisler[24] has shown that increasing the intensity of the lighting environment for night workers resulted in a successful shift in these workers' circadian rhythms. Czeisler placed night workers under 7,000-12,000 lux (651-1116 ft-c) mid-point through an 8-h night shift. After 5 days, he noted that these workers showed a synchronized shift in their circadian rhythms. Other studies have implied that physical fitness and psychobiological maintenance, improved visual awareness, greater eye comfort, and less fatigue occur when the light source simulates the full visible and balanced ultraviolet (UV) spectrum of the solar disc.[25] These same studies have shown that inadequate exposure to UV radiation during winter can significantly impair the body's utilization of calcium.[26] Furthermore, providing artificial light with solar characteristics during long-duration missions may aid against bone demineralization.[27] Therefore, by using artificial illumination equivalent to solar radiation, 270-1500 nm, with a minimum intensity of 2500 lux (232.5 ft-c), these physiological and biochemical responses could be influenced during space flight.

Fluorescent lamps that are currently available offer the relative spectral power distribution of the solar disc. These lamps operate at a color temperature of 5000 K and display a continuous spectrum from 280-900 nm proportional to the spectral distribution of the solar radiation at sea level. Continuous spectrum lamps may, however, be replaced by lamps displaying three prime energy peaks. These peaks closely match the three spectral response peaks of human vision, 400 nm, 540 nm, and 610 nm,[28] and provide the visual environment of continuous spectrum lamps. These lamps do not, however, produce the UV radiation of the continuous spectrum lamps. Several subjective evaluations at NASA have verified reports that this type of lamp does improve the brightness and clarity of visual scenes and enhances the color rendition of objects.

Space-flight and space-based hardware have critical weight and power constraints. Therefore, the benefits achieved by high-energy solar spectrum lighting sources must be viewed against power availability and weight requirements and the illumination levels necessary to provide the crew adequate illumination.

To establish the illumination requirements, one may consult various reference documents, the most authoritative in the United States being the *Illuminating Engineering Society Handbook*. However, the publication represents the industry's recommended illumination levels for industrial facilities and living areas. With each revision of the handbook, the recommended illumination levels have increased. Comparison of the recommended levels in the United States with those of other major countries (Table 9) reveals considerable variation. The primary reason for the difference is the selection criteria used to define acceptable visual performance. Research by Luckish and Moss[29] suggests that preferred light intensities are between 538 lux (50 ft-c) and 1076 lux (100 ft-c). Tinker's analysis[30] shows that preferences are dependent upon adaptation. In his experiment he found that readers adapted to 86 lux (8 ft-c) and chose 129 lux (12 ft-c) for comfort, whereas readers who adapted to 560 lux (52 ft-c) chose the median, 560 lux (52 ft-c). These results would suggest that the human eye will adapt readily to a wide range of illumination levels with no loss of acceptable visual performance.

Experiments performed by Tinker[31] on reading speed and visual acuity showed that both improved very little when the illumination level was increased above 269 lux (25 ft-c). These studies also showed that visual clarity was impaired by 2 h of reading at illumination levels below 32.26 lux (3 ft-c) but was not affected at levels above 32.26 lux (3 ft-c). Therefore, it would appear that those illumination guidelines presently being used on surface and commercial vehicles, rather than the recommended industrial levels, would be appropriate for spacecraft design (Table 10).

Many sources have noted that high illumination is not necessarily pleasant illumination. Also, the best lighting for reducing eye fatigue is diffused or reflected illumination in all directions. The most efficient way to diffuse lighting is to use a diffuser lens on all luminaires and provide a matte finish to all ceilings, walls, and floors.

The primary concerns for design of spacecraft lighting are the luminaire efficiency, diffuse light source, optimum placement of the luminaire, diffused reflection of the spacecraft surfaces (ceiling, walls, floor) and elimination of all glare or flare sources; i.e., specular surfaces, such as instrument bezel and glass. They should be positioned not to shine in crewmembers' eyes or cause serious reflection that would degrade the visual task. All glass surfaces should use antireflector coatings.

XI. Light Sources

The most appropriate light sources for conservation of power are fluorescent lamps. Fluorescent lamps not only use less power (50-70 lm/W) but also operate at a lower radiating temperature, thereby adding less heat load to the environmental control system. Also, fluorescent lamps can be used to provide a whiter or higher Kelvin color, which improves the crewmember's acuity of color discrimination.

The placement of the luminaires and the amount of illumination required for each work area are dependent upon the location of the object to be illuminated and the task to be accomplished within that area, respectively. General illumination within the working and living areas should be evenly distributed to preclude shadows. A medium-level intensity of white lighting is highly recommended, utilizing supplemental task lighting where functionally required. The minimum levels are shown in Table 11. The lighting should cover the entire work area with uniform intensity. It should not shine in crewmembers' eyes, or present serious glare and reflected flare that could degrade the visual scene. Some recommended illumination intensities are shown in Table 12. To provide the greatest visibility and brightness range to the crew, the workstation lighting should be fully adjustable. The controls should be located within the reach envelope of the operator. The luminaires need to be positioned to avoid casting shadows on the work area and reflecting images from the instruments and viewing screens.

XII. Illumination Level

Lighting levels should provide sufficient illumination for the crew to perform all visual tasks without eye fatigue or a power drain from other essential equipment or experimental systems. Conservation of the limited power and minimal weight are also design concerns. Work by Tinker[32] demonstrates that illumination levels above 269 lux are accompanied by modest gains in visual performance or in reduction of eye strain (Fig. 14). Therefore, the lowest recommended illumination level in spacecraft should be those shown in Table 11. The general illumination level of 108 lux (10 ft-c) is recommended with implemented lighting from 269 lux (25

Table 9 Recommended industrial levels of illumination in lux (foot-candles)

TASK	USA [1]	England [2]	France [3]	Germany [4]	Sweden [5]	Finland [6]	Belgium [7]	Switzerland [8]	Australia [9]
Most difficult tasks finest detail work, no contrast	9953-19917 (925-1851)	1592-2980 (148-277)	1592-2980 (148-277)	3981 (370)	1001-1991 (93-185)	1001-1991 (93-185)		968 (90)	1991 (185)
Very difficult tasks fine detail, moderate contrast	4982-9953 (463-925)	699-1592 (65-148)	699-1592 (65-148)	592-1001 (55-93)	301-506 (28-47)	506 (47)	506-1001 (47-93)	301-1001 (28-93)	699-1592 (65-148)
Critical tasks fine detail, moderate contrast	1001-4982 (93-463)	301-699 (28-65)	301-699 (28-65)	258-506 (24-47)	301 (28)	301 (28)	258-506 (24-47)	151-301 (14-28)	301-699 (28-65)
Ordinary tasks moderately fine detail, normal contrast	506-1001 (47-93)	151-301 (14-28)	151-301 (14-28)	118-258 (11-24)	151 (14)	151 (14)	97-258 (9-24)		151-301 (14-28)
Casual tasks service area, washrooms, etc.	204-301 (19-28)	65-151 (6-14)	65-151 (6-14)	54 (5)	32-75 (3-7)	75 (7)	65-75 (6-7)	32-75 (3-7)	65-151 (6-14)
Rough tasks hallways, passages, etc.	97-204 (9-19)	22-65 (2-6)	22-65 (2-6)	22 (2)	11 (1)	32 (3)	11-22 (1-2)		43-65 (4-6)

Extracted from:

1. Illuminating Engineering Society of North America, *IES Handbook*, 3rd. Edit. New York, IES, 1959, pp. 9-53-9-88.
2. Technical Committee of the Illuminating Engineering Society of Great Britain *The I.E.S. Code. Recommendations for good interior lighting.* London, I.E.S, 1962.
3. Association Francaise de L'Éclairage. *Recommendations relatives de l'Éclairage interieur.* Paris, L'Association Francaise des Éclairgistes, Paris, Societé d'editions LUX, 1977.
4. *Deutschen Normenausschuss DIN 5035 5035.* Berlin, 1953.
5. Swedish Lighting Engineering Society, *Luxtabellen*, Stockholm, Swedish Lighting Engineering Society, 1949.
6. Halbertsma, N.A., Jansen, J., Eds. *Proceedings of 12th Session of Commission Internationale d'Eclairage* (CIE), 1951, New York CIE.
7. Comité National Belge de l'Éclairage. *Code Préliminaire.* Brussels, Comité National Belge de l'Éclairage, 1951.
8. Schw. Elekts. Vercein, Leitsatze, 1947.
9. Australian Standards, Code AS 1680.2.0-1990. *Interior lighting: Recommendations for specific tasks and interiors.* Sydney, 1990.

Table 10 Recommended illumination levels for various areas in different vehicles in lux (foot-candles)
(Adapted from: Illuminating Engineering Society of North America. *IES Lighting Handbook, Application Volume.* New York, 1987, pp. 2-5–2-20)

AREA/TASKS	VEHICLES					FACILITIES				SPACE VEHICLES	
	Surface Ships Naval	Submarines	Surface Ships Commercial	Railway Passenger Cars	Commercial Airliner	Hotels	Hospitals	Libraries	Residence	Spacecraft	Long Duration Space Habitat
GENERAL	75 (7)	75 (7)	54 (5)	215 (20)	108 (10)	108 (10)	108 (10)			32-108 (3-10)	54-108 (5-10)
READING	301 (28)	301 (28)	54-323 (15-30)	215-538 (20-50)	269-430 (25-40)	323 (30)	323 (30)	323-753 (30-70)	215 (20)	215-323 (20-30)	>323 (>30)
FOOD PREPARATION		183 (17)	215 (20)	108 (10)	215-323 (20-30)	>323 (>30)	>323 (>30)		>161 (>15)	54 (5)	>215 (>20)
DINING	301 (28)	301 (28)	54 (5)	54 (15)	215-430 (20-40)				54-323 (5-30)	108 (10)	>323 (>30)
SCULLERY	301 (28)	301 (28)	54 (15)	54 (15)		>323 (>30)	>269 (>25)		>108 (>10)	108 (10)	>269 (>25)
RECREATION	301 (28)	301 (28)	323 (30)	215 (20)		108-323 (10-30)	108-323 (10-30)		323 (30)	108 (10)	>323 (>30)
MEDICAL TREATMENT			215-538 (20-50)				538-*1076 (50-100)			323 (30)	753-*1076 (70-100)
PERSONAL HYGIENE	151-484 (14-45)	151-484 (14-45)	54-538 (5-50)	54-323 (5-30)		108-323 (10-30)	323-538 (30-50)		323 (30)	108-215 (10-20)	>269 (>25)
STORAGE	75 (7)	54-75 (5-7)	54 (5)			215 (20)	108 (10)		54-108 (5-10)	32-54 (3-5)	54 (5)
PASSAGE AREAS	75 (7)	75 (7)	54-108 (5-10)	54-108 (5-10)		215 (20)	32-215 (3-20)		54 (5)	11-22 (1-2)	54-108 (5-10)

*The IES Handbook, latest edition, has increased surgical area illumination to 5,380 lux (500 fc).

Table 11   Recommended space vehicle minimum illumination levels

(Adapted from: National Aeronautics and Space Administration. *Man-Systems Integration Standards* Volume I, Rev. A(NASA-STD-3000). Johnson Space Center, Houston, TX., NASA, 1989, pp. 8-47.)

Area or Task	LUX	(fc)
GENERAL	108	(10)
PASSAGEWAYS	54	(5)
Hatches	108	(10)
Handles	108	(10)
Ladders	108	(10)
STOWAGE AREAS	108	(10)
WARDROOM	215	(20)
Reading	538	(50)
Recreation	323	(30)
GALLEY	215	(20)
Dining	269	(25)
Food preparation	323	(30)
PERSONAL HYGIENE	108	(10)
Grooming	269	(25)
Waste management	164	(15)
Shower	269	(25)
CREW QUARTERS	108	(10)
Reading	323	(30)
Sleep	54	(5)
HEALTH MAINTENANCE	215	(20)
First aid	269	(25)
Surgical	1076	(100)
IV treatment	807	(75)
Exercise	323	(30)
Hyperbaric clinical lab	538	(50)
Imaging televideo	538	(50)
WORKSTATION	323	(30)
Maintenance	269	(25)
Controls	215	(20)
Assembly	269	(25)
Transcribing	323	(30)
Tabulating	323	(30)
Repair	323	(30)
Panels (positive)	215	(20)
Panels (negative)	54	(5)
Reading	323	(30)
NIGHT LIGHTING	21	(2)
EMERGENCY LIGHTING	32	(3)

Table 12 Recommended minimum illumination levels for various tasks (Adapted from: National Aeronautics and Space Administration. Man-Systems Integration Standards, Volume I, Rev. A. NASA-STD-3000, Houston, NASA Johnson Space Center, 1989)

Illumination Levels			
Work area or type of task	LUX* (fc) Minimum	Work area or type of task	LUX* (fc) Minimum
Assembly, general		Inspection tasks, general	
Coarse	325 (30)	Rough	325 (30)
Medium	540 (50)	Medium	540 (50)
Fine	810 (75)	Fine	810 (75)
Precise	1075 (100)	Extra fine	1075 (100)
Bench work		Meters	110 (10)
Rough	325 (30)		
Medium	540 (50)	Work, general	325 (30)
Fine	810 (75)		
Extra fine	1075 (100)	Ordinary seeing tasks	215 (20)
Machine operation (calculator, digital, input)	325 (30)	Reading	
		Large print	110 (10
Console surface		Newsprint	325 (30)
	215 (20)	Handwritten reports	
Circuit diagram		in pencil	325 (30)
	325 (30)	Small type	325 (30)
Dials		Prolonged reading	540 (50)
	215 (20)		
Panels		Repair work	
Front	215 (20)	General	325 (30)
Rear	110 (10)	Instrument	810 (75)

* As measured at the task

ft-c)- 538 lux (50 ft-c) where necessary. Reflected luminance off non-illuminated instruments and function panels should not exceed 17 cd/m^2 (5 fL). Integral lighted panels and instruments should be from 0.34 cd/m^2 (0.1 fL) to 7 cd/m^2 (2.1 fL). It is highly recommended that all displays be self-illuminated and adjustable from high intensity to extinguished. Allowing for low level white lighting of panels eliminates the need for red lighting, which presents visual problems and impairs the efficiency of color coding. Optimum illumination is 269-323 lux (25-30 ft-c) on major work surfaces with the capability to increase the level to 530 lux (50 ft-c), when necessary. The level in general working areas should be 215-269 lux (20-25 ft-c).

XIII. Surface Materials

Different materials and surfaces react differently to the various types of lighting. Slick and glossy materials, instrument bezels and covers, window glass, and painted surfaces can create specular reflection and specular scatter that result

in visual glare, flare, and veiling luminance of the task. The reduction or elimination of these problems requires proper placement of the illumination source and special selection of the reflecting surfaces. Neither the hue nor the shade of surfaces has any significant influence on perception. The reflectance characteristics of the surrounding surfaces has the greatest effect. These surfaces become effective secondary illumination sources when appropriately applied, so it is important that they be matte or diffusing in character. The recommended reflectance magnitude from these surfaces should be 25-45 percent from consoles; 15-25 percent from work benches and tables; 60-80 percent from ceilings and walls; and 30-40 percent from floors. The relative percentages of the surfaces will give a greater diffuse luminous flux, resulting in a more uniform luminous intensity. All glass surfaces should have antireflective coating applied to reduce reflection. All instrument bezels should have anodized finishes. The recommended brightness ratio at the workstations should be 3:2 within a 30° visual angle, 5:1 within a 60° visual angle, and not greater than 20:1 between the light source and the total visual sur-

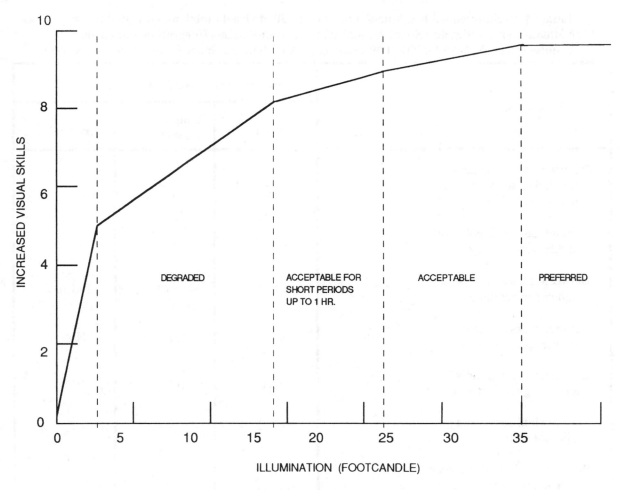

Fig. 14 Visual skills vs. illumination level. (Adapted from: U.S. Office of Naval Research. A Survey Report on Human Factors in Undersea Warfare. Washington, D.C., U.S. Govt. Printing Office, 1949)

rounds. Table 13 shows brightness ratios for some specified visual functions.

XIV. Exterior Viewing

During extended space flight, crewmembers will perform the majority of their visual tasks under artificial lighting. However, there will be periods of operation when sunlight and Earthshine will be the primary source of illumination. This lighting environment is limited to "out the window" tasks and EVA. Many of these visual tasks will also require artificial illumination during nightside operation. Solar light—whether direct sunlight or reflected from clouds—may enter the vehicle window, causing "veiling luminance" or severe sunshafting of the visual scene. Either of these conditions will result in the loss of vision or make it difficult to perform the visual task. Window filters can eliminate or reduce the effects of high-intensity light sources during daylight "out the window" observations. Except for celestial observations during navigation, external artificial lights may be necessary for the crewmember to complete a visual task.

XV. Exterior Illumination

An exterior lighting system may be needed for EVA, acquisition, rendezvous, tracking, and docking operations.

A. EVA Lighting

Lighting for EVA traverse routes and workstations may be provided by either direct or reflected solar illumination, diffused Earthshine, or permanently mounted lights, portable lights, or a combination of these sources. However, darkside operations will require artificial illumination. It is recommended that fixed mounted light sources be used to relieve crewmembers of the burden of transporting lighting systems. The same care should be taken to provide a nonglare, low-brightness ratio to the visual scene, as for interior illumination. Because of the "nonscatter" (no atmosphere) effect of the space environment, there will be little or no scattering of the light sources. Therefore, it is important to utilize the reflective characteristics of the surfaces available. It is recommended that the illumination levels be those shown in Table

Table 13 Recommended brightness ratios for specified visual functions (Adapted from: National Aeronautics and Space Administration. Man-Systems Integration Standards, Volume I, Rev. A. NASA-STD-3000, Houston, NASA Johnson Space Center, 1989, pp. 8–49)

Comparison	Environmental classification		
	Interior	Limited control	Exterior
Between lighter surfaces and darker surfaces within the task	5 to 1	5 to 1	5 to 1
Between tasks and adjacent darker surroundings	3 to 1	3 to 1	5 to 1
Between tasks and adjacent lighter surroundings	1 to 3	1 to 3	1 to 10
Between tasks and more remote darker surfaces	10 to 1	20 to 1	N/A
Between tasks and more remote lighter surfaces	1 to 10	1 to 20	N/A
Between luminaires and adjacent surfaces	20 to 1	N/A	N/A
Between the immediate work area and the rest of the environment	40 to 1	N/A	N/A

14. The brightness ratios should be those of Table 13, for the exterior light source.

B. Rendezvous and Docking

In order to initiate rendezvous of a payload or another vehicle for the purpose of berthing or docking, crews have expressed the need for direct visual reinforcement at a minimum distance of 304.8 m (1000 ft), with object definition at 213.36 m (700 ft) and visual resolution at 152.4 m (500 ft). Several artificial lighting systems can provide accurate information on range, closing perspective, orientation of the object, and alignment for effective berthing or docking during darkside operations.

For long-range search and detection, a flashing white rendezvous light can be placed on the primary approach axis of the payload. The light should have a flash rate of between 50 and 65 flashes a minute. The beam should have as large a cone of radiation as possible. However, for power efficiency,

the beam normally should not be greater than ±60° (120°). The intensity of a flashing beacon should be equal to that of a third-magnitude star at the desired detection distance. Table 15 depicts minimum intensity for various ranges of detection. It is suggested that a flashing white light be used for rendezvous beacons. Blondel and Ray[32] showed that a flashing light at the same intensity and distance as a steady-state light is perceived by the observer as being five times brighter. Also, research on search and detection has shown that a flashing light is a better attention getter than a steady-state light.

Running or orientation lights may be used to provide gross orientation and attitude at distances greater than 427.4 m (1000 ft). These lights should be positioned on the rendezvous vehicle using the international navigational color code. Red on port (-y), green on starboard (+y), yellow or amber on the bottom (+z), white aft (-x), yellow/white forward (+x). For optimum visual orientation, it is recommended that the lights be mounted orthogonally. Their intensity is dependent upon the visual distance desired for color recognition. Standard

Table 14 Recommended minimum illuminance levels for EVA tasks (Adapted from: National Aeronautics and Space Administration. Man-Systems Integration Standards, Volume I, Rev. A. NASA-STD-3000, Houston, NASA Johnson Space Center, 1989, pp. 8–24)

EVA Tasks	Minimum illuminance	
	Lux	fc
Astronaut movement to and from worksite. Cargo transfer operation	55 - 110	5 - 10
Station Worksite Area	215	20
Satellite Servicing: hand tool utilization for simple, nonhazardous repair missions	269	25
Satellite Servicing: Complex tools, nonhazardous	377	35
Satellite Servicing: Complex tools and hazardous tasks	538	50

Table 15 Intensity of a flashing light to be detected at various distances

Light Intensity BCPS (beam candle power seconds)	Visual range	
	Kilometers	Nautical mile
45	28.2	20
65	35.2	25
80	42.2	30
120	50.7	36
140	56.3	40
200	67.5	48
295	84.5	60
420	98.6	70
750	140.8	100

distances for visual detection of orientation lights is 1609 m (1 mile), and for color recognition, 900 m (3000 ft).

The final berthing/docking maneuver requires precision alignment and accurate ranging and closing perspective. This visual information is presented only by a three-dimensional view of the approaching vehicle. Therefore, artificial flood lighting will need to be provided. These systems can be mounted either to the object being retrieved or to the primary spacecraft to illuminate the contact interface of the approach-ing payload. If docking or grapple aids are to be used, it is important that the lighting system appropriately illuminate these aids with sufficient intensity for good visual acuity. For the majority of payloads it is recommended that the illumination level on the surface be a minimum of 16.5 lux (1.5 ft-c) at a distance of 427.4 m (1000 ft).

On the daylight side, illumination from the solar disc or Earthshine will provide sufficient lighting to perform the majority of visual tasks. Most spacecraft, payloads, and other man-made orbiting objects provide excellent reflectance. Because their surfaces are designed to provide good heat exchange, they reflect a high percentage of the incident sunlight. They also exhibit medium contrast against the luminous Earth background. However, for "close in" visual tasks, especially under sunlight conditions, experience at Johnson Space Center indicates that supplemental artificial lighting will aid in providing the fill illumination necessary for good visual performance in the space environment. This is because the Sun's rays are nearly parallel and there is no atmospheric scattering of the natural light source.

In conclusion, based on present spacecraft and submarine experience, it is recommended that illumination levels not exceed those used in present day surface or commercial vehicles. Based on this recommendation, lighting levels for future space vehicles should be specified to achieve the most pleasing living and working environment, with the proper correlation between illumination and visual acuity, decoration, surface reflectance, source dispersion, and the power and weight allocation.

References

[1]Boff, K.R., and Lincoln. J.E. Effects of environmental stressors. In: Engineering data compendium: Human perception and performance. AAMRL, Wright-Patterson AFB, Ohio, 1988, p. 2057.

[2]Sanders, M., and McCormick, E. Noise. *Human Factors in Engineering and Design.* Sixth edition, New York, McGraw-Hill, 1987, p. 466.

[3]National Aeronautics and Space Administration. Natural and induced environments. NASA-STD-3000, vol. 1, rev. A, Washington, D.C., NASA Hq., pp. 5-43.

[4]Bluth, B.J., and Helppie, M. Soviet space stations as analogs. Second edition, NAGW-659, Washington, D.C., NASA Hq., 1986. p. I-146.

[5]Sutherland, L.C., and Cuadra, E. Preliminary criteria for internal acoustic environments of orbiting space stations. NASA TM 69-2, 1969, p. 16.

[6]Yamada, S.; Ichinose, K.; Kamiya, H.; Watanabe, T.; and Kosaka, T. Occurrence and effects of low-frequency noise. *Internoise '83,* 1983, p. 859.

[7]Sandberg, U. Combined effect of noise infrasound and vibration on driver performance. *Internoise '83,* 1983, p. 887.

[8]Jones, D., and Broadbent, D. Noise. In: Salvendy, G., Ed. *Handbook of Human Factors,* New York, John Wiley & Sons, 1987. p. 641.

[9]Bruel and Kjaer Instruments. *Human Vibration.* DK BR 0456-11, Denmark, K. Larsen & Sons, 1988, p. 2.

[10]Matikainen, E.; Leinonen, H.; Juntunen, J.; and Seppalainen, A.M. The effect of exposure to high and low frequency hand-arm vibration on finger systolic pressure. *European Journal of Applied Physiology,* 1987, vol. 56, pp. 440-443.

[11]Sen, R.N. Incidence of Raynaud's phenomenon in workers using vibrating tools. *Vibration at Work—Abstracts of the Papers and Posters,* Third International Symposium of the ISSA for research and prevention of occupational risks, Apr. 19-21, 1989, Vienna, Austria, p. 26.

[12]Radwin, R.G.; Armstrong, Y.J.; and Chaffin, D.B. Power hand tool vibration effects on grip exertions. *Ergonomics,* 1987, vol. 30, no. 5, pp 833-855.

[13]Poirer, J.L., and Clere, J.M. Low-frequency mechanical vibration and the vascular system. *Vibration at Work— Abstracts of the Papers and Posters,* Third International Symposium of the ISSA for research and prevention of occupational risks, Apr. 19-21, 1989, Vienna, Austria, p. 21.

[14]Kjellberg, A., and Wikstrom, B.O. Acute effects of whole-body vibration: stabilography and electrogastrophy. *Scandinavian Journal of Work and Environmental Health,* 1987, vol. 13, pp. 243-246.

[15]Ruppe, K., and Blankenburg, H. Peripheral nerve disorders in the case of exposure to high-magnitude whole-body vibration. *Vibration at Work—Abstracts of the Papers and Posters,* Third International Symposium of the ISSA for research and prevention of occupational risks, Apr. 19-21, 1989, Vienna, Austria, p. 22.

[16]Ezzedine, H., and Angue, J.C. Visual information pickup by men exposed to low-frequency rotation. In: *Vibration at Work—Abstracts of the Papers and Posters,* Third International Symposium of the ISSA for research and prevention of occupational risks, Apr. 19-21, 1989, Vienna, Austria, pp. 33-34.

[17]Leatherwood, J.D.; Clevenson, S.A.; and Hollenbaugh, D.D. Evaluation of ride quality prediction methods for helicopter interior noise and vibration environments. NASA TP-226, NASA, 1984.

[18]Lengel, R.C. Vibroacoustic noise source data, literature survey results. JSC-24148, Houston, NASA Johnson Space Center, 1990, p. F-56.

[19]Lengel, R.C., and Wheelwright, C.D. Vibroacoustic monitoring system requirements and concept overview. *Proceedings of the 20th Intersociety Conference on Environmental Systems,* SAE Technical Paper 901442, 1990, p. 3.

[20]Hannaford, B., and Rosar, W.H. Effects of vibration on grasp control. *NASA Technical Briefs,* 1989, vol. 12, p. 90.

[21]Rader, W.P.; Barantono, J.; Bandgren, H.; and Erwin, R. Noise in space. *Proceedings of the 89th Meeting of the Acoustical Society of America,* 1975, pp. 4-7.

[22]Rochon, A., and Scheer, S.A. Crew activity and motion effects on space station. In: Structural dynamics and control interaction of flexible structures, NASA Conference Publication 2467, Part 2, Huntsville, Ala., NASA Marshall Space Flight Center, 1986, pp. 1095-1160.

[23]Hughes, P.C. An examination of the beneficial action of natural light on the psychobiological system of man. In: Illuminating Engineering Society (IES) of North America. *IES Handbook,* vol. 2, New York, 1978, pp. 74-77.

[24]Czeisler, C.A.; Johnson, M.P.; Duffy, S.F.; Brown, E.N.; Ronda, S.M.; and Kronauer, R.E. Exposure to bright light and darkness to treat physiologic maladaptation to night work. *New England Journal of Medicine,* May 1990, vol. 322, pp. 1253-1259.

[25]Maas, J.B.; Jayson, J.K.; and Kleiber, D.A. Effects of spectral differences in illumination on fatigue. *Journal of Applied Psychology,* vol. 59, no. 4, 1974, pp. 524-526.

[26]Neer, R.M.; Clark, M.; Friedman, V.; Belsey, R.; Sweeney, M.; Buonchristiani, J.; and Potts, J.R., Jr. Environmental and nutritional influences on plasma 25-hydroxy-vitamin D concentration and calcium metabolism in man. In: Norman, A.W., Ed. *Vitamin D: Biochemical, Chemical, and Clinical Aspects Related to Calcium Metabolism,* Berlin, N.Y., Walter de Gruyter, 1977.

[27]Wurtman, R.J. The effects of light on the human body. *Scientific American,* vol. 233, no. 1, 1975, pp. 68-77.

[28]Thornton, W.A. The high visual efficiency of prime color lamps. *Lighting Design and Application,* 1975, pp. 35-39.

[29]Luckish, M., and Moss, F. K. *The New Science of Seeing.* Cleveland, Ill., General Electric Co., 1934.

[30]Tinker, M.A. Effect of visual adaptation upon intensity of light preferred for reading. *American Journal of Psychology,* 1941, vol. 54, pp. 559-563.

[31]Tinker, M.A. Illumination intensity preferred for reading with direct lighting. *American Journal of Optometry and Archives of the American Academy of Optometry,* 1944, vol. 21, pp. 213-219.

[32]Tinker, M.A. Review of M. Luckish, light, vision and seeing. *Journal of Applied Psychology,* 1945, vol. 29, pp. 252-253.

[33]Blondel, A., and Ray, J. Perception of light flashes at their limit of range. *Journal de Physique,* 1911, pp. 531-536.

Chapter 6

Clothing and Personal Hygiene of Space Crewmembers

A. N. Azhayev, A. A. Berlin, G. A. Shumilina, J. D. Villarreal, and P. F. Grounds

I. Clothing

In everyday life, clothing protects us from adverse environmental conditions, such as high and low temperatures, rain, snow, wind, and dust. In the spacecraft cabin, where the environment is controlled and essentially unperturbed, clothing plays a somewhat different role. Its auxiliary functions become more important: it is used to restrain the body in a fixed position so that it will not float in weightlessness, to attach training devices, and to secure various kits and tools. To accommodate these functions, space clothing must be designed with pockets and retention devices that may be utilized for a myriad of tasks. Figure 1 illustrates the use of the Shuttle astronaut's shorts to restrain food trays; the shorts have a removable pocket containing utensils. Even with numerous Velcro™ patches, snaps, zippers, and pockets, space clothing must still be comfortable and not hamper movement. It has been said that the best clothing is so unobtrusive that one is not even aware that he/she has it on, and this is certainly true in space.

Every aspect of space clothing is designed to contribute to the success of mission objectives and to the safe return of the crew. For example, one of its most critical functions is to protect the crew from the inherent dangers of hazardous chemicals and propellants in an enclosed and isolated environment. Thus, the materials from which garments are fabricated must be carefully selected and designed.

Garments worn daily, such as intravehicular activity (IVA) clothes and underwear, may be either disposable or reusable. Disposable clothes are worn for a certain period of time and then discarded into the waste management system, or restowed and returned to Earth for disposal. Nondisposable clothes are cleaned and worn again.

Both types have advantages and disadvantages. The use of disposable clothing, which does not require a laundry system, simplifies the design of the spacecraft cabin, clothing fabric, and water recovery system. A laundry system would require that fabrics be compatible with the water and detergents and that the materials not release any products incompatible with the water recovery system.

With larger crews and longer flights, stowage of disposable clothing becomes a problem. Nevertheless, in present-day Russian space programs, preference is given to disposable clothes. On NASA Space Shuttle missions, which typically have crews of eight or fewer and durations of 10 days or less, clothing is returned for cleaning and reuse. On NASA's permanently manned space station, however, clothing will be cleaned in flight because of the extended mission durations and limited stowage space.

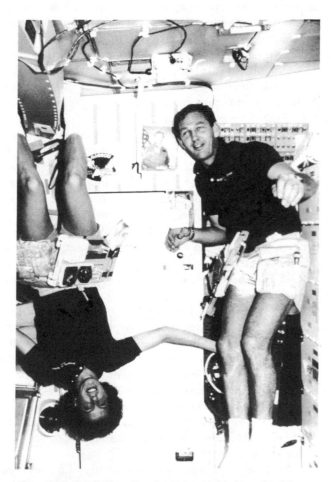

Fig. 1 On the Shuttle, shorts are equipped with detachable pockets and Velcro® strips to restrain food trays. (NASA photograph S32-14-26)

The Russian material in this chapter was translated into English by Galina Tverskaya and Lydia Stone.

Space clothing includes underwear, garments worn inside the cabin for IVA, and special thermal garments. Russian thermal suits are worn in emergency situations (e.g., landing in a hot or cold area or failure of the air-conditioning system in the spacecraft cabin). On launch and reentry, cosmonauts wear pressurized suits that do not have thermal suits as integral parts. NASA's clothing ensemble includes undergarments, IVA clothing, and expedition-weight thermal underwear in place of the Russian thermal suit. NASA's "thermals" are worn in conjunction with a launch and entry suit, which incorporates protective measures for an emergency landing or a bailout (see Chapter 14). Sleepwear includes sleep shirts and sleeping bags with inserts that serve as linens.

Russian space station crews also wear constant loading suits to compensate for the long-term effects of the absence of gravity. (These effects are discussed in Volumes III and IV of this work.)

A. Underwear

Since underwear contacts the skin directly, the primary requirement for such garments is nonirritability. Underwear should be durable enough for long-term use, and, in the Russian program, for supporting the attachment of biotelemetric sensors. Washing and various types of sterilization procedures should not alter the characteristics of the fabric. It should be lightweight and elastic and should not prevent heat transfer or evaporation from the body surface. Underwear should protect the body from cold and dirt; cleanse it of sweat, fat, and desquamated epidermis; and prevent these by-products from entering the cabin environment.

Underwear fabric must be moisture-absorbing to facilitate its hygienic function, which is especially important in light of the limited hygienic measures available in flight. When dampened, the underwear should not cling to the skin and absorbed moisture should readily dissipate into the environment.[2] Fabrics with wicking properties are preferred.

Because of limitations on bathing and washing in space, absorbent fabrics should be used for underwear. Underwear fabric with high wicking capacity can effectively absorb skin secretions; this becomes increasingly important with increasing mission durations.

Underwear can be made from cotton, silk, synthetics, or blends, although cotton has the best hygienic properties. Cotton underwear easily absorbs moisture from the body surface. Its moisture regain (hygroscopicity) is approximately 7–12 percent at a relative humidity of 65 percent. Cotton manifests high air permeability, ranging from 13.9–36 $cm^3/cm^2 \cdot s$ at a pressure of 49 Pa (0.007 psi) and a fabric thickness of up to 0.3 mm (0.012 in), and readily removes moisture from the body. The moisture conduction of cotton ranges from 53–68 $g/m^2 \cdot hr$ (0.25–0.33 $lb/ft^2 \cdot hr$).

The moisture regain and air permeability of fabrics used in underwear and the first layer of clothing should be no less than 7 percent and 10 $cm^3/cm^2 \cdot s$, respectively.[3,4]

The Apollo astronauts wore underwear manufactured of porous knitted cotton. This was a mass produced fabric, which demonstrated high air permeability and moisture regain, as well as the ability to absorb bodily secretions. Subsequent U.S. space programs have consistently used commercially available cotton underwear for astronauts. Cosmonauts have worn underwear made primarily from cotton (70 percent) and linen (30 percent), designed in either one or two pieces. Because of their good hygienic properties, these fabrics were the first to be considered by the designers of space clothing.

Cotton-linen fabric has the following characteristics: air permeability of 30–35 $cm^3/cm^2 \cdot s$ at a pressure of 49 Pa (0.007 psi); moisture capacity of 1.5–2.9 grams (0.0525–0.1015 oz); and moisture regain of 7 or 13 percent at relative humidity of 65 or 100 percent, respectively. To improve their wear-resistance, cotton and linen are used in combination with other, more durable fibers. This is especially important for underwear worn under space suits.

The structure of the fabric is also an important consideration in the design of underwear. The need to make the underwear as compatible as possible with the next layer of clothing (IVA or space suit), and thus to minimize folds and seams, led to the use of knitted fabric in the Soviet space program. Knitted underwear fits the body smoothly, with few seams and folds. Knitted fabric for underwear includes synthetic fibers—acetate and viscose rayon, polyesters, and others. However, supplementing cotton with synthetic fibers decreases the moisture regain of the fabric by 10 percent.[3]

Physiological-hygienic and physical-chemical investigations of various knitted materials for use as underwear for cosmonauts concluded that cotton/viscose rayon knit produced by means of circular-knitting, spring-needle machines was most suitable. This fabric has a high air permeability of no less than 40–60 $cm^3/cm^2 \cdot s$ at a pressure of about 5 mm (0.20 in) of water, and a high vapor permeability with resistance of about 1 mm (0.04 in) of air. The moisture regain is no less than 7 percent at a relative humidity of 60 percent. This fabric demonstrates sufficient strength with a 50-mm (2 in) band able to withstand at least 20 kg (44 lb).

The cotton/viscose rayon knitted underwear worn by cosmonauts does not hamper them in donning space suits, nor does it cause any unpleasant sensations even when worn for as long as 10 days. Space suit blowers assist in providing adequate aeration of the skin.

Successful demonstration of the underwear ensemble on Vostok flights led to its selection for use beneath the space suit.[5] This ensemble included a thermal shirt, seamless socks, and thermal pants equipped with a special flap in the perineal area, which permitted the use of a waste management system.

Microbial contamination of the skin is a particular problem for long-term space flights. Use of antimicrobial fabrics can reduce contamination of the skin and underwear; however, such fabrics are very difficult to manufacture. Moreover, it is hard to select effective combinations of bactericidal (bacteriostatic) preparations and synthetic fibers and at the same time avoid dysbacteriosis.

B. IVA Suit

Depending on the flight profile and program, cosmonauts wear either an IVA or space suit. For long-term missions on the Russian space station, the IVA suit has included components designed to exert pressure on the body and simulate gravitational loading (Fig. 2). U.S. Shuttle crewmembers wear a Launch and Entry Suit (LES) and then change into their IVA clothing in orbit. The LES is configured to facilitate emergency egress and landing operations and improve adaptation to the attendant harsh conditions imposed therein. NASA's IVA clothing is designed to feel like traditional clothing worn on Earth, while optimizing safety, productivity, and comfort.

An IVA suit must neither limit freedom and range of movement nor decrease work capacity. It should allow rapid, unassisted donning and doffing, and permit the use of a waste management system. The clothing should be loose enough for adequate air circulation and compatible with the underwear and thermal suit. Its thermal properties should be optimal for the temperature regimen of the spacecraft cabin.

The Russian IVA suit was designed to accommodate biotelemetric sensors. No physiological sensors are used with NASA's IVA clothes, with the exception of a personal dosimeter. The use of electrodes is limited to specific experiments and medical emergencies (personal interview with D. Rushing on January 16, 1991). In orbit, skin-surface electrodes are used on these occasions. During launch and reentry, physiological parameters can be monitored through a biomedical instrumentation port in the LES. Use of the port, however, is also limited to experiments and medical emergencies.

Both the Russian and U.S. IVA garment designs accommodate work in microgravity by incorporating numerous pockets, snaps, or Velcro™ to restrain or tether tools, personal articles, etc.

Engineers have spent decades developing materials that meet the stringent performance criteria required for space. Materials are evaluated for flammability, offgassing of products upon exposure to a vacuum, odor, comfort, electrostatic and hygroscopic properties, wrinkle/shape recovery, linting, chemical stability, aesthetics, flexibility, and permeability. The selected materials must also be resistant to abrasion, wear and tear, shrinkage, and stretching.

Fabric used for IVA suits must be light; soft; elastic; and wear-, fire-, and dust-resistant. The 100 percent wool knit used in the Russian IVA suit has the following characteristics: air permeability of 15–17 $cm^3/cm^2 \cdot s$; moisture regain of 10.9 or 16.6 percent at a relative humidity of 65 or 100 percent, respectively; and moisture capacity of 1.2–2.5 grams (0.042–0.0875 oz). These characteristics meet hygienic requirements for woolen fabrics.[3]

The evolution of fire-retardant fabrics for the U.S. space program has spanned more than 25 years. Scientists often resort to blending or spinning fibers with the desired qualities into the host fabric. The result is a blend of the premium qualities of each fiber. In the United States, pairing combina-

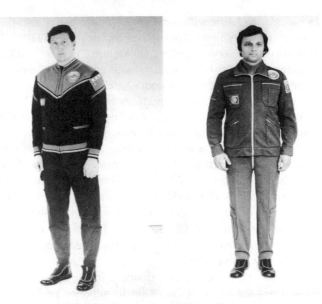

Fig. 2 Cosmonaut IVA suits.

tions of fabrics such as Nomex™, commercial flame-resistant cotton, polybenzimidizole (PBI), and Kevlar™ has proven highly successful in the development of a commercial, nonflammable product. Another technique used to improve the performance characteristics of a pure fiber or woven material is the application of chemical treatments.

Nomex™ aramid was introduced during NASA's Gemini Program. After the fire on the launch pad during a preflight test of Apollo I, increased emphasis was placed on fire resistance in space-flight clothing.[6] The Apollo cabin atmosphere was 100 percent oxygen, making flamability even more critical. Thus, Beta (a fiberglass fabric) and Teflon™ (polytetrafluoroethylene), both of which are inherently nonflammable, were selected for use on subsequent Apollo missions.[6]

The long duration of the Skylab missions necessitated an emphasis on comfort, as well as flame resistance. Durette™, which was developed by Monsanto under a NASA Johnson Space Center contract, was chosen for use on Skylab. PBI, which was developed by the U.S. Air Force in conjunction with Celanese Corporation, was modified by Johnson Space Center to produce knit shirts for the Skylab crews.[6] Because of the halogenation (introduction of bromine) of these fabrics, they came in a golden brown color only. With the arrival of the Space Shuttle era, NASA sought an aesthetically pleasing fabric that was still compatible with flammability and comfort requirements. This led to flame-resistant cotton in "NASA blue." In 1990, the Shuttle garments were updated to a darker, royal blue, still of flame-resistant cotton.

Johnson Space Center, in conjunction with Cotton Incorporated, modified commercial flame-resistant cotton, further increasing its flame-inhibiting properties.[1] This fabric is now used for the entire flight ensemble of Space Shuttle crews. Commercially available (unmodified) flame-resistant cotton is used in the production of flame-retardant sleepwear for infants and uniforms for firefighters, steelworkers, and forest rangers.[1] Commercial grade flame-resistant cotton is produced by treating the fabric with commercial phosphonium salts [i.e., tetrakis (hydroxymethyl) phosphonium hydroxide (THPOH), or tetrakis (hydroxymethyl) phosphonium chloride (THPC)], and then curing the fabric with gaseous ammonia[1] to increase its comfort. This basic "ammonia cure" treatment is insufficient in itself to inhibit flammability to comply with NASA standards. Consequently, a second application using diammonium phosphate (DAP)/urea is added. The process continues by curing and afterwashing the fabric before the final finishing treatment. Dicyandyamide, in solution form, is applied in the final step to inhibit flame propagation (personal interview with F. S. Dawn on January 18, 1991). After the fabric is dried, it is treated with an antilint finish to minimize the generation of fibrous lint in flight. The result is a material proven to be resistant to ignition, sustained combustion, and excessive linting.

The chemical treatments involved in the production of flame-resistant cotton do not alter its superior performance characteristics. It retains a moisture regain of 12 percent at a relative humidity of 65 percent (personal interview with F. S. Dawn on January 18, 1991). Like untreated cotton, the fabric is highly permeable to air and extremely comfortable.

NASA's flame-resistant cotton garments are dry cleaned to preserve the performance characteristics of the fabric. Flammability tests performed after 5, 10, and 25 home washings indicate that exposure to water, detergents, and agitation degrades the effectiveness of the chemical treatments. The treated cotton material passes an upward propagation test after 5 and 10 washings but fails after 25 (White Sands Test Facility test results, ID number 80-13461). In order to preserve the integrity of the flame-retardant treatments, flame-resistant cotton garments are never washed in water.

Naturally, fabric selected for use in IVA suits must be strong and wear resistant, properties characteristic of synthetic fibers.[7] Most synthetic fibers are durable and easily cleaned.[5] However, if overheated, because of the presence of trace quantities of monomers with toxic properties, synthetic polymers can offgas toxic volatiles and be potentially hazardous. Offgassing of monomers and particles with low molecular weights, and production of fibrous debris may also result from degradation processes. Although all debris (e.g., lint, food particles, and hair) is collected in cabin air filters that circulate and clean the air, it is desirable to prevent lint formation to minimize the crew time required to vacuum the cabin air filters.

The electrostatic charge generated by synthetic fibers is a concern in selecting flight materials. Clothes made from acetate, rayon, or silk, as well as footwear made from plastics, were found to generate strong electrostatic charges. In some cases, the electrostatic charge induced unpleasant or even painful sensations. Since electrostatic charge facilitates the accumulation of dirt, only materials that generate electrostatic fields of less than 20 kW/m (66 kW/ft) can be considered hygienically acceptable for space flight.[4]

Overall, the significant disadvantages of synthetic materials (i.e., poor moisture regain, offgassing, and electrostatics) lend preference to natural materials.

One concern for the flight garment designer is the maintenance of the body's thermal balance in space (i.e., prevention of both excessive heat transfer and excessive heat buildup). The use of two clothing layers has been successful in maintaining thermal balance over a range of ambient temperatures and heat production rates.

The environmental parameters in the spacecraft cabin are maintained within comfortable limits: ambient temperature of 18–23 °C (64.4–73.4 °F), air movement velocity of 0.05–0.5 m/s (0.165–1.65 ft/s), and relative humidity of 40–65 percent. Since astronauts and cosmonauts generally are either at rest or performing tasks involving only light exertion, their normal clothes should provide thermal insulation of about 1–1.2 Clo (1.137–1.37 ft^2·h °F/Btu). One Clo = 0.155 m^2 °C/W(0.880 ft^2·h °F/Btu) and is a measure of thermal resistance. This insulation allows the skin temperature to remain in the range of 32–34 °C (89.6–93.2 °F) at rest and 34–35 °C (93.2–95 °F) under mild exertion. In this case, the body surface temperature is 3–4 °C (5.4–7.2 °F) higher than the air temperature beneath the clothing.

The thermal protection properties of the Russian IVA suit have been designed to accommodate the selected temperature profile of the spacecraft cabin. When the ambient temperature rises above the preassigned values, cosmonauts are advised to remove their jackets or wear only their underwear. When the ambient temperature falls below 18 °C (64.4 °F), it is recommended that cosmonauts don their thermal suit (over the IVA suit), woolen socks, and woolen hat or helmet. When exercising, cosmonauts wear an exercise suit over their underwear. The shipset also includes socks (cotton-linen and wool), gloves (leather and knit), ankle boots, fur socks, helmet, earphones, and a sleeping bag with a cambric insert used as a sheet.

The IVA clothing ensemble for Shuttle astronauts includes a pair of trousers, shorts, jacket, removable pocket, and an assortment of commercially available shirts selected by the individual crewmember. The Shuttle shipset also includes cotton socks, T-shirts, sleep shirts, gloves (Nomex™ and deerskin leather), wool slipper-socks with leather soles, athletic supporters, underwear, and brassieres. All shirts, socks, and undergarments are procured from a commercial vendor. The IVA garments may be worn in any combination. Crewmembers usually prefer shorts and a lightweight shirt for exercising. Lined sleep restraints, eye shades, and pillows that strap to the head are provided for sleeping.

During launch and reentry, the LES is worn in conjunction with the thermal underwear, flight boots, helmet, gloves, communications carrier, harness, and emergency oxygen system. The coveralls once used by Shuttle crewmembers have been replaced by the LES and the IVA garments.

In preparation for a mission, the number of crewmembers and the flight duration are taken into account before clothing quantities are calculated and packed. NASA Shuttle astronauts are given one or more lockers or bags, depending on the stowage configuration, into which he or she may pack as

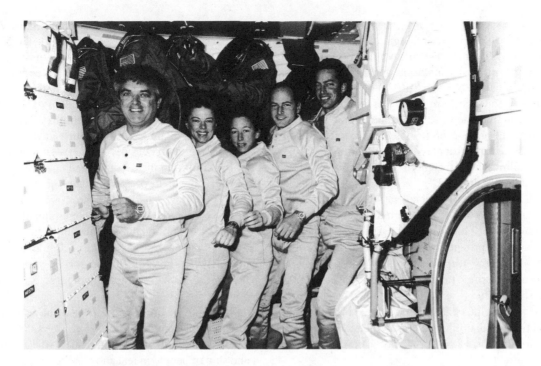

Fig. 3 The crew of STS-32 is outfitted in expedition-weight, thermal undergarments in the Shuttle middeck cabin. (NASA photograph S34-03-26)

many items as will fit. Recommended Shuttle use rates are as follows: trousers, two pairs per mission; shorts, two pairs per mission; underwear, one set per day; shirts, one per day; socks, one pair per day. Cosmonauts have an opportunity to change their underwear and sheets every 7–10 days.

As a part of flight preparation, the clothing articles, footwear, headgear, gloves, helmet, LES, and all EVA gear are fitted to the individual crewmember. After the gear is tailored, it is packed into modular stowage lockers or bags to be integrated into the space vehicle. As a part of the training process for Shuttle missions, the crew has an opportunity to review the contents of each locker, to become familiar with the stowage configuration for the mission, and to make last-minute changes.

C. Thermal Suit

As previously mentioned, the purpose of the Russian thermal suit is to provide protection and comfort if the spacecraft cabin temperature drops (which may occur in an emergency) or after egress during landing (or splashdown). The thermal suit is not used on a regular basis; nevertheless, a cosmonaut must be able to locate and don it quickly. Requirements for its design and construction are very similar to those for the suits of aircraft pilots.

NASA utilizes off-the-shelf, expedition-weight thermal underwear instead of the thermal suit worn by cosmonauts. The astronauts' "thermals" are worn in conjunction with the LES to maintain the body temperature for the same contingency situations described above. Figure 3 shows the crew of STS-32 wearing the thermal garments in the Shuttle middeck cabin.

Effective thermal protection depends on the rational use of different layers. When designing a package of thermal protective clothing, it is important to use strictly specialized layers.

It is usually considered that winter clothing should consist of the following four layers:

1) An outer layer (or shell) protects the other layers and determines the appearance of the suit. The outer layer should be durable and constructed of tough, wear- and crease-resistant material. It must be weather resistant and should not fade.

2) The second, wind-resistant layer should provide low air permeability to maintain heat protection in windy weather. This layer should have air permeability in the range of 0.7–4 $cm^3/cm^2 \cdot s$ (depending on weather conditions) and be lightweight, flexible, relatively durable, and vapor permeable.

3) The thermal layer provides warmth. It can be made from cotton or wool blend batting, or cotton wadding. Occasionally, synthetic materials (e.g., dacron and orlon) are used. This layer should keep its shape and be damage resistant; it should be relatively permeable to air and water vapor. It also should provide adequate moisture conduction [at least 40 $g/m^2 \cdot h$ (0.195 $lb/ft^2 \cdot h$)]. It should be lightweight, tough, wear resistant, and smooth surfaced.

4) The inner liner should have a moisture regain of no less than 7 percent and air permeability of no less than 10 $cm^3/cm^2 \cdot s$ (see Ref. 3).

The configuration of the four layers may be varied as long as adequate heat insulation is maintained. In the Russian thermal suit, the shell also serves as the thermal layer. The NASA Johnson Space Center combines the protection afforded by the LES and the thermal undergarments to provide total heat insulation.

The heat insulation properties of flight clothing should be no less than 2 Clo (2.28 ft$^2 \cdot$h °F/Btu), which corresponds to the heat insulation typical of transitional and winter garments. Ideally, at least 1.6 Clo (1.82 ft$^2 \cdot$h °F/Btu) of heat insulation should be provided for each 1 cm (0.4 in) of thickness[4]; however, it is very difficult to achieve this value in practice. Heat insulation of 4–5 Clo (4.55–5.68 ft$^2 \cdot$h°F/Btu) requires a layer 3 cm (1.2 in) thick; unfortunately, this thickness hampers mobility and explains why the thermal properties of flight clothing have had to be limited.

The thermal properties of special garments are strongly influenced by the curvature of the thermal layer and by the air trapped between the clothing layers. Thermal properties can be significantly improved by utilizing the heat insulation properties of "dead air." Improvements of the fabric itself can only improve thermal properties of the garment by a maximum of 16 percent.[8]

All of these facts emphasize the importance of design and materials selection in the production of adequate, flight-qualified thermal clothing.

II. Personal Hygiene

Medical support of space missions involves optimizing the sanitary-hygienic characteristics of the internal spacecraft environment and facilitating compliance with personal hygiene guidelines by the crewmembers. Personal hygiene, including proper skin care, plays an important role in maintaining the health and high performance of the crew. Therefore, it is justifiable to view personal hygiene measures as crucial and necessary components of flight programs.

Normal conditions of the skin and mucosa can be characterized by a number of parameters, the most important of which are: 1) the chemical composition of sweat gland secretions; and 2) the state of the skin, including the antimicrobial properties needed to maintain the qualitative/quantitative composition of an individual's commensal micro-organisms. The personal hygiene measures developed for use in space are intended to normalize the state of the skin and mouth.

Prolonged and continuous confinement of space crewmembers in a closed cabin makes it extremely important to maintain the cabin environment within comfortable and healthy limits. This requirement is a challenge in microgravity, which precludes the automatic purification of the air that normally occurs on Earth, where aerosol particles settle because of the gravitational force. In microgravity, dust remains in the cabin air and slowly builds up because of the action of electrostatic forces behind the interior shields and on various instruments, such as fans. Continuous air circulation constantly returns the dust to the cabin.

The major sources of dust in the spacecraft cabin include humans themselves and their skin, food, and clothing, as well as various instruments and hardware. Epidermis desquamation occurs continuously due to skin-clothing friction and spontaneously through skin keratinization. At 1-g, when an individual changes his clothes, approximately 5×10^6 epidermis squamae can be released into the air, 5–10 percent of which carry viable bacteria. Many authors claim that this condition increases the probability of infectious diseases.[9-15] When walking at a normal speed, an individual sheds as many as 1×10^4 squamae per minute. This value may increase, reaching 2×10^5 squamae per minute or 3×10^8 squamae per day. These squamae are 4–25 μm in size.[16] In space, the desquamation process develops at a greater rate.

In addition to the desquamated epidermis, which reaches an average weight of approximately 3 grams (0.105 oz) per person per day, other endogenous contaminants are present in the spacecraft cabin. These contaminants, including volatile products formed through decomposition of perspired and excreted compounds, amount to 100 grams (3.5 oz) per man per day.[17,18] Therefore, it is important to prevent contamination of the air with aerosols and gaseous compounds of endogenous origin.

Problems of life support in space have made it necessary to carry out comprehensive (e.g., physiological, biochemical, hygienic, and microbiological) studies of the mouth, hair, and skin of people in real and simulated space flights.[11,19-26] These studies have demonstrated that extended confinement of humans in the small enclosed space of an actual spacecraft or a mockup causes physiological changes, the pattern and scope of which are largely dependent on the individual's baseline health status and duration of confinement.

Changes in the mouth include inhibition of salivation, which interferes with natural cleansing processes, increase of salivary residue, and dental plaque and tartar formation. These changes in the mouth, in turn, modify microbial conditions, leading to an increase in microbial count and the occurrence of areas carrying pathogenic *Staphylococci* and *Candida* fungi.[27]

Skin changes have also been observed during real and simulated space flights. During 90-day confinement studies, the desquamation rate of the keratinized epidermis was found to increase by approximately 47 percent.[28] It should be noted here that hypokinesia per se did not increase the epidermis desquamation rate.[18] In addition to desquamation rate changes, effects on other skin parameters were detected, as summarized in Table 1.

As early as 5 days into a 90-day confinement study, subjects reported skin greasing, itching, and desquamation, all of which were especially noticeable on the scalp. These sensations grew stronger during exercise sessions and periods of ambient temperature rise. After the 30- and 45-day confinement studies, the male subjects demonstrated not only subjective but also objective changes (e.g., increases in the concentration of saturated C_{14}–C_{19} fatty acids and palmitic acid in skin fat). Lipids isolated from all the examined skin sites contained greater amounts of C_{16} fatty acids, whereas those isolated from the face contained greater amounts of palmitoleic acid.[28] These skin changes may exert an unfavorable effect on the health and psychological status of crews. Increased concentrations of micro-organisms on the skin and

Table 1 Skin parameters of male subjects confined in a closed environment (n = 76)[29]

Parameter	Day 1 before confinement	Period of confinement, days 1–10	Period of confinement, days 40–50	Period of confinement, days 80–90
Time for mark on skin to disappear, days*	—	8.1±0.5	6.9±0.4	4.3±0.2
pH, units	5.3±0.1	5.7±0.1	6.24±0.1	6.4±0.1
eH, mV	280±15	238±7.1	223±11	230±9.1
Lipids on 25 cm² of skin, mg	—	1.26±0.16	—	2.23±0.26
Epidermis desquamated from 25 cm² skin per swab, mg	—	1.06±0.10	—	1.76±0.16

*Inversely related to desquamation rate.

clothing may aggravate epidemiological conditions in the cabin.

The potential for human indigenous microflora to act as pathogens increases in space, making it important that personal hygiene procedures be used not only to clean the skin but also to maintain microflora at appropriate levels. The latter measures may help to decrease the number of micro-organisms released into the environment and, consequently, to reduce the probability of microbial buildup in the spacecraft cabin and microbial transfer among crewmembers.[9]

Major requirements for personal hygiene measures are that they be 1) completely safe for regular and prolonged use; and 2) compatible with life support systems.[18,24] The second significantly limits the use of many personal hygiene products available today, and makes it necessary to develop such products specially for space crews.

Specific features of the personal hygiene methods used in the NASA and Soviet (Russian) space programs have been dictated by microgravity and power, water, weight, and size constraints. Personal hygiene methods utilized during space flight should meet several basic requirements. All the procedures should 1) make the body and mouth feel clean, 2) normalize the chemical composition and physical-chemical properties of the secretions of the sweat and sebaceous glands, and maintain the qualitative/quantitative composition of indigenous microflora, and 3) reduce contamination of the air with endogenous aerosols and gases and deodorize the cabin environment.

Personal hygiene products should be of minimal weight and size and easy to use. Hygienic procedures should require as little time and consume as little power as possible. The number of procedures will depend not only on the flight duration, number, and gender of crewmembers but also on the flight program. When selecting specific procedures, primary attention should be given to flight duration and the equipment onboard the spacecraft or space station. However, regardless of flight duration, crewmembers should be provided the means to care for their skin, hair, and mouth.

Space missions can be subdivided into four categories on the basis of their duration: 1) flights of 24 h or less; 2) flights of 24 h to 30 days; 3) flights of 30 days to 180 days; and 4) flights longer than 180 days (interplanetary flights).

The category of flight influences the selection of personal hygiene items. Normally, crewmembers have used various wipes impregnated with different compounds, as in the Gemini, Apollo, and Space Shuttle programs. These were packed together in the ration, medical, personal hygiene, or survival kits. Cosmonauts on the Vostok, Voskhod, and Soyuz spacecraft, as well as the Salyut and Mir space stations, used dry and wet wipes and towels sealed in plastic bags and packed in color-coded plastic packages. Color codes were used to identify wipes and towels with various purposes, some of which are shown in Fig. 4.

It has been demonstrated that lotion-impregnated wipes and towels can efficiently remove metabolites and dirt from human skin. For example, one wipe can remove an average of 99 mg (0.0035 oz) of chlorides, 105 mg (0.0037 oz) of ammonium compounds, and 0.7 mg (0.00024 oz) of nitrites from the face and hands. After use, a single wipe has been found to contain 1060 mg (0.0371 oz) of organic compounds and a large number of micro-organisms. Wipes and towels show good cleansing action, are refreshing, and help to maintain normal skin functions. The lack of any signs of skin pathologies in the Soyuz or Salyut crewmembers demonstrates the effectiveness of these products.

The type and scope of hygienic procedures used differ from flight to flight, naturally. On very short flights (up to 24 h), cleansing the skin and the inside of the mouth with a wipe is sufficient. On longer flights (up to 30 days), crewmembers need to clean the whole body with wet towels, to care for the hair and nails, and to shave. On still longer flights (over 30 days), the crewmembers should supplement these procedures with showers and daily washing of the face and hands. The items contained in cosmonauts' personal hygiene kits are listed in Table 2.

Cotton wipes impregnated with various hygienic lotions are packed in a plastic bag and are intended for use by a single cosmonaut to clean his face, hands, feet, armpits, and groin

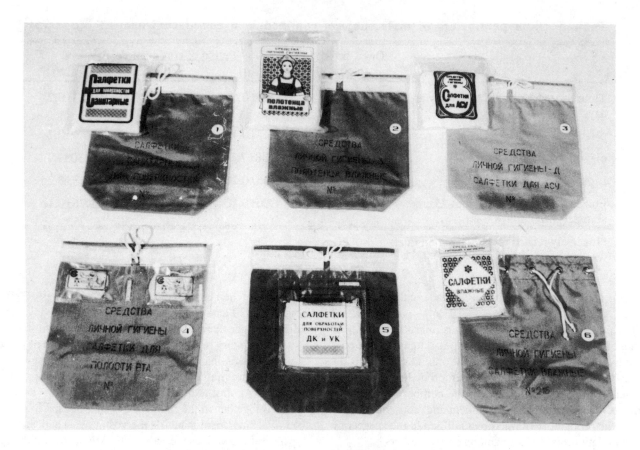

1. Wipes treated with disinfectant for interior cabin surfaces
2. Moist towels
3. Wipes to clean waste management system surfaces
4. Wipes to clean the mouth
5. Wipes to mop the shower stall and wash basin
6. Moist wipes

Fig. 4 Packages containing Soviet personal hygiene aids.

over a 24-h period. Dry and lotion-impregnated towels are used to wipe the body. Typically, towels are used daily after exercise and before changing the underwear. Wipes and towels should be made of soft, light, absorbent materials that do not produce dust.

Special emphasis should be given to oral hygiene. Gemini astronauts used a toothbrush, toothpaste, and chewing gum. Apollo astronauts had small tubes of toothpaste, toothbrushes, and dental floss. The crewmembers were advised to brush their teeth after each meal to prevent dental plaque and gingivitis.[18]

Early space flights demonstrated that changes in the mouth were associated with changes in salivation, which, in turn, may have resulted from psychological stress. These changes inhibited the natural cleansing of the mouth and led to abundant plaque formation and unfavorable microbial changes. Oral examinations, which were performed for the first time in space on Salyut 7 crewmembers, revealed disorders similar to those seen during flight simulations. However, these disorders were transient and corrected by hygienic procedures.

The effectiveness of various regimens of hygienic procedures was evaluated in 35 Soviet cosmonauts who remained in a spacecraft mockup for 16–90 days. During the study, the following parameters were measured: leukocyte migration from the mucosa, salivation parameters, saliva pH, saliva protein, and plaque. The state of the mouth was assessed using a hygiene score and that of the gums with the Schiller-Pisarev periodontal score.[30] Microbial counts included the total number of bacteria, as well as counts of *Staphylococci*, including pathogenic forms, and *Candida* fungi.

These investigations demonstrated that chewing gum for 10 min after meals increased the salivation rate from 0.88 ± 0.07 to 1.34 ± 0.09 mL/min, with the increase being most significant in those subjects with low initial salivation rates. The concentration of plaque in the saliva decreased from 5.7 ± 0.73 to 2.46 ± 0.15 percent. These results supported a recommendation to chew gum in order to stimulate salivation and facilitate cleansing of the mouth for subjects remaining in a

Table 2 Personal hygiene items used by cosmonauts on space flights of different categories

Item	Recommended use	Number per crewmember	Size, mm	Weight, g	Flight category*
Wipes:					
— Moist gauze	For daily wiping of the face, neck, and hands after shaving	4–9 pre day	330 × 225	12	1, 2, 3
— Dry gauze	For wiping the face and sweaty areas of the body; wiping dishes and utensils	1–4 per day 4 per day	330 × 225	4	1, 2, 3
— Gauze swab	For the teeth and mouth	2 per day	8 × 5	5	1, 2, 3
— Gauze moistened with lotion	For wiping the hair and scalp (to control itching and greasiness)	1–3 every 3 days	330 × 255	12	2, 3
Towels:					
— Moist honeycomb fabric	For wiping the head and body on changing underwear after work in the spacesuit	1 every 3 days	1000 × 350	200	2
— Dry honeycomb fabric	For drying the head and body after using the moist towel, for drying the hands and face after washing	1 every 3 days	1000 × 350	80	2
— Terrycloth	For drying the body after showering	1 every 7 days	1000 + 350	200	3
Sponges:					
— Honeycomb fabric	For washing the hair and body while showering	1 per shower	500 × 95	55	3
— Terrycloth	For washing the hair and body while showering	1 per shower	500 × 95	120	3
Packet with detergent	For washing the face and hands at the washstand	8 per day	90 × 60	7	3
Honeycomb fabric mitt	For wiping the interior surfaces of the washstand and shower cabinet	1 per shower and 1 per day for washstand	180 × 150	40	3
Towel treated with disinfectant	For disinfecting the interior surfaces of the cabin	1–4 every 7 days	500 × 350	100	1, 2, 3
Personal hygiene kit: — Comb, — Hairbrush, — Nail file, — Toothpicks, — Chewing gum	For caring for hair, teeth and nails	1 kit	220 × 150 × 50	400	1, 2, 3

* 1 = 1 day or less; 2 = 1 day to 30 days; 3 = 30 days or more.

closed environment for an extended time.

Thus, recommendations to cosmonauts for proper care of the mouth in space include cleaning the teeth twice a day (in the morning after breakfast and in the evening before bed) for 3 min using a toothbrush and a medicinal toothpaste selected on the basis of an individual cosmonaut's dental parameters. Chewing gum, mouthwash, and toothpicks are also recommended. The regular use of these measures helps to improve values of hygienic and inflammatory indices and stabilize carious and poorly mineralized areas of the teeth.

Prime and backup Skylab 2, 3, and 4 astronauts participated in preflight and postflight oral health studies[31] to assess the effects of their missions on population dynamics of oral microflora, secretion of specific salivary components, and clinical changes in oral health.

The Skylab crews brushed their teeth twice a day with an ingestible toothpaste and flossed once a day during the flights. Results of this study suggested that the microgravity environment is relatively nonhazardous from an oral health standpoint. Subsequently, Space Shuttle crews have been allowed a little more latitude in oral hygiene procedures, although it is still recommended that they brush their teeth after each meal and floss once a day. The astronauts are allowed to select toothbrushes with varying bristle stiffness based on their personal preference, and the toothpaste used is a commercial brand.

On short-term flights, crewmembers use a comb, hairbrush, and wet towels to clean the scalp and hair. They have shaved with electric or mechanical razors equipped with a special device to collect hair; however, it was found that razor blades and shaving cream suit them best. On Soyuz and Apollo flights, crewmembers used razor blades and applied cream with their fingertips; the cream was good for the facial skin and could be removed without water. After shaving, the crewmember cleaned the razor with wet wipes.

On Soviet (Russian) missions, each crewmember is supplied with personal hygiene kits, as well as wipes and towels (see Fig. 5). The kit consists of a soft plastic bag with seven pockets to hold such items as a comb, toothpicks, nail files, toothbrush, hair brush, and chewing gum. The kit for female cosmonauts also includes a powder box, medicinal lipstick, individually selected skin cream, and deodorant. The bag and pockets have fasteners that prevent the contents from escaping. Each bag is labeled with its owner's name and a listing of the items within.

U.S. astronauts use similar kits for personal hygiene.[32,33] The Shuttle kit contains toothbrush, toothpaste, comb, hairbrush, deodorant, skin emollient, shaving razor, shaving gel, nail clippers, dental floss, contact lens kit, styptic pencil, chapstick, disposable gloves, and shampoo. These items are held in the kit by elastic bands.

Missions longer than 10 days require all the items listed above, in addition to instruments for trimming crewmembers' hair and nails. Skylab and Soviet space stations provide a vacuum cleaner to collect hair and nail debris while preventing cabin contamination.[33] U.S. Skylab astronauts reported

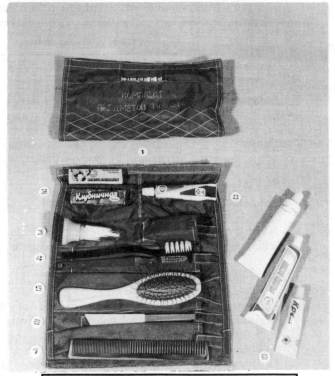

1. Toilet items in a bag
2. Chewing gum packs
3. Toothpicks in a container
4. Toothbrushes
5. Hair brush
6. Nail file
7. Comb
8. Tube of toothpaste
9. Tubes of multipurpose skin cream

Fig. 5 Soviet spacecraft hygienic kit.

"subjectively and without taking measurements, that the fingernails and toenails tended to grow a little bit slower in flight. Rather than trimming them once a week it was on the order of once a month or so."[31]

Onboard showers increase crew comfort. This measure is especially important for extended orbital and interplanetary missions because, as previously mentioned, the rate of desquamation of keratinized epidermis increases significantly on long-term flights. If the skin is rubbed for a long time with wipes and towels, the keratinized layer becomes thinner and the skin may be easily injured.

Shower units were used for the first time on the Salyut and Skylab flights. The collapsible units consisted of a zippered bag, ceiling and floor section, and water heating and supply systems. However, their setup and cleaning were difficult. It should be noted that members of the third Salyut-6 expedition showered approximately once a month.[34] Skylab astronauts were permitted to take showers once a week, if they wished. In actuality, the use rate of the shower was dependent upon individual preferences. The crew reported satisfaction with the shower equipment, but they indicated that

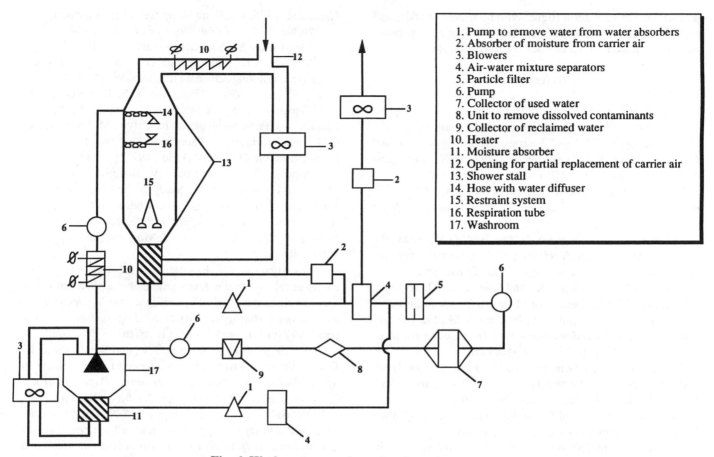

1. Pump to remove water from water absorbers
2. Absorber of moisture from carrier air
3. Blowers
4. Air-water mixture separators
5. Particle filter
6. Pump
7. Collector of used water
8. Unit to remove dissolved contaminants
9. Collector of reclaimed water
10. Heater
11. Moisture absorber
12. Opening for partial replacement of carrier air
13. Shower stall
14. Hose with water diffuser
15. Restraint system
16. Respiration tube
17. Washroom

Fig. 6 Wash water supply and reclamation system.

an excessive amount of time was required to vacuum the collected water and dry the shower after use.[31] On Mir, the "Kvant" module was equipped with a rigid shower stall connected with the wash-water reclamation system. A block diagram of the system is shown in Fig. 6. The entire showering procedure takes approximately 30 min in space: 10–15 min to wash and 15 min to dress (the washing procedure also includes cleaning the shower stall). After a shower, the stall can be treated with catamine AB solution (alkyl dimethyl benzyl ammonium chloride—a detergent and bactericide)[35] or dried and heated to 60 °C (140 °F). The stall walls can be pretreated with iodine and then heated for 2 h.[36] Water can be heated to 38–43 °C (100.4–109.4 °F) according to cosmonauts' preferences.

At the present time, a cosmonaut on an orbital station is allowed 10 liters of wash water per shower, which is twice as much as the normal minimum. The U.S. Space Station crewmembers will be allocated 3.8–5.5 liters. Detergent for showers can either be applied to a sponge or washcloth in advance or delivered by a dispenser.[37] The shower process leads to the formation of an air-water mixture consisting of used wash water, dirt, detergent, and exogenous contaminants of the carrier air. Prior to water reclamation, the air must be removed from the water by an air/water separator. The water is forced from the separator into the reclamation system, and the air is returned to the spacecraft cabin. The shower stall is supplied with fresh air. This removes carbon dioxide from the carrier air and saturates it with oxygen.[36]

Water reclamation is described in detail in Chapter 12 of the present volume. The only thing that should be noted here is that in the Soviet, now Russian, space program water has been preserved using silver at a concentration of 0.6–2 mg/L. Testing of a prototype shower system under development for the U.S. Space Station has shown that the water can be preserved using iodine and heating the water to 85 °C (185 °F) for 3 h.[36] Before use, water would be passed through ion-exchange resins to remove the iodine.

After showering, crewmembers dry themselves using a disposable towel and don clean underwear. After use, underwear, towels, and wipes are placed into a waste collector. (Currently, there are no washing machines onboard space stations.)

For washing the hands and face, a cosmonaut is allowed 0.3 liter of water supplied from a 1-liter dispenser, which should be an ample amount. Each cosmonaut is supplied with one towel to dry himself for 3 days. Because the wash basin is cleaned once every 24 procedures, or at least every 24 h, microbial contamination is not a problem.

Ground-based tests have shown that a modular design can best meet requirements for providing wash water in space flight. Modules might include a shower, a washstand, a washbasin to wash the hair or feet, etc., depending on the flight program, environment, number and gender of crewmembers, and so on. On long-term flights with no access to additional supplies, the personal hygiene or housekeeping system should be supplemented with a clothes washing module.

References

[1]Dawn, F.S., and Morton, G.P. Cotton protective apparel for the Space Shuttle. *Textile Research Journal*, 1979.

[2]Koshcheyev, V.S., and Kuznets, Ye.I. *Physiology and Hygiene of Individual Protection at High Temperatures.* Moscow, Meditsina, 1986 (in Russian).

[3]Del, R.A.; Afanasyeva, R.F.; and Chubarova, Z.S. *Clothing Hygiene.* Moscow, Legkaya Promyshlennost, 1979 (in Russian).

[4]Cheka, V.N.; Akimenko, V.Ya.; Bey, G.V.; Shandala, M.G.; and Rapoport, K.A. *Hygienic Characterization of Synthetic Clothing.* Kiev, Zdorovye, 1982 (in Russian).

[5]Popov, I.G.; Savinich, F.K.; and Krichagin, V.I. Hygienic evaluation of the garments worn beneath the space suits used in the second group flight. In: Sisakyan, N.M., Ed. *The Second Group Space Mission (Biomedical Investigations)*, Moscow, Nauka, 1965, pp. 17–22 (in Russian).

[6]Grick, S., and Godwin, D. Space station clothing development study. NASA Contract NAS9-16589, Houston, NASA Lyndon B. Johnson Space Center, Nov. 1984.

[7]Kiryukhin, S.M., and Dodonkin, Yu.V. *Fabric Quality.* Moscow, Legpromyshizdat, 1986 (in Russian).

[8]Burton, A., and Edholm, O. *Man in a Cold Environment.* London, Hafner, 1955.

[9]Zaloguyev, S.N.; Viktorov, A.N.; and Startseva, N.D. Sanitary-microbiological aspects of habitability. In: Nefyodov, Yu.G., Ed. *Sanitary, Hygienic, and Physiological Aspects of Habitable Spacecraft, Problems of Space Biology, Vol. 42*, Moscow, Nauka, 1980, pp. 80–120 (in Russian).

[10]Lechtman, M.D., and Nachum, R. Microbiological aspects of space flight. *American Journal of Medical Technology*, 1967, vol. 33, no. 6, pp. 515–623.

[11]Gurovskiy, N.N., Ed. *Results of Medical Research Performed on the Salyut-6-Soyuz.* Moscow, Nauka, 1986 (in Russian).

[12]Dubinin, D.M.; Popov, I.G.; Viktorov, A.N.; and Shumilina, G.A. The state of man's skin in an enclosed environment. *Kosmicheskaya Biologiya i Aviakosmicheskaya Meditsina*, 1988, vol. 22, no. 5, pp. 68–71 (in Russian).

[13]Konstantionova, I.V., and Antropova, Ye. I. Immunological reactivity of the human body in an enclosed environment. In: Nefyodov, Yu.G., Ed. *Sanitary, Hygienic, and Physiological Aspects of Habitable Spacecraft, Problems of Space Biology, Vol. 42*, Moscow, Nauka, 1980, pp. 191–213 (in Russian).

[14]National Academy of Sciences. Infectious diseases in manned spaceflight. Washington, D.C., National Academy of Sciences, 1970.

[15]Nefyodov, Yu.G.; Zaloguyev, S.N.; and Viktorov, A.N. Microbiological aspects of life support systems in long-term spaceflights. *Kosmicheskaya Biologiya i Aviakosmicheskaya Meditsina*, 1975, vol. 9, no. 4, pp. 19–23 (in Russian).

[16]Noble, W.C. *Microbiology of the Human Skin.* London, Lloyd-Luke Medical Books, Ltd., 1981, p. 493.

[17]Mattoni, R.H., and Sullivan, G.N. Sanitation and personal hygiene during aerospace missions. WADD-MRL-TDR-62-68, Wright-Patterson AFB, Ohio, U.S. Air Force, 1962.

[18]Finogenov, A.M.; Azhayev, A.N.; and Kaliberdin, G.V. Clothing and Personal Hygiene. In: Calvin, M., and Gazenko, O.G., Eds. *Foundations of Space Biology and Medicine, Vol. III*, Washington, D.C., NASA Hq., 1975, pp. 111–131.

[19]Popov, I.G.; Borschenko, V.V.; Savinich, F.K.; Kozar, M.N.; and Finogenov, A.M. Study of the human skin under conditions of limited washing. In: Chernigovskiy, V.N., Ed. *Work Performance Issues of Habitability and Biotechnology, Problems of Space Biology, Vol. 7*, Moscow, Nauka, pp. 413–420 (in Russian).

[20]Sevastyanov, A.V. Evaluation of the state of man's oral cavity in relation to the development and application of personal hygiene measures in spaceflight. In: *Important Problems of Space Biology and Medicine, Paper Abstracts*, Moscow, 1977, vol. 1, pp. 83–85 (in Russian).

[21]Ivaschenko, G.M.; Nikitina, T.V.; and Neumyvakin, I.P. Dental support of cosmonauts in long-term space flights. In: *Space Biology and Aerospace Medicine, Paper Abstracts*, Moscow-Kaluga, 1972, vol. 2, pp. 50–52 (in Russian).

[22]Nefyodov, Yu.G., and Zaloguyev, S.N. The present and future of hygienic support of manned space missions. *Kosmicheskaya Biologiya i Aviakosmicheskaya Meditsina*, 1981, vol. 15, no. 2, pp. 30–36 (in Russian).

[23]Nefyodov, Yu.G.; Borschenko, V.V.; and Shumilina, G.A. On the development of methods that may help maintain high performance and tolerance of man to adverse effects of extended space flights. In: *Problems of Aviation and Space Biology and Medicine, 5th Gagarin Lectures*, Moscow, 1975, pp. 184–193 (in Russian).

[24]Levashov, V.V. New aspects of personal hygiene. In: Sisakyan, N.M., Ed. *Problems of Space Biology, Vol. 4*, Moscow, Nauka, 1965, pp. 165–168 (in Russian).

[25]Berry, C.A. Summary of medical experience in the Apollo 7 through 11 spaceflights. *Aerospace Medicine*, 1970, vol. 41, no. 5, pp. 500–519.

[26]Zaloguyev, S.N.; Borschenko, V.V.; Viktorov, A.N.; Prishchep, A.G.; and Shumilina, G.A. Research into sanitary-hygienic support of space missions of up to two years in duration. In: *VIth National Conference on Space Biology and Aerospace Medicine, Paper Abstracts*, Kaluga, June 5–7, 1979, Moscow-Kaluga, 1979, Pt. 2, pp. 110–113 (in Russian).

[27]Zaloguyev, S.N.; Viktorov, A.N.; Shumilina, G.A.; and Dubinin, D.M. Criteria for evaluating the physiological-hygienic state of cosmonauts' skin. In: *Problems of Aerospace Biology and Medicine, 15th Gagarin Lectures*, Moscow, 1985, pp. 31–32 (in Russian).

[28]Zaloguyev, S.N.; Dubinin, D.M.; and Naydina, V.A. Examination of man's skin using gas chromatography. *Kosmicheskaya Biologiya i Aviakosmicheskaya Meditsina*, 1985, vol. 19, no. 6, p. 69–73 (in Russian).

[29]Berlin, A.A. Characteristics of the functional state of human skin in small closed environments. *Kosmicheskaya Biologiya i Aviakosmicheskaya Meditsina,* 1990, vol. 24, no. 2, pp. 51–54 (in Russian).

[30]Fedorov, Yu. A., and Koren, V.I. *Fundamentals of Oral Hygiene.* Leningrad, Meditsina, 1973 (in Russian).

[31]Johnston, R.S., and Dietlein, L.F., Eds. *Biomedical Results From Skylab.* NASA SP-377, Houston, NASA Lyndon B. Johnson Space Center, 1977.

[32]National Aeronautics and Space Administration Office of Public Affairs. Skylab news reference. Washington, D.C., NASA Hq., Mar. 1973.

[33]Nicogossian A. E.; Huntoon, C.L.; and Pool, S.L., Eds. *Space Physiology and Medicine.* Second Edition, Philadelphia, London, Lea & Febiger, 1989.

[34]Zaloguyev, S.N.; Viktorov A.N.; Shumilina, G.A.; and Kondratova, I.V. Sanitary and housekeeping support. In: Gurovskiy, N.N., Ed. *Results of Medical Research Performed on the Salyut-6-Soyuz,* Moscow, Nauka, 1986, pp. 46–53 (in Russian).

[35]Berlin, A.A. Rationale for sanitary-hygienic procedures. *Kosmicheskaya Biologiya i Aviakosmicheskaya Meditsina,* 1989, vol. 23, no. 2, pp. 21–25 (in Russian).

[36]Verosto, C.E.; Price, D.F.; and Garcia, R. Test results of a shower water recovery system. *17th Intersociety Conference on Environmental Systems,* Seattle, Washington, July 13–15, 1987.

[37]Manovtsev, G.A., and Zhuravlev, V.V. Evaluation of man's functional capabilities in an extreme environment. In: Chernigovskiy, V.N. *Sanitary, Hygienic, and Physiological Aspects of Manned Spacecraft, Problems of Space Biology, Vol. 42,* Moscow, Nauka, 1980, pp. 171–190 (in Russian).

Chapter 7

Design of Interior Areas

Chris Perner and William Langdoc

Success in the quest to establish new space frontiers requires special habitats that are compatible with extremely harsh environments and are conducive to human productivity over very long periods of time. Thus, habitat design is not just the creation of an environmentally protective shell but the development of a reliable, multipurpose system that serves as a shelter for people, equipment, and supplies and as an efficient workstation and safe haven.

As mission durations and crew sizes increase, habitability issues become more important. Added emphasis must be placed on formulating complete, applicable requirements for the basic habitability elements, including architecture, environmental control, personal hygiene, waste management, food, clothing, communication, housekeeping/maintenance, mobility aids/restraints, and recreation. When considering extended-duration missions, one cannot assume that the crewmembers will readily adapt to the new ambiance; and, therefore, the design of spacecraft interiors must be conducive to physical comfort, psychological well-being, and enhanced productivity.

In order to properly design spacecraft interiors, it is necessary to understand humans and human performance capability, the effect of the environments in which they must operate, and the principles of human engineering. While it is not possible in these few pages to cover all these topics—along with the elements of habitability—to the depth required, it is possible to give an appreciation for the most significant or unique space-flight factors that should be of concern to the human-systems designer of the inhabited areas of a manned spacecraft.

In its totality, manned space flight involves a range of acceleration environments from high-g during launch and entry/landing, to microgravity under orbital or transplanetary flight, to partial-g on extraterrestrial surfaces. Each of these acceleration conditions involves unique design problems and solutions. In this chapter, though, only the microgravity condition will be addressed. Also, the contents of this chapter are limited to intravehicular activities (IVA); i.e., non-pressure-suit, "shirtsleeve" conditions. Extravehicular activity (EVA) design considerations, which are unique and significantly dif-

ferent from those of IVA, are addressed elsewhere. Likewise, the many human factors considerations that are no different in a space flight setting than they are in 1-g are not covered here, although they are still of great importance to the overall design of a successful space vehicle.

The spacecraft and all crew equipment must be designed to fit the user's body size and range of motion, so a few words on anthropometry are in order. Typically, the user size range is defined as the 5th to 95th percentiles of a given design population. In past space programs, the user population has been relatively small and fairly uniform in size, but the projected user populations for future spacecraft include international crews of both males and females, so the body size range becomes much larger. For example, on the U.S. Space Station, the design population is from a 5th percentile Japanese female to a 95th percentile U.S. male. This equates to a range of stature from 148.9 cm to 190.1 cm. Such a large range must be considered in all space station designs; and, if a single design does not provide enough accommodation, then adjustments or multiple sizes must be provided.[1]

There are several anthropometric effects of microgravity. These changes, which involve posture, stature, and body circumference and mass, are summarized in Table 1. The microgravity neutral body posture, which results from the muscles and joints moving to their minimum energy configuration, is shown in Fig. 1. (Note that in Fig. 1, the segment angles shown are means. Values in parentheses are standard deviations about the mean. The data were developed in Skylab studies and are based on the measurements of three subjects.) Effort is required for the crewmember to assume any other body posture, and fatigue and discomfort may result if such a posture must be held for a long period of time. As a result, accommodating the correct posture is particularly important for any crew workplace.

Some of the design criteria that result from neutral body posture are as follows: 1) foot restraints should be sloping and placed in front of the torso; 2) work surfaces must be located higher than in 1-g, since the effective height of the crewmember is between a normal Earth sitting and standing height and the shoulders/arms assume a higher flexion; and 3) primary displays should be mounted lower than for Earth applications, since the head is tilted forward and downward, depressing the line of sight.

The authors would like to thank A.G. Uspenskiy, of NPO Energiya, for the valuable information he provided concerning design of spacecraft interiors in Russia. Russian information was translated by Lydia Stone.

Table 1 Anthropometric changes in weightlessness

Parameter	Anthropometric change		
		Long-term mission (more than 14 days)	
	Short-term mission (1—14 days)	Premission vs. during mission	Premission vs. postmission
Height	Slight increase during first week (~ 1.3 cm or 0.5 in). Height returns to normal *R+0 Increases caused by spine lengthening	Increases during first 2 weeks then stabilizes at approximately 3% of pre-mission baseline. Increases caused by spine lengthening	Returns to normal on R+0
Circumferences	Circumference changes in chest, waist, and limbs. Changes due primarily to fluid shifts.		
Mass	Postflight weight losses average 3.4%; about 2/3 of the loss is due to water loss, the remainder due to loss of lean body mass and fat. Center of mass shifts headward approximately 3–4 cm (1–2 in)	In-flight weight losses average 3–4% during first 5 days, thereafter, weight gradually declines for the remainder of the mission. Early in-flight losses are probably due to loss of fluids; later losses are metabolic. Center of mass shifts headward approximately 3–4 cm (1–2 in)	Rapid weight gain during first 5 days postflight, mainly due to replenishment of fluids. Slower weight gain from R+5 to R+2 or 3 weeks
Limb volume	In-flight leg volume decreases exponentially during first mission day; thereafter, rate of decrease declines until reaching a plateau within 3–5 days. Postflight decrements in leg volume up to 3%; rapid increase immediately postflight, followed by slower return to premission baseline.	Early in-flight period same as short missions. Leg volume may continue to decrease slightly throughout mission. Arm volume decreases slightly.	Rapid increase in leg volume immediately postflight, followed by slower return to premission baseline.
Posture	Immediate assumption of neutral body posture	Immediate assumption of neutral body posture	Rapid return to premission posture

* Recovery day plus postmission days.

I. General Interior Architecture

A. Volume Required

Crew size, mission objectives, and flight duration combine to dictate the amount of habitable volume required. Work by Fraser indicates that a volume of 0.7–3.5 m³/person is needed for space missions of 7–10 days by a motivated, well trained crew, and that 4.24 m³/person appears to be adequate for flights as long as 30 days.[2] American flight experience substantiates these numbers and seems to indicate that, with larger crew sizes, cramped volumes lead to crew inefficiencies.[3] Also, as the mission length increases, there is a greater tendency for the crew to feel confined or cramped.[4]

These data are very tentative, especially in cases where the crew is flying on a multipurpose space station with high freight traffic and a great deal of scientific instrumentation. Thus, for example, the pressurized cabin of the Mir main module was 130 m³, providing from 13 to 65 m³ per crewmember for crews numbering 2 to 10. However, there were still problems associated with stowage of the scientific instrumentation and consumables brought by the transport vehicle. Only after the main module had docked with the Kvant 2 and Kristall scientific modules, increasing the total volume of the station to 270 m³, was it possible to put everything in order and diminish the stress on the crew. The total volume of the American Skylab station was also about 270 m³ for a crew of three.

Microgravity allows the use of spaces and access to places that would not be possible in 1-g. This fact, coupled with a desire to use work space more efficiently by sharing it for multiple purposes, generally allows more activities to be accommodated in a smaller volume aboard a space vehicle than would be possible in a terrestrial design. Care should be taken, though, not to place excessive value on the use of accessible overhead space in microgravity. Experience in the Skylab

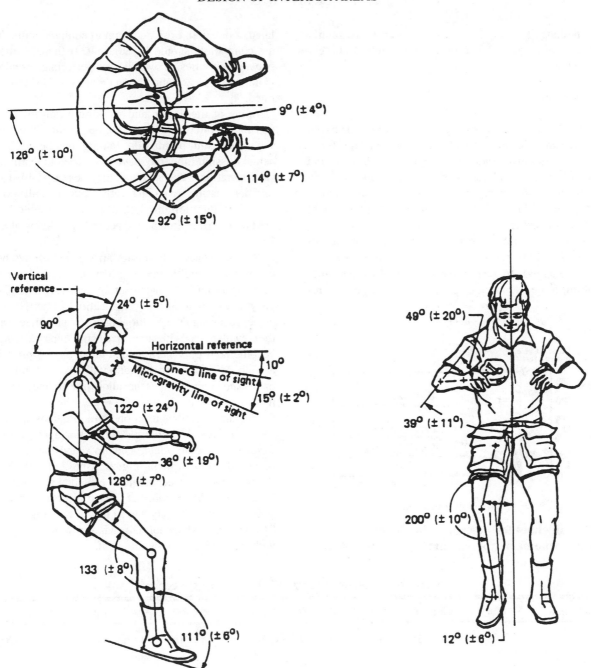

Fig. 1 Neutral body posture.[6]

Orbital Workshop showed that crew utilization of space in the habitable compartments was not much different than on Earth. The crew was not normally inclined to use the volume above tables, over consoles, or in general above shoulder level.[5]

Figure 2 gives guidelines for total habitable volume per crewmember.[6] Within this total value, adequate volume must be allocated for each crew station or activity area to allow the full size range of crewmembers to perform the necessary activities without undue restrictions. Loftus has summarized the volumes of American spacecraft to date, as shown in Table 2. He also notes that more volume for each occupant will en-

hance both operating efficiency and habitability.[3]

Given the fixed and generally small volume of a spacecraft, design features that tend to foster the perception of spaciousness and thereby provide a feeling of reduced crowding and increased privacy must be relied upon. Light, pale colors on the interior walls enhance the perception of spaciousness more than dark, saturated colors. Windows also serve to "open up the environment and increase its perceived size."[7] Nixon notes that an interior that is configured "horizontally" is more effective than a "vertical" arrangement at "accentuating and stimulating crew perception of internal spaciousness and perspective due to the absence of visually-restrictive intermediate floors."[8] For a given volume, irregularly shaped areas are perceived as roomier than equivalent regularly shaped areas.[4]

B. Arrangement

Compartments and crew station layouts should be based upon detailed analyses that consider the following[6]: 1) functional and operational allocations; 2) frequency, duration, and sequence of functions and operations; 3) isolation or privacy needs; 4) safety or special environmental factors; and 5) linkage with other modules of the systems to optimize weight and length of the cable network.

Adjacency, separation, and the transit time required between related activity centers also must be considered. Figure 3 provides a guide to the relative location of various functions that might be found on a space vehicle. In general, re-

lated, sequential, or shared support equipment functions that are compatible should be adjacent. If there is interference between activities, or overall crew performance and/or safety is improved by isolation, then crew stations should be separated.

Some of the design and working arrangements that are possible in microgravity cannot be practically duplicated in 1-g. As a result, premission training may be ineffective and actual mission time may have to be used to learn the necessary operations. This situation may be reasonable for a long-duration mission but could greatly reduce overall performance on a short-duration mission; therefore, it should be considered in the arrangement of spacecraft for flights of a week or less.

To date, spacecraft interior arrangements have been very compact and multipurpose. Most spacecraft have been essentially a single compartment. In such a setting, relative privacy and separation (or identification) of activity areas are achieved through the positioning of equipment, restraints, and the crewmember. With larger spacecraft, separate work, housekeeping, and personal hygiene areas can be provided. The Skylab, Mir, U.S. Space Station all have multiple compartments and bounded areas that allow true architectural arrangements.

The arrangements used on some previous spacecraft are shown in Figs. 4-7. Figure 4 shows the layout of the Apollo Command Module, which accommodated three crewmembers in a single compartment. Figure 5 shows the Skylab Orbital Workshop's lower deck, which provided the living quarters for the three crewmembers. Figure 6 shows the Salyut 6 space station, which normally had a crew of two. Figure 7 shows a Space Shuttle, which normally has a crew of five but has flown with crew sizes from two to eight.

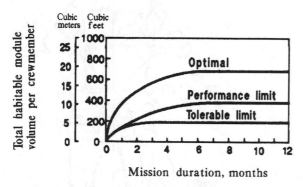

Fig. 2 Guidelines for determination of total habitable volume per person in the space module.[6]

Table 2   Interior sizing of American spacecraft[3]

Characteristic	Mercury	Gemini	Apollo CM	Apollo LM	Skylab	Apollo-Soyuz	Shuttle Orbiter
Volume (habitable), m^3 (ft^3)	1.02 (36)	1.56 (55)	5.94 (210)	4.53 (160)	[a]5.94 (210)	[a]5.94 (210)	35 (1300)
Pressurized volume less volume of equipment, m^3 (ft^3)					[b]344.98 (12,190)	[c]3.1 (109)	
Duration (max.), days	1-1/2	13-3/4	12-1/2	3	84	9	7–30
Crew size	1	2	3	2	3/5	3	2–7

[a]Command module.
[b]Orbital workshop.
[c]Docking module.

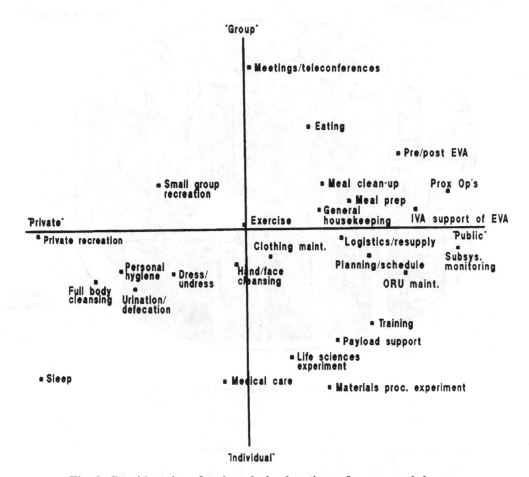

Fig. 3 Considerations for the relative locations of space module functions based on the results of functional relationships analysis.[6]

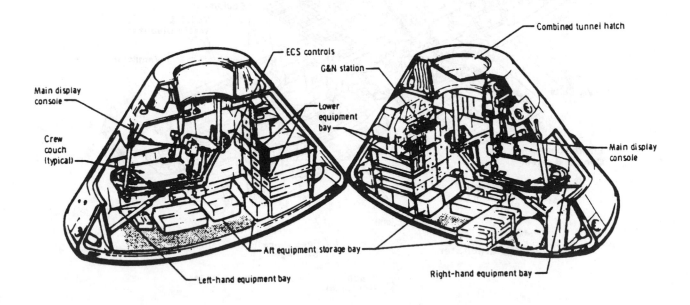

Fig. 4 Apollo Command Module crew station arrangement.

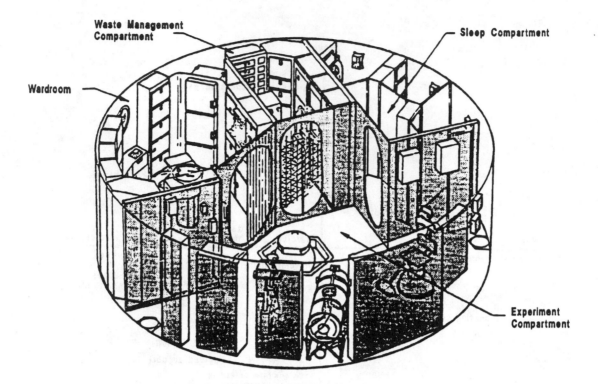

Fig. 5 Skylab crew quarters/experiment deck.

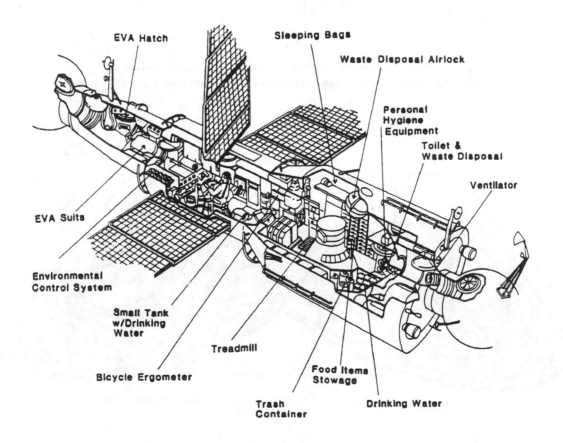

Fig. 6 Salyut-6 Space Station.

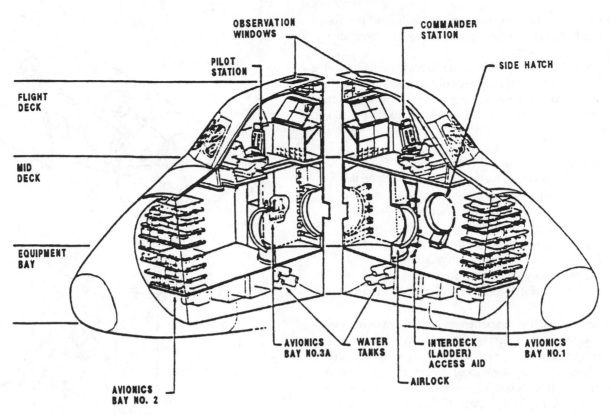

Fig. 7 Shuttle crew module.

Some of the specific arrangement requirements that have been established for a space station are the following[9]: 1) separate work, sleep, exercise, and eating areas will be provided; 2) entry and exit from private crew quarters will not disturb others; 3) commodes and personal hygiene areas will be located away from food preparation and dining areas, and near crew sleeping quarters; 4) the galley/dining area will be separated from crew sleeping quarters; and 5) a maintenance work area capable of being isolated from the remainder of the vehicle will be provided.

C. Orientation

On Earth, orientation is generally not a problem. "Up" and "down" are clearly established by gravity. In microgravity, the human working position is arbitrary. "Up" and "down" are defined through the crewmember's eyes. The top of the field of view plus visual cues from the surroundings define the local vertical. While microgravity greatly expands the possibilities for the number of work surfaces, some crewmembers have reported disorientation if there is no consistent orientation reference within their field of view, or if the view is inconsistent with their mental image of what is normal in 1-g.

Skylab contained interior areas with distinctly different design orientations. Since there were areas with both consistent and inconsistent local verticals, it was a good testbed for determining what differences, if any, result from a 1-g (consistent) or a microgravity (inconsistent) orientation. The mul-

tiple docking adapter (MDA) was the primary area with a microgravity design. It was a cylindrical volume in which equipment, lighting, and crew restraints were mounted in various orientations. As reported in the Evaluation of Skylab IVA Architecture:

The crewmen's reactions to the MDA's microgravity orientation were mixed. Some of them were vociferous in disliking the lack of a "visual gravity vector," while others thought that it was good. Those who liked it thought that it was a more efficient use of the volume than a 1-g orientation could have presented. Those who disliked it felt that it was too confusing to orient themselves and that it was difficult to establish traffic patterns through the area without bumping equipment and each other. All the crewmen, even those who liked the MDA, agreed that the rather hodge-podge equipment orientation was confusing and created difficulty in finding the various stowage lockers or equipment locations.[10]

Experience on Shuttle flights has also yielded mixed opinions on the need for a consistent orientation. The crews, in general, are either ambivalent or in favor of a consistent local vertical. A few crewmembers have also reported that their sense of "up and down" has changed after a few days on orbit. Initially, the floors of the middeck and flight deck were both clearly "down" in their minds; but, after about 4 days of operating in microgravity, the common bulkhead that forms the middeck ceiling and the flight deck floor became "down" for either compartment.

Lebedev has observed that while Salyut maintained a 1-g design orientation in the working compartment, the connecting compartment had a microgravity orientation and the crew positioned themselves however necessary to do the task at hand.

> Any position can be considered normal here. Whether you stand on the ceiling, or walk on the walls, to adjust your mental image you just have to say to yourself that the wall is the floor and everything above is ceiling, you have to look straight ahead and accept this new interior. Now when you place everything in order in your mind, you re-orient yourself and do not feel any inconvenience at walking on the wall or the ceiling.[11]

The result of all these experiences has led to a design guideline for American spacecraft that each crew station should have a definite, consistent orientation; and, while there should also be a generally consistent local vertical throughout a compartment or module, adjacent crew stations may have different orientations if there is a clear, definable demarcation between the two stations.[6]

D. Traffic Flow

Design for the traffic flow within a spacecraft is based upon the number of crewmembers, crew station locations, and the tasks to be performed. Traffic flow design must consider the frequency of the traffic, the size and type of packages to be moved, the need to minimize congestion, potential impingements or obstructions, and emergency egress.[9] Translation in microgravity is generally done either head first or in the upright, neutral body posture. Standard passageways should be designed to accommodate a shirtsleeve crewmember translating in the upright position with a modest size package. Low usage, secondary passageways, or passthroughs are designed for only head-first travel from one point to another. Figure 8 gives the minimum dimensions for translation paths that are now used to design American spacecraft.[6]

Congestion and "bottlenecks" occur on all spacecraft with more than one crewmember and enough room to move around. The nature of spacecraft, with limited volume and lots of equipment, causes traffic problems. Skylab crews reported several areas of congestion; for example, one of the crewmembers on each flight had to crawl over the other two to reach his food in the galley.[10] Shuttle crews also report congestion during missions with seven or eight crewmembers at times of eating, change of shifts, or when several crewmembers need to get to their clothing lockers at the same time.

Experience shows that handrails along translation routes are not normally used for hand-over-hand translation, but

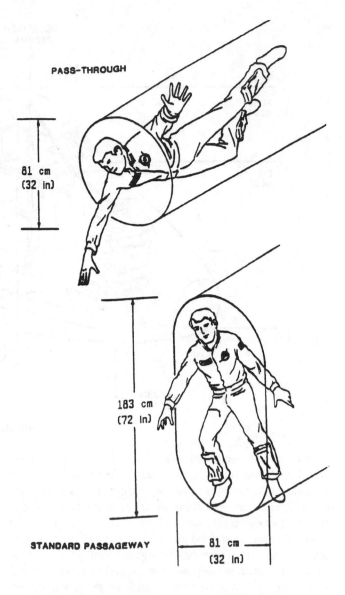

Fig. 8 Minimum translation path dimensions for microgravity, one crew member in light clothing.[6]

rather to aid in the control of body speed, attitude, and stability. Data collected on Skylab show translation rates of 0.4–0.6 m/s for normal translations, 0.15–0.3 m/s for moving large or massive equipment, and 1.8 m/s for a maximum rate.[12]

Walls, ceilings, control panels, or any other surface or piece of equipment may, and will, be used as mobility aids or points to start or stop a translation movement. It is very important to recognize this fact of life in microgravity and to design accordingly.

E. Color and Decor

Interior decor should provide an aesthetic and psychologically satisfying environment for the crew, while maximizing lighting efficiency and meeting the need for easily cleanable and maintainable surfaces. To date, the latter two points have been the primary drivers for spacecraft decor. All American

Table 3 Functional considerations for location of windows

Window functions	Location considerations
Proximity operations	
• Coordination of docking and berthing of other modules	• Near module workstations with communications, control displays, video backup, etc.
• Monitoring and support of EVA personnel	• Location to provide a clear, stereoscopic view of EVA operations
• Teleoperation of EVA equipment	
Earth/celestial observations	
• Discovery and documentation of unpredicted features and events	• Near scientific workstations
• Scientific research and experimentation	• Away from high traffic volume
Support of crew morale	
• Offset claustrophobic effects of tightly confined, long-term isolation	• Near recreational, socialization areas
• Provide recreational and awe-inspiring experiences	• Near areas of boring, monotonous tasks (exercise, for instance)
• Enable photography	• Near private quarters
• Provide educational benefits	• Location to provide view of Earth (if possible) or other interesting celestial sight
• Provide a psychological link to the home planet	
• Afford natural illumination and day/night cycles	

spacecraft have had interiors that are primarily shades of gray or off-white, with accent colors used for markings and color coding.

The interiors of Soviet spacecraft are also painted in subdued colors, neutral shades of yellow, green, and grey. One of the criteria for selecting paint color has been the need to ensure high quality color reproduction for video transmissions.

Research has indicated that, for short-duration confinement with all male crews occupied with meaningful work, "attractive" surroundings add little value. However, as the crews become mixed and the amount of work decreases, the importance of decor increases; and it is assumed that it will become even more important as mission length increases.[13] All three members of the Skylab 4 crew, which had the longest on-orbit stay of any of the Skylab missions, commented that they grew bored with the neutral gray and white shades that were used extensively for interior surfaces and equipment and that they would have liked more variation.[10]

Experiments have established that different colors have different degrees of attractiveness and evoke different emotions. Blue, green, and violet tints are cool, quiet, and conducive to rest. Red, orange, and yellow tints stimulate psychophysiological functions and should be used for work or recreation areas.[14] Use of dark or saturated colors should be limited to small accent areas. A frequently occupied compartment should not be of a single uniform color, and when different colors are used to enhance the decor, no more than five should be used in a given area.[6] Colors in grooming and eating areas should be selected to enhance the appearance of the crew's skin and food.

Varying the textures on surfaces and walls can add another significant variable to the decor through both visual and tactile stimulation. For spacecraft, fine, regular patterns are preferable over gross irregular patterns.[15] Rough surfaces, while aesthetically interesting, soil easily in microgravity and are difficult to clean.

White lighting should be used for most living and working areas. The lighting should be designed to minimize glare or hot spots. Ambient flood lighting that provides general interior illumination should be supplemented with task lighting where required. In Chapter 5 of this volume, Wheelwright et al. cover spacecraft illumination in detail.

F. Windows

Windows are one of the most important—and often controversial—aspects of spacecraft architecture. They are essential for providing direct views to support operational, scientific, and recreational objectives; but, at the same time, they create a variety of engineering problems. Windows are heavy; expensive; subject to breakage and scratches; transmit undesirable light, infrared, and ultraviolet energy into the vehicle; and require special covers and/or coatings to keep them usable. Even with these shortcomings, however, windows are considered invaluable for crew well-being and should be included in all spacecraft designs.[5] Skylab crews reported that looking through their wardroom window was their primary leisure activity.[16] Lebedev's diary is full of comments on window observations, making it clear that window viewing was a major activity on his mission and made a significant impression upon him.[11]

Table 3 shows the primary use and location considerations for spacecraft windows. General window design consideration includes the following:

1) Match the window size, location, and effective thickness with the total field-of-view requirements for the anticipated tasks.

2) Provide adequate space around the windows to accommodate the observer in a neutral gravity posture, along with necessary equipment.

3) Provide proper microgravity restraints to allow the observer to remain in position for extended periods of time.

4) Provide shades, filters, and covers to both protect the window surface and control unwanted light and heat.

The shape of the window is also subject to much debate. Round windows are favored by structural engineers, but flight experiences have shown that a straight window edge provides the viewer with valuable orientation cues when being used for proximity operations in which the attitude of a target is important.[17]

Because windows are subject to both internal and external contaminants that can interfere with their use, special precautions need to be taken to protect them. Windows that are not covered during launch will have collected contamination by the time the vehicle achieves orbit. Interior window surfaces are particularly susceptible to fingerprints, hair smudges, urine, food and drink spills, and other floating contaminants. Protective covers, antifog provisions to preclude breath condensation, and a means to clean the window surface should be provided.

II. Activity Centers

"Activity center" is the term used for the various areas or compartments of a spacecraft that support space crews in their work or daily living. The definition of what is or is not an activity center, as well as the grouping of functions that make up an activity center, is somewhat arbitrary and depends upon the mission and crew for a given spacecraft. The activity centers covered here are workstations; personal hygiene and body waste facilities; sleep accommodations; food preparation and dining facilities; and stowage, housekeeping, and recreation areas.

A. Workstations

The term "workstation," as used here, is limited to display and control stations. Most of the requirements and design practices for 1-g workstations also apply to microgravity workstations and will not be reiterated. The guiding principles for workstation designs, display and control panel layouts, and human-computer interfaces are the same as those required for good human factors designs in terrestrial applications. The significant differences in spacecraft workstations are because of the acceleration range that needs to be accommodated and the requirement that a crewmember in a pressure suit must be able to operate interior controls.

The development of space technology has compelled changes in the concept of workstations. There has been a consistent increase in the number of consoles in the central control post of manned spacecraft (for example, from 1 on Vostok to 19 on Mir).

Analysis shows that, compared to the first manned spacecraft, there has been an increase in the total surface area of the face of control consoles, whereas the volume allocated to the consoles has increased only slightly. The number of consoles could be reduced by sharing their use for a number of purposes through signal switching and interchangeable templates on the console faceplate and by coding commands in matrix or digital form.

As mentioned earlier, for a microgravity workstation, the single most important factor to bear in mind is the neutral body posture (Fig. 1), which dictates a raised control surface and a depressed line of sight for display monitoring when compared to normal aircraft or 1-g designs. The layout of a workstation should be designed for a specific operator attitude based upon either the requirements for direct visual monitoring associated with workstation operations or for consistency with the orientation of the surrounding area.

Microgravity restraints for the operator and for checklists, pens, tape recorders, and other loose items are also a significant consideration. Acceptable restraints include foot restraints, waist tethers, and microgravity leg restraints. Any design combining restraints and a workstation must adjust to accommodate the full range of the user population. The magnitude of this range is shown in Fig. 9, which shows a 95th percentile American male and a 5th percentile Japanese female at a space station workstation.

One workstation restraint that does not function very well in microgravity is a chair and a lap belt. Skylab used such a restraint with the solar telescope workstation. Although one

95 PERCENTILE MALE, 20 INCH EYEPOINT

5 PERCENTILE FEMALE, 16 INCH EYEPOINT

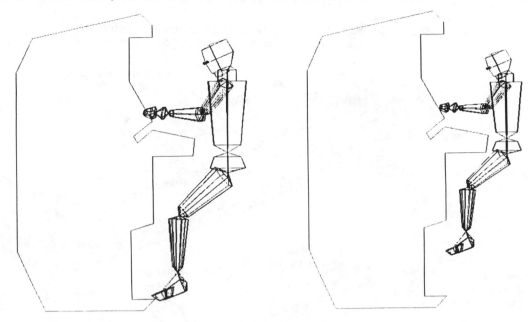

Fig. 9 Space station user population range.

of the crewmembers used it successfully in conventional 1-g fashion, the others found it to be unnatural for microgravity and to cause uncomfortable pressure points.[18]

Controls for operating external hatches, airlocks, and atmosphere/pressure control systems, which may have to be operated to recover a pressurized module following a repair for depressurization, must be designed to meet spacing, force, and handle/knob size requirements for pressure suit operation. In general, this will cause these controls to be larger, spaced farther apart, and have higher, more discernible operating forces and throws.

B. Personal Hygiene and Body Waste Facilities

As Connors et al. pointed out, "the hygienic and waste management facilities of early spaceflight must be considered, at best, primitive."[13] Hygiene and waste collection facilities on Skylab were a significant improvement, but even these had problems. The Skylab 3 crew reported that they used the shower only three times in 59 days because of the time required for preparation and cleanup, and that the water dispenser in the waste management compartment was usable for hand and face washing only if one was very careful.[19] The Shuttle has no shower or hand/face washer, and the commode was a major source of problems for most of the early flights. All in all, there is still much that must be done to provide long-duration space missions with fully satisfactory personal hygiene and waste collection facilities.

In general, the facilities that need to be provided are those for whole and partial body washing; body waste collection; oral hygiene; grooming; and, on longer missions, hair cutting. The detailed design requirements for these types of fa-

cilities are beyond the scope of this chapter, but a few general considerations are worth noting. Ease and comfort of use, privacy, fast cleanup, and control of odor and microbes are all necessities.

Cleanup of both the individual and the equipment associated with personal hygiene functions is much more time-consuming and complicated in microgravity than similar tasks in 1-g. As a result, any design that reduces cleanup effort and time is well worth pursuing. The long-term control of microorganisms and a means to prevent cross-contamination among crewmembers sharing facilities are also required.

Earth's gravity plays a significant role in controlling water flow, separating human wastes from the body, and helping to collect debris such as hair or soapy water. In microgravity, some other method must be provided to perform these same functions. In theory, and in current practice, air flow entrainment can be utilized, but implementation of the design has proven difficult and not always successful, since the forces available from air flow are relatively small for the job, even in microgravity.

C. Sleep Accommodations

The volume allocated for and the design of sleep accommodations depend on the mission duration and whether single- or dual-shift operations are being conducted. Longer mission durations or multishift operations require private and sound and light isolatable sleeping quarters,[6,20] although this has not been observed in every case. Certain crewmembers experience a feeling of isolation and need to keep their fellow crewmembers in sight at all times. Crewmembers have shared sleeping quarters (a hot-bunk) on short-duration, dual-shift

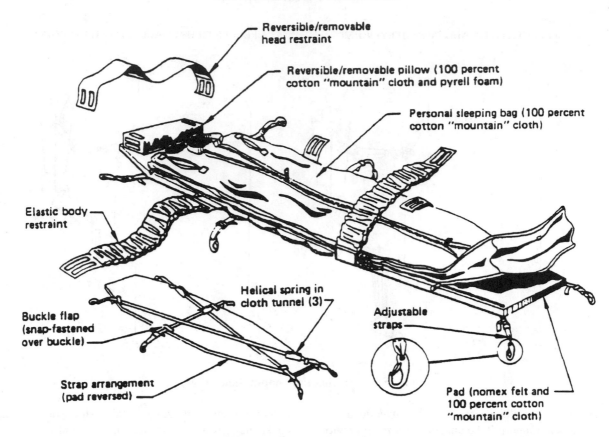

Fig. 10   Typical sleep restraint.

missions; but, for long missions, each crewmember should have his or her own personal space.

Sleep accommodations on early spacecraft were rudimentary to nonexistent. Early space crewmembers slept in their couches, and at least one Mercury crewman reported that he hooked his thumbs under the helmet restraint cables to keep his hands from floating and accidentally activating any switches. He also said that he always had the sensation of sleeping sitting up.[20]

Skylab was the first American spacecraft to provide individual sleep quarters for each astronaut. These sleeping accommodations worked very well and the crews felt that such individual, private quarters would be needed for any long-duration mission.[20] A private sleep compartment requires at least 1.5 m^3 for sleeping and 0.63 m^3 for stowage of personal equipment.[6]

Since crewmembers' requirements for cabin facilities and sleep accommodations differ as a function of psychological characteristics, it is obviously desirable to offer some selection in facilities. For example, a portable folding "bed" equipped with lighting, ventilation, and a sleeping bag that becomes a tent at the head can be set up within the cabin according to individual tastes. When a visiting crew is on the station, this bed may be installed in any other area of the spacecraft. A folding bag may be used for storage of personal items and other accessories and attached to one cabin wall.

Sleep accommodations should include the means to assist the control of body temperature and to restrain a sleeping crewmember. There is much individual preference and variation in the necessary sleep restraint, as Shuttle mission crew reports attest.[16,21-31] Some prefer just to float free and have no restraints. Others want only a simple tether to keep them restrained. Still others prefer to have their head secured or their whole body strapped down to be comfortable. Initially, some crewmembers have reported difficulty with sleeping vertically against a wall or on the ceiling of a sleep compartment, but all have said that the difficulty passed after a few days in microgravity.[26,32] A blindfold and ear plugs have also been used by some to mask sleep-disturbing light and sounds. Figure 10 shows a typical sleep restraint, such the one used on the Shuttle, with the capability for a variety of adjustments to accommodate individual desires.

D. Food Preparation and Eating

Food preparation and eating in microgravity are complicated by three factors. First, traditional food preparation techniques, such as boiling and convection heating, do not work in microgravity. Second, powdery, flaky, or crumbly foods create such a mess in space that they must be avoided (sticky foods or foods in a heavy sauce are acceptable, since they remain in open containers without floating away). Third, spills and food particles do not settle as they do on Earth, complicating cleanup.

Several different methods of food preservation are appropriate for manned spacecraft. Rehydratable foods have been

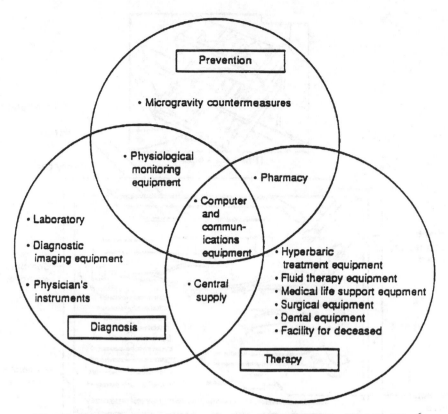

Fig. 11 Function and equipment related to a space medical facility.[6]

the primary type utilized. Thermostabilized, refrigerated, and frozen foods have also been used, but few spacecraft have had a refrigerator or freezer. The commander of the Skylab 4 mission summarized the opinion of most crewmembers when he said, "the frozen food was the best and the thermostabilized food the next best. We would certainly suggest that for extended missions, the rehydratables should be minimized."[33]

Menu selection is, and has been, an important issue with flight crews. A variety of foods and the freedom to make menu changes are considered strong requirements for any long mission. Crews have found a pantry style food stowage and selection system more desirable than a preflight menu selection and stowage of complete meals in a sequence.[22,23,33] Both American and Soviet crews have reported changes in taste in microgravity compared to the ground, noting that food in flight seems blander and less tasty.[33,34]

The following equipment is required for satisfactory food preparation and eating in microgravity[6]:

1) An ambient stowage system (pantry) that is easily accessible, with all food packages clearly marked, provides a means to rapidly review and update the inventory.

2) A means to store, chill, or freeze foods.

3) A means to rehydrate food and drinks.

4) A means to heat food and drinks to at least 66 °C in less than 30 min.

5) Serving and eating utensils.

6) A table where all crewmembers can eat at one time.

7) A means to collect, contain, and stabilize wet and dry trash.

8) Supplies and equipment to clean and sanitize food preparation equipment and reusable utensils.

E. Exercise and Medical Facilities

Exercise and medical equipment are required to support and maintain the health and well-being of the crew.

Exercise capabilities are provided aboard spacecraft to assist in maintaining physical conditioning, to counteract the physiological effects of microgravity, and to provide a recreational outlet. To date, exercise facilities on spacecraft have been limited to those that provide the most benefit for the least volume and weight. Skylab initially provided a bicycle ergometer and an isometric device and later added a treadmill and a spring tension minigym.[13] Salyut and Mir exercise equipment has included a bicycle ergometer, a treadmill that can be used in the active or passive mode, and an elastic and spring exerciser.[34] A passive treadmill is carried on all Shuttle flights. Whatever the devices, the general requirement is that exercise equipment is desirable for all space flights and mandatory for all missions lasting 10 days or longer.[6]

The exercise facility needs to provide an isotonic strength device to exercise the muscles of the upper arm, forearm, thigh, lower leg, and trunk, as well as aerobic exercise equipment for the cardiovascular system. The facility also needs to provide special cooling and ventilation for the increased metabolic load during exercise, noise and vibration control to minimize disturbances to other onboard activities, a means to minimize boredom while exercising, and a means to monitor and

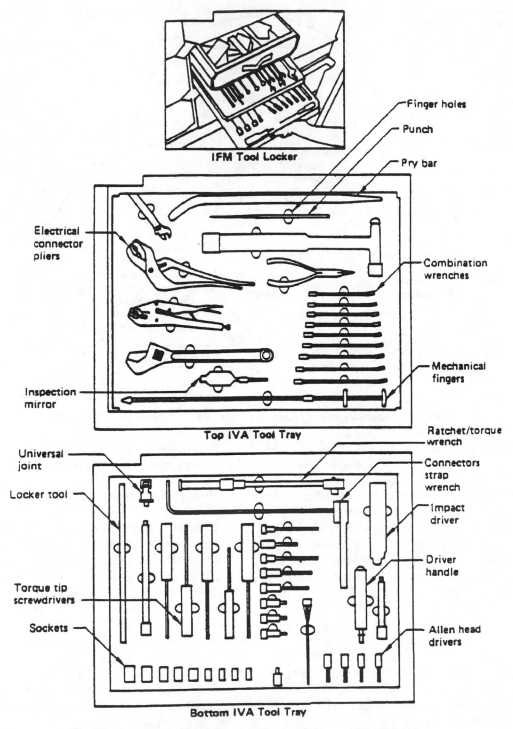

Fig. 12 Examples of IVA hand tools, stowage, and identification.

display exercise physiological data.[6]

Medical equipment is needed aboard a spacecraft to aid in the prevention, diagnosis, and treatment of illness or injuries. The type of medical equipment required is dependent upon the health, age, and number of crewmembers; the duration of the mission; the nature of mission activities; and the level of medical support available both onboard and on the ground. For missions of more than 14 days and for which outside medical treatment is not available upon short notice, a medi-

cal facility should be provided aboard the spacecraft.[6] Figure 11 shows the relationship between the medical functions and the equipment required.[35]

F. Stowage

There never seems to be enough volume to temporarily place things until they are needed. This situation exists in homes, offices, warehouses, boats, planes, and in just about every place that requires a large accumulation of loose items. A manned spacecraft is no exception; and the problem is compounded by weight limitations, severe gravity loading during launch and entry, standardization requirements for equipment interfaces, and a very complex microgravity environment. Growth in stowage requirements can be expected with increased emphasis on long-duration missions, scientific and applications experiments, and the additional equipment to support these activities.[3]

Stowage of loose items for a space flight is a challenge for three reasons. First, they must be packed securely enough to withstand acceleration and vibration during launch. Second, individual items must be packed so that they do not float free when their container is opened but, at the same time, not so tightly that they are difficult to remove or restow. Third, the several thousand stowed items typically carried on a space mission must be arranged logically enough that they are easy to find and can be removed without requiring crewmembers to sort through or remove many other items. Typically systems of lockers, drawers, and bags—each with straps, nets, bungees, or form-fitting foam cushions—have been used to solve these problems.

To contend with these anticipated operational demands, some basic design guides can be followed to optimize stowage configurations. Since the efficient use of crew time is paramount, items should be stowed as near as possible to their point of planned use. This distributed stowage arrangement can make inventory tracking difficult; but, in most cases, from the user's standpoint, it is better than a centralized stowage system. A combination of central and distributed stowage should be considered in the case of the galley, where food for several meals is stowed in the pantry, while the main food supply is stowed in a central facility.[6]

Because of the effort to fully utilize all available space, some customized stowage compartments will endure; however, standardization of stowage containers, compartments, and racks should be the design goal. All stowage locations and stowed items should be coded, using an arrangement compatible with the general space vehicle inventory management system, to allow for quick and easy location, replacement, or inventory review.

Latching devices, containers, and container covers should be of common design, and any associated stowage retainers should be designed for one-hand operation without tools. Stowed items must be secured within any given container so that the item remains in the container/enclosure when the container is opened. Removal of retention devices should not release unneeded items.[6] Tools and maintenance aids require a more systematic stowage approach, since they are used repeatedly. Tools should be placed in a stowage container, properly marked for easy location, and arranged in such a way that a missing item is quickly identified. Figure 12 illustrates examples of proper tool stowage.

In all stowage areas, decals and placards with appropriate instructions should be visible to minimize crew training and save time during mission operations.

G. Housekeeping

The importance of housekeeping in a confined, crowded environment cannot be overemphasized, because it directly affects crew health, safety, comfort, morale, and productivity. Long-duration missions will increase the need for effective and efficient housekeeping capabilities and provide the impetus for developing new housekeeping aids.

It is ironic that the beneficiaries of good housekeeping practices (flight crews) are, in fact, the principal sources of microbes, chemicals, and debris that cause housekeeping problems (fingernail clippings, hair, dead skin, fingerprints, perspiration, body oils, clothing lint, food spills, etc.). Microgravity causes this ostensibly unlimited supply of refuse, once released, to migrate and lodge on all surfaces, especially in cracks and crevices that are difficult to reach.

It follows then that a key solution to housekeeping problems begins with a crew compartment design in which materials used for all interior surfaces are selected to minimize particulate and microbial contamination and surfaces are easy to clean (smooth, solid, nonporous). Narrow openings and crevices should be avoided when possible, and closures/closeouts should be provided as needed. Spacecraft contamination control during ground buildup and handling, from manufacturing to launch, must be effectively enforced. Since experience has shown that most particulate matter eventually collects on protective screens and filters, these elements should be easily accessible for replacement or cleaning without the risk of dispersing the trapped material.[6] Although crewmembers have voiced concern about the excessive noise levels, limited suction, and available attachments of vacuum cleaners, they have used vacuum cleaners effectively on Skylab and Shuttle to remove and dispose of dust, lint, liquids, and other debris. Mold and mildew flourish on surfaces that are damp, poorly ventilated, and improperly lit; therefore, personal grooming, dining, and food preparation areas should be designed with proper ventilation and illumination.

Trash management is a critical problem because of the limited space for stowing trash until it can be off-loaded or disposed of, and the fact that, in microgravity, the trash expands to fill the available volume of its container. In addition, trash always occupies more space than the original packaging, compounding the problem. Special care must be taken to design receptacles so that new trash can be deposited without letting old trash escape, or requiring the crewmember to stick a hand into the old trash to deposit a new piece. Wet trash, which can promote bacterial growth, needs to be separated from dry, inert trash and needs to have a vented compartment, biocide, or some other means to control gas and odor buildup.

Food and drink spills can be cleaned with wet rags, but odor-causing debris and waste disposal area cleanup require biocide wipes. A single-step biocide that does not have to be rinsed off is recommended as a time saver. Aerosol biocides may prove useful. It is expected that missions of longer duration with larger crew complements will require increased use of chemical cleansers to handle contamination and odor problems. Care must be taken to ensure that all planned cleansers are compatible with the components of the space vehicle environmental control system.

Properly designed dishwashers and clothes washers can aid good housekeeping, but the tradeoffs between benefits and additional weight, power, and stowage requirements will probably restrict their use to long-duration missions. The same tradeoffs apply to the use of trash compactors. The basic utility of a trash compaction system is very attractive, but the impact in terms of crew time required to gather and sort trash, operate the system, and then properly stow the compacted trash, is unknown. The system may require separation of biologically active and inert trash in order to facilitate safe stowage and disposal.[6] Also, not all trash is compactible and the resulting specialized trash bags may require excessive stowage space. A prototype trash compaction system is being flown on Space Shuttle missions.

H. Provisions for Recreation

Extensive studies pertaining to people living in relative isolation have provided interesting material on preferences for leisure time activity. As one might expect, the order of preference varies significantly, depending on individual personalities, duration of mission, and type of environment; e.g., Antarctica, submarines, space flight, launch sites, and bunkers. There are, however, some focused conclusions that provide meaningful design criteria for space-flight recreation equipment and facilities.

Leisure time contributes to the working efficiency of the crew and, to restore work capacity, there need to be selectable leisure time activities.[34] Individuals in isolation prefer work to inactivity, and they spend almost twice as much time eating as they do under normal conditions. The most popular activities among isolated groups include conversation, reading novels, and watching movies and television.[14]

Table 4, compiled by Eberhart from questionnaires sent to 30 NASA astronauts[14] and Skylab mission reports[16,19] indicate that viewing through windows and listening to taped music were popular activities during leisure periods. Space Shuttle crew reports[21,23] identify the tape player as a preferred recreational device, even though the Space Shuttle missions were relatively short in duration. Physical exercise continues to be a valued leisure time activity and contributes significantly to the well-being of the crew. Valentin Lebedev mentioned several times in his book, "Diary of a Cosmonaut: 211 Days in Space,"[11] that a favorite event was real-time communications with family members. American astronauts have agreed. Special recreational devices, such as darts, playing cards, checkers, chess, puzzles, and model kits designed specifically for use in microgravity, have been made available to cosmonauts and astronauts but did not receive high ratings.

The playing of musical instruments, a pleasing pastime on Earth, presents some problems in space vehicles. Most popular musical instruments, aside from being relatively large and difficult to stow, are enjoyed only by the player and become,

Table 4 Recreation equipment used by 30 astronauts in order of preference[14]

Use of equipment in spacecraft	Importance
Viewing through windows	1
Physical exercise equipment	2.5
Tape recorder, record player	2.5
Books	4
Sports equipment	5
Radio	6
Newspapers	7
Magazines	8
Photographic equipment	9
Radio equipment for personal communication	10
Television	11
Writing equipment	12
Playing cards	13

more often than not, an annoyance to the "captive" audience.

A quick review of the preceding comments would indicate that designs for an effective microgravity recreation facility should include, as a minimum, provisions for reading (electronic reproduction of text is recommended for long-duration missions), physical exercise, listening to music, communications with friends and family on Earth, movies, and looking out a window at space and Earth. General accommodations for adding various microgravity games and supplies for inventing new games should also be considered. Table 5 lists design considerations for a basic recreation facility.

IV. Restraints and Mobility Aids

As spacecraft and space habitats increase in size and complexity, added emphasis must be placed on human and equipment restraints and mobility aids, if human work capacity is to approach comparable Earth levels. The size of compartments, passageways, and workstations is a significant factor in determining the need for and design of restraints and mobility aids. Obviously, smaller volumes that allow fast, convenient crew contact with walls, ceilings, and floors require only a few simple devices, as opposed to surroundings so large that no two surfaces can be contacted simultaneously.

A. Human Restraints and Mobility Aids

Experience reports and comments from crew debriefings indicate that many features of vehicle interior designs (e.g., corners, indentations, gaps, handles, and other protrusions) can and will be used as substitute restraints and mobility aids

Table 5 Recreation facility design considerations based on recreation activity

Recreation activity	Design considerations
Reading	Restraints or seating in isolated locations Adequate illumination at reading surface Quiet for concentration Storage area for books or other reading material
Conversation	Comfortable furnishings arranged to promote social interaction Noise level below speech interference level Reduce illumination Proximity to galley
Observation	Proximity to windows Image enhancements (binoculars, telescope) Reduced illumination
Visual entertainment (movies, tapes, etc.)	Variable illumination Visual entertainment equipment, storage areas, power supplies Arrangement of restraints or seating for visibility
Games—active	Proximity to personal hygiene facilities Adjustable ventilation and thermal controls to accommodate increased activity Clear area and furnishing storage area Padding Storage area for games equipment (including personal protective gear) Acoustical and dynamic isolation from sensitive areas of the module
Music listening	Audio generation equipment, storage location, power Musical selections, storage location Speakers (room or individual)

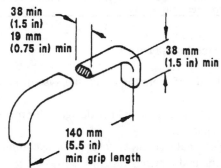

Fig. 13 Example of IVA handhold configuration used in previous U.S. space modules.[6]

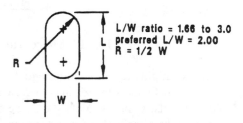

Fig. 14 IVA handhold cross-section.[6]

and should be structurally sound to accommodate this function and avoid inadvertent breakage. While some of these features suffice as impromptu aids, their planned use as such should be discouraged in the interest of both efficiency and safety.

Crew comments from Skylab and Shuttle flights strongly indicate that foot restraints—as opposed to waist, thigh, lower leg, and hand restraints—are the most usable and provide better stability during prolonged operations at workstations.

Some combinations of the different designs have been utilized for unique applications; however, if properly designed workstations are provided with adequate foot restraints, additional body restraints are not required.

Handholds and handrails are favored over all others as the most efficient translation aids but should have standardized dimensions to facilitate gripping and equipment mounting. Figures 13 and 14 show the dimensions and cross-section patterns used on the Apollo, Skylab, and Space Shuttle programs. Distinctive, contrasting colors that are clearly visible under all conditions of illumination should be used to identify structurally secure handholds. Also, commonality for all

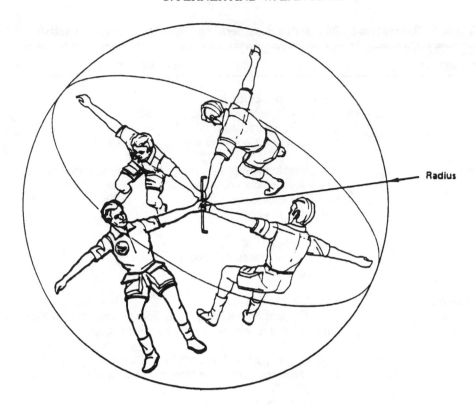

	Radius of fingertip reach boundary
95th percentile male	195 cm (77 inches)
5th percentile female	150 cm (63 inches)

Notes: (Fig. 15)

a. Subjects — These data were generated using a computer-based anthropometric model. The computer model was developed using a sample of 192 male astronaut candidates and 22 female astronaut candidates measured in 1979 and 1980. The 5th percentile stature of the male population is 167.9 cm (66.1 inches), and the 95th percentile male stature is 189.0 cm (74.4 inches). The 5th percentile stature of the female population is 157.6 cm (62.0 in.) and the 95th percentile female is 175.7 cm (69.2 in.).

b. Gravity conditions — Although the motions apply to a microgravity condition, the effects of spinal lengthening have not been considered.

Fig. 15 Microgravity handhold restraint reach boundaries.[6]

restraint devices is a highly desirable design goal.

Figures 15, 16, and 17 show the reach boundaries for foot and handhold restraints. Foot restraints should be designed to withstand minimum loads in tension and torsion of 445 N and 200 N, respectively, with a yield factor of safety of 1.10 and an ultimate factor of safety of 2.0.[6] Basic foot restraint load limits are illustrated in Fig. 18.

General personal restraints, including seat belts; shoulder harnesses; and body, foot, and sleep restraints should comply with the following requirements[6]:

1) Restraint forces should be reasonably distributed over the body to prevent discomfort, and the crewmember should not have to exert a conscious effort to remain restrained.

2) Comfort of the IVA restraint system should allow for a 4-h uninterrupted use.

3) Restraint design should minimize or eliminate muscular tension.

4) All personal restraints should accommodate the spe-

cific population of users for which the system is to be designed.

5) Personal restraints should be designed for microgravity posture compatibility.

6) The personal restraint system should accommodate on-orbit cleaning and repair.

The capability to quickly and effectively restrain loose equipment in microgravity is mandatory. Everything—from large consoles to small nuts and bolts—needs some means of retention at stowage and worksites to keep them from floating free. Skylab and Space Shuttle experience has shown that a wide variety of devices, including duct tape, bungee cords, snaps, Velcro®, straps, tethers, clips, nets, and bags, can be used with some degree of success.

Figure 19 illustrates some commonly used equipment restraints. As a general guide, restraints of this type should be standardized, multipurpose, and easy to use and stow; and no tools should be required to operate them.

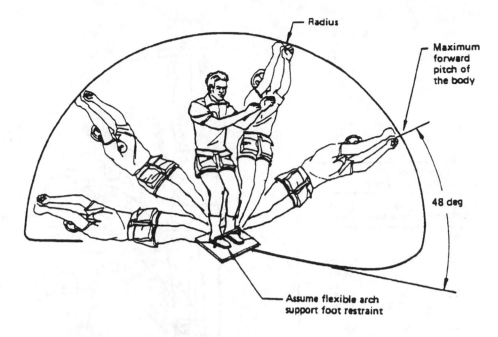

	Radius of reach fingertip boundary in X-Z plane	
	Flexible arch support foot restraint	Fixed "flat" foot restraint
95th percentile male	222 cm (87 in)	212 cm (83 in)
5th percentile female	188 cm (74 in)	172 cm (68 in)

Notes: (Fig. 16)

a. Subjects — These data were generated using a computer-based anthropometric model. The computer model was developed using a sample of 192 male astronaut candidates and 22 female astronaut candidates measured in 1979 and 1980. The 5th percentile stature of the male population is 167.9 cm (66.1 inches), and the 95th percentile male stature is 189.0 cm (74.4 inches). The 5th percentile stature of the female population is 157.6 cm (62.0 in.), and the 95th percentile female is 175.7 cm (69.2 in.).

b. Gravity conditions — Although the motions apply to a microgravity condition, the effects of spinal lengthening have not been considered.

c. Restraint configuration — Two sets of dimensions are given for the fore/aft reach boundary. One set, the larger dimensions, apply to a fairly snug, but flexible, arch support that allows the toes and heels to raise slightly from the floor. The other set of dimensions apply to a foot restraint that secures the feet flat to the floor.

Fig. 16 Microgravity foot restraint reach boundaries—fore/aft.[6]

B. Equipment Mounts and Fasteners

Launch and landing accelerations/vibrations, plus free floating in microgravity while on orbit, combine to make fasteners for equipment essential. Since the launch and landing problems are not unlike well-documented aircraft situations, the emphasis here will be on the microgravity aspects. Fasteners on any spacecraft should be standardized, and the number of types should be minimized to reduce the number of different types of tools required. Even if in-flight maintenance is not planned, it will occur if there is a human on board to help fix a problem. This means that fasteners used on access doors, containers, panels, equipment stowage, covers, restraints, or any replaceable unit should be selected with crew operational capabilities and limitations in mind. To minimize the number of tools required to operate fasteners, the crew workload required in gathering appropriate tools, and the potential for using the wrong tool, tool-actuated and hand-actuated fasteners should also be of a common type and size. Each type of fastener must be readily distinguishable from

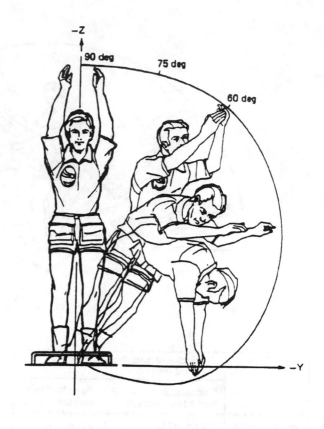

Dimensions of fingertip reach boundary in Y-Z plane			
	Angle (degrees)	Y-axis dimension	Z-axis dimension
95th percentile male	90	0	222 cm
	75	80 cm (31 in)	193 cm (76 in)
	60	110 cm (43 in)	160 cm (63 in)
5th percentile male	90	0	188 cm (74 in)
	75	28 cm (11 in)	175 cm (69 in)
	60	80 cm (31 in)	140 cm (55 in)

Notes: (Fig. 17)

a. The angle is measured between the x-axis and a line drawn from the center of the foot restraint to the reach boundary.
b. The full reach boundary (up to 0 degree angle) will be provided in the next revision of this document.
c. These data were generated using a computer-based anthropometric model. The computer model was developed using a sample of 192 male astronaut candidates and 22 female astronaut candidates measured in 1979 and 1980 (Reference 365). The 5th percentile stature of the male population is 167.9 cm (66.1 inches), and the 95th percentile male stature is 189.0 cm (74.4 inches). The 5th percentile stature of the female population is 157.6 cm (62.0 in.), and the 95th percentile female is 175.7 cm (69.2 in.).
d. Although the motions apply to a microgravity condition, the effects of spinal lengthening have not been considered.

Fig. 17 Microgravity foot restraint reach boundaries—side to side using flexible arch support foot restraint configuration.[6]

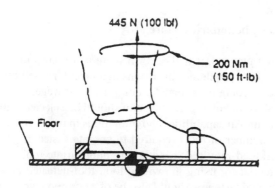

Fig. 18 IVA foot restraint load limits.[6]

all others to minimize the risk of inserting one in the wrong location.

Hand-operated, partial-turn fasteners are always preferred and are mandatory for frequent use applications. Remember, in microgravity, the operator will most likely have only one hand to use (the other being used for position/restraint), and any applied force or torque will be reacted back to the operator. In microgravity, using a screwdriver to loosen a fastener is a very difficult and frustrating task. High-torque applications should use internal hexagonal head designs to keep the tool on the fastener. Figure 20 shows hand torque capabilities for different size fasteners under two different restraint conditions. Table 6 illustrates torque values by knob size for a 5th percentile male.

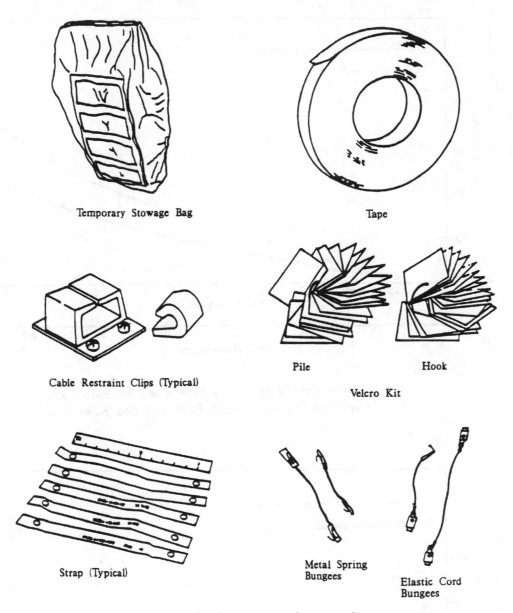

Temporary Stowage Bag

Tape

Cable Restraint Clips (Typical)

Pile

Hook

Velcro Kit

Strap (Typical)

Metal Spring Bungees

Elastic Cord Bungees

Fig. 19 Equipment restraint examples.

V. Miscellaneous Design Considerations

A. Maintainability

When new space ventures are planned with the attendant austere budgets and short lead time schedules, system maintainability all too often appears near the bottom of the priority list. No matter how well a piece of hardware is designed, constructed, tested, and operated, it will eventually need some degree of maintenance. It is prudent to specify, then, that all orbital equipment that will be accessible to crew personnel should be designed to accommodate planned and contingency in-flight maintenance.

In a general sense, this means that consideration must be given, early in the equipment design process, to physical access; visual access; removal, replacement, and modularity requirements; fault detection and isolation requirements; and provisions for a maintenance data management system.

Since crew time is a scarce commodity, preventive maintenance should not require special skills, lengthy training, or complicated tools, and prescribed schedules should be sufficiently flexible to accommodate time changes in other mission activities. If critical systems operations would be interrupted in order to permit planned maintenance, redundant installations should be considered. Effective maintainability is not without time, weight, and volume penalties; therefore, the time and effort involved in corrective maintenance must be weighed against the cost and feasibility of carrying replacement units. Maintainability requirements are provided in Table 7.

A key factor in establishing an in-flight maintenance capability is the selection of the right supporting tools. A generalized approach, used successfully in the Skylab and Space Shuttle programs, is to develop a tool kit based on systems

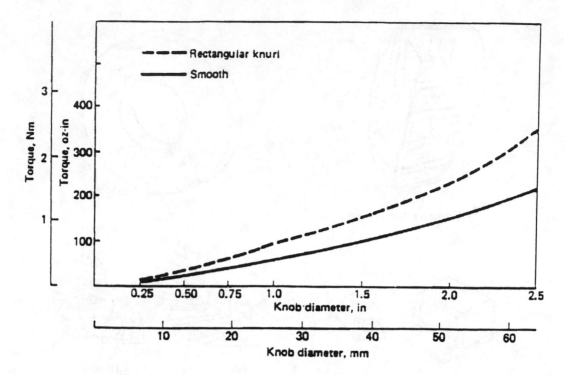

Hand Torque Capabilities When Restrained by Both Feet,
Both Feet and Pelvis, or Both Feet and One Hand (IVA)

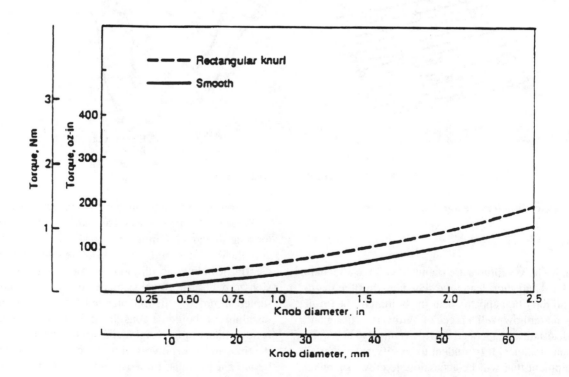

Hand Torque Capabilities When Restrained by One Hand (IVA) [6]

Fig. 20 Hand torque capabilities.[6]

Table 6 Torque by knob size (values for 5th percentile male)[6]

Knob diameter		Rim surface					
		Rectangular knurl		Diamond knurl		Smooth	
cm	in.	Ncm	lb-in	Ncm	lb-in.	Ncm	lb-in
0.3	1/8	2.3	0.2	3.4	0.3	0.3	0.03
0.6	1/4	.8.8	0.6	7.9	0.7	2.3	0.2
1.0	3/8	11.3	1.0	12.4	1.1	4.5	0.4
1.3	1/2	14.7	1.3	17.0	1.5	6.8	0.5
1.6	5/8	22.6	2.0	20.3	1.8	9.0	0.8
1.9	3/4	27.1	2.4	27.1	2.4	15.8	1.4
2.2	7/8	32.8	2.9	32.8	2.9	15.8	1.4
2.5	1	45.2	4.0	40.7	3.6	17.0	1.5
3.2	1-1/4	44.1	3.9	49.7	4.4	22.6	2.0
3.8	1-1/2	63.3	5.6	59.9	5.3	38.4	3.4
4.4	1-3/4	81.4	7.2	83.6	7.4	42.9	3.8
5.1	2	97.2	8.6	91.5	8.1	50.9	4.5
5.7	2-1/4	116	10.3	116	10.3	71.2	6.3
6.4	2-1/2	140	12.4	131	11.6	93.8	8.3
7.0	2-3/4	174	15.4	173	15.3	88.1	7.8
7.6	3	181	16.0	179	15.8	94.9	8.4
8.9	3-1/2	220	19.5	244	21.6	147	13.0
10.2	4	280	24.8	290	25.7	164	14.5
11.4	4-1/2	320	28.3	330	29.2	208	18.4
12.7	5	380	33.6	392	33.8	244	21.6

requirements, tempered with past maintenance/repair experience.

A basic tool kit should include normal multipurpose and multisize tools required for comprehensive usage, as well as special tools required for unique aerospace hardware. Despite the urge to reduce tool kit weight by not including sockets, wrenches, and other tools that have no identified requirements, crewmembers have requested that all sizes be included, since unexpected needs invariably arise for the tool that was left behind.[6] Until a single measurement standard is implemented, both English and metric wrenches and sockets must be included in the tool kit; an appropriate tool coding system should readily distinguish English from metric.

Power tools can be used to accomplish repetitive manual tasks, such as disengaging large numbers of captive fasteners or operating mechanical drive systems. These kinds of tools, although very efficient, can subject the user to specific hazards and stresses. Examples include electric shock, heat, fly-

Table 7   Maintainability design requirements (adapted from Ref. 6)

Item	Requirement
Growth and update	Facilities, equipment, and software design shall allow reconfiguration and growth during the mission.
Independence	Systems and subsystems shall be as functionally, mechanically, electrically, and electronically independent as practical to facilitate maintenance.
Maintenance support services	Maintenance support services (e.g., electrical outlets) shall be accessible at potential problem locations or at a designated maintenance location.
Reliability	Equipment design shall reduce to a minimum the incidence of preventive and corrective maintenance.
Simplicity	Equipment design shall minimize maintenance complexity.
Time requirements	Equipment design shall minimize the time requirements for maintenance.
Equipment	Maintenance equipment and tools shall be kept to a minimum.
Hazardous conditions	System design shall preclude the introduction of hazardous conditions during maintenance procedures.
Critical operations	Critical systems shall be capable of undergoing maintenance without interrupting critical services and shall be maintained.
Noncritical operations	Noncritical systems shall be designed to operate in degraded modes while awaiting maintenance. Degraded mode operation shall not cause additional damage to the system or aggravate the original fault.
Redundancy loss	Notification of loss of operational redundancy shall be provided immediately to the crew.
Connectors	Quick-disconnect connectors shall be used.
Plug-in installation	Plug-in type hardware installation and mounting techniques shall be employed.
Quick-release fasteners	Quick-release fasteners shall be used where consistent with other requirements (e.g., strength, sealing).
Replacement capabilities	Capacity of replaceable or reserviceable items (filters, screens, desiccant units, battery power supplies, etc.) shall be higher than the minimum functional requirements of the system.
Automation	Fault isolation, inspection, and checkout tasks shall be automated to the extent practical.
Restraints	Personnel and equipment mobility aids and restraints shall be provided to support maintenance.
Special skills	Maintenance requiring special skills shall be minimized.
EVA	Maintenance requiring EVA shall be minimized.
Soldering, welding, and brazing	Soldering, welding, brazing, and similar operations during maintenance shall be minimized.

ing particles or sparks, and hazards to the non-operating hand or nearby equipment. Attention must be given to electrical safety precautions and hazardous electromagnetic interference. The designer should review and understand such hazards and remove them whenever possible. When this cannot be accomplished, appropriate warning labels on the tool and/ or properly worded warnings in the instructional material should recommend the use of protective clothing or devices— eye protectors, special grounding devices, and gloves.

Special restraints required to operate the tool during

Table 8 Cover and closeout requirements (adapted from Ref. 6)

Item	Requirement
Sealing	The inaccessible areas shall be sealed to prevent small items from drifting into them.
Removal	Closures shall be quickly and easily removed to allow maintenance of equipment.
Securing	It shall be obvious when a closure is not secured, even though it may be in place.
Loads	Nonstructural closures should be capable of maintaining closure and of sustaining a crew-imposed minimum design load of 451 N (125 lbf) and a minimum ultimate load of 632 N (175 lbf).
Instructions	If the method of opening a cover is not obvious from the construction of the cover itself, instructions (including applicable tool instructions) shall be permanently displayed on the outside of the cover.
Clearance	Bulkheads, brackets, and other units shall not interfere with removal or opening of covers.
Application	An access cover shall be provided whenever frequent maintenance operations would otherwise require removing the entire case or cover or dismantling an item of equipment.
Self-supporting covers	All access covers that are not completely removable shall be self-supporting in the open position.
Ventilation screen access	Where ventilation screens, holes, or grids are used, the ventilation surface shall be accessible for vacuuming in its installed position.

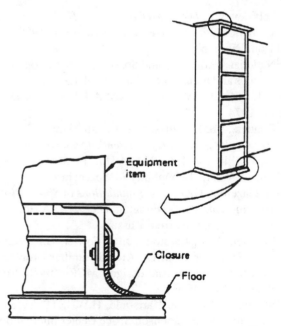

Fig. 21 Example of use of closure.[6]

any given task should be identified as part of the design process. Previous orbital missions indicate that, when properly restrained, crewmembers can perform most manipulative operations on orbit as effectively as on Earth, using standard tools.[6]

B. Closeouts

All systems utilizing electrical power and moving parts require some form of protective closure to protect the equipment and provide a measure of safety for the operators. Well-designed closures and closeouts take on added importance in a microgravity environment because of the presence of floating items. Anything that is not restrained is a potential problem.

Design requirements for all spacecraft equipment housings (e.g., electrical bays, cabinets, lockers, and consoles) should specify that effective closures and covers are necessary to prevent loose items such as small tools, fasteners, and refuse from drifting. Small items cannot be retrieved easily if they migrate into inaccessible locations; they may drift into areas where they could cause damage to mechanical or electrical components or become permanently lost inside an equipment housing.[6] Applicable cover and closeout requirements are listed in Table 8. Figure 21 illustrates a typical console-to-floor closure.

C. Connectors and Cable Management

Connectors are essential for assembling and disassembling equipment during the construction and checkout phase and later during maintenance. The number of different types of connectors used to meet electrical, fluid, and structural design requirements is enormous, and it is not practical for the purpose of this chapter to deal specifically with each configuration. However, the basic human factors considerations relative to connector design can be extensively applied to all configurations.

Connectors, like other mechanical devices, are not totally reliable; and, since most are susceptible to failure, they should be used only where needed to provide fast, easy maintenance, removal, and replacement of components and units. Acceptable connectors should be designed to minimize danger to personnel and equipment caused by content spills, electrical shocks, or damage from the release of stored mechanical energy during mating or demating. Multiple rows of connectors are undesirable; but, if required, the connectors should be staggered.[6]

All connectors, whether operated by hand or tool, should be designed so that they can be mated/demated using one hand. It should be possible to mate/demate or replace individual connectors without having to remove or replace other connectors. Quick disconnects for fluids that are designed to be operated under pressure will not require pressure/flow indicators. Connectors should be selected, designed, and installed so they cannot be mismated or cross-connected. Connectors in a single row should be spaced to allow for hand access during alignment and insertion.[6]

If connectors on the ends of loose electrical cables or fluid hoses are not identical, each end should be uniquely identified to prevent improper usage. The loose ends of hoses and cables should be restrained to prevent them from floating out of reach and to avoid injury to crewmembers and damage to equipment.[6] Connectors should incorporate readily distinguishable identification marks, alignment pins/keys, and any necessary coding to support fast, easy, and safe crew operations.

VI. Conclusion

Human systems is one of the broadest disciplines involved in spacecraft design. Everything a space crewmember can see, touch, hear, taste, or smell is involved, along with all those things with which he or she can interact mentally. The principles of human engineering and crew equipment design for terrestrial applications are well documented, and many apply equally well to the design of spacecraft interiors. Any differences will be the result of the closed, multigravity or microgravity environment. This chapter has attempted to highlight some of the primary effects or concerns when designing inhabited areas for that "different" extraterrestrial environment.

References

[1]National Aeronautics and Space Administration. Man-systems integration standards for Space Station Freedom, Revision A, Vol. IV. NASA-STD-3000, Houston, NASA Johnson Space Center, June 1991.

[2]Fraser, T.M. The effects of confinement as a factor in manned spaceflight. NASA CR-511, Houston, NASA Johnson Space Center, 1966.

[3]Loftus, J. An historical review of NASA manned spacecraft crew stations. Paper delivered at International Conference for Transportation Studies, Amalfi, Italy, Oct. 1983.

[4]Wise, J.A. Quantitative modeling of human spatial habitability. Moffett Field, Calif., NASA Ames Research Center, Dec. 1989.

[5]National Aeronautics and Space Administration. Lessons learned on the Skylab program. Houston, NASA Johnson Space Center internal document, Mar. 1974.

[6]National Aeronautics and Space Administration. Man-systems integration standards, Rev. A. NASA-STD-3000, Houston, NASA Johnson Space Center, Oct. 1989.

[7]Harrison, A.A.; Caldwell, B.; Struthers, N.J.; and Clearwater, Y.A. Incorporation of privacy elements in Space Station design. Final Report to NASA, Moffett Field, Calif., NASA Ames Research Center, May 1988.

[8]Nixon, D. Space station group activities habitability model study. NASA CR-4010, Moffett Field, Calif., NASA Ames Research Center, Nov. 1986.

[9]Lockheed Missiles & Space Co. Space Station human productivity study. LMSC-F060784, NASA report, Nov. 1985.

[10]National Aeronautics and Space Administration. Evaluation of Skylab IVA architecture, Skylab Experience Bulletin No. 18. JSC-09552, Houston, NASA Johnson Space Center, Dec. 1975.

[11]Lebedev, V.V. *Diary of a Cosmonaut: 211 Days in Space.* College Station, Tex., Phyto Resources Research, 1988 (translated from Russian).

[12]National Aeronautics and Space Administration. Translation modes and bump protection, Skylab Experience Bulletin No. 1. JSC-09535, Houston, NASA Johnson Space Center, June 1974.

[13]Conners, M.M.; Harrison, A.A.; and Akins, F.R. *Living Aloft: Human Requirements for Extended Spaceflight.* NASA SP-483, Washington, D.C., NASA Hq., 1985.

[14]Petrov, Yu.A. Habitability of Spacecraft. In: Calvin, M., and Gazenko, O.G., Eds. *Foundations of Space Biology and Medicine, Vol. III.*. Washington, D.C., NASA Hq., 1975, pp. 157–193 (translated from Russian).

[15]Rosener, A.A.; Baratono, J.R.; Fowler, B.F.; Karnes, E.W.; and Stephenson, M.L. Architectural/environmental handbook for extraterrestrial design. MCR-70-446, Martin Marietta Co., Nov. 1970.

[16]Mattingly, T.K., and Hartsfield, H.W. STS-4 crew report. Houston, NASA Johnson Space Center internal document, Aug. 1982.

[17]Haines, R.F. Space station proximity operations and window design. NASA TM 88233, Moffett Field, Calif., NASA Ames Research Center, 1986.

[18]National Aeronautics and Space Administration. Body restraint systems, Skylab Experience Bulletin No. 10. JSC-09544, Houston, NASA Johnson Space Center, Dec. 1974.

[19]Bobko, K.J.; Williams, D.E.; Seddon, M.R.; Griggs, S.D.; and Hoffman, J.A. STS-51D flight crew report. Houston, NASA Johnson Space Center internal document, Jan. 1986.

[20]National Aeronautics and Space Administration. Architectural evaluation for sleeping quarters, Skylab Experience Bulletin No. 3. JSC-09537, Houston, NASA Johnson Space Center, July 1974.

[21]Lousma, J.R., and Fullerton, C.G. STS-3 flight crew report. Houston, NASA Johnson Space Center internal document, Oct. 1982.

[22]Brand, V.D.; Overmyer, R.F.; Allen, J.P.; and Lenoir, W.B. STS-5 flight crew report. Houston, NASA Johnson Space Center internal document, Mar. 1983.

[23]Weitz, P.J.; Bobko, K.J.; Peterson, D.H.; and Musgrave, F.S. STS-6 flight crew report. Houston, NASA Johnson Space Center internal document, 1983.

[24]Crippen, R.L.; Hauck, F.H.; Fabian, J.M.; Ride, S.K.; and Thagard, N.E. STS-7 flight crew report. Houston, NASA Johnson Space Center internal document, Aug. 1983.

[25]Truly, R.H.; Brandenstein, D.C.; Gardner, D.A.; Bluford, G.S.; and Thornton, W.E. STS-8 flight crew report. Houston, NASA Johnson Space Center internal document, July 1984.

[26]Young, J.W.; Shaw, B.H.; Parker, R.A.; and Garriott, O.K. STS-9 flight crew report. Houston, NASA Johnson Space Center internal document, June 1984.

[27]Brand, V.D.; Gibson, R.L.; McCandless, B. II; McNair, R.E.; and Steward, R.L. STS-41B flight crew report. Houston, NASA Johnson Space Center internal document, June 1984.

[28]Crippen, R.L.; Scobee, F.R.; Hart, T.J.; Van Hoften, J.D.; and Nelson, G.D. STS-41C flight crew report. Houston, NASA Johnson Space Center internal document, May 1984.

[29]Hartsfield, H.W.; Coats, M.L.; Mullane, M.; Hawley, S.A.; and Resnik, J.A. STS-41D flight crew report. Houston, NASA Johnson Space Center internal document, Jan. 1985.

[30]Crippen, R.L.; McBride, J.A.; Sullivan, K.D.; Ride, S.K.; and Leestma, D.C. STS-41G flight crew report. Houston, NASA Johnson Space Center internal document, Dec. 1984.

[31]Hauck, F.H.; Walker, D.M.; Allen, J.P.; Fisher, A.L.; and Gardner, D.A. STS-51A flight crew report. Houston, NASA Johnson Space Center internal document, Mar. 1985, NASA.

[32]National Aeronautics and Space Administration. Skylab experiment M487: habitability/crew quarters. JSC-09677, TMX-58163, Houston, NASA Johnson Space Center, Oct. 1975.

[33]National Aeronautics and Space Administration. Food system, Skylab Experience Bulletin No. 19. JSC-09553, Houston, NASA Johnson Space Center, Feb. 1976.

[34]Bluth, B.J., and Helppie, M. Soviet space stations as analogs, second edition. NASA CR-180920, Washington, D.C., NASA Hq., Aug. 1986.

[35]Medical Operations Branch, National Aeronautics and Space Administration. Space Station Health Maintenance Facility status update. Houston, NASA Johnson Space Center internal document, Feb. 1986.

Part II:

Life Support Systems

Chapter 8

Metabolic Energy Requirements for Space Flight

Helen W. Lane

The international space community, including Japan, Germany, the European Space Agency, the Russian Federation (formerly the Soviet Union or U.S.S.R.), and the United States, is preparing for extended stays in space. Much of the research planned for space will be tended by humans; therefore, maintaining adequate nutritional status during long stays in space has become an issue of much interest. Historically, it appears that on space missions of short or moderate duration minimum nutritional requirements have been met.[1-3] Thus far, crewmembers have been able to consume adequate food to maintain nominal performance in microgravity. However, plans call for increases in the duration of certain future flights, including interplanetary missions. This means that special attention must be devoted to the capacity of flight rations to fully meet the nutritional needs of space crews exposed to microgravity and other flight factors. At the same time, it is essential to minimize the weight, size, and power requirements of the life support systems on such flights. These requirements can be based only on experimental data collected on actual space flights.

For this reason, the current review is focused on energy utilization during the Apollo lunar missions, Skylab's extended space laboratory missions, and Space Shuttle flights. Available data include those recorded during intravehicular activity (IVA) and extravehicular activity (EVA), as well as data acquired during microgravity simulation (bed rest). Data on metabolism during flight and bed rest will be discussed, with a followup on the human gastrointestinal function.

The energy expended by humans during many activities in 1-g (Table 1) has been calculated using a variety of methods. Human energy utilization during space flight has been determined indirectly using several methods, including recording food intake (diet history) and studying metabolic balance, food disappearance, and respiratory gas production.[2-5] The most detailed nutritional studies, which were performed during the Skylab missions, included dietary records in combination with metabolic balance studies.[4] The energy levels of Skylab menus were determined directly using bomb calorimetry and indirectly using crewmember records to calculate the amounts of carbohydrates, proteins, and fat consumed (see

Table 2). Energy levels of stools were determined directly by bomb calorimetry, and these data were used to calculate energy availability. Apparent energy intake was calculated as energy in the diet minus the energy found in the urine and stools.

The energy level of food consumed before flight did not differ from that of food consumed during flight (Table 2). The length of the flight had no effect on apparent energy availability from foods consumed. Mean energy available in kcal ($\pm$ SD) was, at 28 days, 2686 $\pm$ 141; at 59 days, 2939 $\pm$ 538; and at 89 days, 2972 $\pm$ 78. For comparison, preflight resting energy expenditure (REE) was also calculated for the Skylab crewmembers using the Harris-Benedict equation (Table 2).[6] Apparent energy intake was about 1000 kcal/day greater than the Harris-Benedict measure of REE.

The type of energy consumed before flight, however, differed from in-flight intake; i.e., carbohydrate intake was significantly higher, and fat intake was significantly lower during flight than before. In an effort to identify the primary substrate for energy utilization, nonprotein respiratory quotients (RQs) were calculated from existing measurements of resting $\dot{V}_{O_2}$ and $\dot{V}_{CO_2}$ levels (J. Leonard, personal communication). These measurements had been taken before, during, and after flight over 5-min periods while the subjects were at rest, at three levels of exercise, and during recovery. Mean RQ values corrected for urinary nitrogen are shown in Table 3. Interestingly, the mean RQ during flight was higher than preflight or postflight RQ for all measurements except exercise level 1. An increase in RQ has been interpreted as reflecting a shift from fat to carbohydrate as the primary substrate for energy utilization (Table 4).[6] Furthermore, an RQ greater than 1.0 implies the occurrence of lipogenesis.[6] The increase in carbohydrate intake during flight and the continued loss of lean body mass,[7,8] taken together, support the conclusion that the Skylab crewmembers increased their utilization of carbohydrates during flight.[9]

Table 5 shows changes in body weight during the Skylab missions. Although Leach and colleagues have estimated a fluid loss of approximately 900 mL,[9-11] some evidence exists that weight loss may include loss of fat and lean body mass as well as fluid.[11] The small but persistent negative nitrogen balance during Skylab flights (Table 5) suggests that the major component of the nonfluid weight change may have

The contribution of Christine Wogan to the preparation of this paper is acknowledged with appreciation.

Table 1 Energy expenditure in selected household, recreational, and sports activities[a]

Activity	Energy expended (kcal·min^{-1}·kg^{-1})	Energy expended (kcal/min) for an 80-kg (176-lb) person	Activity	Energy expended (kcal·min^{-1}·kg^{-1})	Energy expended (kcal/min) for an 80-kg (176-lb) person
Archery	0.065	5.20	Golfing	0.085	6.80
Badminton	0.097	7.80	Gymnastics	0.066	5.28
Basketball	0.138	11.00	Lying at ease	0.022	1.76
Bookbinding	0.038	3.00	Painting, inside	0.034	2.72
Card playing	0.025	2.00	Painting, outside	0.077	6.16
General carpentry	0.052	4.20	Running cross country	0.163	13.04
Circuit training:			Running, 11.5 min/mile	0.135	10.80
Hydra-fitness	0.132	10.56	Running, 7 min/mile	0.228	18.24
Universal	0.116	9.28	Scrubbing floors (F)	0.109	8.72
Nautilus	0.092	7.36	Scrubbing floors (M)	0.108	8.64
Free weights	0.086	6.88	Sitting quietly	0.021	1.68
Cleaning (F)	0.062	4.96	Snowshoeing, soft snow	0.166	13.28
Cleaning (M)	0.058	4.64	Standing quietly (F)	0.025	2.00
Cooking (F)	0.045	3.60	Standing quietly (M)	0.027	2.16
Cooking (M)	0.048	3.84	Table tennis	0.068	5.44
Cycling:			Tennis	0.109	8.72
at 5.5 mph	0.064	5.12	Typing (electric)	0.027	2.16
at 9.4 mph	0.090	7.20	Typing (manual)	0.031	2.48
racing	0.169	13.52	Walking, normal pace		
Drawing (standing)	0.036	2.88	Asphalt road	0.080	6.40
Eating (sitting)	0.023	1.84	Fields and hillsides	0.082	6.56
Electrical work	0.058	4.64	Writing (sitting)	0.029	2.32
Fishing	0.062	4.96			

[a]Adapted from McArdle, W.D.; Katch, F. I.; and Katch, V. L. *Exercise Physiology: Energy, Nutrition, and Human Performance.* 2nd Edition, Appendix D, pp. 642–649, Philadelphia, 1986, Lea and Febiger.

been loss of lean body mass. The concurrent presence of an RQ greater than 1.0 and a negative nitrogen balance suggests that some lean body mass may have been replaced with fat. The Skylab crewmembers tended to lose more weight during the shorter flights than the longer ones. The original explanation for this effect was that inadequate energy had been provided during the earlier, shorter flights. During the longest Skylab flight (84 days), both available energy from food and the length of in-flight exercise increased; mean body weight loss, in contrast, decreased. Exercise and increased energy supplied in food, therefore, appeared to counteract body weight loss. However, the combination of chronic negative

nitrogen balance, maintenance of body weight, and RQ greater than 1.0 suggests that space flight may induce or encourage the replacement of lean body mass with fat.[11,12] These interactions will become still more important as the duration of space flights lengthens and crews undertake the physical work involved in EVA for Space Station construction.

Because the Skylab crewmembers consumed metabolic diets as part of the mission, some quantification of nutrient intake, output, and energy utilization was possible. In contrast, the U.S. Space Shuttle Program has no requirement for monitoring individual intake; therefore, the few data that are available reflect only patterns of food consumption among

Table 2 Nutritional intake of Skylab crewmembers

Subject	Days of study Preflight	Days of study Flight	Carbohydrate[a] Preflight	Carbohydrate[a] Flight	Fat[a] Preflight	Fat[a] Flight	Protein[a] Preflight	Protein[a] Flight	Apparent energy[b] Preflight	Apparent energy[b] Flight	REE[c]
1	30	28	319	376	105	76	103	101	2668	2649	1487
2	30	28	382	402	101	80	108	105	2903	2774	1768
3	30	28	364	394	109	72	110	97	2931	2634	1776
4	20	59	331	426	98	66	95	95	2648	2666	1613
5	20	59	315	368	110	76	112	107	2763	2592	1521
6	20	59	490	565	132	77	163	148	3877	3560	1921
7	26	84	363	398	108	100	121	118	2949	2959	1602
8	26	84	358	395	108	92	113	111	2882	2901	1654
9	26	84	348	385	116	109	127	128	3005	3055	1600
Mean ± SD			363±52	412±60[d]	110±10	83±14[d]	117±19	111±18	2958±367	2865±307	

[a] Grams per day.
[b] kcal per day defined as total energy consumed minus (stool energy + urine energy).
[c] Resting energy expenditure calculated from Harris-Benedict equation.[5]
[d] Preflight intake differed from in-flight values ($p < 0.05$).

Table 3 Respiratory quotient of Skylab crewmembers (N=9)

Time period	5-min pre-exercise rest	Exercise level, (% $\dot{V}_{O_2}$ max) 25%	Exercise level, (% $\dot{V}_{O_2}$ max) 50%	Exercise level, (% $\dot{V}_{O_2}$ max) 75%	5-min recovery postexercise
Preflight	0.887 ± 0.099[a]	0.840 ± 0.081	0.907 ± 0.0501[a]	0.939 ± 00.030[a]	1.201 ± 0.055[a]
In flight	1.041 ± 0.088[b]	0.854 ± 0.056	0.955 ± 0.043[b]	1.021 ± 0.051[b]	1.384 ± 0.116[b]
Postflight	0.901 ± 0.095[a]	0.829 ± 0.056	0.907 ± 0.048[a]	0.976 ± 0.031[a]	1.212 ± 0.072[a]

[a,b] Values in the same column that have different superscripts are significantly different (<0.05) using general linear model procedures and Tukey's Studentized range test.

the crews. Energy requirements are calculated from the Harris-Benedict equation for basal energy expenditure (BEE),[6] which accounts for height, weight, age, and sex. Male crewmembers are judged to require 1.7 times their BEE and females 1.6 times their BEE. Nutrient content is calculated to meet the dietary allowances recommended by the National Academy of Sciences.

Some indirect assessments of energy utilization from Space Shuttle flights are presented in Table 6. Mean dietary intakes during the first eight Shuttle missions were calculated from the disappearance of food from the food lockers;[4] these data were compared to mean atmospheric CO_2 produced during each flight (unpublished data). Mean energy utilization per person ranged from 1910 to 3576 kcal/day; if data from STS-2, during which a large amount of CO_2 was produced, is eliminated, the high end of the range is reduced to 2760 kcal/day. Although these methods are less reliable than those used on Skylab, the energy utilization values are, nonetheless, similar for the Shuttle and Skylab missions.

Energy utilization has also been calculated from metabolic CO_2 production during EVAs on the lunar surface. Energy utilization on the Moon ranged from about 120–400 kcal/h.[13–15] By comparison, preflight EVA training sessions in

the Weightless Environment Training Facility (WETF) at NASA Johnson Space Center tended to require more energy than that required for similar activities on the Moon (Table 7). The energy used in working on the Moon fell within the range for similar activities on Earth. Walking on the Moon and collecting geological samples at 250 kcal/h, for example, is comparable to a brisk walk while lifting light objects on Earth.[6] The energy expended riding in the lunar rover was very similar to that spent driving an automobile on Earth.[6] Energy utilization during Skylab EVA in space was remarkably consistent, ranging from 200–250 kcal/h.[15] These data suggest that one might be able to predict the energy required for performing planetary activities from knowledge of requirements for performing similar activities on Earth.

From studies completed thus far, the total energy intake required to function in space appears to be similar to that required for 1-g activities; i.e., approximately 2000 to 3000 kcal/day, depending on lean body mass and activity level. This conclusion is far from definite, however, because of the sketchy data from Shuttle flights, and because crew activity levels and performance were not assessed in conjunction with these preliminary energy studies. Russian cosmonauts are reported to consume up to 3200 kcal/day; however, they also

Table 4 Thermal equivalent of oxygen for nonprotein respiratory quotient[a]

Nonprotein RQ	kcal/L O$_2$ consumed	Percentage derived from		g/L O$_2$ consumed	
		Carbohydrate	Fat	Carbohydrate	Fat
0.707	4.686	0	100	0.000	0.496
.71	4.690	1.10	98.9	.012	.491
.72	4.702	4.76	95.2	.051	.476
.73	4.714	8.40	91.6	.090	.460
.74	4.727	12.0	88.0	.130	.444
.75	4.739	15.6	84.4	.170	.428
.76	4.751	19.2	80.8	.211	.412
.77	4.764	22.8	77.2	.250	.396
.78	4.778	26.3	73.7	.290	.380
.79	4.788	29.9	70.1	.330	.363
.80	4.801	33.4	66.6	.371	.347
.81	4.813	36.9	63.1	.413	.330
.82	4.825	40.3	59.7	.454	.313
.83	4.838	43.8	56.2	.496	.297
.84	4.850	47.2	52.8	.537	.280
.85	4.862	50.7	49.3	.579	.263
.86	4.875	54.1	45.9	.621	.247
.87	4.887	57.5	42.5	.663	.230
.88	4.899	60.8	39.2	.705	.213
.89	4.911	64.2	35.8	.749	.195
.90	4.924	67.5	32.5	.791	.178
.91	4.936	70.8	29.2	.834	.160
.92	4.948	74.1	25.9	.877	.143
.93	4.961	77.4	22.6	.921	.125
.94	4.973	80.7	19.3	.964	.108
.95	4.985	84.0	16.0	1.008	.090
.96	4.998	87.2	12.8	1.052	.072
.97	5.010	90.4	9.58	1.097	.054
.98	5.022	93.6	6.37	1.142	.036
.99	5.035	96.8	3.18	1.186	.018
1.00	5.047	100.0	0	1.231	.000

[a]Reproduced from McArdle, W.D.; Katch, F.I.; and Katch, V.L. *Exercise Physiology: Energy, Nutrition, and Human Performance.* 2nd Edition, Philadelphia, 1986; Lea and Febiger, p. 127.

exercise strenuously daily.[3] Studies of how exercise affects energy requirements in space are just beginning. Variables such as energy substrates (carbohydrate, protein, and fat), level and type of activity (e.g., exercise countermeasures), and fluid shifts may have a profound effect on energy requirements for space flight. Furthermore, data from Skylab suggest that the relationship of REE to total energy expenditure may differ in space; i.e., energy expenditure at rest may be higher and en-ergy utilization during physical activity may be lower in space compared to 1-g. Studies correlating these potentially confounding factors have yet to be performed.

Horizontal or head-down bed rest is used as a model to mimic microgravity-induced changes in the human musculoskeletal system,[16] the advantage being the capability to collect extensive biochemical data under well-controlled conditions. Shangraw et al.[17] found that 7 days of bed rest did not change blood glucose levels in six healthy men; however, their basal plasma glucagon and insulin were higher during bed rest than during the ambulatory-control period (Table 8). Furthermore, their glucose and insulin responses to glucose tolerance tests were higher during the bed-rest period than during the control period. These results are similar to those of Dolkas and Greenleaf,[18,19] who found higher plasma insulin levels—but not plasma glucose levels—during a glucose tolerance test on day 10 of a 14-day bed rest. These results, which are suggestive of increased carbohydrate utilization during bed rest, are intriguing in light of increased RQ during flight (see above). In one of these studies,[18] isotonic exercise during bed rest diminished the hyperinsulinemia, suggesting that isotonic exercise during flight may ameliorate the effect of microgravity on carbohydrate metabolism. Interestingly, more body weight was lost during bed rest with isotonic exercise than without exercise, demonstrating that significant energy was used during the exercise.[19]

Other investigators from both the U.S. and the U.S.S.R. have reported slight increases in blood glucose early during flight, followed by a decrease.[20,21] In the second expedition of the Salyut 4 orbital station,[21] the crew's blood glucose and lactic acid levels rose slightly after 2 days and 7 days of flight relative to preflight values. Slight increases in blood glucose and insulin have also been noted during bed rest. In another study, Grigoriev and co-workers[22] compared blood, insulin, and free fatty acid levels before, 1 day after, and 7 days after flights of 4 to 14 days. Fatty acid levels were lower and serum insulin levels were higher 1 day after flight than they were before flight; insulin levels remained elevated until 7 days after landing. In contrast, no preflight-to-postflight differences were found in blood glucose, lactic acid, or pyruvic acid. Although these data are inconclusive, it is possible that they may reflect a shift to carbohydrate and protein as primary energy substrates. Alternatively, one might speculate that the increased insulin levels during flight are associated with increased lipogenesis, perhaps reflecting a decrease in the efficiency of energy utilization in space. More in-flight data are needed to explore these speculations.

Energy can also be derived from the metabolism of tissues. U.S. and Soviet scientists have noted decreases in lean body mass during space flight, which implies catabolism of protein. The nitrogen levels of Skylab crewmembers' stools were no different in flight than before flight, indicating that consumed protein was digested normally. In contrast, nitrogen was increased in their urine, suggesting that the nitrogen balance was negative (Table 5). This negative nitrogen balance occurred even during Skylab 4, an 84-day flight, despite adequate to high protein intake (Table 2), as well as an energy intake sufficient to maintain body weight after taking fluid loss into account.[23] The Soviets found elevated serum levels of amino acids at landing;[24] however, it is unclear whether this was a result of cosmonauts' high-protein diet[2] or, perhaps, mobilization of amino acids from tissues to the liver. Furthermore, protein synthesis may be depressed in microgravity.[25] This hypothesis will be studied on U.S. and

Table 5 Body weight changes and nitrogen balance in Skylab crewmembers

Crew-member	Length of flight (days)	Body weight changes in flight (kg)	Nitrogen balance (g/day)[a]	
			Preflight	In flight
1	28	-2.3	2.95	-0.96
2	28	-2.3	3.12	-2.22
3	28	-2.3	3.00	-1.71
4	52	-3.6	3.07	-0.99
5	52	-2.7	3.42	-0.78
6	52	-2.7	4.05	-0.81
7	84	-0.9	3.31	-1.24
8	84	-1.8	2.20	-0.68
9	84	-1.4	2.78	-0.06

[a]Reproduced from Ref. 10.

Table 6 Energy consumed and utilized on U.S. Space Shuttle flights

STS mission	Mean energy calculated from		Difference (%)
	Food disappearance, (kcal/day/person)	CO_2 production (kcal/day/person)	
1	2565	2568	0
2	2200	3576	62
3	1910	2688	41
4	2446	2616	7
5	2322	2712	17
6	1957	2664	36
7	2535	2424	-4
8	2517	2760	10

Table 7 EVA metabolic rates during 1-g training and during flight (Apollo 15)[a]

Activity	Training, 1-g (kcal/h)	EVA, lunar surface (kcal/h)
Maintaining lunar outpost	445	228
Driving lunar rover	203	123
Average of all activities	393	230

[a]Reproduced from Ref. 13.

Table 8 Glucose and insulin responses during 7 days of bed rest[a,b]

	Basal concentrations				Glucose tolerance test			Daily urinary excretion	
Activity	Blood glucose (mg/dL)	Plasma glucagon (pg/mL)	Plasma insulin (μU/mL)	Plasma cortisol (μU/dL)	Glucose area (mg/hr/dL)	Insulin area (μU/hr/mL)	Cortisol (μg/24 h)	Meta-nephrine (mg/24 h)	Normeta-nephrine (mg/24 h)
Control	74±3	109±6	6.7±0.6	15±2	305±27	108±22	44±4	225±22	228±27
Bed rest	74±3	128±7[c]	9.5±1.6[c]	19±1	355±27[c]	155±32[c]	51±4[c]	229±11	245±17[c]

[a]Values are means ± SD for six subjects.
[b]Reproduced from Ref. 18.
[c]Significantly different from control (p <0.05).

European Spacelab flights. In any case, it is clear that crewmembers are using tissue protein for energy. Theoretically, therefore, adjustments in diet and exercise protocols may counteract the loss of lean body mass and the use of body protein as an energy source. However, this supposition requires empirical verification.

Some animal data exist, also, to supplement the minimal human data available from space flight. Unfortunately, access to animals flown in space is frequently delayed for hours to days, and readaptation to 1-g thus confounds interpretation of results. Nevertheless, a few studies of the effects of microgravity on rats have been performed. Two groups of investigators have analyzed body weight, feed intake, and liver enzyme changes in rats that flew on Cosmos 1887 and compared the results to control animals under similar housing, lighting, and feeding conditions.[26,27] Interestingly, these rats lost weight during flight. This result was explained as an increase in energy utilization to compensate for heat loss, since the rats were unable to curl up and decrease their surface area in microgravity. These results, although intriguing, suggest that rodents may not be a valid model for determining energy requirements in humans. In a related study, the activity of three microsomal hepatic enzymes (hepatic aniline hydroxylase, ethylmorphine N-demethylase, and P_{450} cytochrome oxidase) from rats exposed to microgravity was decreased relative to the control rats.[27] Although these enzymes are not related directly to energy metabolism, the possibility is raised that enzyme regulation is also affected by microgravity. The lower T_3, lower thyroxine, and higher corticosterone levels in the microgravity-exposed rats compared to the control rats may suggest endocrinological changes as well.

Energy metabolism can be affected, also, by changes in the gastrointestinal (GI) function, which influences the absorption and metabolism of nutrients. Although neurovestibular adaptation is believed to be responsible for the unpleasant GI effects of space motion sickness, the GI effects themselves tend to depress appetite, which leads to reduced food and fluid intake. Approximately 50 percent of space travelers show some symptoms of space motion sickness during the first few days in flight; some have experienced illness during the entire mission.[28] The decreased GI motility associated with motion sickness, coupled with the

reduced food and fluid intake, can easily affect nutritional status after a relatively short time. The presence of motion sickness symptoms, therefore, can be used as an indirect indicator of potential changes in nutritional status as well as the GI function.

Another rough estimate of the GI function can be made by tracking the number of stools produced and their wet and dry weight over time. None of these parameters changed during Skylab missions (Table 9). It should be noted, however, that stool number or weight provides no information on the availability or absorption of specific nutrients during space flight. A Russian report suggests that intestinal microflora may be affected by space flight;[29] however, far more data are needed before conclusions can be drawn with certainty.

The GI function is also influenced by fluid status and the presence or absence of gravitational vectors.[29–31] The fluid redistribution that occurs during horizontal bed rest has been shown to slow GI transit time.[31] Furthermore, appetite is depressed during periods of reduced GI motility.[32] Thus, although there is no direct evidence of the effect of microgravity on nutrient and micronutrient availability, clearly this area also needs further exploration.

The effect of space flight on fluid-electrolyte metabolism is discussed in detail in Volume III of this series, *Humans in Space Flight*. The present chapter describes only those aspects that determine water balance in humans exposed to space. From a nutritional standpoint, water intake in food and fluid and output in stools, urine, and sweat can be used to calculate how much water is used in metabolism and lost through evaporation. In the Skylab missions, total body water was determined using the isotope (^{3}H) dilution method before and immediately after flight.[9] The three crewmembers on the 84-day flight showed changes in total body water of -900, -600, and -900 mL after flight, as compared to preflight values of 100, 200, and 700 mL, respectively. Mean urinary and stool water losses for two of these crewmembers were similar before and after flight (urine, 1660 ± 161 and 1681 ± 113 mL; stool, 77 ± 26 and 61 ± 81 mL). However, water ingested from foods and fluids was significantly higher before flight than during flight (3293 ± 225 vs. 2953 ± 45 mL/day). Evaporative water losses before and during flight were 1938 ± 69 mL/day and 1597 ± 40 mL/day, respectively;

Table 9 Effect of space flight on stool production in nine Skylab crewmembers

Time	Number of stools/day	Wet weight (grams)	Dry weight (grams)
Preflight	0.72±0.19	81.5±33.6	25.4±4.7
In flight	0.54±0.26	69.9±19.0	23.9±4.8
Postflight	0.55±0.2	51.4±35.4	23.6±6.1

the latter calculation takes the decrease in total body water and water balance during flight into account.[9] In order to correct for weight loss in two of the three crewmembers, evaporative water loss was also calculated in terms of body surface area. These calculations also showed decreased evaporative losses during flight [1096 ± 39 mL/day/m^2 (preflight) and 903 ± 22 mL/day/m^2 (in flight)]. It should be noted that Skylab atmospheric conditions were different than present-day Space Shuttle conditions. However, the decrease in evaporative water loss may be due in part to weightlessness, since sweat remains on the skin in microgravity rather than dripping off. Skylab 4 included a fan, which provided increased air convection; however, as noted above, evaporative losses were still lower in flight than they had been before flight. Much research directed at elucidating the neuroendocrine mechanisms responsible for maintaining water balance in space is underway.

This review has focused on the energy required to live and work in space. Although well-controlled nutritional studies have been few, several conclusions can be drawn from existing data. First, the availability of food and the stool weight during Skylab flights were no different than before flight. It appears that the energy required for performing activities in space is at least as high as for ground-based activities; however, the difference may lie in a change in resting energy utilization in space rather than in the actual energy required to perform work in space. The persistent negative nitrogen balance is puzzling and requires further study to support development and application of appropriate countermeasures. Both American and Russian data suggest that lean body mass may be replaced with fat during flight; this issue needs to be addressed, too. Finally, the results from one Russian study with rats suggest that rodents may not be the best model for determining energy requirements in humans. Water balance studies also performed during Skylab suggest that space flight does not affect total fluid loss in stool and urine, but may decrease fluid intake and evaporative loss.

For the future, research on energy utilization during space flight must include the development of reliable predictions of energy requirements, particularly for long-duration flights. In light of evidence of elevated blood glucose levels and increased RQ during flight, the best balance of substrate (carbohydrate or fat) for maintaining optimal metabolism should be determined. The role of exercise in negative nitrogen balance, and potentially concurrent reductions in strength, must be investigated. Finally, little information is available concerning the role of micronutrients, such as vitamins, in energy utilization. Although significant progress has been made, more research is needed to ensure that, as flights lengthen, space crews can remain healthy and perform optimally in space.

References

[1]Johnson, P.C.; Leach, C.S.; and Rambaut, P.C. Estimates of fluid and energy balances on Apollo 17. *Aerospace Medicine,* 1973, vol. 44, no. 11, pp. 1227–1230.

[2]Calloway, D.H. Basic data for planning life-support systems. In: Calvin, M., and Gazenko, O.G., Eds. *Foundations of Space Biology and Medicine*, Washington, D.C., NASA Hq., 1975, vol. III, pp. 3–21.

[3]Bychko, V.P.; Ushakov, A.S.; Kalandarov, S.; Markaryan, M.V.; Sedova, Ye A.; Sivuk, A.K.; and Khokhlova, O.S. Diet of crew on the Salyut-6 orbital station. *Kosmicheskaya Biologiya i Aviakosmicheskaya Meditsina,* 1982, vol. 16, no. 2, pp. 10–13 (in Russian).

[4]Rambaut, P.C.; Leach, C.S.; and Leonard, J.I. Observations in energy balance in man during spaceflight. *American Journal of Physiology,* 1977, vol. 233, no. 5, pp. R208–212.

[5]Stadler, C.R.; Rapp, R.M.; Bourland, C.T.; and Fohey, M.F. Space Shuttle Food-System Summary, 1981–1986. NASA TM-100469, Washington, D.C., NASA Hq., 1988, p. 335.

[6]Bursztein, S.; Elwyn, D.H.; Askanazi, J.; and Kinney, J.M., Eds. *Energy Metabolism, Indirect Calorimetry and Nutrition.* Baltimore, Md., Williams and Wilkins, 1989.

[7]Thornton, W.E., and Ord, J. Physiological mass measurements in Skylab. In: Johnston, R.S., and Dietlein, L.F., Eds. *Biomedical Results from Skylab,* NASA SP-377, Washington, D.C., NASA Hq., 1977, pp. 175–182.

[8]Thornton, W.E., Hoffler, G.W., Rummel, J.A. Anthropometric changes and fluid shifts. In: Johnston, R.S., and Dietlein, L.F., Eds. *Biomedical Results from Skylab,* NASA SP-377, Washington, D.C., NASA Hq., 1977, pp. 330–338.

[9]Leach, C.S.; Leonard, J.I.; Rambaut, P.C.; and Johnson, P.C. Evaporative water loss in man in a gravity-free environment. *Journal of Applied Physiology,* 1978, vol. 45, no. 3, pp. 430–436.

[10]Leach, C.S. An overview of the endocrine and metabolic changes in manned space flight. *Acta Astronautica,* 1981, vol. 8, no. 9–10, pp. 977–986.

[11]Leonard, J.I.; Leach, C.S.; and Rambaut, P.C. Quantitation of tissue loss during prolonged space flight. *American Journal of Clinical Nutrition*, 1983, vol. 38, pp. 667–679.

[12]Michel, E.L.; Rummel, J.A.; Sawin, C.F.; Buderer, M.C.; and Lem, J.D. Results of Skylab medical experiment M-171 metabolic activity. In: Johnston, R.S., and Dietlein, L.F., Eds. *Biomedical Results from Skylab*, NASA SP-377, Washington, D.C., NASA Hq., 1977, pp. 372–387.

[13]Waligora, J.M.; Hawkins, W.R.; Humbert, G.F.; Nelson,

L.J.; Vogel, S.J.; and Kuznetz, L.H. Apollo experience report: Assessment on metabolic expenditures. NASA Technical Note D-7883, Washington, D.C., NASA Hq., 1975.

[14]Waligora, J.M., and Horrigan, D.J. Metabolism and heat dissipation during Apollo EVA periods. In: Johnston, R.S.; Dietlein, L.F.; and Berry, C.A., Eds. *Biomedical Results from Apollo,* NASA SP-368, Washington, D.C., NASA Hq., 1975, pp. 115–128.

[15]Waligora, J.M., and Horrigan, D.J. Metabolic cost of extravehicular activities. In: Johnston, R.S., and Dietlein, L.F., Eds. *Biomedical Results from Skylab,* NASA SP-377, Washington, D.C., NASA Hq., 1977, pp. 395–399.

[16]Dietrick, J.E.; Whedon, G.D.; and Shorr, E. Effects of immobilization upon various metabolic and physiologic functions of normal man. *American Journal of Medicine,* 1948, vol. 4, pp. 3–36.

[17]Shangraw, R.E.; Stuart, C.A.; Prince, M.J.; Peters, E.J.; and Wolfe, R.R. Insulin responsiveness and protein metabolism in vivo following bedrest in humans. *American Journal of Physiology (Endocrinology and Metabolism),* 1988, vol. 225, pp. E548–E558.

[18]Dolkas, C.B., and Greenleaf, J.E. Insulin and glucose responses during bedrest with isotonic and isometric exercise. *Journal of Applied Physiology,* 1977, vol. 46, no. 6, pp. 1033–1038.

[19]Greenleaf, J.E.; Bernauer, E.M.; Juhos, L.T.; Young, H.L.; Morse, J.T.; and Staley, R.W. Effects of exercise on fluid exchange and body composition in man during 14-day bedrest. *Journal of Applied Physiology,* 1977, vol. 43, no. 1, pp. 126–132.

[20]Leach, C.S.; Alexander, W.C.; and Johnson, P.C. Endocrine, electrolyte, and fluid volume changes associated with Apollo missions. In: Johnston, R.S.; Dietlein, L.F.; and Berry, C.A., Eds. *Biomedical Results of Apollo,* NASA SP-368, Washington, D.C., NASA Hq., 1975, pp. 163–184.

[21]Tigranyan, R.A.; Popova, I.A.; Belyakova, M.I.; Kalita, N.F.; Tuzova, Ye G.; Sochilina, L.B.; and Davydova, N.A. Results of metabolic studies on the crew of the second expedition of the Salyut-4 orbital station. *Kosmicheskaya Biologiya I Aviakosmicheskaya Meditsina,* 1977, no. 2, pp. 48–53 (in Russian).

[22]Grigoriev, A.I.; Popova, I.A.; and Ushakov, A.S. Metabolic and hormonal status of crewmembers in short-term space flights. *Aviation, Space, and Environmental Medicine,* 1987, vol. 58, no. 9, pp. A121–125.

[23]Rambaut, P.C., and Johnson, P.C. Nutrition. In: Nicogossian, A.E.; Huntoon, C.L.; and Pool, S.L., Eds. *Space Physiology and Medicine*, Philadelphia, Lea and Febiger, 1989, pp. 202–213.

[24]Popov, I.G., and Latskevich, A.A. Effect of 140-day flight on blood amino acid levels in cosmonauts. *Kosmicheskaya Biologiya i Aviakosmicheskaya Meditsina,* 1983, vol. 17, no. 2, pp. 23–30 (in Russian).

[25]Schonheyer, F.; Heilskov, N.S.C.; and Olesen, K. Isotopic studies of the mechanism of negative nitrogen balance produced by immobilization. *Scandanavian Journal of Clinical Investigations,* 1954, vol. 6, pp. 178–188.

[26]Grindeland, R.E.; Popova, I.A.; Vasques, M.; and Arnaud, S.B. Cosmos 1887 mission overview: Effects of microgravity on rat body and adrenal weights and plasma constituents. *FASEB Journal,* 1990, vol. 4, pp. 105–109.

[27]Merrill, A.H.; Hoel, M.; Wang, E.; Mullins, R.E.; Hargrove, J.L.; Jones, D.P.; and Popova, I.A. Altered carbohydrate, lipid, and xenobiotic metabolism by liver from rats flown on Cosmos-1887. *Federal Proceedings,* 1990, vol. 4, pp. 95–100.

[28]Homick, J.L., and Vanderploeg, J.M. The neurovestibular system. In: Nicogossian, A.E.; Huntoon, C.L.; and Pool, S.L., Eds. *Space Physiology and Medicine.* Philadelphia, Lea and Febiger, 1989, pp. 154–166.

[29]Smirnov, K.V., and Lizko, N.N. Problems of space gastroenterology and microenvironment. *Die Nahrung,* 1987, vol. 31, pp. 563–566.

[30]Nimmo, W.S., and Prescott, L.F. The influence of posture on paracetamol absorption. *British Journal of Clinical Pharmacology*, 1978, vol. 5, pp. 348–349.

[31]Groza, P. Digestive reactions to simulated and real space flight. *Physiologie,* 1988, vol. 25, pp. 207–231.

[32]Meyer, J.H. Motility of the stomach and gastroduodenal junction. In: Johnson, L.R., Ed. *Physiology of the Gastrointestinal Tract,* 2nd edition, New York, Raven Press, 1987, pp. 613–629.

Chapter 9

Air Regeneration in Spacecraft Cabins

A. S. Guzenberg

Air regeneration is one of the major aspects of space crew life support. In pressurized spacecraft cabins the air regeneration subsystem scrubs the atmosphere of carbon dioxide, harmful trace contaminants, and water vapor until their levels meet acceptability criteria. Air regeneration also provides the crew with oxygen by maintaining acceptable levels in the cabin atmosphere.

In an emergency, humans can survive without food for more than a month and without water for several days, but a crew cannot remain conscious in a pressurized cabin for more than a few hours after the air regeneration subsystem stops functioning, even when the cabin is comparatively large.

On Earth humans are but a single component of a complex ecological system with human waste products being assimilated by the biosphere and transformed into the substances required for life. Creating an analogous biological cycle on a spacecraft would be an extremely complicated undertaking given the low energy efficiency of natural processes, their unreliability in a small volume, and the high launch weight of the required equipment. For this reason, the gas cycle is supported on spacecraft through special physicochemical methods of substance regeneration. For short-term flights, air regeneration can rely on stored supplies of gases and chemicals. Systems of this type are extremely simple and reliable, and use only a few watts of power. However, their weight increases in direct proportion to flight duration and crew size. Thus for flights of very long duration, subsystems must be developed to regenerate oxygen from human waste products. These subsystems are complex, consume power in amounts up to several hundred watts, and have significant fixed weight. For example, given the need to provide backup subsystems and ensure a high level of reliability, their weight can reach over 150 kg for a crew of three. The weight of regenerative subsystems, however, is virtually independent of flight duration (the only stores these subsystems need are replacements for components).[1,2,3]

Between the extremes of these two air regeneration subsystems, exists a third alternative that combines features of both. These are the semiregenerative or partially closed subsystems with various degrees of closure, such as are used on

current manned space flights. Such subsystems remove carbon dioxide using regenerable absorbers and produce oxygen through electrolysis of purified condensates of atmospheric moisture, or crew urine, or through partial conversion of carbon dioxide (CO_2) to obtain oxygen (O_2) through the Sabatier reaction.

The need to increase the efficiency of long-term space stations in Earth orbit, to minimize costs of delivering cargo to orbit, and particularly to develop interplanetary spacecraft will stimulate more complete closure of the air regeneration cycle. For flight durations beyond a certain period, supplies of substances and chemicals will be stored only as backups.

The schematic diagram of air regeneration in Fig. 1 depicts both of the structural principles that can underlie air regeneration subsystems; i.e., use of stored supplies or of a closed substance cycle. The hierarchical structure of air regeneration subsystems is presented in Fig. 2.

This chapter describes various physicochemical methods and hardware for regenerating air. It considers nonregenerative methods for disposing of CO_2 and water vapor and for producing O_2 through the use of stored supplies of substances, as well as regenerative methods for disposing of water vapor, and methods for eliminating CO_2 using regenerable adsorbents. It also discusses the design principles underlying such subsystems, and ways of estimating and regulating changes in partial CO_2 pressure in the air of a pressurized cabin when absorbers are being used. One section describes a closed cycle for regeneration of O_2 from CO_2 and water. Another section describes the configuration of the major types of subassemblies and units of air regeneration subsystems. It provides their mass and energy characteristics and compares a number of subsystems for air regeneration using regenerative principles with those based on stored supplies. The chapter concludes with examples of regenerative subsystems used on actual spacecraft and a discussion of pertinent future developments. Methods for disposing of toxic trace gases are not considered, since Chapter 2 covers this issue.

The discussion of pressurized spacecraft cabin air in this chapter is based on the ideas in Chapter 1 of this volume. The source data on crew vital processes were derived from Chapter 8.

Integrated physicochemical life support systems, which include the kind of air regeneration subsystems analyzed in

The Russian original of this paper was translated by Lydia R. Stone. Technical editing was provided by Timothy J. Sharpe and Edward J. Stone.

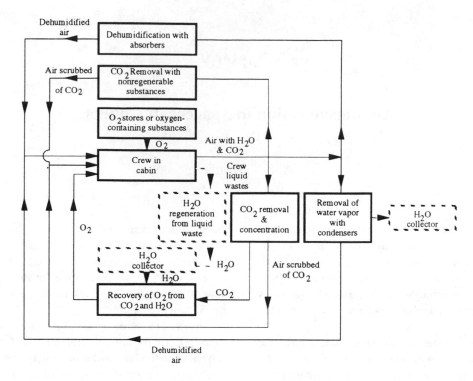

Fig. 1 Air regeneration.

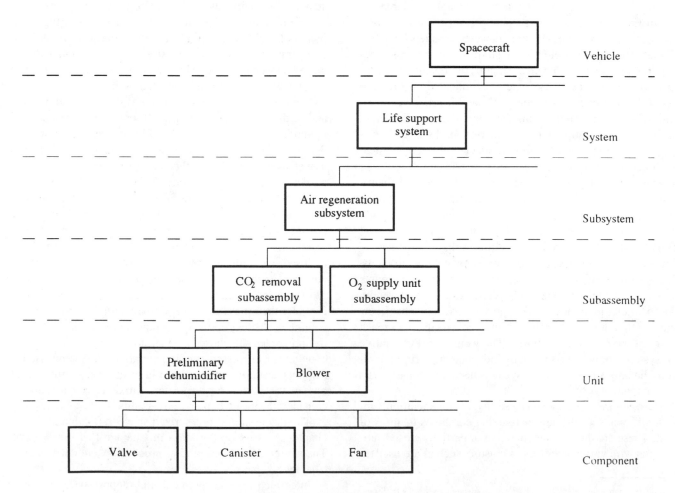

Fig. 2 Hierarchy of air regeneration subsystems.[2]

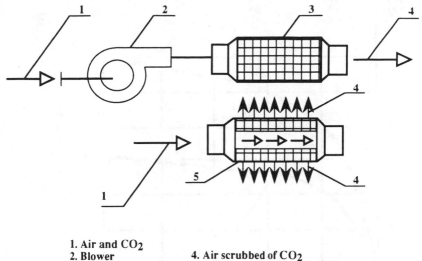

1. Air and CO_2
2. Blower
3. Canister with LiOH
4. Air scrubbed of CO_2
5. Canister with LiOH, extended absorbent bed

Fig. 3 Flow diagram of CO_2 removal subassembly using the nonregenerable absorbent LiOH.

this chapter, are discussed in Chapter 15. Chapter 16 considers biological life support systems that incorporate a number of the subassemblies of physicochemical air regeneration subsystems considered here.

I. Scrubbing Carbon Dioxide from the Air of Pressurized Environments

The acceptable levels of CO_2 concentration in the air of inhabited pressurized cabins are very low (only a few mm Hg), whereas the amount of CO_2 exhaled by a human reaches almost 1 kg/day (the computed value is 0.96 kg/day per person). Scrubbing CO_2 from cabin air is, therefore, a critical requirement for the air regeneration subsystem.

Both regenerative and nonregenerative methods may be considered for removing CO_2 from the air. Since most of the mass of such a subsystem comes from consumables, it is proportional to flight duration and crew size. Therefore regenerative methods based on stores of nonregenerable sorbents are used on short-term flights and regenerative methods utilizing regenerable sorbents, diffusion methods, and freezing are most desirable for long-term flights; these methods can be used not only to scrub CO_2 but also to concentrate it for subsequent regeneration of O_2.

A. Nonregenerative Methods for Removing Carbon Dioxide

The simplest method for removing CO_2 involves the use of hydroxides of alkali and alkali earth metals [LiOH, KOH, $Ca(OH)_2$, NaOH]. All reactions of these compounds with CO_2 are exothermic.

The most widely used method for removing CO_2 from the air of pressurized, isolated, or poorly ventilated environments uses a lime chemical absorbent, 75 percent (by weight) of which is calcium hydroxide $Ca(OH)_2$.

$$Ca(OH)_2 + CO_2 \longrightarrow CaCO_3 + H_2O$$

This chemical is comparatively cheap and it is mass-produced in many nations. However, its efficiency—the amount of CO_2 absorbed per 1 kg weight of the chemical—is comparatively low (no greater than 130 L/kg), since the atomic weight of Ca (42) is high.

Since the launch weight of equipment and consumable materials plays a decisive role, the best absorbent for supporting space flight is lithium hydroxide.

$$2LiOH + CO_2 \longrightarrow Li_2CO_3 + H_2O + 89 \text{ kJ/mole}$$

The low atomic weight of lithium (7) makes this absorbent highly efficient: 350–400 liters of CO_2 are absorbed by 1 kg of lithium hydroxide.

A CO_2 absorber based on lithium oxide (Li_2O) is even more efficient than the one based on lithium hydroxide; its absorbing capacity reaches 450 L/kg, and the amount required is only 1.1 kg/day per person. Binders are added to the hygroscopic alkaline substances, which are then shaped into granules or blocks. This increases the consumption of the absorber by approximately 25 percent above the stoichiometric ratio. Absorption of 1 kg of CO_2 by LiOH, requires lithium canisters weighing 2.1 kg (including canister weight) providing an efficiency ratio = 0.4); when Li_2O is used, the required canister weight drops to 1.8 kg per kg of CO_2.

Figure 3 presents a flow chart of a subassembly for removing CO_2 from the air using a LiOH-based absorber.

A blower moves air from the pressurized cabin through the absorber canister, which is connected to the blower by a flexible pipeline. The granulated absorbent is held in the canister by a screen. The capacity of the absorbent determines the mass required; the dimensions of the bed depend on both absorbent capacity and rate of absorption, i.e., the kinetics of the process determine the size and shape of the bed. (Design

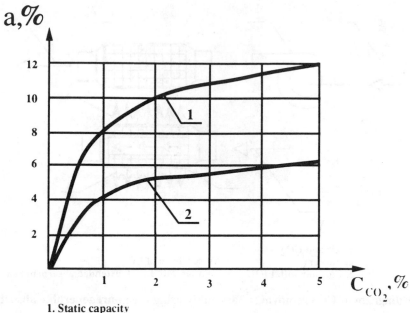

1. Static capacity
2. Dynamic capacity at flow rate of 0.1 m/s, length of 1 m

Fig. 4 Isotherms of CO_2 absorption using industrial zeolites (CaA) at 293° K.[2]

issues are considered in more detail below in a separate section.) The kinetics of the process determine the loading on a cross section (L/min × cm^2) and the bed length required. To ensure that the absorber bed is long enough and does not have an unnecessarily large diameter, a so-called expanded bed is frequently used in which the absorbent in the canister is sandwiched between two cylindrical surfaces (cf. Fig. 3).

Since the rate of absorption of CO_2 decreases when the absorber has been used for too long and results in failure to maintain the required level of CO_2, it is desirable to insert a new canister while the previous one is still functioning, thus they are both in use simultaneously for a period of time.

Substances based on superoxides and ozonides of alkali metals absorb CO_2 as they release O_2. These substances are considered in the section devoted to O_2 supply. The CO_2 absorption capacity of absorbers containing KO_2 can be as high as 180 L/kg; while for absorbers containing NaO_2 it can reach 260 L/kg.

Subassemblies using stores of nonregenerable absorbents are reliable and simple, and use minimal power (no more than 10 watts).

B. Removal of Carbon Dioxide with Regenerable Absorbers

Since the removal of CO_2 through nonregenerative methods requires consumable absorbents with significant mass, increases in the duration of space flight and the development of orbital space stations compel the development of subassemblies that do not have this problem. The most suitable physicochemical method for removing CO_2 involves the use of solid regenerable absorbers, or adsorbents. This method is widely used in industry for purifying gas and fractionating

gas mixtures.[4-7]

The capacity of the adsorbent at a given level of pressure and temperature can be derived from equations of statics. An equation of isothermic adsorption can be derived for each specific temperature (Fig. 4). There are a number of theories of adsorption, each of which has its own isotherm equation,[4,8-14] and depending on the complexity of the process, each can be applied with certain assumptions to sorption of different substances by various types of sorbents. In a convex adsorption isotherm (characteristic of isotherms of adsorption and chemisorption of CO_2 by the majority of solid sorbent substances in use), the rate of uptake increases with increasing pressure until capacity is reached, reflecting saturation of the surface, (after which further pressure increases effect no further uptake) (see Fig. 4, Ref. 2). When temperature increases, adsorption capacity drops, and the isotherms enter an area of decreased capacity. It thus follows that an adsorber may be regenerated from the adsorbed gas either by increasing its temperature through heating, decreasing its pressure through evacuation, or a combination of these methods. These processes are termed thermal, vacuum, and thermovacuum regeneration, respectively.

Currently the major regenerative sorbents of CO_2 are physical adsorbents—activated charcoal, zeolites, solid chemisorbents, and liquid absorbers.[4,6] The adsorbents used are solid capillary porous substances with an internal surface ranging from hundreds to thousands of square meters per 1 gram material. Their static capacity may reach hundreds of liters of adsorbed gas per 1 liter of sorbent.[2] However, the capacity of the adsorbents at room temperatures with partial CO_2 pressure suitable for breathing is substantially below this value.

One of the most widely used CO_2 adsorbents is activated

Table 1   Adsorption of carbon dioxide (3.2 Å) on potassium, sodium and calcium zeolites (T=20 °C)[1]

pCO$_2$, mm Hg	Capacity, % mass		
	KA (3.3Å)	NaA (4.0Å)	CaA(5.0Å)
3	1.32	5.70	7.50
6	1.76	7.05	9.70
15	2.20	8.80	12.70

charcoal. Its dynamic capacity to absorb CO_2 at partial pressure of 7.6 mm Hg and standard temperature does not exceed 0.5 percent by mass, while its capacity by bulk (mass of gas uptake per unit volume of sorbent) does not exceed 0.4 kg/L. CO_2 gas and moisture are removed from the charcoal through special addition of heat at standard temperatures. The sorption isotherm of water vapor by charcoal is concavo-convex up to a relative humidity of 40 percent. Under these conditions only small quantities of water vapor are adsorbed. In air with an elevated concentration of O_2, the use of charcoal is not recommended because of the fire hazard. The disadvantages of most charcoals result from their high pore size variability. However, at the present time a whole class of fine-pored charcoals is being produced, making charcoal competitive with zeolites.

The most promising adsorbents for space flight are zeolites, aluminum silicate sorbents with a regular crystal structure, the most finely porous of all the sorbents known. Static capacity of zeolites for CO_2 at partial pressure of 7.6 mm Hg and standard temperature reaches 6 percent (by mass). The capacity by bulk of zeolites is 0.7–0.8 kg/L.

Thermal, thermovacuum, and vacuum regeneration of zeolites from CO_2 are all possible. In cyclical vacuum regeneration, given the conditions described above, dynamic capacity can reach 3 percent. Zeolites are not harmed by a pure O_2 atmosphere; they can undergo many thousands of cycles of operation with virtually no alteration in their adsorptive and mechanical properties. However, they have the major disadvantage of requiring the use of dry air [with a dew point temperature not exceeding -60 °C (213 K)], since they absorb water vapor preferentially over CO_2, causing their CO_2-absorbing capacity to drop sharply. For example, after the zeolite NaX has absorbed 1 percent moisture, its capacity for CO_2 decreases by 40 percent. To regenerate zeolite from moisture it must be heated to 350–400 °C, a method unacceptable from the standpoint of power use. For this reason, a zeolite subassembly must pump air through a bed of a regenerable water vapor absorber to dry the air before it reaches the zeolite bed.

Zeolite's porous structure may be represented schematically in the form of pore spaces, which are the size of molecules and more or less spherical in shape, connected to each other by narrower openings, or "windows." Only molecules that are smaller than these windows can enter the pore space of the crystals and be adsorbed by them. This explains the selectivity of various types of zeolites. Zeolite granules produced industrially (1–5 mm in diameter) consist of crystalline powders and binder (up to 20 percent). The binder binds the crystals into granules from 1 to several millimeters in size and forms a secondary porous structure. According to M. M. Dubinin's data,[15,16] the equivalent radii of the secondary porous structure range from tens to hundreds of thousands of angstroms. The coefficient of diffusion in the secondary pores is a function of the conditions of zeolite granulation.

Adsorption of CO_2 gas on potassium, sodium, and calcium zeolites at 20 °C is presented in Table 1 (Ref. 1). The data in Table 1 show that the capacity to adsorb CO_2 is a clear function of the size of the windows of elementary pore space of the crystal structure. Water, with molecule size of 2.6 Å, selectively displaces CO_2 from all these zeolites.

CO_2 may also undergo chemisorption by sorbents containing potash or soda formed into beds or blocks. Sorption is based on the reaction

$$K_2CO_3 + CO_2 + H_2O \longrightarrow 2\,KHCO_3$$

The heating temperature for regeneration must be as high as 150–200 °C. In a cycling operation, because of the slow kinetics, the duration of a sorption cycle is no less than several hours. The dynamic capacity of these solid regenerable absorbers for CO_2 is high—reaching 20–30 percent by weight at standard temperatures. A problem with such chemisorbents is their short life (no longer than a few months) when used in a cycling operation. Chemisorption using metal oxides, such as silver, manganese, and iron is also of some interest. The capacity of these oxides for CO_2, although significantly lower than that of zeolites, can reach several percent.[17] Special chemisorbents can be produced from these compounds that can undergo vacuum regeneration at normal temperatures.

Sorbents based on ion exchange resins, which can be regenerated by heated water vapor, are of great practical interest.[39]

One promising group of absorbers is the combined chemisorbents, which are solid porous carrier substances (of the silica gel type) specially treated with liquid chemisorbents. This treatment produces sorbents that are regenerable in a vacuum without heating and last for several years, as well as sorbents of the amino silica gel type with a dynamic capacity for CO_2 of up to 5 percent (by mass) for CO_2 concentrations in cabin air of 7.6 mm Hg.[22]

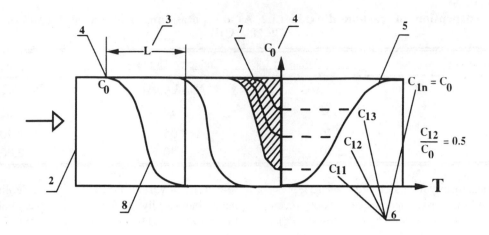

1. Air from the cabin containing CO_2
   at concentration C_0
2. Adsorption bed
3. L—length of the bed
4. Initial concentration of CO_2 in air

5. Yield curve
6. Concentrations of CO_2 on exit from the canister
7. Unused capacity of the adsorption bed
8. Concentration front moving along the bed as the capacity is used up

Fig. 5 Flow diagram of movement of adsorption waves through the absorbent canister.[4,7]

Liquid regenerable chemisorbents, including monoethanolamine, monoethylene diamine, and alkacydes, which are used in ground facilities, can be regenerated at temperatures above 110 °C (383 K). Their dynamic capacity for CO_2 reaches 10–15 percent (by mass). The major problems with using these liquid sorbents in spacecraft are associated with the separation of the gas and liquid phases in weightlessness.

All these chemisorption processes absorb water vapor in addition to CO_2.

Absorption processes are exothermic in physical and chemical sorption, and regeneration of the sorbent requires input of the quantity of heat that was emitted in sorption (neglecting losses). The process of regenerating a sorbent typically requires high temperatures, substantially increasing the mass of the air scrubbing subassembly.

The rate of sorption of CO_2 from air by zeolites is determined by the rate at which air is pumped into the sorption bed, since the process of adsorption itself is several orders of magnitude faster.

References 19–21 describe studies of the rate of adsorption of gases in detail. References 22 and 23 discuss the kinetics of adsorption of CO_2 by zeolites.

Figure 4 shows that the adsorption capacity of the industrial zeolite CaA reaches 7 percent (by mass) at standard temperatures and acceptable partial pressure of CO_2 in the air of a pressurized cabin. This is the maximum static capacity, which is attained under conditions of unlimited duration of contact between the gas being adsorbed and the adsorbent. Since the rate of the adsorption process is limited by external and internal diffusion, complete saturation cannot be attained. An air stream with an initial CO_2 concentration C_0 enters the sorbent bed. As it passes through the bed (L), the CO_2 is partially adsorbed and its concentration in the gas stream de-

creases from C_0 to 0. A saturation curve forms, which is displaced, without changing shape, along the bed until CO_2 begins to be released into the cabin air. The change in concentration of effluent CO_2 is called the yield curve (cf. Fig. 5, Refs. 4,7). Since the appearance of CO_2 in effluent gas (breakthrough) marks the beginning of a rapid decrease in rate of absorption, the process must be designed so that the relative concentration of CO_2 on output does not exceed 50 percent. Since this means that a portion of the zeolite's capacity will remain unutilized, the actual capacity of the adsorbent bed, [its dynamic capacity (a_d)] is always below its static capacity (a_0). A. A. Zhukovskiy, Ya. L. Zabezhinskiy, and A. N. Tikhonov[24–26] obtained an asymptotic solution in analytical form for the stage of parallel transfer of the sorption front. An analytical semiempirical solution to a system of equations for dynamic sorption of CO_2 by zeolites has also been obtained.[27–29] The approximate solution for sorption of CO_2 by zeolites for a mixed form of external and internal kinetics[30] is of some interest.

A schematic for an air scrubbing subassembly using regenerable adsorbents is presented in Fig. 6.

To provide continuous CO_2 sorption, two parallel canisters are employed, one of which is adsorbing while the other is being regenerated. The blower pumps air from the cabin through a moisture-absorbing canister, where it is warmed as the moisture is absorbed, and then through a regenerative heat exchanger, where it is cooled and then fed into the CO_2 adsorber. Scrubbed of CO_2, the air is heated in the regenerative heat exchanger and heated again before entering another moisture absorber (or the absorbent bed itself is heated) and the moisture is returned to cabin air; this is the so-called "blowback" method. Meanwhile, the other CO_2 adsorbent canister is vented into the vacuum of space and is regenerated. Before

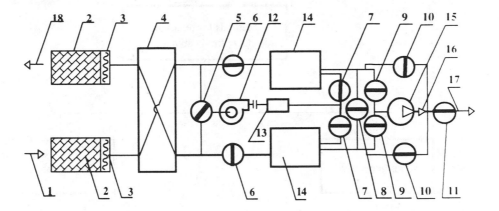

1. Air from the cabin
2. Desiccant
3. Heater
4. Regenerative heat exchanger
5. Valve for switching desiccants
6. Inlet valve for adsorbent canister
7. Discharge valve for adsorbent canister
8. Bypass valve
9. Vacuum pump valve
10. Valve for venting into space
11. Emergency vacuum valve
12. Blower
13. Flow rate sensor
14. Adsorbent canister
15. Vacuum pump
16. Air venting into cabin
17. Venting of CO_2 into space
18. Venting of air scrubbed of CO_2 into the cabin

Fig. 6 Schematic of CO_2 removal subassembly using regenerable absorbers.

this occurs, the air is pumped out of the CO_2 adsorber into the cabin, to minimize air losses.

Vacuum regeneration may either be accompanied by heating (the thermovacuum method) or used alone (the adiabatic vacuum method). The heat needed for desorption of CO_2 from the adsorber is generated as a result of change in the heat content of the adsorber itself. After completion of the cycle, the valves are switched so that air is fed into the regenerated moisture absorber and the regenerated CO_2 adsorber, while the other moisture absorber and the CO_2 adsorber that had been in the sorption mode enter the regeneration mode. The longer the duration of the cycle, the greater the amount of adsorbent and desiccant required and the greater the mass of the subassembly. This increased mass is associated with increased hydraulic resistance and increased power consumption. When the switching cycle duration is decreased, the required amounts of desiccant and adsorbent decrease, but the power used increases somewhat because of losses from heating the canister, and the useful life of the valve decreases. In thermovacuum regeneration, decrease in cycle duration is limited by the time required to heat and cool the canister; and in vacuum regeneration, by the time required for that process to occur and the time required to heat the desiccant.

The possibility of sorption with a heated sorbent bed without preliminary cooling is of significant interest as a means to decrease the duration of the cycle. Keltsev[6] demonstrated that during the nonisothermal process, thermal and sorption waves arise, and their motions are interrelated. When the rate of the thermal wave is greater than the rate of motion of the isothermal front, all the heat emitted in adsorption is removed by the air stream and adsorption takes place on a cold sorbent (single thermal wave mode). In subassemblies with a single

thermal wave, the sorbent bed does not have to be cooled after its thermal regeneration, decreasing the duration of the cycle.

To accommodate a single individual exhaling 20 liters of CO_2 per hour with partial CO_2 pressure of 4–5 mm Hg, the flow rate of the air stream must be 6–6.5 m^3/hr, allowing for possible surges in emission. The power consumed in vacuum regeneration of the absorber does not exceed 300 watts. This subassembly for scrubbing CO_2 from the air involves virtually no consumable resources, with the exception of air lost during vacuum regeneration. Since the air is first pumped out into the pressurized cabin, its loss may be held to a level not exceeding 50 L/day. The subassembly requires only regular replacement of the blower, vacuum pump, and valve units.

Possible methods for CO_2 removal are summarized in Fig. 7.

C. Regulation of Changes in Concentration of Carbon Dioxide in the Pressurized Cabin Atmosphere

For absorption of CO_2 (and also generation of O_2 in subassemblies with superoxides) air must be pumped through the canister in an amount sufficient to maintain CO_2 concentrations in the requisite range in the face of potential fluctuations in its emission by humans.

The cabin has the property of equilibration of partial CO_2 pressure; i.e., as time passes, partial CO_2 pressure reaches a new steady state without the need for an automatic regulator. The steady state concentration of CO_2 in the pressurized cabin may be derived from the equation[31]

$$C_0 = \dot{V} CO_2 / g + C_1$$

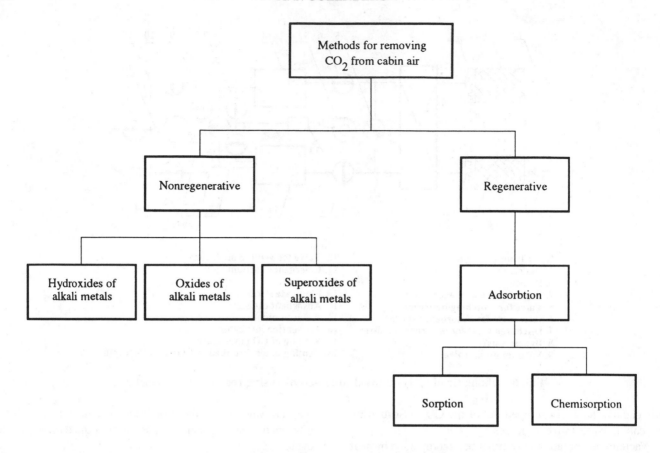

Fig. 7 Methods of removing CO_2 from cabin air.

where $\dot{V}CO_2$ is the volume of CO_2 generated by a human being, g is the flow rate of air through the subassembly, and C_0 and C_1 are concentrations of CO_2 upon intake into the scrubbing canister and outflow, respectively.

The major parameters responsible for the stability of CO_2 concentration in the pressurized cabin air under conditions of unstable CO_2 emission rate by crewmembers are 1) the ratio of rate of CO_2 emission to rate of air flow through the absorbent canister, and 2) the ratio of the free volume of the pressurized cabin to the same rate of air flow. The latter ratio is called the time constant (T_0) of the pressurized cabin with respect to concentration of CO_2 and, if one neglects effluent concentration from the sorbent bed, $T_0 = V/g$. If the ratio of concentrations at exit and entry ($C_1/C_0 = K_{reg}$) is taken into account, the time constant is expressed as $T_1 = V/g \cdot (1-K_{reg})$, where K_{reg} is called the coefficient of regulation.

The presence of CO_2 in effluent gas (called breakthrough) degrades the performance of the regulation subassembly, since it increases both the time constant ($T_1 = T_0/(1-K_{reg}) > T_0$) and the static deviation ($C_1 = C_0/(1-K_{reg}) > C_0$).

Since the duration of the transient is equal to three times the time constant,[32] to evaluate the time required to achieve a steady state one may use the equations

$$t_y = 3V/g \quad \text{and} \quad t'_{y1} = 3V/g(1-K_{reg})$$

respectively. The greater the time constant, the more slowly

the concentration of CO_2 in the pressurized atmosphere changes in response to changes in CO_2 exhaled by the crew. From the standpoint of regulation, to decrease this constant we must increase the rate of air flow through the CO_2 scrubbing subassembly.

To determine the steady state concentration of CO_2 supported by the pressurized cabin air scrubbing subassembly when CO_2 is emitted at a constant rate, it is convenient to use the equation $C_0 = \dot{V}CO_2 /g(1-K_{reg})$. The equation holds if the relative effluent concentration of CO_2 from the sorbent layer is constant.

The amount of CO_2 exhaled by the crew may change by a factor of nearly 10 as a function of physical work performed. In accordance with the above equation, the concentration of C_0, given a constant flow rate g, will change when emitted CO_2 changes. If the subassembly's flow rate was designed for a certain mean level of CO_2 emission, and if physical workload increases, the CO_2 concentration in pressurized cabin air will increase, just as it will decrease while the crew is sleeping. The scrubbing subassembly must be designed to support regulation of CO_2 concentration in cabin air within acceptable limits, whatever the rate of CO_2 emission by the crew.

As the equations show, an increase in the flow rate through the subassembly decreases the steady state concentration of CO_2 in the air of the pressurized cabin, regardless of its level of emission. However, if the flow rate is to be increased to

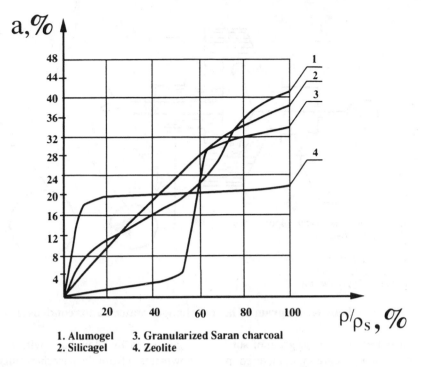

1. Alumogel   3. Granularized Saran charcoal
2. Silicagel   4. Zeolite

Fig. 8 Isotherms for sorption of water vapor from regenerable desiccant.[4]

handle greater CO_2 concentrations, either the regeneration cycle time has to be decreased or inefficiently large quantities of sorbent must be used. The most effective subassembly, especially for small volumes, is a subassembly in which the flow rate and operating cycle are regulated on the basis of effluent CO_2 concentrations.

II. Methods of Dehumidifying and Regulating Humidity

The humidity in pressurized cabin air is attributable primarily to the crew's emission of moisture through respiration and transpiration; this amount can be as high as 1500 grams/day per person. Additional moisture enters the air as a result of the operation of a number of subassemblies (such as a CO_2 absorption subassembly using hydroxides of alkali metals and the O_2 regeneration system) and as a result of crew washing procedures. Moisture entering from other sources does not exceed a few percent.

The operation of an O_2 supply subassembly that uses superoxides of alkali metals must be regulated by partially dehumidifying the incoming air stream. Air entering a system for scrubbing and concentrating CO_2 must be thoroughly dehumidified to permit the adsorbents to function and to prevent moisture loss from the cabin during vacuum and thermovacuum regeneration.

Electrochemical methods of O_2 supply or absorption subassemblies for removing CO_2 require the air to be dehumidified and moisture to be collected within the subassembly. Aside from the need to minimize mass and power consumption, it is critical, because of the possibility of condensation, that this process be highly reliable in weightlessness.

Whether nonregenerative or regenerative dehumidifying methods are used is dependent on space-flight duration. Nonregenerative methods involve the use of stores of nonregenerable absorbents or chemisorbents (primarily oxides, peroxides, and superoxides of alkali and alkali earth metals) which enter into a chemical reaction with water or form crystalline hydrates (salts of the type LiCl, $CaCl_2$, $ZnCl_2$, and others). The moisture capacity of LiCl, for example reaches 70 percent by mass. The principles of chemisorbents action are described in the section on CO_2 scrubbing.

Regenerative methods use regenerable adsorbents and involve cooling the air below the dew point. Such adsorbents include activated charcoal, alumogels, and silica gels.[4] Activated charcoals are described in the section on methods of CO_2 scrubbing. The capacity of charcoal increases significantly (reaching 30 percent by mass) at relative humidity greater than 50–60 percent, when capillary condensation occurs (Fig. 8). As discussed above, the use of charcoal allows a self-regulating method for supporting relative humidity in the cabin.

Alumogels are sorbents consisting of a mixture of normal hydroxides of aluminum Al_2O_3 and polyhydrates of aluminum. These substances have the advantage of thermal stability and moisture resistance, although, as desiccants, they are inferior to silica gels. The bulk density of alumogels is as high as 0.8 kg/L. Their porous surface reaches 300–400 m^2/g. Their moisture capacity, at 100 percent relative humidity and standard temperatures, reaches 40 percent by mass (Fig. 8).

Among the most active regenerable adsorbers of moisture are silica gels. These are solid, highly porous substances based on silica dioxide (SiO_2), characterized by a well-developed internal surface of pores and containing up to several hun-

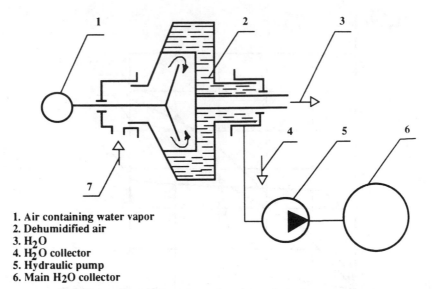

1. Air containing water vapor
2. Dehumidified air
3. H_2O
4. H_2O collector
5. Hydraulic pump
6. Main H_2O collector

Fig. 9 Schematic diagram of heat exchanger-water vapor condensor.

dred square meters of surface area in a single gram of substance (up to 700 m^2/gram). Silica gels are manufactured in the form of pellets or granules of irregular shape, 0.2–7.0 mm in size. Their major advantages are their low regeneration temperature (no higher than 200 °C, 473 K) and the fact that the power requirements for their regeneration are lower than for such sorbents as alumogels and zeolites. As a function of pore size, they can be classified as fine-pored (bulk density of up to 0.7 kg/L), large-pored (bulk density of up to 0.5 kg/L), and mixed-pored (intermediate between fine and large). The moisture capacity of fine-pored silica gels at a relative humidity of 100 percent and a temperature of 20 °C reaches 28 percent by mass; while that of large-pored gels, reaches 40 percent. The silica gel used most extensively in spacecraft subassemblies is coarse-grained and fine-pored, modified to increase its strength and moisture resistance. Unlike the pores in charcoals, the pores in silica gels are uniform in size and homogeneously distributed. The gel, in addition, is nonflammable. When the process is set up properly, after passing through a silica gel bed, effluent air humidity corresponding to a dew point of up to -60 °C (213 K) may be obtained. Isotherms of water vapor on silica gels are convex (Fig. 8).

Zeolites were discussed above as adsorbers of CO_2, but they are also highly effective desiccants. Their capacity at a standard temperature is less than that of silica gels (reaching 20 percent by mass, cf. Fig. 8), but their drying capacity is higher, since the dew point temperature of air after passing through a zeolite bed may drop to -70 °C (203 K) and below. When zeolites are used as desiccants, water displaces all other adsorbed substances. The water regeneration temperature for zeolites can reach 350–400 °C (623–673 K). However, an acceptable level of regeneration may be attained with some zeolites at lower temperatures. The zeolite Ka, which has a negligible CO_2 capacity, may be used as a desiccant in subassemblies for removing and concentrating CO_2. Desiccants

regenerated by blow-back with dry gas scrubbed of CO_2 downstream from the adsorber canister, fed on exit from the desiccator, is the major method used in subassemblirs of CO_2 removal and concentration using regenerable adsorbents.

The most expedient and economical method for removing moisture while maintaining the humidity of pressurized cabins is direct condensation of water on chilled surfaces. In this method heat and moisture are removed from the air by a single component, a combination heat exchanger and water vapor condenser. The major advantages of this method are: 1) required mass and volume do not depend on duration of use; 2) the operation of the dehumidifier is simple and reliable; and 3) some portion of the soluble toxic contaminants is removed from the air along with the water vapor. A shortcoming is the comparative complexity of further separating the gas-liquid mixture formed by condensation in weightlessness. A schematic of a condenser is provided in Fig. 9.

A blower circulates cabin air through the space around the heat exchanger pipes, which circulate a liquid coolant at 5–7 °C (278–280 K). Air passing over the chilled surfaces of the heat exchanger is cooled, and the water vapor it contains precipitates in the form of a liquid film (the condensate). In weightlessness, the film of condensate that accumulates increases the thermal resistance of the process of heat transfer from the air to the surface and thus must be removed. The heat exchanger and dehumidifier contain hydrophilic wicks, which, as a result of the capillary force of the water, draw the condensate into an intermediate collector filled with a capillary-porous hydrophilic absorbent. The water is pumped from this collector to the main condensate collector which is also filled with moisture-absorbing porous material. The air, captured when the liquid is pumped from the intermediate collector, is separated from water droplets after passing through the main collector and recirculated to the cabin.[2]

Two methods are used in air regeneration subsystems to separate the liquid and gas phases in weightlessness: 1) a

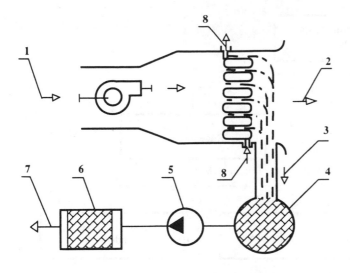

1. Electric drive
2. Liquid
3. Dehumidified air
4. H_2O
5. Hydraulic pump
6. H_2O collector
7. Air with water vapor
8. Thermoregulation system

Fig. 10 Schematic of centrifugal gas: liquid phase separator.[2]

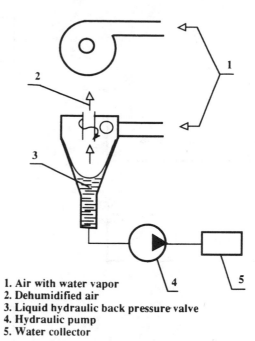

1. Air with water vapor
2. Dehumidified air
3. Liquid hydraulic back pressure valve
4. Hydraulic pump
5. Water collector

Fig. 11 Schematic of cyclonic gas: liquid phase separator.[2]

method of semipermeable porous membranes; and 2) a method based on centrifugal force. The first uses capillary membranes of hydrophilic and hydrophobic material, with specific capillary sizes. By selecting relatively small capillaries, it is possible to create a stable surface to separate liquids and gas independently of the magnitude and direction of gravity. Hydrophilic membranes include the majority of materials (asbestos and metals). Hydrophobic membranes are polymers (e.g., Teflon®). These semipermeable membranes make it possible to separate gas and liquid in weightlessness by feeding a two-phase stream into a narrow space between membranes of the two types. When there is excess pressure, the liquid will flow through the hydrophilic membrane and the gas through the hydrophobic one. This method may be used for condensation or evaporation, and is extremely efficient with respect to mass and power. However, its widespread use is limited by the short service life of the membranes, particularly when they are used with contaminated liquids.[2]

Centrifugal methods of separation do not have this limitation. When liquids are rotated, centrifugal forces replace the force of gravity. The principle of action of a centrifugal separator is shown in Fig. 10. The gas-liquid mixture, after entering the rotating drum of the separator, achieves angular velocity. The liquid, under the influence of the centrifugal force, is thrown to the periphery of the disc, forming a ring-shaped "liquid-gas" interface. The dehumidified gas is vented and the liquid is pumped out through a drain in the centrifuge. A condenser and evaporator can be constructed according to this design.

There are, however, problems with this type of subassembly, including: the complexity of the design; the need for rotating parts and dynamic seals, and for a special power drive

and, thus, additional power use; and the difficulty of maintaining the hydraulic seal, especially during stopping and starting.

Cyclonic separators, which do not have moving parts, are significantly simpler structurally (cf. Fig. 11). Vortex motion of the gas-liquid mixtures in the separators occurs as a result of the initial kinetic energy of the gas-liquid stream entering the separator. In the cyclonic separator the mixture stream enters the conical compartment of the separator at a tangent to the circumference of the top of the cone. The liquid, under the influence of centrifugal force, is thrown to the walls of the separator, and the gas is vented through a central pipe. In the narrow lower portion of the separator cone, the velocity of the vortex flow of gas increases and static pressure decreases correspondingly. As a result of this drop in pressure, the liquid film moves toward the narrow end of the cone, where, under the influence of surface tension, it forms a liquid hydraulic seal for the gas. The liquid is pumped out of the narrow end of the compartment. Disadvantages of vortex separators include the difficulty of maintaining a stable hydraulic seal when the flow rate of the gas-liquid mixture fluctuates and the need for a special servomechanism to support a constant level of liquid in the hydraulic seal.[2]

Figure 12 presents a summary of methods for dehumidifying the air and separating gas-liquid mixtures as applied to the air of pressurized cabins and air regeneration subsystems.

III. Sources of Oxygen: Methods for Storage and Metered Delivery

Chapter 8 of this volume cites the mean daily O_2 consumption by a human as 0.86 kg/day. The need to supply such

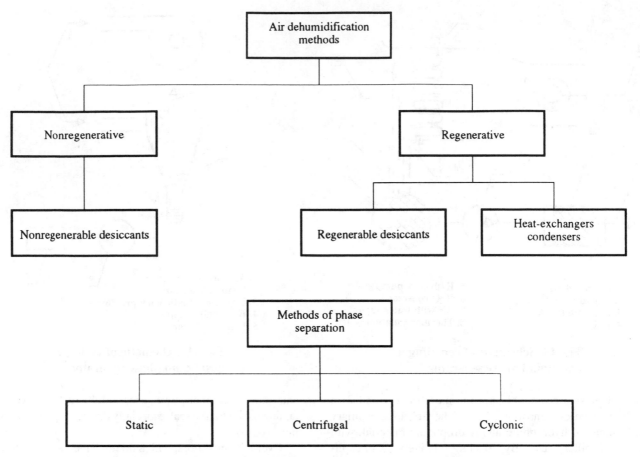

Fig. 12 Methods of air dehumidification and liquid: gas phase separation.

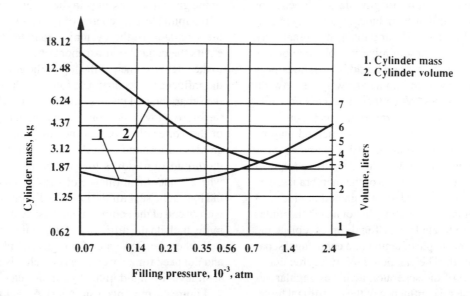

Fig. 13 Mass and volume of steel spherical oxygen cylinders as a function of filling pressure.[1,34]

a substantial amount of gas per crewmember per day can make it difficult to comply with mass limits when flight duration and crew size are increased.

In space flight, O_2 may be stored in gaseous or liquid form, or in the form of oxygen-containing substances. Each method has its own advantages, disadvantages, and areas of use.

A. Gaseous and Liquid Oxygen

At normal temperature and pressure, O_2 is a colorless gas without odor or taste, somewhat heavier than air, with density at pressure of 760 mm Hg of 1.43 kg/m^3 at 0 °C (273 K) and 1.33 kg/m^3 at 20 °C (293 K). When O_2 is cooled at atmo-

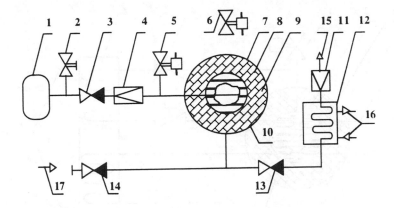

1. Cylinder with pressurization gas at high pressure
2. Cylinder filling valve
3. Check valve
4. Reducer
5. Pressure relief cock
6. Pressure relief valve
7. Cryogenic Dewar
8. Liquid oxygen
9. Vacuum screen insulation
10. Elastic expulsion tank
11. Flow rate regulator
12. Heat exchanger
13. Check valve
14. Filling nozzle
15. Oxygen outlet
16. Thermoregulation (system loop)
17. Oxygen for filling

Fig. 14 Schematic diagram of cryogenic oxygen supply subassembly.

pheric pressure to -183 °C (90 K) it is transformed into a transparent bluish liquid with density of 1.13 kg/L. When it is further cooled to a temperature of -218.7 °C (54.3 K), it passes into a solid state with density of 1.46 kg/L. One kilogram of liquid O_2 evaporated at 20 °C and pressure of 760 mm Hg yields 750 liters of gaseous O_2.[33]

Storage of O_2 in the form of gas at high temperatures is the simplest and most reliable type of O_2 supply subassembly. The general approach to the design of such a subassembly involves determining the appropriate relationships between gas pressure and the volume and mass of the cylinders. Figure 13 shows that optimal mass is attained at a pressure of 200–220 atm, while the combination of mass and volume will be optimal at a pressure of 500–700 atm.

When O_2 is stored in cylinders at high pressure, and when the cylinders are designed efficiently, 2 kg of cylinder weight is required for every 1 kg of O_2. The specific density of O_2 stored in this manner does not exceed 0.3 kg/L; to safely withstand high pressures during storage, the cylinders must have thick walls.

Since the density of liquid O_2 is more than 3.5 times that of compressed gaseous O_2, it is expedient to store supplies of O_2 in liquid form. In this approach, the low pressure at which liquid O_2 can be stored makes it possible to decrease the structural weight of the tanks. The major engineering problems in creating subassemblies for storing liquid O_2 are associated with limiting heat inputs to the O_2 and ensuring homogeneous bleed-off of O_2 vapors from the tanks in weightlessness. Because of the large temperature differential between the environment and liquid O_2, the heat input to the tanks must be restricted by special methods. The rate of evaporation of O_2 from the tank must not exceed the required flow rate of O_2

for crew breathing, $V_i < P_{O_2} \times K$. On the other hand, $V_i = A/b_{O_2}$ from which it follows that $A < b_{O_2} \times P_{O_2} \times K$, where A is the heat input to the tank, $b_{O_2} = 210$ kJ/kg is the specific heat of evaporation of O_2, $P_{O_2} = 36$ g/hr is the mean hourly consumption of O_2 by an individual, and K is crew size.

The acceptable heat input derived from these equations is only 2 watts per person. If heat input exceeds this level, a portion of the O_2 is wasted. To ensure low heat inputs, the outer surfaces of the tanks are provided with special thermal insulation, known as vacuum shield insulation, with low thermal conductivity. This insulation consists of a series of layers of metallic film with low emissivity ε under vacuum conditions. Vacuum shield insulation operates on the principle of multiple reflection of the radiant flow of heat.

Aside from the difficulties described above with regard to storage of liquid O_2, such subassemblies pose the problem, as yet unresolved, of reliable bleed-off of gas phase and metering of the amount of O_2 in the tank. To store 1 kg of O_2, given the appropriate optimal design, requires 0.25 kg tank weight, so that the weight ratio is 0.25 (Ref. 34).

A schematic of an O_2 supply subassembly is presented in Fig. 14. In this subassembly, O_2 is expelled from the cryogenic tank by an elastic bladder within the tank shell, into which gas (helium or nitrogen) is fed under pressure. The reliability of this subassembly is determined primarily by the strength of the expulsion bladder after multiple deformations. Input of heat to all the surfaces of O_2 must be uniform, or else local boiling and gas formation may occur.[1] In two-phase storage without an expulsion bladder, O_2 bleed-off is very difficult because of the need to separate the phases. In addition, the O_2 may shift in the tank, under the influence of surface tension and the hydrophilic tank walls, and vapor may

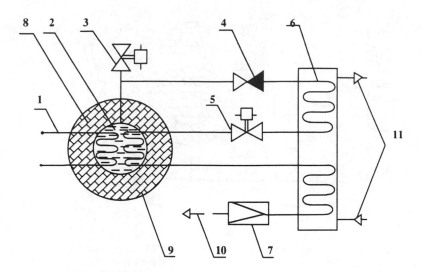

1. Additional heat source
2. Supercritical oxygen
3. O_2 drainage and pressure relief valve
4. Stop valve
5. Heat delivery regulator valve
6. Heat exchanger

7. Pressure regulator
8. Vacuum screen insulation
9. Internal heat exchanger
10. Oxygen vent to cabin
11. Thermoregulation system loop

Fig. 15 Schematic diagram of supercritical oxygen supply subassembly.[1]

leak through the drainage bleed-off nozzle, etc.

The best solution to all these problems is to store O_2 in a supercritical state under pressure and at temperatures that are above critical levels. In the region of critical points at $T_{cr} = -118.8$ °C (154.2 K) and $P_{cr} = 49.7$ atm (4.87 MPa), the liquid and gas phases of O_2 are in a homogeneous, uniform state with a rather high density of 0.43 kg/L. The weight ratio of tanks to O_2 in supercritical storage of O_2 is 0.3–0.7, depending on the density of the O_2 fed into the tank.[35] A flow chart of an O_2 supply subassembly using supercritical O_2 is presented in Fig. 15. O_2 is expelled from the tank in this subassembly by increasing pressure through internal input of heat. This subassembly does not require phase separation and can be used without difficulty in weightlessness.[1]

The disadvantages of cryogenic subassemblies for supplying spacecraft crews with O_2 include the difficulty of filling and storing before launch due to large O_2 losses, the difficulty of storing O_2 in flight, and the loss of O_2 during intervals between crew flights when the spacecraft is unmanned or crew size is diminished. To prevent losses of O_2 during storage in the absence of a crew, a special refrigeration machine is included in the subassembly. For this reason O_2 supply subsssemblies that involve cryogenic storage are used only for short-term flights, and then only when O_2 is used primarily for supporting the operation of the power supply system.

A problem with all O_2 subassemblies, especially those using high pressure, is the hazard of explosion if there is contamination by organic compounds, oil, or other substances. This requires special processing of the structural components and observation of safety precautions for working with O_2.

Metered delivery of O_2 into the cabin air is triggered in all

these subassemblies by a command delivered to the electric delivery valve by a gas analyzer sensitive to atmospheric O_2.

B. Oxygen Supply Using Oxygen-Containing Substances

The use of chemically bound O_2 has a number of advantages with regard to simplicity of structure and use and long-term storage. This is particularly true for substances in the solid state. At present, three groups of such substances have been identified. The first includes substances based on superoxides, peroxides, and ozonides of alkali metals. The second includes chlorates and perchlorates of alkali metals. The third group comprises liquid O_2-containing substances, including hydrogen peroxide, nitrogen dioxide, and water. The major characteristics of O_2-containing substances are listed in Table 2 (Refs. 3, 34).

The most efficient sources of O_2, which simultaneously absorb CO_2, are superoxides and ozonides of alkali metals. The use of superoxides and ozonides is based on the following exothermic reactions (using potassium compounds as an example):

$$4 KO_2 + 2 H_2O \longrightarrow 4 KOH + 3 O_2$$

$$4 KO_3 + 2 H_2O \longrightarrow 4 KOH + 5 O_2$$

The alkali formed is an active absorber of CO_2, and for this reason the second stage of the reaction proceeds as follows:

$$4 KOH + 2 CO_2 \longrightarrow 2 K_2CO_3 + 2 H_2O$$

Table 2   Major properties of oxygen-containing substances[3]

Oxygen-containing substance	Chemical formula	Specific emission of O_2, kg/kg substance	Density, kg/L
Lithium superoxide	LiO_2	0.610	
Sodium superoxide	NaO_2	0.436	
Potassium superoxide	KO_2	0.338	0.655
Calcium superoxide	$Ca(O_2)_2$	0.460	
Lithium peroxide	Li_2O_3	0.347	2.140
Sodium peroxide	Na_2O_2	0.205	
Potassium peroxide	K_2O_2	0.145	
Lithium ozonide	LiO_3	0.730	
Sodium ozonide	NaO_3	0.563	
Potassium ozonide	KO_3	0.460	
Lithium perchlorate	$LiClO_4$	0.601	2.430
Sodium chlorate	$NaClO_3$	0.451	2.260
Hydrogen peroxide	H_2O_2	0.471	1.420
Nitrogen dioxide	NO_2	0.720	
Water	H_2O	0.890	1.0

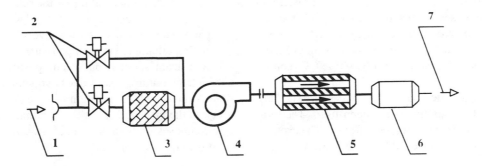

1. Air stream inlet
2. Shut-off valves
3. Desiccator (with LiCl)
4. Blower
5. Regenerator
6. Charcoal filter
7. Outlet of air stream scrubbed of CO_2 and enriched with oxygen

Fig. 16   Schematic of an oxygen regeneration subassembly with KO_2.[34,36,37]

$$2 K_2CO_3 + 2H_2O + 2CO_2 \longleftrightarrow 4 KHCO_3$$

The ratio of the amount of CO_2 emitted and the amount of O_2 consumed by an individual is called the respiratory quotient, and its mean value is 0.8. To support the gas balance in the atmosphere, an O_2 subassembly must generate 1.25 liters of O_2 for every liter of CO_2 it absorbs.

The stoichiometric ratio in the reactions above dictates that when carbonate is formed, the ratio of the volume of released O_2 to the volume of absorbed CO_2 is 1.5, and when hydrocarbonate is formed, this ratio is 0.75. If carbonate alone is formed in the reaction, there will be a constant increase in partial O_2 pressure in the cabin. To regulate the process of O_2 release, there must also be a reaction that forms bicarbonate. This reaction begins to dominate when the rate of delivery of water vapor to the surface of the KO_2 decreases. Thus, by

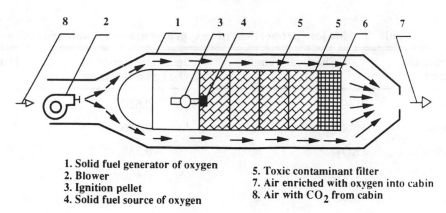

1. Solid fuel generator of oxygen
2. Blower
3. Ignition pellet
4. Solid fuel source of oxygen

5. Toxic contaminant filter
7. Air enriched with oxygen into cabin
8. Air with CO_2 from cabin

Fig. 17 Schematic of an oxygen supply subassembly using a solid fuel source—lithium perchlorate.

regulating the delivery of water vapor, it is possible to attain the requisite mean ratio of 1.25 between the volume of O_2 released and that of CO_2 absorbed.

A schematic of an air regeneration subsystem using stored KO_2 is presented in Fig. 16 (Refs. 34, 36, 37). Air from the pressurized cabin, containing CO_2 and water vapor, is moved by a blower into a canister containing a KO_2-based substance, where it is scrubbed of CO_2 and enriched with O_2. The temperature in the reaction zone may reach 200 °C (473 K). The same canister destroys bacteria and partially removes toxic contaminants. The final scrubbing of toxic contaminants from the air occurs in a charcoal canister, after which the air enters the cabin. The release of O_2 is regulated in the subassembly by a distribution valve and an air-drying subassembly. If partial O_2 pressure increases, in response to a signal from the gas analyzer, the distribution valve shuts off the flow of gas through the KO_2 canister and directs it into this canister through the dehumidifying subassembly, while CO_2 continues to be absorbed.

O_2 supply subassemblies based on solid sources of O_2, chlorates, and perchlorates have also been used. The most efficient of these sources is lithium perchlorate. The exothermic reaction involved is expressed by the equation

$$LiClO_4 \longrightarrow LiCl + 2\,O_2 + Q$$

Here the temperature in the reaction zone can reach 700 °C. The product decomposes as a result of "flameless combustion". A diagram of the subassembly is presented in Fig. 17. The $LiClO_4$ substance is formed into cylindrical pellets which are placed in cartridges. The top pellet contains additives facilitating ignition. Each cartridge is designed to supply one person with O_2 for 1 day (no less than 600 liters). The cartridge is placed in a generator for decomposition, ignited with an igniter, and "burned" for no more than 20 minutes. The outer shell of the generator is cooled by forced air from a blower. This air impels the O_2 leaving the generator through the scrubbing filter, mixes with it, and, after cooling, the O_2 enters the cabin. After it cools, the spent cartridge is removed from the generator and a new one inserted. The mass of one cartridge is 2.2 kg; the fixed mass of the subassembly

(mass of the solid fuel generator) is no greater than 10 kg. The weight ratio for this subassembly is 0.55.

The major advantages of subassemblies utilizing solid O_2 containing substances are: ease of storage, simplicity of design, high reliability, high energy efficiency compared with other subassemblies, and minimal servicing time. The major disadvantage is the significant variable weight of the subassembly.

Hydrogen peroxide occupies a special place among the substances listed in Table 2. Hydrogen peroxide is a liquid with density of 1.42 kg/L and concentration of 95 percent by mass (the remaining element is water). Concentrated hydrogen peroxide freezes at temperatures ranging from -3 to -1 °C (270–272 K) depending on the admixture of water, and boils at a temperature of 157 °C (430 K). It decomposes into O_2 and water at temperatures above 127 °C (400 K). At normal temperatures hydrogen peroxide is stable; there is only insignificant spontaneous decomposition, which increases with temperature. Losses due to spontaneous decomposition are limited with the addition of special substances, stabilizers. In the presence of silver or platinum catalysts, peroxide decomposes without additional heating and releases a significant quantity of heat:

$$2\,H_2O_2 \xrightarrow{\text{catalyst}} 2\,H_2O + O_2 + 3300\ kJ/kg$$

All products of the reaction may be used in life support systems based on stored supplies. Obtaining the necessary quantity of O_2 (0.86 kg/day for a single person) requires 1.9 kg of 95 percent H_2O_2. At the same time more than 1 kg/day of water is formed, which can be used as potable water after appropriate purification. Since hydrogen peroxide is stored at low pressures, the relative mass of the cylinders is less than for the storage of gaseous O_2 (the coefficient is no greater than 0.25). Consumption of mass for O_2 supply is 1.35 kg/day per person, which is close to that for cryogenic storage. The advantage of hydrogen peroxide, as compared with cryogenic O_2, is the simplicity of its storage. A schematic of such a subassembly is presented in Fig. 18.

Hydrogen peroxide is stored in an expulsion tank with an

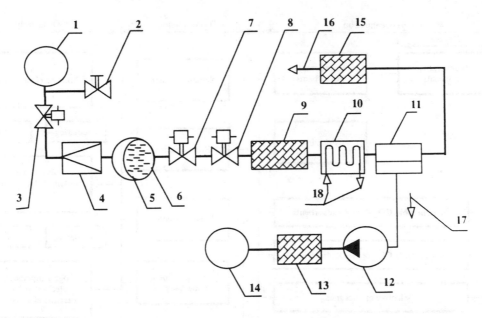

1. Cylinder with compressed inert gas (nitrogen)
2. Fill valve
3. Stop valve
4. Reducer
5. Flexible membrane
6. Tank with H_2O
7. Valve
8. Metering valve
9. Catalytic canister

10. Heat exchanger-condenser
11. Separator
12. Hydraulic pump
13. H_2O cleaning filter
14. H_2O tank
15. Oxygen scrubbing filter
16. Oxygen outlet
17. Water
18. Thermoregulation system

Fig. 18 Schematic of oxygen supply subassembly using stores of hydrogen peroxide.

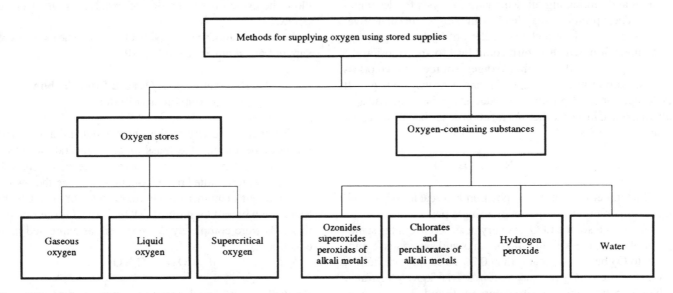

Fig. 19 Methods for supplying oxygen using stored supplies.

elastic bladder separating the liquid and inert gas, the expellant (nitrogen), which is fed from a cylinder. While the subassembly is operating, the hydrogen peroxide delivery valve opens and peroxide enters the reactor containing the catalyst through a special metering valve, and decomposes. Released heat transforms the water produced into vapor, forming a vapor-gas O_2 mixture at a temperature of 600 °C (873 K); the mixture subsequently cools in the heat exchanger and condenser and enters the drinking water tank through a purification filter, while O_2 passes through a purification filter into the cabin. The hydrogen peroxide delivery valve may be controlled by an automatic gas analyzer sensitive to partial O_2 pressure.

The major disadvantage of the use of hydrogen peroxide is the need for a high degree of cleanliness of the surfaces in

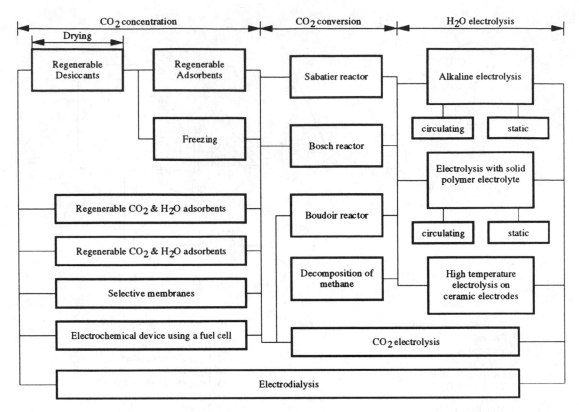

Fig. 20 Methods of regenerating oxygen.[38]

contact with it to ensure the absence of traces of organic substances and lubricating oil, which are catalysts for decomposition. Their presence may lead to an abrupt emission of vapor-gas as a result of a chain reaction of hydrogen peroxide decomposition, which in turn could lead to an explosion.

Nitrogen dioxide, another oxygen source, is a colorless liquid, boiling at 21 °C (294 K), and a brown toxic gas. It decomposes in the presence of catalysts containing oxides of alkali metals, in an exothermic reaction described by the equation

$$2\,NO_2 \longrightarrow N_2 + 2\,O_2 + Q$$

The temperature at decomposition can reach 900 °C, and up to 99 percent decomposes in a single pass.

Water, as a source of O_2, is very desirable from the standpoint of mass, the weight ratio of tanks and associated equipment to O_2 being no greater than 0.2. To supply one human with 0.86 kg of O_2 per day requires 1.16 kg/day of water, which is better than the parameters for liquid O_2. However, water is an extremely stable compound, requiring significant input of energy for decomposition. Of the existing methods for decomposing water (thermal decomposition, radiolysis, etc.), the most desirable is electrolysis of water at normal temperatures. Even in the adiabatic process of electrolysis, the power consumed to supply one person with O_2 is 220–230 watts. In addition, the water electrolysis subassembly is a very complex electrochemical system requiring special safety procedures. Although water electrolysis can produce

O_2, it is currently used in O_2 supply subassemblies only to close the cycle of regeneration of exhaled air, as discussed below.

Possible methods of supplying O_2 through the use of stored supplies are summarized in Fig. 19.

IV. Regeneration of Oxygen from Carbon Dioxide and Water

The opening section of this chapter stated that the major means of decreasing the mass of air regeneration subsystems on long-term space flights is to regenerate O_2 from the CO_2 and water emitted by crewmembers. Since the respiratory quotient of humans is approximately 0.8 (see Chapter 8), for each liter of O_2 utilized, 0.8 liters of CO_2 is emitted. If this CO_2 were completely decomposed, as expressed in the equation

$$CO_2 \longrightarrow C + O_2$$

this method would produce only 80 percent of the O_2 required. The remaining 20 percent (0.17 kg/day per person) could be obtained from 0.19 kg of water, through the reaction

$$2\,H_2O \longrightarrow 2\,H_2 + O_2$$

Theoretically, the excess water given off by the crew ("metabolic water") could be used to achieve complete closure of the water and O_2 cycles. In practice, however, because of the incomplete regeneration of water from urine and

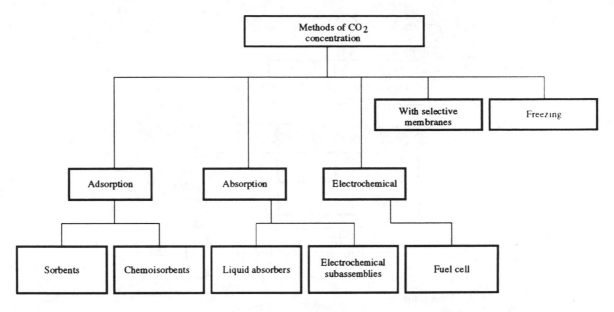

Fig. 21 Methods of CO$_2$ concentration.

the complex technology required to recover water from solid wastes, some of the water for closing the O$_2$ cycle must be obtained from stored supplies.

The design of O$_2$ regeneration subassemblies requires: 1) the development of methods for regenerating substances and 2) the development of hardware to implement these methods in space. The methods must provide maximal regeneration of substances, be very intensive (to minimize mass), energy efficient, reliable, and stable, and produce O$_2$ that meets medical standards. Such methods are difficult to develop. Generation of O$_2$ through direct decomposition of CO$_2$ and water in accordance with the reactions cited above is virtually impossible, since this requires input of thermal energy at a temperature of several thousand degrees. Increase of water temperature to 2000 K induces only 4 percent decomposition, and CO$_2$, at the same temperature undergoes only 13 percent decomposition.[2]

In general, the process of regeneration of O$_2$ may be divided into three stages: the concentration of CO$_2$, the conversion of CO$_2$, and the electrolysis of water. However, there are methods that combine these stages. Figure 20, based on a paper by Ingelfinger and Secord,[38] presents a taxonomy of methods of O$_2$ regeneration.

A. Methods for Concentrating Carbon Dioxide

A taxonomy of these methods is provided in Fig. 21. The best developed method is concentration of CO$_2$ that has been removed from the air by adsorbents. The configuration, underlying theory, and principles of operation of subassemblies using this method are analogous to those for scrubbing CO$_2$ using adsorbents considered above. The configuration in Fig. 7 must be supplemented with a unit for evacuating and collecting CO$_2$. Such a subassembly would include a vacuum pump for evacuating CO$_2$ from the adsorber, a compressor,

and a tank for collecting the CO$_2$. The efficiency of this configuration depends, to a large extent, on the specific adsorbents used (their capacity, kinetics, moisture resistance, and operational stability), the parameters of the adsorber units, and technological process (cross section and length of the bed, air flow rate, regeneration temperature, etc.).

This method does not require preliminary drying since the adsorbents utilized have virtually unchanged CO$_2$ absorption capacity from humid air. Such substances include solid amines (based on silica gels and solid amino acid compounds). A schematic of a subassembly utilizing solid amines is presented in Fig. 22 (Ref. 39). Air from the pressurized cabin is blown into the heat exchanger and condenser to impart the requisite temperature and relative humidity and then fed into the absorbing canister. The scrubbed air is returned to the cabin through a second heat exchanger and condenser. The adsorbing canisters are regenerated with heated water vapor. Water from a tank is fed through a heater and evaporator (heat is input by the liquid-containing loops of the thermoregulation subsystem). Streams of heated vapor enter the adsorber canister, releasing CO$_2$, which is then pumped into a tank after passing through a moisture collector. Water from the collector enters a tank and then a desiccator. A temperature sensor at the outlet of the adsorbing canister reacts to a surge in the vapor stream and signals the end of the regeneration process. This subassembly can use two or three canisters cyclically.

A method for concentrating CO$_2$ using liquid absorbers (absorbents) is promising from the standpoint of power consumption. Absorbents may be regenerated by heating to temperatures above 100 °C (373 K) or by electrochemical processes. One type of subassembly based on this principle has the configuration of a closed loop, including an absorber and a desorber through which monoethanol amine, for example, circulates. Another type of subassembly using liquid

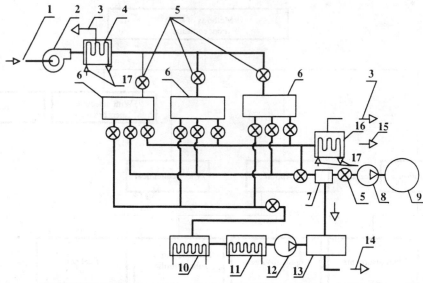

1. Air from cabin
2. Blower
3. H_2O in water regeneration subsystem
4. Heat exchanger-condenser
5. Cocks
6. Absorbing canisters
7. Moisture trap
8. Compressor
9. CO_2 collector

10. Heater
11. Evaporator
12. Hydraulic pump
13. H_2O tank
14. H_2O for water regeneration subsystem
15. Purified air into cabin
16. Condenser-heat exchanger
17. Interface with thermal control system

Fig. 22 Schematic diagram of subassembly for concentrating CO_2 using solid amines.[39]

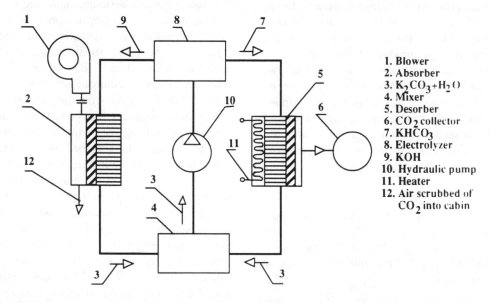

1. Blower
2. Absorber
3. $K_2CO_3 + H_2O$
4. Mixer
5. Desorber
6. CO_2 collector
7. $KHCO_3$
8. Electrolyzer
9. KOH
10. Hydraulic pump
11. Heater
12. Air scrubbed of CO_2 into cabin

Fig. 23 Schematic of CO_2 concentration subassembly with electrochemical regeneration of liquid absorbent.

absorbents entails two-stage electrochemical regeneration.[1] When alkaline chemical absorbents, for example, are used in the absorber unit, CO_2 from the air is chemically bound by the liquid absorbent (Fig. 23):

$$2\,KOH + CO_2 \longrightarrow K_2CO_3 + H_2O$$

The potassium carbonate and water that are formed are fed by a hydraulic pump into an electrochemical reactor, where

the K_2CO_3 is dissociated into $2\,K^+$ and CO_3^{--} ions. At the cathode, potassium ions interacting with water increase the concentration of the alkali KOH, which is fed back into the CO_2 absorber. CO_3^{--} and HCO_3^{-} are concentrated at the anode and form potassium bicarbonate, which is fed into the desorber, where it is heated so that it decomposes and releases CO_2:

$$2\,KHCO_3 \longrightarrow K_2CO_3 + H_2O + CO_2$$

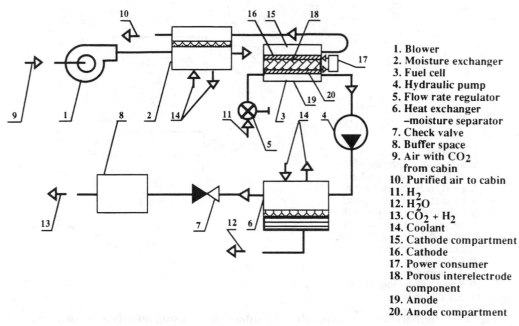

Fig. 24 Schematic of CO_2 concentration using a fuel cell.[1,40]

1. Blower
2. Moisture exchanger
3. Fuel cell
4. Hydraulic pump
5. Flow rate regulator
6. Heat exchanger –moisture separator
7. Check valve
8. Buffer space
9. Air with CO_2 from cabin
10. Purified air to cabin
11. H_2
12. H_2O
13. $CO_2 + H_2$
14. Coolant
15. Cathode compartment
16. Cathode
17. Power consumer
18. Porous interelectrode component
19. Anode
20. Anode compartment

The CO_2 thus produced is fed into a collector, while the potassium carbonate and water enter a mixer along with K_2CO_3 from the absorber and are again pumped into the electrochemical reactor. In this manner the subassembly is in continuous operation. Theoretically, this method has many advantages: lack of complicated valves, capacity for continuous operation, production of extremely pure CO_2, the relative ease with which heat can be input, low mass, and insignificant heat losses. However, its practical implementation presents a number of problems, such as the need to regulate the moisture content of the air pumped through the absorber (to maintain the necessary concentration of absorbent), loss of absorbent, the complexity of the two-phase process in the absorber, and the inadequate lifetime of the absorber and electrochemical elements, etc. This method is widely used on the ground where most of these practical problems can be solved easily.

An industrial process for concentrating CO_2 using an electrochemical O_2-hydrogen fuel cell is of significant interest from the standpoint of acceleration of chemisorption processes,[40] since mass exchange processes depend, to a great extent, on the rate of the electrochemical process. A schematic configuration of the fuel cell is presented in Fig. 24 (Refs. 1, 40). The cell consists of two compartments–one for air and one for hydrogen–separated by a diaphragm consisting of a carbonate electrolyte in a porous asbestos matrix sandwiched between two porous electrodes. The following chemical reaction occurs in the cell:

$$O_2 + CO_2 + 2\,H_2 \longrightarrow 2\,H_2O + CO_2 + Q$$

Moist air from the spacecraft cabin, containing CO_2, circulates through the cathode compartment. At the cathode, the O_2 interacts with the water, forming hydroxyl ions (OH^-),

which combine with CO_2 in the gas passing over the cathode, thereby producing moist air with diminished CO_2 concentration. Carbonate ions (CO_3^{--}) formed at the cathode are displaced toward the anode, where H_2 interacts with OH^- ions forming H_2O.

The number of OH^- ions forming in the electrolyte is deficient, causing the CO_3^{--}/CO_2 equilibrium to shift, and CO_2 to form. The flow from the anode contains CO_2 mixed with H_2.

One of the problems with this process is the need to remove the water generated as a result of the chemical reaction. A flow chart of a CO_2 concentrator using a fuel cell is shown in Fig. 24. As Fig. 24 shows, the air stream is moved by the blower through a moisture and heat exchanger and then through the cathode compartments of an electrochemical reactor. Air scrubbed of CO_2 enters the cabin through the moisture and heat exchanger. A second blower directs the stream of hydrogen through the anode compartments, where it mixes with CO_2, then passes through the heat exchanger and condenser to the CO_2 and H_2 collector. The moisture and heat exchanger serve as a stabilizer for the fuel cell with respect to temperature and electrolyte concentration. The gas mixture produced may then participate directly in the CO_2 conversion. The advantage of this method is the simplicity of the process. The disadvantages are the need to regulate humidity, the short service life of the electrochemical element, and the presence of a CO_2 and H_2 mixture, necessitating specific methods of conversion.

A promising method for concentrating CO_2 is the use of membrane technology for separating gases.[2] This technology is based on diffusion of gases through membranes selectively permeable by one of the gases of the initial mixture. The process of diffusion is controlled by the differential in partial gas pressure created on the membrane. A number of

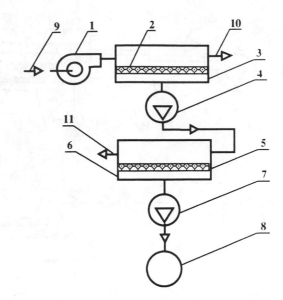

1. Blower
2. Selective membrane of the
   first stage gas exchanger
3. First stage gas exchanger
4. First stage vacuum pump
5. Selective membrane of the
   second stage gas exchanger
6. Second stage gas exchanger
7. Second stage vacuum pump
8. CO_2 collector
9. Air with CO_2
10. Scrubbed air into cabin
11. Air into cabin

Fig. 25 Schematic of CO_2 concentrating subassembly using selective membranes.[2]

polymer materials have high permeability for CO_2, but lower permeability for O_2 and N_2. Membrane selectivity is quantitatively described by the selectivity factor

$$K_s = K_{cd}/K_a$$

where K_{cd} and K_a are permeability constants for CO_2 and air (cm^3/cm^2s mm Hg). The volume concentration of CO_2 gas (C_1) in the mixture after it passes through the membrane as a function of initial concentration (C_0) and selectivity factor (K_s) may be expressed as:

$$C_1 = C_0 K_s /(C_0 K_s - C_0 + 1)$$

It is obvious from this equation that as K_s increases, so will concentration C_1 after passage through the membrane. The coefficient of selectivity of typical polymer materials is no greater than 5–10 for CO_2. However, by modifying the structure of the polymer by inoculating it with alkali groups, it is possible to increase the coefficient of selectivity to 100 and higher. When $K_s = 100$ and the initial concentration of $C_0 = 0.01$, after passage of the mixture through the second stage of separation $C_1 = 0.99$.

A schematic diagram of a two-stage subassembly is presented in Fig. 25 (Ref. 2). Air from the pressurized cabin is directed into the membrane gas exchanger, where it passes above the surfaces of the selective membranes. During this process, pumped by a vacuum pump, the CO_2 and some of the air diffuse through the membrane into the compartment while air scrubbed of CO_2 is pumped into the pressurized cabin. The gas mixture enriched with CO_2 is propelled by a vacuum pump through the second stage gas exchanger; after the mixture passes through the selective membranes, the resulting concentrated CO_2 is pumped into a collector. This method is very simple and energy efficient. However, highly

selective reliable membranes have to be produced to enable the process to occur in two or three stages using gas exchangers of acceptable size.

At a temperature of -56.6 °C (216.4 K) and pressure of 5.28 kg/cm^2, CO_2 becomes a solid, bypassing the liquid phase. Freezing is used as a method of CO_2 concentration on the ground. However, its use on spacecraft presents significant problems, although there may also be some advantage if it is possible to use the coolant loop of the thermoregulation subsystem. Construction of such a loop is difficult because of the changing orientation of the spacecraft, and its use also presents insulation problems. The use of a refrigeration machine and the creation of a loop consume significant power. At present, this method is not considered competitive for use in a spacecraft air regeneration subsystem.

B. Methods for Converting Carbon Dioxide

In a CO_2-H_2 gas system at a temperature interval of 200–1000 °C (473–1273 K) three basic reactions are thermodynamically possible:

$$CO_2 + H_2 \longrightarrow CO + H_2O$$

$$CO_2 + 2 H_2 \longrightarrow C + 2 H_2O$$

$$CO_2 + 4 H_2 \longrightarrow CH_4 + 2 H_2O$$

The third reaction, the Sabatier reaction, which produces methane and water, is of greatest practical interest.[1,2] This reaction occurs at a relatively low temperature 250–300 °C (523–573 K) in the presence of a catalyst (nickel) and emits heat, maintaining the requisite temperature without additional power consumption. One of the major advantages of the methane reaction is the possibility of a conversion rate of close to

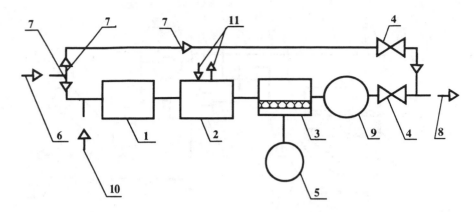

1. Sabatier reactor
2. Heat exchanger-condenser
3. Separator
4. Regulator
5. Water collector

6. CO_2 from the concentrator subassembly
7. CO_2
8. Jettisoning of $CH_4 + CO_2$
9. CH_4 collector
10. H_2 from electrolysis subassembly

Fig. 26 Schematic of a CO_2 conversion subassembly using a Sabatier reactor.[2]

1 for a long period of time without catalyst regeneration. In addition to the reaction products listed, the water forming as a result of the reaction contains a small amount of contaminants. The water that forms undergoes electrolysis to produce O_2. The hydrogen that forms in electrolysis is returned to the Sabatier reactor for CO_2 hydration, closing the regeneration cycle. However, closure is not complete, since half of the initial hydrogen is bound in the methane. In principle, it would be possible to recover this hydrogen from the methane by methane pyrolysis in the presence of a catalyst, through the chemical reaction

$$CH_4 \longrightarrow C + 2H_2$$

However, the high temperature of this reaction, 1030 °C (1303 K), and the difficulty of regenerating the catalyst from the crystalline hydrogen precipitated on it, make it difficult to implement during space flight. Nor is recovery of hydrogen from methane practical through other reactions under these conditions. The simplest way to close the cycle of the O_2 reaction is to electrolyze additional supplies of water to produce the 50 percent hydrogen lost in this reaction. Electrolytic decomposition of the total quantity of water produces half of the total O_2 needed. The other half of the total quantity of water comes from the Sabatier reactor, and the stoichiometric ratio indicates that this uses 60 percent of the total amount of CO_2 emitted in a day. The remaining 40 percent of the CO_2 and the methane that forms may be used in the engineering systems of the spacecraft or jettisoned. Thus, an additional amount of water, comprising 0.5 kg/day per person, is consumed. The flow diagram of the conversion of CO_2 with a Sabatier reactor is provided in Fig. 26 (Ref. 2). CO_2 from the CO_2 collector of the concentration subassembly is fed into the Sabatier reactor, and the methane-water vapor mixture that forms is fed into the heat exchanger and condenser and then into the water separator. The water then

enters an electrolysis cell and, after its decomposition, hydrogen is fed into the reactor; while the methane, along with a portion of the CO_2, is jettisoned. Depending on the ratios between the gases in the reactor, some quantity of hydrogen may also be jettisoned. The recommended mass ratio of CO_2 and hydrogen is 9:1 (stoichiometrically 5.45:1), at which ratio the efficiency of hydrogen conversion is approximately 98.5 percent.

The (two-stage) Bosch-Boudoir reaction may also be used for decomposing CO_2. This reaction may be summarized as:

$$CO_2 + 2H_2 \longrightarrow C + 2H_2O$$

A single-stage Bosch reaction producing water and carbon in the presence of an iron catalyst occurs at a temperature of 540–600 °C (813–873 K) and converts up to 30 percent CO_2 in a single pass. However, the dense carbon that forms adheres to the catalyst in the form of a solid deposit. For this reason it is desirable to use the two-stage process, in which porous carbon is formed in the second stage:

$$CO_2 + H_2 \longrightarrow CO + H_2O$$

$$2CO \longrightarrow C + CO_2$$

Implementation of the first stage of this process does not present any special problems (with the exception of the recirculation process when there are traces of air in the CO_2) and can occur through plasmochemical as well as chemical hydration of CO_2. The major advantages of the plasmochemical hydration method are the simplicity of the equipment needed, the insignificant mass of the plasmochemical reactor, and the production of extremely pure water.[1]

The major implementation problems in the second stage, the Boudoir process, involve removal of the carbon, some consumption of the catalyst, and a change in the rate of the

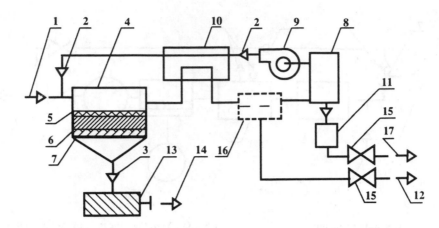

1. CO_2 from the concentrator subassembly
2. CO_2
3. O_2
4. CO_2 electrolyzer
5. Porous cathode
6. Solid electrolyte
7. Porous anode
8. Boudoir reactor
9. Blower

10. Regenerative heat exchanger
11. Carbon collector
12. Hydrogen for venting
13. Scrubbing filter
14. Oxygen to cabin
15. Drainage valve
16. Separator of hydrogen from the palladium membranes
17. Carbon to jettison

Fig. 27 Schematic conversion subassembly using CO_2 electrolysis.[2]

process as carbon accumulates. The catalyst used in the Boudoir reactor is low carbon steel and the process occurs at a temperature of 500 °C (773 K), forming carbon with a "fleecy" structure and density no greater than 0.25 kg/L, which can be removed with relative ease. The main (and probably only) advantage of the Bosch-Boudoir process is the recovery of all the O_2 from the CO_2. Closure of the O_2 regeneration process requires additional decomposition of 0.17 kg/day of water per person.

One of the most promising methods for creating closed processes for regenerating O_2 is that of direct decomposition of CO_2 by means of high temperature electrolysis of CO_2 on solid ceramic electrolytes.[41,42] In this process carbon monoxide forms at the anode, and O_2 at the cathode. The second stage of the process, the Boudoir reaction, involves the formation of solid carbon and CO_2 from CO. The electrolysis process occurs at a temperature of 800–900 °C (1073–1173 K). The electrolyte is a composite material of zirconium oxide (approximately 90 percent) and scandium or ytrium oxides. The electrodes are metal ceramic based on platinum and zirconium oxides. The CO_2 electrolysis cell contains a ceramic membrane with walls 0.5–1.0 mm thick,[2] coated on both sides with a layer of porous platinum (or palladium), serving as the electrode, and at the same time, as catalyst for the CO_2 decomposition process.

Figure 27 depicts the configuration of the CO_2 electrolysis unit.[2] CO_2 from the CO_2 collector of the condenser subassembly enters the electrolytic cell and forms O_2, which is fed into an O_2 collector. CO is fed into the regenerative heat exchanger and then the Boudoir reactor. The CO_2 from the Boudoir reactor passes through the regenerative heat exchanger and electrolysis starts, while the carbon enters the

carbon collector and is then jettisoned. Thus, this method provides the complete recovery of O_2 from CO_2, bypassing the stage of water generation. The 0.17 kg of H_2O per day per person that is still needed for O_2 balance may enter the electrolysis process in the CO_2 electrolytic cell. In this case the hydrogen forming must be removed from the loop by a separator made of palladium membranes with high selectivity for hydrogen (depicted in Fig. 27 by a dotted line). Because of the increased efficiency of the electrolytic cell at high temperatures, the electrical power used by this subassembly is minimal.

Still another variant of the method of CO_2 conversion is the electrolysis of salt solutions with ion-exchange membranes, a process called electrodialysis. The use of ion exchange membranes in electrochemical devices for O_2 regeneration make it possible to construct a unit that performs several functions at once: production of O_2 and hydrogen, scrubbing of CO_2 from the air, and CO_2 concentration.[1] This method makes it possible to construct a single-stage air regeneration subsystem. This type of subsystem is extremely complex and requires the development of a reliable electrodialysis cell and ways to structure the processes of separation of liquid electrolytes. Development of such a subsystem would require extensive experimental investigation.

C. Methods of Water Electrolysis

Water decomposition is the most power consuming process in air regeneration subsystems. Because of the need to maintain the balance of O_2 consumption and CO_2 emission, this process will be essential for any type of subsystem for air regeneration, if only to supply the 20 percent of O_2 still re-

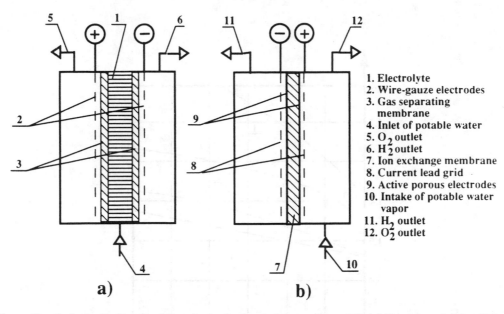

Fig. 28 Schematic of electrolysis cell of the electrolyzing subassembly with (a) liquid and (b) solid electrolytes.

1. Electrolyte
2. Wire-gauze electrodes
3. Gas separating membrane
4. Inlet of potable water
5. O_2 outlet
6. H_2 outlet
7. Ion exchange membrane
8. Current lead grid
9. Active porous electrodes
10. Intake of potable water vapor
11. H_2 outlet
12. O_2 outlet

quired for balance. Since water is easily stored, has a high density, and contains 89 percent O_2, as noted above, it may readily be used as a stored supply for any partially closed subsystem. The most well-developed technique for decomposing water is electrolysis at normal temperatures.[2] In its pure form, water has very low electrical conductivity and salts or bases are added to it to produce an electrolyte.

Theoretically, the minimal difference in potential required for water decomposition to occur is 1.23 V. In the actual process, the difference in potential on the electrodes of the electrolytic cell must be significantly higher because of the electrical resistance of the electrolyte and the polarization of the electrodes when they interact with the electrolyte and products of the electrochemical reaction. The least amount of energy consumed in water electrolysis will correspond to a voltage of 1.48; thus, to produce the 0.86 kg/day of O_2 needed by a single individual requires 176 watts. The actual power consumed by electrolysis depends to a large extent on the design of the electrolytic cell, the materials of which the electrodes are made, and the type of electrolyte and electrolyzer.

Maintenance of the stability of the electrolysis process requires good contact between the electrolyte and the electrodes, separation of the product gases from the electrolyte, separation of hydrogen and O_2 from each other, maintenance of the requisite concentration of the electrolyte and of the water level, and heat removal. In microgravity, these requirements compel new approaches to designing and structuring the processes. Rotating electrolyzers cannot be used because of their complexity and unreliability. The most practical technique for structuring the electrolysis process is acknowledged to be the use of capillary porous elements, with the subsequent separation of the products from the electrolyte in dynamic as well as static separators.

Analysis of electrolysis components has shown that alkaline electrolytic cells (KOH electrolyte) use less electricity

than the analogous acid ones.

A schematic configuration of electrolysis cells is presented in Fig. 28. Power loss is greatest from cells with liquid electrolyte and wire-gauze electrodes because of the high ohmic resistance of the electrolyte. Porous electrodes instead of wire-gauze ones improve this parameter.

Two types of electrolyzers can be distinguished on the basis of how the water is fed in: those with circulating electrolytes, and those with static feeding of water. With a circulating electrolyte it is easy to solve the problems of homogeneity of electrolyte concentration in the cell and heat removal. Static feeding significantly simplifies the process, as well as equipment design, since it does not require gas-electrolyte separators, water circulation circuits, etc. For static feeding, a porous matrix impregnated with the electrolyte is located in the inner compartment of the cell, with electrodes tightly affixed to both sides. Water is fed through a porous membrane. As it evaporates from the surface of the membrane, it enters the cathode compartment, and from there, the matrix.[39]

The most efficient type of electrolytic cell uses a solid electrolyte made of ion exchange membranes and electrochemically active electrodes.[2,43] The cation-exchange polymer membranes that have been developed for this purpose have high electric conductivity for H^+ ions and may be made thin enough (up to 0.25–0.5 mm) to significantly decrease electrical resistance. Active electrodes are manufactured from platinum, with palladium coating on the surface of the ion exchange membrane in the form of porous layers with highly developed surfaces. Voltage is supplied to the electrodes by attaching metal grids (conductors) to them. The water may be delivered through a circulation loop or statically in the vapor phase, producing dry O_2 of high purity. A comparison of the volt-ampere characteristics of the cells (Fig. 29) shows that the use of a polymer electrolyte decreases power consumption by 20–30 percent.[2] However, this method requires

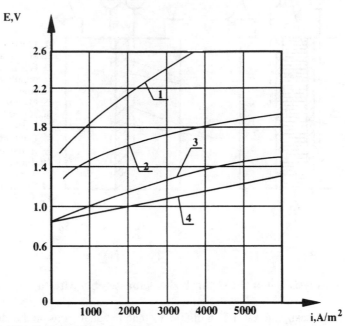

1. With liquid alkaline electrolytes
2. With polymer electrolyte
3. High temperatures electrolyzer with electrolytic membrane 1 mm thick
4. As above but with membrane thickness of 0.5 mm

Fig. 29 Volt-ampere characteristics of electrolyzer types.

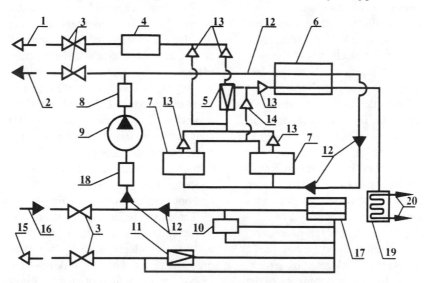

1. Oxygen into cabin	11. H_2 pressure regulator
2. Water into water regeneration subassembly	12. H_2O
3. Stop valve	13. O_2
4. O_2 scrubbing filter	14. $H_2 + H_2O$
5. O_2 pressure regulator	15. Hydrogen for jettisoning
6. Heat exchanger	16. Water from the water regeneration subsystem
7. Electrolyzer	17. Separator
8. Ion exchange filter	18. Filter
9. Circulation pump	19. Heat exchanger
10. Pressure differential regulator	20. Thermoregulation system

Fig. 30 Schematic of water electrolysis subassembly with circulation loop using solid ion-exchange electrolyte.[43]

water of extremely high purity.

High temperature electrolysis of water in electrolytic cells with solid ceramic electrolytes (considered in the discussion of CO_2 electrolysis) is of interest. Such cells have the best power and mass parameters, since losses due to electrolyte resistance and polarization are minimized and high current densities can be achieved.

The design of electrolyzers usually includes 10–15 cells connected in series, with common collectors to input water and output O_2 and hydrogen, forming an electrolyzing battery. The mass of the battery is proportional to the working surface of the electrolytic cells, which becomes smaller as the current density increases. However, when the density of the current increases, so does loss of electric power, and for this reason the optimal current density must be selected as a function of electrolytic cell design. Current density in well designed electrolyzers reaches several thousand A/m^2 (Ref. 2).

A schematic diagram of an electrolyzer using an ion-exchange electrolyte with a circulation loop is presented in Fig. 30 (Ref. 43). Water circulates continuously in the subassembly through the hydrogen (cathode) compartments of the electrolytic cells, ensuring production of "dry" O_2. Excess heat produced by electrolysis is transmitted by a heat exchanger to the hydraulic loop of the thermoregulation subsystem. The hydrogen generated is separated from water in separators and jettisoned, while the water returns to the circulation circuit. A pressure differential regulator in the circulation loop supports the pressure differential in the separator. The water circulation loop contains an ion-exchange filter for removal of contaminants in the incoming water. After passing through a charcoal filter, the O_2 generated is vented directly into the pressurized cabin.

A method for electrolyzing moisture that enters the electrolytic cells in humid cabin air makes it possible to combine O_2 regeneration with regulation of atmospheric humidity. This involves the use of an electrolysis cell that contains an electrolyte layer in bound form sandwiched between permeable electrodes.[44]

The explosion safety of electrolysis subassemblies is of particular concern because of the presence of O_2 and hydrogen. To ensure safety, the O_2 level in the hydrogen and the hydrogen level in the O_2 must be monitored using special gas analyzers. In addition, electrolyzer subassemblies should contain cylinders of inert gas (nitrogen) to purge the subassemblies before they are turned on and after they are turned off.

V. Weight-Energy Characteristics of Subassemblies and Subsystems

Table 3 compares the mass characteristics and power consumption of major air regeneration subassemblies and subsystems, noting the spacecraft on which they are used. Figure 31 shows the mass of these subsystems as a function of flight duration.

It is clear that air regeneration subsystems have an advantage in terms of mass for a crew of three for flights not exceeding 1 month. From the standpoint of energy consumption, however, air regeneration subsystems are significantly less efficient than those using stored supplies. In addition, the heat generated in the components of the subsystem must be removed using the thermoregulation subsystem loops. For this reason, air regeneration subsystems should be compared to an equivalent mass including, aside from their own mass, that of the power supply systems and thermoregulation subsystems. If solar arrays are used as an energy source, then the specific mass of the electric power supply system may be approximately 200 kg/kW, while the specific mass of the thermoregulation subsystem is 50 kg/kW.[2] The curves of this function, adjusted for equivalent mass, are shown in Fig. 31 by dotted lines (numbering of lines corresponds to entries in Table 2), and are juxtaposed with equivalent curves for subsystems using stored supplies, for which these corrections are less than 10 kg. As the curves show, these adjustments do not significantly affect the results of the comparison of subsystems: after no more than 2 months, the regenerative air supply subsystems, and even individual subassemblies, have the advantage over subsystems using stored supplies. In practice, the possible dimensions of solar arrays, even on existing orbital space stations, enable the use of a closed-cycle subsystem for air and water regeneration. A more efficient power source would also expand these capacities.

VI. Use of Air Regeneration Subsystems on Spacecraft

Because of the short duration of the first manned space flights, cabin air regeneration subsystems were based on stored supplies. Air was regenerated on the Soviet Vostok, Voskhod, and Soyuz spacecraft by blowing cabin air through a regenerator containing a substance based on potassium superoxide. The configuration of the air regeneration subsystem on Vostok was analogous to that depicted in Fig. 16. On Soyuz spacecraft, humidity was not regulated when air was fed into the KO_2 regenerators; however, flow rate was changed using special rubber stoppers to alter the size of the outlet cross section when crew size changed or when the regeneration canister began to wear out. Humidity in the Soyuz cabin was controlled by the heat exchanger and condenser.

Air regeneration on the American Mercury, Gemini, and Apollo spacecraft used lithium hydroxide canisters in a subassembly similar to the subassembly depicted in Fig. 3 to absorb CO_2. O_2 was supplied on Mercury from cylinders with compressed O_2 (pressure 527 kg/cm^2). On Gemini and Apollo, O_2 was provided from supplies of cryogenic O_2 stored in the tanks of the power supply system, with additional reserve supplies on these spacecraft and O_2 for the Apollo lander stored in compressed gas cylinders. The Space Shuttle uses an improved air regeneration subsystem based on the Apollo subsystem. The Soyuz-T transport spacecraft has an air regeneration subsystem using lithium hydroxide (analogous to the configuration in Fig. 3) and stores of gaseous compressed O_2. A regenerator with KO_2 is intended only to be used as a

Table 3   Mass characteristics and power consumption of air regeneration subassemblies and subsystems

Number/Subassembly or subsystem	Constant weight, kg	Weight of expendables, kg[a] Power use (W)			Space craft
		O_2 recovery	CO_2 removal	Total	
1. Gaseous O_2 and chemical sorbent	< 15	7.8 —	6.3(5.4) < 10	14.1(13.2) 10	Mercury, Soyuz T
2. Solid O_2 source and chemical sorbent	< 15	6.6 —	6.3(5.4) < 10	12.9(12) 10	Mir
3. Potassium superoxide and chemical sorbent	< 15	10.8 < 20	0.9 < 10	11.7 20	Salyut
4. Supercritical O_2 and chemical sorbent	< 20	4.2 < 20	6.3 (5.4) < 10	10.5(9.6) 30	Gemini, Apollo, Shuttle
5. Hydrogen peroxide and chemical sorbent	< 50	4.2 —	6.3(5.4) < 10	10.5(9.6) 10	
6. Liquid O_2 and chemical sorbent	< 20	3.6 —	6.3(5.4) < 10	9.9(9.0) 10	
7. Sodium superoxide	< 15	8.4 —	—	8.4	
8. Gaseous O_2 and regenerable absorbent	< 150	7.8 —	0.6 < 300	8.4 300	
9. Solid O_2 source and regenerable absorbent	≤ 150 b< 200	6.6 —	0.6 < 300	7.2 300	Mir + Kvant
10. H_2O electrolysis and regenerable absorbent	≤ 450 b700	4.2 < 750	0.6 < 300	4.8 1050	Mir + Kvant 2
11. Hydrogen peroxide and regenerable absorbent	≤ 200 b< 270	4.2 —	0.6 < 300	4.8 300	
12. Concentrator—regenerable absorbent, Sabatier reactor, and H_2O electrolysis	≤ 300 b< 600	1.8 < 750	— < 550	1.8 1300	Space Station (design)
13. CO_2 concentrator, fuel cell, CO_2 and H_2O electrolysis, and Boudoir reactor	≤ 200 b< 550	0.6 < 750	— < 550	0.6 1300	

[a]For the chemical sorbents, data is for lithium hydroxide (with data on lithium oxide in parentheses).
[b]Equivalent weight, counting power consumption.

backup after landing under contingency conditions.

Analysis shows that an air regeneration subsystem based on separate stores of absorbers and O_2 is the most practical for transport spacecraft with flight duration of up to 30 man-days, although with respect to mass, such a subsystem suffers somewhat compared to one using potassium superoxide. Separate stores of O_2 make such a subsystem operationally more flexible, since it can be used for pressurizing in contingency situations, for working in space suits in an unpressurized cabin, etc.

In both the Soviet Union and the United States, extensive ground research was conducted to test experimental regenerative subassemblies for air regeneration subsystems. In the late 1960s a Soviet ground-based experimental subsystem, including a subassembly for concentrating CO_2 with zeolites and silica gel, a conversion subassembly using a Sabatier reactor, and an electrolysis subassembly with a circulation loop, was tested through long-term inhabitation with human subjects. In 1970, the United States conducted a 90-day test with human subjects, involving analogous subassemblies, as well as an adsorption subassembly for concentrating CO_2 with solid amines regenerated with water vapor.[39] These tests were the basis for further design of Soviet and U.S. air regeneration subsystems. From 1973–1974, a partially regenerative subassembly for removing CO_2 with zeolites was used successfully for the first time on board Skylab.[45] This subassembly

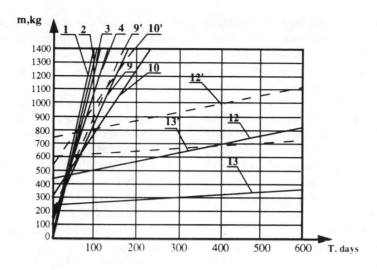

1. Numbering corresponds to Table 3.
2. Dotted lines represent curves of equivalent mass, counting power consumption, and thermoregulation.

Fig. 31 Mass of the air subsystems and regeneration subassemblies as a function of flight duration (crew size of three).

contained two zeolite canisters, each of which had two adsorbent layers; the first was composed of type 13X zeolite for drying and the second layer of zeolite 5A for CO_2 scrubbing. The sorption cycle was equal in duration to the regeneration cycle (15 minutes). Adsorbent regeneration from water and CO_2 used the vacuum method. High temperature thermovacuum regeneration lasting a number of hours was supposed to be performed every 28 days. In actuality this process was performed less frequently, i.e., four times in 171 days.

A subassembly for removing CO_2 and water using solid amines regenerated in a vacuum without special heating was also designed for the Space Shuttle.[46] However, this subassembly was not installed in the spacecraft.

The Salyut station, which first flew in 1970, had an improved air regeneration subsystem based on the subsystem in the Soyuz transport spacecraft. It included regenerative subassemblies with KO_2 and highly efficient subassemblies for absorbing CO_2 using lithium oxide. To optimize functioning, the regeneration and absorption canisters worked in an overlapping mode; for a period after fresh canisters were inserted, air continued to be pumped through the old ones.

The Mir complex began operating in orbit in 1986; it had an air regeneration subsystem using CO_2 absorption lithium oxide canisters, while O_2 was supplied by solid sources based on lithium perchlorate. Additional O_2 was delivered in cylinders by the Progress cargo vehicles.

After the Kvant module docked with the Mir complex in the first quarter of 1987, adsorption was successfully performed by a subassembly using a special adsorbent that could be regenerated in the vacuum of space without heating. Before entering the adsorption canister, the air passed through desiccant canisters containing silica gel in a blow-back pro-

cedure. This subassembly could operate in several modes and provided life support for two to five crewmembers. After the Kvant 2 module docked with the Mir complex in December 1989, a water electrolysis subassembly with a circulating electrolyte loop began to operate. This subassembly provided life support for three crewmembers. Water was fed into it from the subassembly that regenerated water from urine.

VII. Air Regeneration Methods of the Future

At the present time, the first subassemblies of a semiregenerative air regeneration subsystem are functioning successfully on the Mir complex. To further close the cycle, the subassembly that removes CO_2 will have to be converted into a concentrating subassembly, and a CO_2 conversion subassembly will have to be added. The use of such a subsystem under conditions of actual space flight will provide the experience required to further improve air regeneration subsystems and select the most appropriate regeneration methods.

The United States is continuing to develop and test a series of air regeneration subassemblies, primarily for use on Space Station.[47–58] Developmental work, which was conducted actively in the 1970s, again received financial support after the adoption of the space station program.

Recently, further development of this type of subassembly has been emphasized by Japanese scientists and engineers.[59–61] A four-canister design using zeolites and desiccants, a subassembly using amines regenerated with water vapor, and an electrochemical method with a fuel cell are being considered as a method for concentrating CO_2 on Space Station. A method based on Sabatier and Bosch reactions is being investigated for CO_2 conversion; and static methods, using liquid and solid polymer electrolytes, are under consideration for water electrolysis. For the future, methods of high-temperature electrolysis of CO_2 and water, based on solid ceramic electrolytes are being considered. Also under consideration is a method for electrolysis of water vapor taken directly from the air of the pressurized cabin.

Analysis of the mass characteristics of regenerative subassemblies shows that the fixed mass of the subassembly is not a critical selection criterion. The first regenerative subassemblies have had fixed mass of up to 150 kg, including backup, redundancy, reserves, etc. However, when methods are improved, this mass will be decreased by a factor of 2–2.5. Even the power consumption of these subassemblies is not a critical selection criterion; the power consumption for CO_2 concentration will be 5–12 W/L of CO_2, depending on the efficiency of the method and equipment. Analogously, power consumption in water electrolysis will be 8–12 W/L of O_2. CO_2 conversion will not require power consumption (or only minimal power if heat loss is considered). These figures do not include power consumed by the blowers, compressors, hydraulic pumps, and control elements. The decisive selection factors are the magnitude of variable (consumable) mass due to the lack of complete closure of the substance cycle, the useful lifetime of individual components, and the reliability and stability of the subassembly in operation. Furthermore, one of the most important factors is the design reliability of the method.

Adsorption subassemblies for concentrating CO_2 might be considered from the following standpoint. As noted above, the major shortcoming of a subassembly using zeolites is the significant decrease in the CO_2 adsorption capacity when zeolites come into contact with water, requiring thorough dehumidification of incoming gas. If moisture gets in the zeolites, as a result of failure of the preliminary dehumidification device or crewmember error, for example; the concentration subassembly may cease to function. For this reason it may be expedient to use adsorbents whose absorbing capacity is not altered through contact with water, such as solid amines or amino silica gels, which also have a lower regeneration temperature.

However, a disadvantage of solid amines is that they change volume during sorption-regeneration cycles, and probably also have an inadequate useful life. In addition, the adsorption capacity of these sorbents is inferior to that of zeolites. One promising direction may be the synthesis of adsorbents that are not spoiled by water and have a capacity of up to 3–5 percent at partial CO_2 pressure of approximately 4 mm Hg (if possible with a convex isotherm in this region). These substances should also have the potential for regeneration in the vacuum of space if the CO_2 concentration or conversion units break down. A concentration method based on this type of hydrophilic adsorbent with the potential for CO_2 venting in the vacuum of space appears promising and reliable.

The development of highly selective membranes and reliable gas exchangers may make the diffusion method of CO_2 concentration promising.

Advantages of adsorbents include their capacity to function without interruption and the purity of the CO_2 they produce. Their disadvantages are that the useful life does not exceed several months, air humidity must be regulated, and the absorber is complex.

An electrochemical concentration subassembly using a fuel cell has the same disadvantage as the absorption one; i.e., its performance depends on the humidity of the air stream. Another problem is creating electrochemical batteries with the necessary useful life. Analysis by Wynveen and Quattrone[40] suggests that an electrochemical concentrator offers advantages in mass over absorption concentrators if the partial CO_2 pressure in cabin air is below 3 mm Hg.

There are other potential types of electrochemical concentrators that operate without loss of O_2 and accumulate CO_2 that is not mixed with hydrogen. These subassemblies have a number of advantages, but the problem of electrode corrosion is very difficult.

The method for converting CO_2 using a Sabatier reactor has a significant advantage from the standpoint of design reliability, i.e., the reaction takes place in a single pass at moderate temperatures. All other methods based on recycling present an explosion hazard because of the nature of the gases that accumulate in the loop. The method of electrodialysis is also highly complex and has not yet been developed to a sufficient level. The major disadvantage of a Sabatier reaction is the use of only 60 percent of the CO_2 emitted, requiring a daily additional supply of O_2 in the amount of 260 grams, or 300 grams of water, to meet human metabolic needs. It would hardly be desirable to further complicate the method by adding high temperature decomposition of methane. The Sabatier reactor would have additional advantages if O_2 produced by electrolysis of water supplies could used to fill the cylinders of EVA suits. Hydrogen forming through this process may significantly increase the percentage of CO_2 utilized. The method based on the Sabatier reactor will be the method of choice for a first-generation closed subsystem of air regeneration.

Although reliable electrolyzers with an alkali circulating loop exist, a major disadvantage is their potential for leakage of the alkalis into the cabin if the equipment fails. An electrolyzer with static feeding of water with an alkali matrix appears preferable, but requires improvements in reliability and longevity. The most promising is an electrolyzer using solid polymer electrolytes; such a subassembly functions with a large pressure differential at the membrane, maintains constant electrolyte concentration, precludes contamination of the generated gases or cabin air with electrolytes, is energy efficient, and has a useful life of several years.

To develop second-generation air regeneration subsystems, it will be desirable to consider subassemblies for electrolysis of CO_2 and water vapor using ceramic electrolytes at high temperatures. Such subassemblies could prove to be relatively simple condensers if their useful life were improved. A subassembly for electrolysis of water vapor from the air stream would be a desirable backup component of the subsystem.

An analysis by Kubasov, et al.[62] has demonstrated that in the coming decades this type of physicochemical closed subsystem would be desirable on lunar bases and Mars missions. When the size of space crews increases to several dozen members and space stations are substantially enlarged, biological air regeneration subsystems based on photosynthesis may be considered. Even here, however, because of the inadequate predictability of the course of biological processes in small spaces under conditions of zero-g or microgravity, physicochemical air regeneration subsystems will probably be used as backups. In addition, reliable, small, energy efficient, closed air regeneration subsystems developed for space flight may be used successfully to create closed ecological cycles on the ground or under the sea.

References

[1]Grishayenkov, B.G. Air conditioning and regeneration. In: Calvin, M. and Gazenko, O.G., Eds. *Foundations of Space Biology and Medicine*. Washington D.C., NASA, 1975, Vol. III, chapter 3, pp. 56–111 (translated from Russian).

[2]Serebryakov, V.N. *Design Principles for Crew Life Support Systems and Space Flight Vehicles*. Moscow, Mashinostroyeniye, 1983, chapter 2, pp. 35–76; chapters 4 and 5, pp. 101–153 (in Russian).

[3]Ivanov, D.I. and Khromushkin, A.I. *Man-rated Life Support Systems at High Altitudes and During Space Flights*. Moscow, Mashinostroyeniye, 1968, chapter 4, pp. 60–84 (in Russian).

[4]Serpionova, Ye.N. *Industrial Adsorption of Gases and Vapor*. Moscow, Vysshaya Shkola, 1969, part 1, chapters 2 and 3, p 9–47, part 2; chapters 3 and 4, pp. 60–97 (in Russian).

[5]Romankov, P.G. and Lepilin, V.N. *The Continuous Adsorption of Vapor and Gases*. Leningrad, Khimiya, 1968, chapters 1 and 2, pp. 11–75; chapter 6, pp. 139–154 (in Russian).

[6]Keltsev, N.V. *Principles of Adsorption Technology*. Moscow, Khimiya, 1984, chapters 1 and 3, pp. 16–115; chapter 6, pp. 138–151; chapter 8, pp. 167–203 (in Russian).

[7]Rachinskiy, V.V. *Introduction to Common Theories of Dynamic Sorption and Chromatography*. Moscow, Nauka, 1969, chapters 1–4, pp. 5–105 (in Russian).

[8]Dubinin, M.M.; Zhukov, Z.A.; and Keltsev, N.V. The applicability of potential theory to adsorption of vapor and gases by synthetic zeolites. In: Dubinin, M. M. and Serpinskiy, M., Eds. *Synthetic Zeolites*. Moscow, U.S.S.R. Academy of Sciences, 1962, pp. 7–17 (in Russian).

[9]Trepnel B. *Chemisorption*. Moscow, Inostrannaya Literatura, 1958, p. 148 (translated into Russian).

[10]Dubinin M.M. and Chmutov, K.V. *Physical and Chemical Principles of Protection from Toxic Gases*. Moscow, Voyennaya Akademiya Chimzashity, 1939 (in Russian).

[11]Dubinin, M.M. *Porous Structures and Adsorbent Properties of Activated Charcoal*. Moscow, Voyennaya Akademiya Chimzashity, 1955 (in Russian).

[12]Kiselyov, A.V. The nature of adsorption by zeolites. In: *Zeolites, Their Synthesis, Properties and Use*. Moscow-Leningrad, Nauka, 1965, pp.13–25 (in Russian).

[13]Avgul, N.N.; Guzenberg, A.S.; Kiselyov, A.V.; Kurdyukova, L.Ya.; and Ryabkin, A.M. Calculation of adsorption of CO_2 by nonporous and small-pored crystalline adsorbents at various pressures and temperatures using virial equations. *Zhurnal Fizicheskoy Khimii*, 1971, vol. 45, p. 442 (in Russian).

[14]Guzenberg, A.S.; Kurdyukova; and L.Ya, Ryabkin, A.M. Use of virial equations to describe adsorption of CO_2 by zeolites. In: Dubinin, M.M. and Serpinskiy, V.V., Eds. *Fundamental Aspects of Theories of Physical Adsorption*. Moscow, Nauka, 1970, pp. 398–400 (in Russian).

[15]Dubinin, M.M. Adsorption properties and structures of silica and alumogels. *Doklady Akademii Nauk SSSR*, 1949, vol. 69, no. 2, p. 209 (in Russian).

[16]Dubinin, M.M.; Vyshnyakova, M.M.; Zaverina, E.D.; Zhukovskaya, E.G.; and Sakharov, A.I. Investigation of the adsorption properties of secondary porous structures of adsorbents acting as molecular sieves. *Izvestiya Akademii Nauk SSSR, Otdel Khimicheskikh Nauk*, 1961, pp. 1387–1395 (in Russian).

[17]Guzenberg, A.S.; Nakhalov, V.V.; Ryabkin, A.M.; and Savelyev, G.G. Chemisorption of CO_2 on metal oxides. *Izvestiya Tomskogo Gosudarstvennogo Universiteta*, 1973, p. 198 (in Russian).

[18]Danilychev, I.A.; Strelko V.V.; Burushkina, T.I.; Cherkasov, V.K.; Avetisyants, B.L.; and Menshova, V.M. Aminosilica gels—regenerable sorbents for the absorption of CO_2, H_2S and water vapor. *Kosmicheskaya Biologiya i Meditsina*, 1971, no. 3, pp. 77–79 (in Russian).

[19]Todes, O.M. and Bikson, Ya.M. On the dynamics of sorption on an actual granular adsorbent. *Doklady Akademii Nauk SSSR*, 1950, vol. 75, p. 727–750 (in Russian).

[20]Bikson, Ya.M. On the evaluation of the length of the sorbent bed in the dynamics of sorption on an actual granular adsorbent. *Zhurnal Fizicheskoy Khimii*, 1953, vol. 27, p. 1530 (in Russian).

[21]Bikson, Ya.M. The role of diffusion kinetic factors in dynamic sorption. Dissertation, 1950 (in Russian).

[22]Abakumov, Ye.P.; Guzenberg, A.S.; Ryabkin, A.M.; and Sabelyev, G.G. Internal diffusion kinetics of CO_2 on zeolites. *Izvestiya Tomskogo Politekhnicheskogo Instituta*, 1970, 251 (in Russian).

[23]Timofeyev, D.P. *Kinetic Adsorption*. Moscow, U.S.S.R. Academy of Sciences, 1962, chapter 2, pp. 31–70; chapters 7–8, pp. 184–249 (in Russian).

[24]Zhukhovitskiy, A.A.; Zabezhinskiy, Ya.L.; and Tikhonov, A.N. Absorption of gas from an air stream by a layer of granular material. I. *Zhurnal Fizicheskoy Khimii*, 1945, vol. 19, p. 253 (in Russian).

[25]Zhukhovitskiy, A.A.; Zabezhinskiy, Ya.L.; and Tikhonov, A.N. Absorption of gas from an air stream by a layer of granular material. II. *Zhurnal Fizicheskoy Khimii*, 1945, vol. 20, p. 113 (in Russian).

[26]Zhukhovitskiy, A.A.; Zabezhinskiy, Ya.L.; and Tikhonov, A.N. Absorption of gas from an air stream by a layer of granular material. III. *Zhurnal Fizicheskoy Khimii*,1949, vol. 23, p. 198 (in Russian).

[27]Yiru, P.; Rolek, P.; and Grubner, O. Methods for designing adsorbents with molecular sieves. In: Dubinin, M. M. and Plachenov, T. G., Eds. *Zeolites: Their Synthesis, Properties and Applications*. Moscow, Nauka, 1965 (in Russian).

[28]Fenelonov, V.Ye.; Fenelonova, L.Ye.; Satyukov, A.N.; and Mazin, V.N. The kinetic and dynamic sorption of gases and vapor on synthetic zeolites. In: Dubinin, M.M. and Plachenov, T.G., Eds. *Zeolites: Their Synthesis, Properties, and Applications*. Moscow, Leningrad, Nauka, 1965 (in Russian).

[29]Jackson, J.K. and Blakely, R.L. Application of adsorption beds to spacecraft life support system. Douglas Aircraft Co., SAE TPS, 67842, 1967.

[30]Guzenberg, A.S. On the intradiffusional kinetics of sorption of CO_2 by zeolite. In: Dubinin, M. M. and Radushkevich, L. V., Eds. *The Kinetics and Dynamics of Physical Adsorption*. Moscow, Nauka, 1973, pp. 247–248 (in Russian).

[31]Bykov, L.T.; Yegorov, M.S.; and Tapasov, P.V. *High-altitude Equipment for Aircraft*. Moscow, Oborongiz, 1958, chapter 7, pp. 201–218 (in Russian).

[32]Popov, Ye. N. *Automatic Regulation and Control*. Moscow, Fizmatgiz, 1962, chapters 1 and 2, pp. 14–100 (in Russian).

[33]Ishkin, I.P. and Kaganer, M.G. *Oxygen*. Moscow-Leningrad, Goskhimtekh-izdat, 1949, vol. 2, p. 35 (in Russian).

[34]Voronin, G.I. and Polivoda, A.I. *Crew Life Support Systems for Spacecraft*. Moscow, Mashinostroyeniye, 1967, chapters 1 and 2, pp. 15–80 (in Russian).

[35]Manned Spacecraft Center Cryogenic Symposium. Houston, NASA, May 1971, (MSC-04, 312).

[36]Voronin, G.I.; Polivoda, A.I.; and Vinogradov, Ye.A. Spacecraft life support systems. *Aviatsiya i Kosmonavtika*, 1966, no. 9, pp. 44–47 (in Russian).

[37]Genin, A.M.; Gurovskiy, N.I.; Yemelyanov, M.D.; Saksonov, P.P.; and Yazdovskiy, V.I. *Man in Space*. Moscow, Medgiz, 1963 (in Russian).

[38]Inglefinger A.L. and Secord, T.C. Life support for a large space station. AIAA Paper no. 68-1032.

[39]Mills, E.S.; Linzey, T.T.; and Marker, I.F. Oxygen recovery for the 90-day Space Station simulator test. ASME publication no. 71-Av-18.

[40]Wynveen, R.A. and Quattrone, P.D. Electrochemical carbon dioxide concentrating system. ASME publication no. 71-Av-21.

[41]Elison, L.; Merris, J.P.; Wu, C.K.; and Sounders, C.C. 160-day life test of solid electrolyte system for oxygen regeneration. ASME publication no. 71-Av-32.

[42]Weissbart, J.; Smart, W.H.; and Wydeven, T. Design and performance of a solid electrolyte oxygen generator test module. ASME publication no. 71-Av-8.

[43]Nuttal, L.J. and Fetterington, W.A. General Electric Company solid polymer electrolyte water electrolysis system. ASME publication no. 71-Av-9.

[44]Celino, V.A. and Wydeven, T. Development status of the water vapor electrolysis system. ASME publication no. 71-Av-24.

[45]Hopson, G.D. Skylab life support and habitability system requirement and implementation. Paper presented at the XXIInd International Aeronautic Congress, Brussels, 1971.

[46]Boehm, A.M. The development and testing of a regenerable CO_2 and humidity control for the Shuttle. ASME publication, San Francisco, 1977.

[47]Boyda, R.B.; Lance N.; and Schwartz, M. Electrochemical CO_2 concentration for the Space Station program. 1985, SAE TPS, 851341.

[48]Wagner, R.C.; Carrasquillo, R.; Edwards, J.; and Holmes, R. Maturity of the Bosch CO_2 reduction technology for Space Station application. 1988, SAE TPS, 880995.

[49]Isenberg, A.O. and Cusick, R.J. Carbon electrolyte cells for oxygen recovery in life support system. 1988, SAE TPS, 881040.

[50]Forsythe, R.K.; Verostko, C.E.; Cusick, R.J.; and Blakely, R.L. A study of Sabatier reactor operation in zero "G". 1984, SAE TPS, 840936.

[51]Miller, C.W. and Hoppner, D.B. Space Station environmental control/life support engineering. 1985, SAE TPS, 851375.

[52]Fortunato, F.A. and Burke, K.A. Static feed electrolyzer technology advancement for space application. 1987, SAE TPS, 871450.

[53]Spina L. and Lee, M.C. Comparison of CO_2 reduction process-Bosch and Sabatier. 1987, SAE TPS, 851343.

[54]Noyes, G.P.and Cusick, R.J. Initial development and performance evaluation of a process for formation of dense carbon by pyrolysis of methane. 1985, SAE TPS, 851342.

[55]Ericson, A.C.; Puskar, M.C.; Zagaija, I.A.; and Miller, P.S. Performance evaluation of SPE electrolyzer for Space Station life support. 1987, SAE TPS, 871451.

[56]Chullen, C.; Heppner, D.B.; and Sudar, M. Advancements in water vapor electrolysis technology. 1988, SAE TPS, 881041.

[57]Nason, I.R. and Tremblay, P.G. High pressure water electrolysis for the Space Station. 1987, SAE TPS, 871473.

[58]Nocheff, M.S.; Chang, C.H.; Colombo, G.V.; and Cusick, R.J. Metal oxide regenerable carbon dioxide removal system for an advanced portable life support system. 1989, SAE TPS, 871595.

[59]Ishida, H.; Yamashiro, H.; Fujita, S.; Masuyama, K.; Kondo, S.; Mitsuda, S.; Watanabe, T.; and Shoy, T. Study of advanced system for air revitalization. 1989, SAE TPS, 891575.

[60]Otsuji, K.; Hanabusa, O.; Etoh, T.; and Minemoto, M. Air revitalization system study for Japanese Space Station.

1988, SAE TPS, 881112.

[61]Otsuji, K.; Hanabusa, O.; Sawada, T.; Satoh, S. ; and Minemoto, M. An experimental study of the Bosch and the Sabatier CO_2 reduction processes. 1987, SAE TPS, 871517.

[62]Kubasov V.N.; Zaitsev, Ye.N.; Korsakov, W.A.; Guzenberg, A.S.; and Lepsky, A.A. Regenerative life support system development problems for the Mars missions. *Acta Astronautica*, 1991, vol. 23, pp 271–274.

Chapter 10

Maintenance of Thermal Conditions in Pressurized Spacecraft Cabins

A. S. Guzenberg

On space flights, thermal conditions in the pressurized cabin as a whole and in each of its separate parts must be maintained throughout all legs of the flight. Specifically, this includes rejection of the heat generated by the crew and equipment to the vacuum of space, maintaining an appropriate ambient temperature in the inhabited modules, and ensuring temperatures required for the equipment and structural elements of the cabin.

When the spacecraft is on the launch pad, thermal conditions in the cabin are maintained by ground-based facilities. During launch, the spacecraft is generally protected from aerodynamic heating by the booster rocket and also by special heat-resistant materials applied to the outer surfaces of the spacecraft. The pressurized cabin is similarly protected for landings on planets with atmospheres. This chapter will, however, focus on the maintenance of thermal conditions during the orbital leg of a flight.

As is well known, humans can work normally for extended periods only in a rather narrow range of ambient temperatures, 15–30 °C (288–303 K), with an optimal temperature of 18–23 °C (291–296 K).

The flow velocity of the cabin air must be within the limits of 0.1–0.3 m/s, crewmembers should be able to adjust airflow for personal comfort.

Under these conditions each crewmember generates a mean of 100–150 Kcal/hr (115–175 W). This heat is transferred to the cabin air mainly by convection. Another source of internal heat generated is the equipment in the cabin. Virtually all of the electrical power used by the equipment is transformed into heat. At the same time the exterior surface of the cabin is subjected to several types of radiant energy.

Thus, the general goal of maintaining thermal conditions may be divided into two basic subgoals: internal and external control. The internal task involves removing heat from the atmosphere and equipment of the cabin to an intermediate heat transfer agent by either convective, conductive, or radiative heat transfer. The external task involves ensuring radiative heat transfer to the vacuum of space. The whole thermal control system is a collection of transfer devices that regulate internal and external heat transfer.

During the early years of spacecraft development, flight times were short and internal heat loads did not exceed tens of watts, therefore, it was possible to use a thermal control system involving only thermal control coatings of the surfaces and insulation. Later, as flight time, weight, and power increased and it became necessary to support more stable thermal environments, semipassive methods were employed. These techniques use a combination of passive methods with consumable refrigerants. Semipassive thermal control methods subsequently developed into the closed loops used on many current space vehicles. Given the heat loads to which spacecraft are currently subject, approximately 5–10 kW, heat removal occurs at low temperatures, with the temperature of the thermal radiator below that of the cabin air. However, further increases in spacecraft power will require bigger radiators and to minimize their area, heat removal will occur at higher temperatures. If traditional liquid loops continue to be used, support of thermal conditions for future spacecraft with heat loads greater than 10 kW will require significant increases in the power of refrigerant pumps, in the internal volume of the system, and in system mass and power requirements. It would, therefore, seem promising to develop highly effective thermal control systems based on two-phase loops (i.e., using a closed evaporation-condensation cycle).

A diagram of radiative thermal fluxes affecting a spacecraft is presented in Fig. 1. The structural hierarchy of thermal control systems is presented in Fig. 2.

The present chapter is devoted to a description of various means and methods for maintaining thermal conditions. It covers internal and external heat transfer, various passive and active methods, configurations of subsystems and liquid coolant loops based on these methods, and classification and selection of thermal control systems. The chapter closes with some examples of the use of thermal control methods in existing spacecraft and future development of thermal methods.

The initial data on the requisite thermal conditions for a crew are based on material from Chapter 3. The internal heat transfer subsystems and subassemblies analyzed in this chapter are also considered as components of integrated physico-chemical and biological life support systems in Chapters 15

The author expresses his appreciation to Ye. P. Belyavskiy for his aid in preparing material for this chapter. The original Russian text of this chapter was translated by Lydia R. Stone. Dr. John Keller acted as technical editor of the translation and Dr. Edward J. Stone provided additional technical consultation.

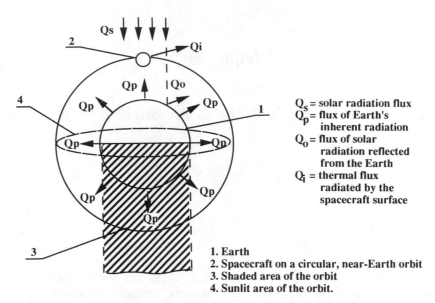

Q_s = solar radiation flux
Q_p = flux of Earth's inherent radiation
Q_o = flux of solar radiation reflected from the Earth
Q_i = thermal flux radiated by the spacecraft surface

1. Earth
2. Spacecraft on a circular, near-Earth orbit
3. Shaded area of the orbit
4. Sunlit area of the orbit.

Fig. 1 Diagram of heat fluxes affecting a spacecraft in near-Earth orbit.

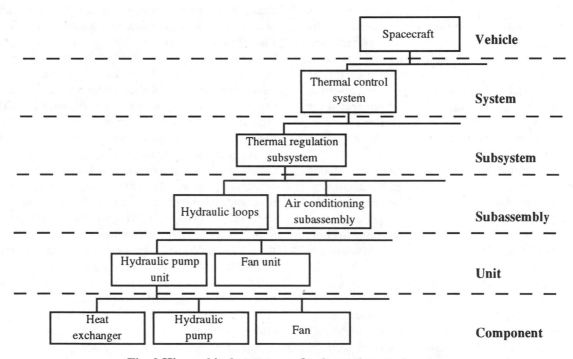

Fig. 2 Hierarchical structure of a thermal control systems.

and 16. Material in this chapter was derived from Soviet and other sources.[1–4]

I. External Heat Transfer

In space, the major type of heat transfer between a spacecraft and the space surrounding it is radiative. The energy thermal balance of the surface of the spacecraft has the form

$$m \cdot cp \cdot dT/dt = \alpha_s Q_s \cdot AF_1 + \alpha_s Q_o \cdot AF_2 + \varepsilon Q_p \cdot AF_3 + Q_I + Q_E - Q_i$$

where m, cp, and T are the mass of a unit surface of the spacecraft, its heat capacity, and temperature, respectively; t is time; σ is the Stephan-Boltzman constant; α_s is the solar absorptivity; ε is the infrared emissivity; A is the spacecraft surface area; F_1, F_2, and F_3 are view factors; $Q_i = \varepsilon \cdot \sigma \cdot AT^4$ is the radiative heat flux emitted by the spacecraft's surface; Q_s, Q_o, and Q_p are radiant fluxes of solar radiation, solar radiation reflected from the planet, and intrinsic thermal emission of the planet itself, respectively; Q_E is the heat from the exterior of the spacecraft; and Q_I is the heat from internal generation.

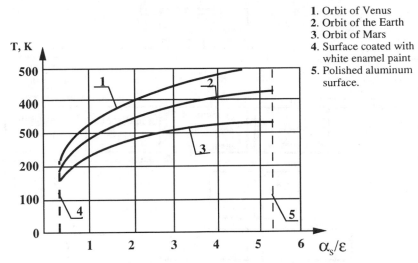

Fig. 3 Temperature of a heat-conducting sphere as a function of α_s/ε as distance from the Sun increases.[4]

The major component of external heat input is solar radiation, the density of which–called the solar constant–is inversely proportional to distance from the Sun. Solar radiation reflected from the Earth does not exceed 20 percent and the intrinsic thermal emission of the Earth itself, $Q_p = 0.15 \cdot Q_s$ (for near-Earth orbits of 200–300 km).

This equation shows that, in the absence of the Q_I and Q_E terms, the steady state temperature of the spacecraft surface when it is illuminated by the Sun depends only on the ratio α_s/ε (solar absorptivity/infrared emissivity).

In the shaded portions of the orbit the temperature of the spacecraft surface, in the absence of thermal fluxes Q_I and Q_E, is determined only by the coefficient ε.

Figure 3 shows that the steady state temperatures of bodies in space may have very different values, depending on the properties of the surface and distance from the Sun.[4] For a sphere made of polished aluminum ($\alpha_s/\varepsilon = 5.2$) with no Q_I or Q_E heat terms, the equilibrium temperature is 150 °C (423 K); for the same sphere covered in white enamel paint ($\alpha_s/\varepsilon = 0.19$), the equilibrium temperature is -89 °C (184 K).

For nonspherical bodies this temperature depends, to a significant extent, on the orientation of the body with respect to solar rays as well as the ratio between the absorbing and radiating surfaces. Coatings are conventionally divided into four groups:

1) Solar reflectors ($\alpha_s \approx 0$, $\varepsilon \approx 1$)
2) Solar absorbers ($\alpha_s \approx 1$, $\varepsilon \approx 0$)
3) True reflectors ($\alpha_s \approx 0$, $\varepsilon \approx 0$)
4) True absorbers ($\alpha_s \approx 1$, $\varepsilon \approx 1$)

Altering the α_s/ε ratio causes the external heat transfer of the spacecraft surface to vary. The values of the ratios of absorbing and radiative properties of coating attainable today vary from $0.15 < \alpha_s/\varepsilon < 8.0$.[2]

Appropriate thermal conditions can be maintained solely through use of coatings only if heat generation is low and a wide range of temperature fluctuations is acceptable.

This means that a whole series of other control methods must be used. An effective technique for regulating the temperature of a spacecraft surface is changing its orientation in space with regard to the incident thermal flux. However, this method is used mainly in contingency situations, since performance of the major tasks of the flight mission usually requires a specific orientation.

Another technique for regulating radiant heat transfer is to use adjustable screens, called louvers, to expose or close off portions of the surface with various radiative characteristics as dictated by temperature of the surface. The effectiveness of the louvers is limited by the radiative characteristics of their coatings and the reliability of the mechanical drive controlling their movement.

An effective method is the use of special radiative surfaces, heat exchangers, separated (insulated) from the spacecraft body. In such systems the external heat transfer is regulated by altering the thermal linkages between the radiative surfaces and the interior. The temperature of such a surface changes as a function of the quantity of heat it radiates. Radiators are located on the surfaces of the spacecraft in areas of minimal external thermal fluxes and covered with coatings with a maximal degree of emissivity and a minimal coefficient of solar absorptivity (α_s).

An additional external thermal control method is the use of multiple layers of screens. When there are several screens with the same emissivity, the thermal flux radiated by the surface into space is decreased by a factor of $N + 1$, where N is the number of layers. The most effective method is vacuum screening insulation—packets of foil or metallic film screens several microns thick, grooved or interleaved with glass netting to reduce physical contact. The weight of a unit of thermal resistance of such insulation is 1/10–1/5 that of porous material. It should be noted that vacuum screening insulation also fosters equilibration of the temperature field between the illuminated and nonilluminated surfaces of the spacecraft shell.

An alternative approach to rejecting heat to the vacuum of space is to employ evaporative coils. Here, the heat generated by the vehicle is used to vaporize a liquid, which, in

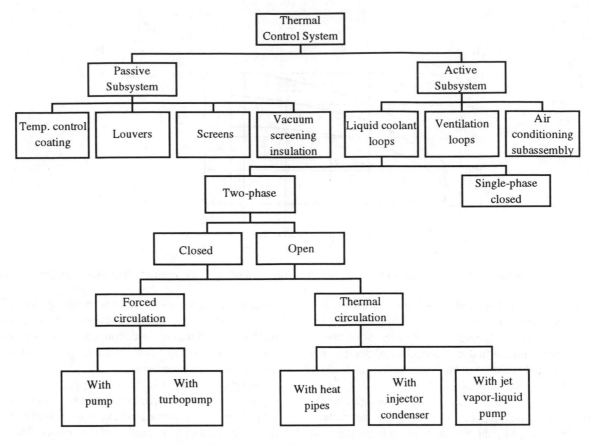

Fig. 4 Taxonomy of thermal control systems.

turn, is vented to space. One of the main working fluids used in such subassemblies is water, since it has a high heat of vaporization.

II. Internal Heat Transfer

Internal thermal control systems must remove heat generated by the crew and equipment and transfer it to external radiative surfaces. They also must redistribute heat among the spacecraft components. The simplest method is radiative heat transfer. To foster radiative heat transfer, the interior surface of the spacecraft has an emissivity, ε, near 1. For a 1 K temperature differential at a temperature of 300 K, radiative heat transfer is close to 5.5 W/m^2. If the equipment density is high, this method is insufficient and special metal thermal bridges (heat pipes) are needed to increase heat transfer over greater distances. For large pressurized cabins, especially inhabited ones, there must be air movement to equalize the temperature of the atmosphere and structural elements; in other words, ventilation is required. To remove heat from powerful sources and maintain their temperature in an acceptable range, liquid cooling is used. The working fluid circulates through heat transfer elements in the equipment that generates heat or else this equipment is mounted on thermostatically controlled plates through which the fluid circulates. Hydrocarbons, silicone fluids, freons, water solutions of ethylene glycols, water, and other fluids serve as the coolant.

Heat pipes may be used to transfer heat over large distances (10 m) from sources with high heat generation density. Working fluids used in heat pipes include water, freons, and ammonia. The density of the heat flux transferred can reach tens of watts per square centimeter cross section of a heat pipe.

Removal of heat from the cabin atmosphere can be achieved by the same component that removes the moisture generated by the crew, a condensing heat exchanger, the configuration and operation of which are covered in Chapter 9.

III. Classification, Selection, and Use of Thermal Control Systems

A taxonomy of thermal control systems is presented in Fig. 4. Thermal control systems are a collection of loops, subassemblies, equipment, and components controlling the external and internal heat transfer for a spacecraft. Thermal control systems may be divided into two subsystems: passive thermal control subsystems and active thermal control subsystems. The thermal control systems of manned spacecraft and the majority of unmanned spacecraft use a combination of passive and active subsystems with single-phase, closed liquid coolant loops. (The only two-phase loops are the heat pipes.)

Passive means of thermal control provide the surfaces of the spacecraft with the required optical characteristics to minimize unregulated heat transfer between the spacecraft and surrounding space. These subsystems include components maintaining parameters of radiative heat transfer and thermal conductivity using temperature control coatings, screens, thermal bridges, and thermal insulation. Active thermal control subsystems regulate the release of excess heat generated by equipment and crew into space and also maintain the temperature of components of the spacecraft structure. Active thermal control subsystems may include an air loop with ventilation subassemblies, a liquid coolant loop with heat exchangers and heat flow controllers, and active radiative heat transfer controllers.

The major factors in the selection of a thermal control system are the flight region, thermal requirements, amount of internal heat generation, and orientation and design characteristics of the spacecraft.

External heat input to the surface of an orbital station in near-Earth space is determined primarily by the solar constant, which at Earth orbit is approximately 1400 W/m^2.

Revolving around the Earth, a space vehicle periodically enters its shadow, where the sole external heat source is the intrinsic radiation of the Earth. The time a station in circular orbit spends in the Earth's shadow depends on the angle between the plane of orbit and the direction to the Sun, the height of the orbit, and the period of revolution. Because of the Earth's revolution around the Sun and the precession of the orbit, this angle periodically changes from minimum to maximum, and the amount of time the spacecraft is in the shadow of the Earth changes accordingly (see Fig. 1).

In a spacecraft with a large mass and thus large heat capacity, fluctuations in temperature of the structure associated with passage into the Earth's shadow are not great. Here thermal conditions may be estimated from the equilibrium temperature, using the mean thermal flux for a single orbit. In the case of a spherical spacecraft in near-Earth orbit in the absence of internal heat generation, temperature control coat-

ings should be selected with an α_s/ε that maintains a hull temperature of 10–40 °C (283–313 K). If there is constant thermal generation, still lower hull temperatures are needed.

If the shape of the spacecraft diverges from spherical, then, through imparting rotation to it about an axis perpendicular to the direction to the Sun, thermal control coatings can be used to maintain a relatively even distribution of external heat fluxes on its surface and to provide acceptable temperatures.

Thermal control systems in which thermal conditions are supported by a passive subsystem based on temperature control coatings are widely used in small satellites generating only a small amount of heat. Figure 5 provides α_s and ε for temperature control coatings and materials for flights up to 1 year in duration.[2] Where the heat generated by the spacecraft fluctuates widely or temperatures must be maintained in a narrow range, external heat transfer may be controlled actively using screens or louvers. Louvers were used on the small Elektron-1 and Elektron-2 satellites and the first Vostok manned satellites, etc.

From the point of view of reliability, active thermal control subsystems with closed fluid loops and insulated radiative surfaces are preferable to louvers. Such subsystems, combined with passive thermal control using vacuum screen insulation of spacecraft surfaces, are especially effective since they minimize uncontrolled heat transfer with space to a minimum. The sum of maximal prolonged internal heat generation and the maximum value of unregulated heat input must be less than the heat removal capacity of the radiative surface. On the other hand, the sum of the minimal internal heat generation and the maximal amount of unregulated heat losses must be positive to avoid overcooling of the spacecraft.

All modern manned spacecraft and large, unmanned spacecraft have thermal control systems with insulated surfaces and an active single-phase liquid coolant thermal control loop. As Fig. 6 shows, the heat rejection capacity of the radiator depends on its optical coefficients and quickly decreases as

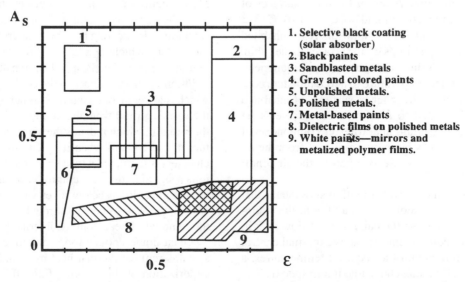

1. **Selective black coating (solar absorber)**
2. **Black paints**
3. **Sandblasted metals**
4. **Gray and colored paints**
5. **Unpolished metals.**
6. **Polished metals.**
7. **Metal-based paints**
8. **Dielectric films on polished metals**
9. **White paints—mirrors and metalized polymer films.**

Fig. 5 Temperature control coatings and material for long-term (1-year) use.[2]

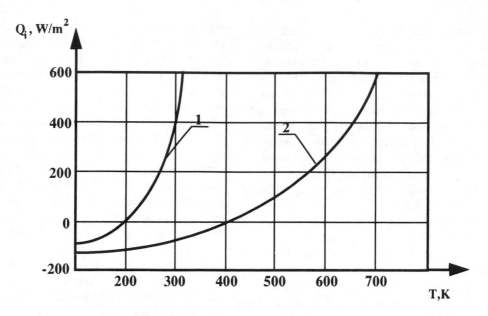

1. Radiative heat exchanger covered with white enamel ($\varepsilon = 0.95$)
2. Radiative heat exchanger—with polished aluminum surface ($\varepsilon = 0.05$)

Fig. 6 Specific heat rejecting capacity of a radiative heat exchanger as a function of its mean temperature.[4]

its temperature drops. A radiator of polished metal with low radiative characteristics ($\varepsilon = 0.05$) at temperatures below 180 °C (453 K) has negative heat rejecting capacity (the amount of solar heat it absorbs exceeds the amount of heat it radiates into space). A radiator covered with white enamel paint ($\varepsilon = 0.95$) has significantly greater heat rejecting capacity; however, this value decreases to zero at a temperature of –70 °C (203 K). The lower the temperature level at which it is necessary to remove heat from the spacecraft, the larger the surface and mass the radiator must have.[4]

As has already been stated, the temperature in the inhabited cabins must be maintained in a range of 18–23 °C (291–296 K). In addition, relative humidity must be kept between 30 and 70 percent, and temperature of the outer surfaces of the equipment and components should not exceed 40 °C (313 K). The presence of humidity in the atmosphere of inhabited modules requires the temperatures of all surfaces in the cabin, including the surface of the hull, components, and equipment, to be above the dew point temperature to avoid moisture condensation. For this reason, the exterior surfaces of inhabited modules must be insulated to minimize unregulated heat losses. Typically, the gas-liquid heat transfer components of the modules simultaneously condense moisture from the atmosphere (see Chapter 9) and are also part of the air conditioning subassemblies.

In large pressurized modules, ventilation subsystems that include ducts and fans are required. In addition, the equipment must be arranged so that the cabin air can flow over it.

There are special requirements for active thermal control subsystems. First, to maintain the required temperatures, a subsystem's working fluid must have maximum specific heat capacity, thermal conductivity, and density. To ensure safety,

especially in inhabited cabins, it must be nontoxic, nonflammable and nonexplosive. Finally, with respect to performance it must have a low freezing temperature, low viscosity, low corrosivity, high antifriction properties, and have a long working life. Water solutions of ethylene glycol and certain freons are used as working fluids.

Experience with Salyut and Mir flights indicates that since the temperature of an insulated radiative surface may be significantly below 233 K, the working fluid in the external loop must have a freezing point below 173 K if it is to reject heat at an orbital altitude of 200–300 km. The internal and external loops transfer heat through a liquid/liquid heat exchanger. The configuration of a liquid coolant single-phase loop of an active thermal control subsystem is shown in Fig. 7. Heat from the cabin passes through the internal heat exchangers (including desiccating heat exchangers) and is transferred to the coolant, which is circulated through the internal loop by a hydraulic pump. The heat is then transferred through the liquid/liquid heat exchanger to the coolant in the external loop, which is lower in temperature. Another hydraulic pump moves the working fluid from the liquid/liquid heat exchanger into the radiator, which radiates the heat into space. The temperature of the coolant when it is fed into the internal heat exchangers is regulated with a temperature sensor, which transmits a signal to the flow controller for the coolant. When the temperature drops below a set value, the flow control decreases the flow of coolant through the radiator, diminishing the removal of heat from the internal loop.[4]

Open liquid coolant loops of active thermal control subsystems remove thermal heat by utilizing the latent heat of vaporization of the working fluid, followed by venting the vapor into space. Loops containing substances in different

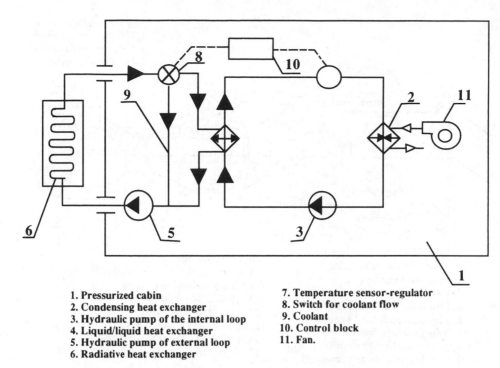

1. Pressurized cabin
2. Condensing heat exchanger
3. Hydraulic pump of the internal loop
4. Liquid/liquid heat exchanger
5. Hydraulic pump of external loop
6. Radiative heat exchanger

7. Temperature sensor-regulator
8. Switch for coolant flow
9. Coolant
10. Control block
11. Fan.

Fig. 7 Configuration of a single-phase active thermal control subsystem.

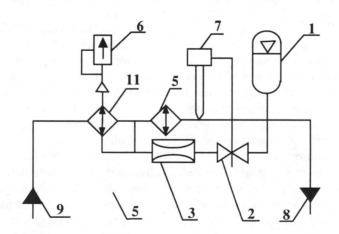

1. Container for coolant storage
2. Coolant feed valve
3. Coolant dispenser
4. Evaporative heat exchanger
5. Radiative heat exchanger

6. Constant temperature differential valve
7. Temperature regulator block
8. Internal loop
9. Internal loop

Fig. 8 Configuration of combined (closed and open) liquid coolant loop of active thermal control subsystem.[2]

phases have high performance characteristics and can remove a great deal of heat from a given surface area. These loops can be used effectively only on short duration flights or only for particular operations on board spacecraft because of the need for large stores of coolant. A loop of this kind was used as a backup on Vostok. Such loops are also used in individual life support systems in extravehicular activity (EVA) suits. Open, active thermal control subsystems may be used along with single-phase, closed loops. In this case, the majority of heat removal is performed by a radiative heat exchanger, and peak heat loads are decreased by changes in the phase of the

coolant and jettisoning of mass. A diagram of a loop of this type of combined active thermal control subsystem is presented in Fig. 8.[2]

In interplanetary space the intensity of solar heat flux changes inversely with the square of distance from the Sun. Accordingly, the temperature of a surface obtaining energy only from the Sun varies in inverse proportion to the square root of the distance from the Sun (Fig. 3). Spacecraft flying to Mars or Venus use solar arrays constantly oriented to the Sun; for this reason the distribution of external heat fluxes on the surface of these spacecraft is constant, which simplifies

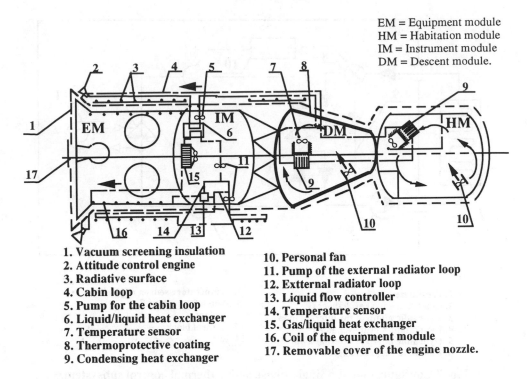

EM = Equipment module
HM = Habitation module
IM = Instrument module
DM = Descent module.

1. Vacuum screening insulation
2. Attitude control engine
3. Radiative surface
4. Cabin loop
5. Pump for the cabin loop
6. Liquid/liquid heat exchanger
7. Temperature sensor
8. Thermoprotective coating
9. Condensing heat exchanger

10. Personal fan
11. Pump of the external radiator loop
12. Extternal radiator loop
13. Liquid flow controller
14. Temperature sensor
15. Gas/liquid heat exchanger
16. Coil of the equipment module
17. Removable cover of the engine nozzle.

Fig. 9 Configuration of the thermal control system of Soyuz.[1]

regulation of thermal conditions.

Constant orientation to the Sun enables radiative surfaces to be oriented so that the flux of solar radiation does not fall on them, whereas the surfaces that are illuminated by the Sun are protected with insulation. For a spacecraft moving toward the orbits of the remote planets of the solar system, upon reaching the orbit of Jupiter, the solar heat flux would be so small that special sources of heat (for example, isotopes) would have to be used to stabilize temperatures.

The thermal boundary conditions of components on the exterior of the spacecraft are determined by the sum of heat fluxes, orientation of the component, and the radiative characteristics of its surface. Since the heat capacity of these components is usually small, their temperature changes significantly when the spacecraft enters the shade of the Earth or is shaded by other portions of the spacecraft structure. At heights of 500 km or less above the surface of the Earth, the temperature of exterior components does not drop below −120 °C (153 K) for any orientation of the spacecraft, because the flux of the intrinsic thermal radiation of Earth falls on virtually its whole surface.

Design of thermal conditions for spacecraft and spacecraft components is a difficult problem, which is solved using modern computer technology. This involves designing the balance of external and internal heat fluxes; the ventilating and coolant loops of the active thermal control subsystem; the temperature and humidity conditions of the cabin atmosphere; the temperature of the spacecraft exterior surface, its radiative heat exchangers, vacuum screening insulation, and support of thermal conditions inside and outside of the spacecraft pressurized cabins, etc. There are special works devoted

to the thermal design of various spacecraft.[2,6]

Actual thermal control system configurations are more complex and contain, as a rule, several internal and external liquid coolant loops because of the significant variation in the thermal conditions required by various systems, spacecraft equipment, and the crew.

As an example, Fig. 9 depicts the configuration of the thermal control system for Soyuz.[1] This system consists of a passive subsystem with vacuum screening insulation and an active subsystem with insulated radiative surfaces and a single-phase, closed liquid loop. Heat from the descent and habitation modules generated by the equipment and crew enters the single-phase, liquid loop of the inhabited modules, the pipes of which heat the components of the attitude control engines. The inhabited modules' loop is linked with the exterior radiator loop through a liquid-to-liquid heat exchanger to allow removal of heat from the descent and habitation modules. The exterior radiator loop also collects heat from the instrumentation module, heats the unpressurized module, and controls the release of heat into the vacuum of space through insulated radiative surfaces. The quantity of heat released by the radiative surfaces is regulated by a flow controller, which allows the liquid of the main interior line of the external radiator loop to enter the radiative surface and maintains the temperature of the liquid on input into the liquid/liquid heat exchanger within the bounds of 5–9 °C (278–282 K). The temperature of the working fluid before entering the condensing heat exchangers is maintained within a range of 7–12 °C (280–285 K).

The temperature of the cabin is controlled by the flow of gas through a condensing heat exchanger. The blower in this heat exchanger also circulates air through the modules. In addition, the inhabited areas have cooling fans that the crews can turn on as desired. To minimize uncontrolled heat transfer, the surfaces of the modules are covered with vacuum screening insulation. The surface of the descent module has thermal screening to protect it from aerodynamic heating during reentry in the Earth's atmosphere, while temperature conditions are maintained inside by the heat capacity of interior structures and equipment.

The thermal control system on Skylab was rather complex. The major parts of the heat regulation system included a passive subsystem, liquid coolant cooling loops for the airlock module, water cooling loops for the space suits, water cooling loops for the scientific apparatus connected to the cooling loop of the descent module by intermediate heat exchangers, components for regulating air temperature inside the station, a self-contained cooling loop for the galley refrigerators, and local surface heaters. The thermal control system maintained temperatures in the station during manned flight within the comfortable limits of 19.3–23.1 °C (292.6–296.4 K). In addition, heat pipes were added for local heating to prevent moisture condensation in certain areas of the inhabited modules.[7–9]

Heat pipes are closed volumes with a porous capillary structure inside, filled with a working medium in a two-phase state. Some of this working medium is in the gas phase and some is in the liquid phase, the latter permeating the porous capillary structure. At high temperatures the working medium evaporates; while at low temperatures it condenses. Because of differences in pressure, the vapor from the evaporation area is displaced into the condensation area. The use of phase change in heat pipes makes them highly thermally efficient.

The requisite safe life and reliability of the thermal control systems are ensured by having backups for the liquid coolant loops of the active thermal control subsystems. It should be noted that the reliability of radiative heat exchangers (their protection from depressurization, for example, due to meteorite hits) may be increased by using heat pipes. The Mir orbital space station complex uses heat pipes in the radiator panels in addition to single-phase liquid coolant loops.

IV. Future Development of Thermal Control Systems

For spacecraft that have heat loads of up to 10–15 kW, it is desirable to use a thermal regulation system that does not rely on the latent heat of vaporization. However, as thermal loads increase further, increases in the mass, energy, and size requirements for the system (associated with the increase of the amount of single-phase working fluid consumed in its liquid coolant loops) become so great that it becomes imperative to use heat of vaporization. The creation of two-phase heat transfer systems to handle such heat loads is a high priority task. Plans for Space Station call for inclusion of this type of system.

To ensure long-duration operation, the first thing that must be done is to remove components with moving parts (i.e.,

electric pumps). The use of electrohydraulic pumps, which have a working life limited only by the lifetime of their electronic components, is promising. The principle of action of electrohydraulic pumps is based on the interaction of unipolar charged dielectric liquid with an electric field created in a system of electrodes varying in curvature. These pumps are silent since they have no moving parts and their output is easily regulated by changing the power voltage. The lifetime of the radiative heat exchanger can be extended by the use of heat pipes with regulated delivery.

The use of thermostats with anisotropic porous structures is promising for the development of heat exchanger components, evaporators, and condensers. The major characteristic of the structure of two-phase thermal control systems is that they use a closed evaporation-condensation cycle in which heat transfer from the heat load to the working fluid and vapor formation occurs in the evaporators, whereas heat transfer to the radiative heat exchanger takes place in the condensers. Transport of vapor from the evaporator to the condenser occurs as a result of the difference in the temperatures of the source and release of heat, whereas return of the liquid is performed by electric or capillary forces. High heat transfer coefficients and the heat of a phase change material makes it possible to have low temperature differentials and low consumption of working fluid in the loop. Because of these advantages, data obtained by the present author indicate that it is possible to decrease the weight of the active thermal control subsystem by 25–50 percent and energy consumption by an order of magnitude or more, compared with a single-phase, active thermal control subsystem.

Two-phase, active thermal control subsystems may be classified on the basis of how the temperatures of heat loads are supported and how the evaporated liquid is delivered. A variant of the subsystem–in which the temperature of the evaporators associated with the thermal load is maintained by regulating the flow of the working fluid in the gas phase through the condenser (bypass line, flow controller, and mixing chamber)–was developed in projects of Goddard Space Center and the European Space Agency for the Columbus Space Module. This two-phase active thermal control subsystem was designed for transfer of 20 kW at 20–25 °C at a distance of up to 15 m.[10] A shortcoming of this approach is the design complexity of the mixer, which not only has to maintain temperature at a certain level but also has to ensure that the liquid remains in a single phase when it enters the pump. In a second type of two-phase, active thermal control systems the temperature and pressure of the vapor in the condenser are maintained through regulating the area of the heat elimination surface by feeding neutral gas into the inner chamber of the condenser or by insulating a portion of the heat transfer surface with a working medium, which has been forced out of the liquid coolant reservoir. Such configurations were used in the Thermal Control System project designed by Johnson Space Center[11] and the firm of Martin Marietta for heat loads of 25–30 kW. The principles underlying the operation and design of the heat

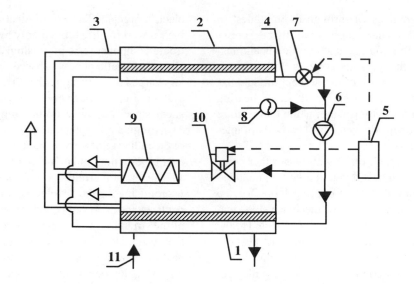

1. Evaporator
2. Condenser
3. Vapor line
4. Liquid coolant loop
5. Control unit
6. Electrohydrodynamic pump

7. Flow regulator
8. Hydraulic accumulator
9. Heater
10. Shutoff valve
11. Heat-exchanger loop

Fig. 10 Configuration of the two-phase liquid coolant loop of an active heat control subsystem.

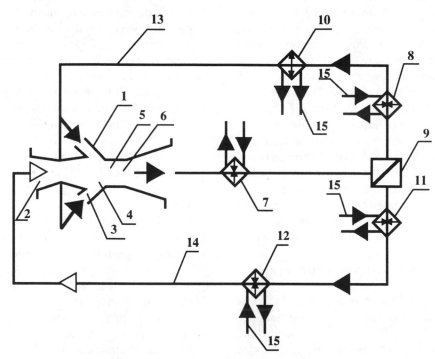

1. Injector-condenser
2. Nozzle
3. Injector
4. Mixing chamber
5. Area of mixture deceleration
6. Area of mixture expansion
7. and 8. Heat exchanger for removing
   heat from equipment

9. Stream separator
10. Radiative condensing heat exchanger
11. Heater
12. Evaporative heat exchanger
13. "Cold" loop
14. "Hot" loop
15. Internal loop

**Fig. 11 Configuration of the two-phase liquid coolant loop of
an active heat control subsystem with an injector-condenser.**

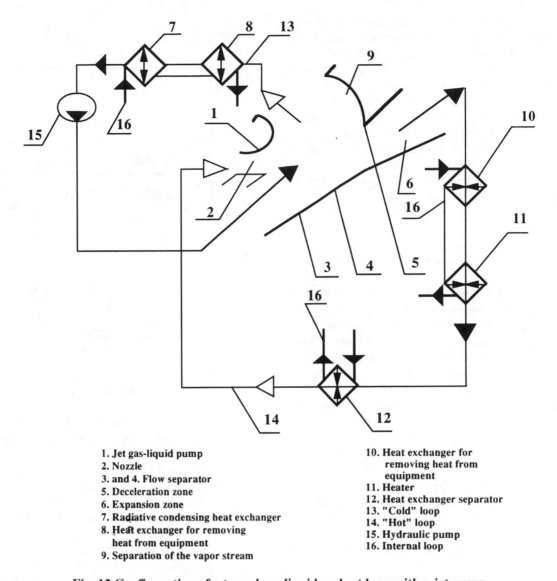

1. Jet gas-liquid pump
2. Nozzle
3. and 4. Flow separator
5. Deceleration zone
6. Expansion zone
7. Radiative condensing heat exchanger
8. Heat exchanger for removing
   heat from equipment
9. Separation of the vapor stream

10. Heat exchanger for
    removing heat from
    equipment
11. Heater
12. Heat exchanger separator
13. "Cold" loop
14. "Hot" loop
15. Hydraulic pump
16. Internal loop

Fig. 12 Configuration of a two-phase liquid coolant loop with a jet pump.

transfer components (condenser and evaporator) are described in detail in Chapter 9. [4–15]

A two-phase loop works as follows (see Fig. 10). When it operates under a full heat load, the liquid flow controller is fully open, creating pressure in the vapor line equal to the upper limit of the range. As a result of the pressure head created by the pump, the working fluid is forced out of the liquid loop into the evaporator with the flow rate corresponding to the heat load. As a result of heat transfer, the liquid is evaporated and the difference in temperature pushes the vapor through the line into the condenser. The liquid forming through condensation is pumped through the porous element of the condenser into the liquid pipe, and from there, again enters the evaporator. When vapor pressure decreases below the highest setting, a flow regulator creates resistance between the condenser and the pump sufficient to pump the liquid from the reservoir into the condenser. This leads to an increase in vapor pressure and maintains the temperature. A decrease in vapor pressure to the lower limit of the range causes the flow controller to close completely so that the liquid enters the evaporator only from the reservoir. The loop contains an electric heater with a cutoff valve that prevents the working fluid from freezing in the condenser when the heat loading decreases. The evaporators are heat pipes filled with an anisotropic porous material.

Another promising development in thermal control systems is a two-phase circulation loop in which the working fluid is moved by jet pump which is powered by external thermal energy generated in the presence of a temperature differential between the heat source and the surface of the radiative heat exchanger. The use of these so-called thermal circulatory loops decreases both mass and energy consumption by taking advantage of change of phase. This makes it possible to have a pump without moving parts that operates virtually indefinitely, as well as to divide a single circulatory loop into a number of separate automatic loops, solving the problem of reliability in the event of depressurization.[2,16,17]

In an active thermal control subsystem with a heat circulation loop, some of the heat removed from hot equipment in a direct cooling cycle is used to circulate the working fluid. Here the liquid coolant loop, with an energy transformer, heat sources, and radiative panels, becomes a thermal mechanism that transforms the low-potential heat input to the coolant into work to overcome hydraulic resistance in moving the working fluid. In such loops it is desirable to use jet pumps without moving mechanical parts, allowing the subsystem to have a virtually unlimited useful life, depending only on the life of the material of which it is made and the working fluid. A control system is only required when the loop is turned on, to start the flow of the coolant, and to input and output heat. For a given range, the active thermal control subsystem loop is self-regulating.

The pressure head that can be created in systems with jet pumps and low volumetric flow rates makes it possible to increase the rate of heat transfer by increasing the speed at which the coolant flows through the channel in the thermal plates, which significantly decreases the weight of the metal components required. Because of the reserve pressure head, passive flow controllers (cavitating Venturi tubes and devices) can be installed in the branches of the system to render it insensitive to where heat loading is applied in the system. In an active thermal control subsystem using jet pumps, there are no limits on the orientation of the thermal plates in the presence of gravity.

For the cooling cycle to operate, the heat rejection temperature has to be decreased, which requires some increase in the area and mass of the radiator. The radiator is in the form of a plate for high reliability and system autonomy.

The heat circulating loop may be designed to include energy transformers of various types. Loops that include an injector-condenser and a jet gas-liquid phase separator pump are the most effective for maintaining temperature in a given range.[2,16,17]

In the injector-condenser (Fig. 11) a stream of vapor or vapor mixed with liquid comes out of the nozzle at a high speed, mixing with cold liquid in the mixing chamber, where the vapor loses its impulse and condenses. The mixture abruptly slows in the narrow end of the diffuser and smoothly regains its pressure as the diffuser widens. When it exits the injector-condenser, it enters the stream separator, where some of it is directed into the radiative heat exchanger for cooling and then is injected into the mixing chamber through the injector nozzle. The rest is directed into the heater and then into the evaporator where, at a constant temperature, it cools the hot equipment of the spacecraft through partial evaporation of the coolant. After leaving the heat exchangers, the cold and hot streams enter the injector-condenser. The operation of the injector-condenser produces a pumping effect. The advantage of this system is its design and engineering simplicity. Additional liquid may be added to the loop to remove heat generated by instruments and equipment, if necessary. Its major shortcoming is that the cooling cycle can not use the full available temperature differential, since the heat in the working fluid is removed in the mixing heat exchanger.

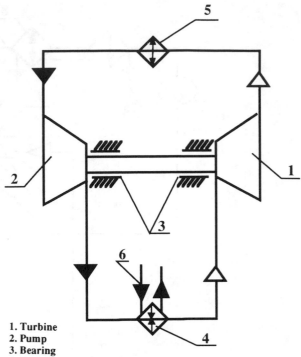

1. Turbine
2. Pump
3. Bearing
4. Heater
5. Radiative condensing heat exchanger
6. Internal loop.

Fig. 13 Configuration of a two-phase loop with a turbopump subassembly.

The liquid coolant loop of the jet phase separator pump may have the configuration shown in Fig. 12. The loop has two main branches: the hot side containing the working liquid, which removes heat from the hot equipment, and the cold side containing the vapor, which transfers the heat from the equipment to the radiative heat exchanger. The superheated vapor-liquid mixture is fed into the nozzle where it accelerates and expands, causing adiabatic cooling. In the dynamic separator, the liquid and vapor separate because of inertia, while the speed of the liquid is maintained. The liquid is fed into a slot in the diffuser in which it recovers its pressure. The movement of the working fluid through the hot loop is analogous to its movement in the injector-condenser loop. An increase in the pressure of the liquid is due to a temperature differential. As in the case of the injector-separator, additional heat exchangers can be added to input or output heat not participating in the cooling loop. After leaving the separator pump, the vapor condenses on the radiative panels of the condenser; then, to ensure stable operation, it is cooled in the heat exchanger. The cycle is more efficient for a given temperature if a jet separator pump rather than an injector-condenser is used. However, in the jet separator pump configuration, external energy must be added to the loop to overcome hydraulic resistance in the cold line. The work required to recover the condensate is no greater than 10 percent of the work to pump the working fluid through the heat removal loop. An auxiliary jet pump may be used to reinject the condensate, allowing the working fluid to be pumped through the entire loop without any mechanical devices. Use of a jet separator pump instead of an injector-condenser increases the pressure head, decreases required temperature differential on the radiative heat exchanger, and thus decreases the surface and mass it must have or, alternatively, allows the loop to handle additional heat load.

The same cycle may be effectively implemented in a forced circulation loop with a turbopump component (Fig. 13). In this case mechanical moving parts have to be used. Power for pumping the working fluid is obtained through partial utilization of the heat that has been extracted and no external power sources are needed. A turbopump is a pressurized subassembly consisting of a turbine and a pump on a single shaft. Pressure of the liquid coolant increases in the pump. The liquid is then partially heated or completely evaporated in the heater, and the vapor expands in the turbine and enters the radiative heat exchanger, where it condenses and is recooled. The cycle is closed by feeding condensate into the pump. The use of hydraulic bearings provides a turbopump subassembly with a long working life. Introduction of a turbopump subassembly into the loop significantly increases heat rejection.[2]

Combination of a heat circulating loop with transformers of both types or a heating circulating loop with a turbopump subassembly are promising future directions for spacecraft thermal control systems.

References

[1]Feoktistov, K.P., Ed. *Spacecraft*. Moscow, Voyennoye Izdatelstvo, 1983, pp. 197–215 (in Russian).

[2]Malozemov, V.V.; Rozhnov, B.V.; and Pravetskiy, V.N. *Support Systems for Flight Vehicle Crews*. Moscow, Mashinostroyeniye, 1986, Section III, pp. 235–391 (in Russian).

[3]Voronin, G.I. and Polivoda, A.I. *Life Support of Spacecraft Crews*. Moscow, Mashinostroyeniye, 1967, pp. 61–66 (in Russian).

[4]Serebryakov, V.N. *Principles of Designing Life Support Systems for Spacecraft Crews*. Moscow, Mashinostroyeniye, 1983, pp. 21–23, 70–76 (in Russian).

[5]Grishayenkov, B.G. Air regenerating and conditioning. In: Calvin, M. and Gazenko, O.G., Eds. *Foundations of Space Biology and Medicine*. Washington, D.C., NASA Hq., 1975, Volume III, pp. 57–58.

[6]Zaletayev, V.M.; Kapinos, V.Yu.; and Surguchev, O.V. *Designing Heat Transfer for Spacecraft*. Moscow, Mashinostroyeniye, 1979, pp. 7–176 (in Russian).

[7]Hopson, G.D.; Littler, I.W.; and Patterson, W.S. Skylab environmental and life support system. Paper presented at SAE/ASME/AIAA Life Support and Environmental Control Conference, 1971, Jul. 12–14, San Francisco.

[8]Hanlon, W.H. and Hevnus, P.E. Skylab habitability evolution. AIAA Paper No. 71-872, 1971.

[9]Hopson, G.D. Skylab life support and habitability system requirements and implementation. Paper presented at XXIInd International Astronautical Congress, Brussels, 1971, Sep. 20–25.

[10]Maller, P. and Kred, H. Advanced thermal control technologies for European space station modules. SAE TPS 85-1366.

[11]Sadunas, J.A. and Lehtinen, A. Spacecraft active thermal control subsystem design and operation considerations. AIAA Paper 86-1277, 1986.

[12]Cullimar, B.A. and Epper, R.C. Thermostatic control of two-phase spacecraft thermal management systems. AIAA Paper 86-1246, 1986.

[13]Edestein, F. and Brown, R. Design and test of two-phase monogroove gold plate. AIAA Paper 85-0918, 1985.

[14]Sweder, J. and Gallucio, R. Space Shuttle environmental and life support system. SAE Paper 86-1420, 1986

[15]Allario, J. The shared flight experiment–an advanced heat pipe radiator for space station. AIAA Paper 86-1297, 1986.

[16]Karvsyov, E.K. A jet vapor pump for circulation in the evaporative loop of a water-boiler reactor. In: *Issues in Atomic Science and Technology*. Raketostroyeniye Series, Moscow, 1979, vol. 25, pp. 3–9 (in Russian).

[17]Gorbenko, G.A. and Frolov, S.D. Study of surface separators of jet liquid pumps with a carrier gas. In: *Issues of Gas Dynamics in Power Installations*. Kharkov, 1975, vol. 2, pp. 68–96 (in Russian).

Chapter 11

Crewmember Nutrition

I. G. Popov and V. P. Bychkov

I. Introduction

From the days of the first short-term spaceflights, providing a high-quality, balanced diet to space crews has been an important issue. Crew diet has received serious attention as one of the most important prerequisites for maintaining good health and high levels of mental and physical performance, as well as providing enjoyment to crewmembers. A nutritionally adequate diet has become increasingly important as spaceflights have grown increasingly longer and more autonomous, mission tasks have become more arduous and critical, and stressful situations have arisen more frequently. To meet these challenges, all the constituents of the onboard food supply system (which is an essential component of the life support system) have evolved from one spaceflight to the next. At the present time, onboard food supply systems, especially for relatively long-term flights, are advanced technological systems comprising, in addition to food for the crews, an "infrastructure" that allows safe storage, preparation, and consumption of food under the specific habitability conditions of the spacecraft cabin.

The initial phase of work on the problem of feeding crews in space was hampered by a lack of experience in supporting spaceflight. Previous experience with high-altitude aircraft flight, as well as simulation of spaceflights in ground-based anechoic and pressurized isolation chambers of restricted size yielded only a tentative understanding of the caloric and nutritional needs of space crews during flight. It was also necessary to solve a number of sanitary and hygienic problems relating to storage, preparation, and consumption of food in weightlessness. Furthermore, information on the functioning of the gastrointestinal tract and other human physiological systems during prolonged weightlessness was totally inadequate, since it was impossible to simulate weightlessness of appreciable duration on the ground.

The task of feeding crews during the first space flights was simplified by their short duration. Crewmembers ate a balanced diet during the preflight period, and this precluded any clinically significant levels of quantitative or qualitative deficiencies, such as lack of vitamins, protein, or minerals.

The first orbital flights clarified our understanding of the physiology and technology of feeding crews in weightlessness and ensuring the safety of the food supply. These flights also provided the first information concerning human caloric and nutritional requirements in space. This focused and facilitated further development of onboard food supply systems.

Today, scientists have accumulated a great deal of practical information about feeding space crews on flights of up to 1 year. In addition, progress has been made with regard to the theoretical principles underlying the physiology of nutrition in space, questions of sanitation and food safety, and the technology for preparing and packaging space rations.

A number of heterogeneous medical, biological, technological, and design problems that had never been encountered on the ground have had to be solved. Onboard food supply systems are closely linked with other life support systems, especially water supply, human waste disposal, power supply, and air conditioning. At the same time, a number of serious scientific and practical problems must be solved to support future long-term autonomous flights to Mars and other planets of the solar system. Information on the dynamics of human metabolism on long-term space flights is still inadequate, in part, because of the methodological difficulties of conducting biochemical studies in flight. Complex technical problems relating to retention of the nutritive properties of food products on long-term flights remain unsolved. In addition, techniques must be developed to produce nutritionally adequate food in flight through physicochemical and biological processing of human wastes and the by-products of technological processes. Thus, a food supply system involving consumption of stored food brought from Earth will have to be replaced by systems generating food, including nontraditional sources of food, onboard. Further improvements are needed in the in-flight monitoring of space crew nutritional status in flight, including prescription of therapeutic nutritional measures, when indicated. Finally, it is becoming increasingly critical to develop rations in which food values are tailored to take account of the nature of crew psychophysical workloads and the physiological idiosyncrasies of individual crewmembers.

For purposes of discussion, the problem of feeding crews in space may be divided into the following categories:

1) Feeding space crews during short-term flights (a few

This chapter was translated from the original Russian by Lydia Razran Stone.

days to 1 month)

2) Feeding space crews on flights of moderate duration (from 1 month to 1 year)

3) Feeding space crews on long-term autonomous flights (over 1 year)

The first two types of space crew food supply systems have already been developed and used. However, there is no doubt that there is room for further improvement. Scientists are beginning to work on the problem of providing food to space crews on long-term flights. National programs to prepare for flights to Mars and other planets will have to intensify the research devoted to this area.

The space food supply systems developed in the United States and the Russian Federation (formerly the U.S.S.R.) have differed in their specific features as a result of differences in spacecraft and crew mission tasks; however, they share a number of characteristics, especially with respect to determining the nutritional requirements of space crews, that arise from a shared understanding of human physiology, biochemistry, and nutritional science. Exchange of scientific ideas within the framework of international collaboration on problems of space exploration has undoubtedly played a significant role in successful work on problems of space nutrition.

This chapter incorporates material we previously presented in Chapter 2, "Provision of Food and Water," of the first edition of *Foundations of Space Biology and Medicine* (Moscow-Washington, 1975), and is supplemented by reports on recent research conducted by Russian and U.S. scientists.

II. Food Supply Systems on Short-Term Flights

Food supply systems for relatively short-term flights, ranging from hours to several days, were naturally made as simple as possible, considering the sanitary and technical constraints on flight vehicles with restricted habitable areas and the need to limit the launch weight and volume of food and water supplies.

When food supply systems were developed for the first space vehicles (Vostok, Voskhod, and Mercury), it was unclear how such physiological acts as chewing, swallowing, and defecation would be affected by weightlessness. Would taste sensations alter in flight? What would be the effects of flight conditions on energy expenditure, metabolism, digestion, and human requirements for water and nutrients? How would the physiological mechanisms that regulate intake of food and water function in space?

Even for short-term flights, providing crews with a sufficient quantity of nutritionally balanced and safe food requires that food supply systems meet a number of specific criteria.

1) The rations (daily or for an entire flight) must compensate for the energy expended by the crewmembers and, to the extent possible, contain nutrients (proteins, fats, carbohydrates, vitamins, and minerals) in quantities necessary to support metabolic processes at an optimal level. This is especially true with regard to the so-called "essential" nutrients, which are not synthesized in the human body or are synthe-

sized in inadequate quantities (these include a number of amino acids, unsaturated fatty acids, and vitamins). The products must be palatable enough to be acceptable to the space crews.

2) Unabsorbable substances in the diet must be held to a minimum to avoid putting a strain on the gastrointestinal tract, to decrease the need for waste disposal, and to make the rations more compact.

3) The volume and weight of the food products must be minimized to decrease the launch weight of the food and water supplies.

4) Crews must be able to consume their rations conveniently in weightlessness within the restricted space of the cabin. The possibility must be considered that the crewmembers may have to eat while wearing full pressure suits or while confined to their couches.

5) Food products should not require further culinary preparation, slicing, and (if possible) heating or rehydration in flight.[1,2]

6) For food supplies on short-term flights, it is preferable to use only products that can be consumed as soon as they are removed from the packaging with no further preparation. This helps to minimize the number of component parts necessary for the food supply system, limiting them to 1) an assortment of food products; 2) a container for storing them; 3) devices for preparing and consuming food (a can opener, table utensils, and a container for storing them); 4) a receptacle for disposing of and storing food wastes and packaging; and 5) a means of cleaning utensils and hands before and after eating (sterile wipes or gauze napkins moistened with disinfectant).

During short-term spaceflights, when potable water is brought from Earth, it is expedient to use standard canned food with normal water content for crew rations.

The first U.S.S.R. and U.S. spaceflights in the Vostok, Voskhod, and Mercury programs provide examples of successful compliance with the above specifications.

During preparations for the first manned spaceflights, the United States and U.S.S.R. conducted research on nutrition under conditions simulating crew work/rest schedules in flight, as well as a number of parameters of the living environment (temperature and humidity conditions, atmospheric composition) in the spacecraft cabin. This made it possible to specify space crew energy expenditure and need for the basic nutrients, and to establish the food value of flight rations. At the same time, various types of food products, methods of packaging and storage, and techniques for consuming food in weightlessness were tested.[1,3,4]

In stipulating nutritional requirements for space rations, nutritionists had to consider national recommended dietary allowances. During preparations for the first Soviet flights, the recommendations of the Nutrition Institute of the U.S.S.R. Academy of Medicine, adopted in 1951, were used. Dietary allowances recommended for adults engaging in sedentary work (the so-called first occupational category) were considered to be most appropriate for the living conditions of the Vostok and Voskhod crews. Energy expended by males, age

18 to 40, in this category at that time was estimated to be 3000 to 3200 kcal/day, and there were also recommendations with regard to needs for protein, fat, carbohydrates, and a number of vitamins and minerals.[4] These dietary allowances were refined during simulation tests on volunteer subjects and cosmonaut candidates. As a result, it was concluded that an acceptable caloric value for the first flights on Vostok spacecraft was 2500 to 2700 kcal/day.[1]

Since it was inevitable that some food would remain in the aluminum tubes used as the primary food container after the cosmonauts had finished eating, especially when the food was sticky in consistency, the caloric value of the daily ration was increased to 2800 kcal per day (available kilocalories). To facilitate assimilation of nutrients and provide uniform loading of the digestive tract, recommendations called for four meals per day, at intervals of 4 to 5 hours during the period the crew was awake.[1] An analogous meal schedule is recommended in the U.S.S.R. for the majority of the population.

For short-term flights, it was considered desirable to maintain the ratios of the basic nutrients (proteins, fats and carbohydrates) within the range recommended by the Nutrition Institute of the U.S.S.R. Academy of Medicine (1:1:3) for individuals not engaging in physical labor. The rations for the first Vostok flights contained approximately 100 g of protein, 120 g of fat, and 300 g of carbohydrates.

To prevent vitamin deficiencies associated with reliance on canned products and, possibly, increased utilization of vitamins by the body under exposure to the stress factors associated with flight, a tablet containing a multivitamin complex (C—100 mg; B_1, B_2, B_6—2 mg each; niacin—15 mg; bioflavenoids—50 mg; pantothenic acid—10 mg; vitamin E /α-tocopherol/—5 mg)[1] was taken twice a day as a supplement. There were no direct indications that there was a risk of vitamin deficiencies developing on short-term flights.

The ration constituents were tested during cosmonaut flight training in anechoic and barochambers. The caloric value of the food actually eaten in these tests ranged from 2500 to 2750 kcal/day. Assimilation of the food was estimated to be 95 percent. Convenience of packaging and taste were evaluated positively. Biochemical parameters of metabolism (protein, fat, and carbohydrate) that were typically measured to evaluate nutritional status in humans, did not differ significantly from the baseline in subjects consuming a diet of these rations.[1]

The fact that food had to be consumed under conditions of weightlessness required the resolution of a number of physiological questions. The most serious of these were 1) whether weightlessness would interfere with the processes of chewing and swallowing, 2) whether taste sensations would be altered, and 3) whether there would be significant changes in the processes of digestion and defecation. Some of these questions were answered through studies during parabolic flights of laboratory aircraft that created conditions of short-term (30-40 s) weightlessness. It was established that swallowing liquids and well-chewed food presented no difficulties in weightlessness.[5,1] These data provided a rationale for the use of only pureed products in the first Vostok flights.

Other limitations on product selection and packaging were associated with the fact that the food generally had to be consumed without additional culinary processing, such as heating. Finally, the difficulty of providing clean dishes (plates, glasses, etc.) for every meal made it desirable to use food products that could be eaten directly from their packages using only a set of utensils (spoon, fork, and knife). Thus, products had to be packaged in individual portions and divided into bite-size pieces before packaging. Eating utensils were kept clean through regular wiping with sterile wipes, either dry or moistened with a disinfectant solution (alcohol). Some limitations were imposed on selection and packaging of food to avoid contamination of the cabin atmosphere by particles of food and fragments of packaging, which, "floating" in weightlessness, could get into the respiratory tract and eyes, with undesirable consequences.

Because of the sanitary limitations noted above, cosmonaut rations for flights on Vostok 1 and Vostok 2 included only pureed and liquid products packed in aluminum tubes and subjected to thermal sterilization. Each tube contained approximately 160 g of food. The food could be eaten directly from the package and did not require heating. The following set of products was used: 1) pureed preserved food—sorrel puree with meat, meat-vegetable puree, meat, meat with grain, and prune purees; 2) pates—meat and liver; 3) juices—plum, black currant, apple, gooseberry; 4) processed chocolate-flavored cheese; 5) a chocolate dessert; and 6) coffee with milk. This large assortment made it possible to provide the varied meals necessary to maintain crew appetite and prevent crewmembers from growing tired of their food. In addition to the products in tubes, the rations contained vitamin tablets (composition listed above).

As an experiment, during the earliest flights the food container also held samples of solid foods—bread, smoked sausage, and pastry—all in bite-size pieces.[1,2]

The food system comprised an opener for removing the stoppers of the tubes, a set of sterile gauze wipes for cleaning the spout of the tubes and hands, a polyethylene bag for uneaten food, and a metal food container in which the remaining components of the system were stored according to a specified system. The food container was filled on the launch pad 1 day before launch, when the spacecraft was already attached to the booster rocket.

Yu. A. Gagarin's flight on Vostok 1 continued for 108 min (one orbit around the Earth). There was no real need for him to eat on such a short flight. However, in accordance with the research program, during min 30 of the flight, the cosmonaut consumed foods of a variety of consistencies. His conclusion was that "In weightlessness, I ate and drank, and everything proceeded just the same as at home on Earth."[1] This suggested that it would be possible to use food products varying in consistency on space flights.[1-3]

During his Vostok 2 flight, cosmonaut G. S. Titov provided more extensive information on eating in weightlessness. During a 25-h flight, he consumed his entire daily ration from tubes and tested the feasibility of consuming solid food products in a variety of packages under conditions of weightlessness.

Overall, both cosmonauts positively evaluated the food supply system. They did not experience any difficulties consuming food of a variety of consistencies or in using the packaging. No changes in taste sensitivity were noted. The short durations of the flights, of course, did not allow sufficient testing of the nutritive content of the rations with respect to the physiological needs of the cosmonauts. Gagarin's body weight decreased only slightly during the flight but did not return to normal until day 6 postflight. Titov's body weight was 1.8 kg below preflight at 9 h and 27 min after landing, and returned to normal only after 9 days.[1] It could not be established whether the decrease in body weight in both cosmonauts was caused by dehydration or dietary inadequacy.

The approach of U.S. specialists to providing astronauts with food on short-term flights in the Mercury program was analogous to the Soviet approach in many respects. The system for feeding the crews during the earliest flights was simplified as much as possible. The two astronauts participating in suborbital Mercury flights on May 15, 1961, and May 21, 1962, did not eat at all. On subsequent flights, food was consumed, in part for experimental purposes.

In the United States, initial recommendations also called for predominant use of liquids and pureed food on short-term flights. The caloric value of the ration was approximately 2500 kcal/day.[6]

Various packaging types and eating techniques were tested in weightlessness. Astronaut Glenn tested a method of eating pureed food from squeezable elastic tubes. Astronaut Carpenter tested a method for eating solid food formed into bite-size cubes. The crumbliness of solid products led to the development of an edible film coating.[7-9]

During Mercury flights on February 20, 1962, May 24, 1962, and October 3, 1962, the functioning of the gastrointestinal tract was observed when a number of meals were eaten. Rehydrated food was first tested during a Mercury flight on May 15 and 16, 1967.[10]

The studies mentioned above allayed fears that weightlessness would adversely affect processes of chewing and swallowing food.[3]

The rations for the Mercury spacecraft consisted primarily of pureed products packaged in aluminum tubes and samples of solid products. Sterile food in tubes with a net weight of 156 g each, used by Glenn, Carpenter, and Schirra on the first three manned Mercury flights, had been developed previously for pilots of the U.S. Air Force and successfully used on high-altitude aircraft flights. It is interesting that, in contrast, in the U.S.S.R., analogous products in tubes began to be used for pilots after testing in space. The Mercury astronauts consumed semiliquid meat (in tubes) and fruit (apple and peach) sauces.[11] The food was squeezed through a polysterene straw 8.75 cm in length. If the faceplate of the helmet was down, the straw was inserted in an opening in the helmet to enable eating and drinking.

Samples of solid food included compressed cubes or cakes of dry food mixtures. Malted milk tablets, cubes made of a mixture of grains, and freeze-dried fruits were also tested. The cubes were covered in gelatin. Grain and fruit cakes covered with an edible coating were also tested.

While the astronauts ate, the packaging containing the products was attached to the walls of the cabin and other free surfaces with pieces of Velcro® (a self-adhering flexible material manufactured in the United States).

During the fourth manned Mercury flight by Astronaut Cooper, the products were packed in an MA-9 container, allowing rehydration of the food. On occasion the contents leaked out into the cabin atmosphere when the container was used in flight.[12]

The rations for Cosmonaut A.G. Nikolayev (Vostok 3, August 11, 1962), P.R. Popovich (Vostok 4, August 12, 62), V.F. Bykovskiy (Vostok 5, June 14, 1963), and V.V. Tereshkova (Vostok 6, October 12, 1964), aside from the previously tested pureed and liquified products in tubes, contained a variety of solid products formed into bite-size portions and vacuum-packed in plastic pouches. The rations for the initial days of the flight of Vostok 4 and 5 contained fresh products with relatively short storage lives. Their taste was rated favorably by the cosmonauts. However, a whole series of additional measures had to be taken to maintain the quality of the products when they were manufactured, transported, and stored on the spacecraft.[2,13,14]

The caloric values of rations on Vostok 3 and 4 for the 3 days of the flight were 2480, 2846, and 2255 kcal/day, respectively. During the first and third days, the caloric value was decreased in consideration of the high-calorie diet consumed preflight and postflight. The rations contained 105-150 g protein, 64-112 g fat, and 290-325 g carbohydrates.[13] Twice a day, each cosmonaut took a multivitamin tablet: C—100 mg; B_1, B_2, B_6—2 mg each; niacin—15 mg; bioflavenoids—50 mg; E (α-tocopherol)—50 mg, and pantothenic acid—10 mg. V. Tereshkova's appetite was depressed in flight, especially for sweets.[14]

Eight hours after landing, the weight of the Vostok 4 cosmonaut was depressed by 1.8 kg and that of the Vostok 3 cosmonaut by 2.1 kg. However, 1 day later the weight loss had diminished to 0.8 kg for the latter. The rapid recovery of weight, especially in the case of the Vostok 3 cosmonaut, suggested that dehydration processes during flight had been the primary cause.[2,13] The rations used for Vostok 5 and 6 did not differ substantially from those on Vostok 3 and 4.

The flight rations of crews of Voskhod featured greater variety. The rations actually consumed by the crew of Voskhod 1 (October 12, 1964) contained approximately 3600 kcal, 150 g of protein, 130 g of fat, and 430 g of carbohydrates. Good appetites were maintained. Immediately after landing, the cosmonauts experienced intense thirst and drank avidly. Crewmembers' body weights decreased during the flight by 1.9 kg, 2.9 kg, and 3.0 kg. The short duration of the flight and the high food value of the rations makes it unlikely that the weight loss was the result of dietary deficit. The intense thirst experienced after landing, analysis of fluid balance, and results of postflight fluid loading tests indicated that water loss during flight was not adequately compensated. [2,15,16]

The crew of Voskhod 2 (March 18, 1965) also rated the onboard feeding system favorably. However, since they landed in a remote region, their postflight nutritional status could not be evaluated immediately.[2,17]

The longer orbital flights in the Gemini, Apollo, and Soyuz programs required further improvement and expansion of the space food supply systems.

The majority of Gemini flights lasted 14 days. Increased rations were needed to meet the nutritional requirements of space crews on these longer flights. It was necessary to coordinate requirements for nutritional adequacy and acceptable taste with continued strict requirements concerning weight and volume.

Work performed at the behest of NASA starting in the fall of 1963 included standardization of products and manufacturing processes and materials and designs of packages and containers. Specifications for food quality, criteria for aesthetic properties, storage life, moisture contents, tendency of fats to become rancid, physical characteristics, and microbiological specifications were developed. Optimal combinations of various types of food were also determined.

Analyses of commercial and experimental products and experience with Mercury astronauts supported the conclusion that specially prepared natural food products (particularly those with decreased moisture content, requiring subsequent rehydration) were the most stable and promising for flight conditions.[18]

Special attention was devoted to the caloric value and the levels of protein, calcium, and fluid in the rations. Here the recommendations of the National Academy of Sciences/National Research Council's Council on Food and Nutrition[19] were adopted as fundamental. In establishing minimum daily requirements and optimal ratios among amounts of protein, fats, and carbohydrates in the rations, nutritionists utilized the results of studies by Sargent and Johnson[20] and Calloway[10] concerning the physiological rationale for the diet in therapeutic nutrition. Experimental testing of prototypes of the astronaut rations in two different laboratories had positive results.[1,21,22] The U.S. Air Force also tested experimental rations on high-altitude flights.[23,24]

In the creation of an onboard system for rehydrating food,[19,23] emphasis was placed on creating convenient packaging for dehydrated products that would ensure their safe rehydration and consumption. An original package was developed in the form of a plastic bag equipped with a valve through which a tube could be inserted, which had reliability of 95 percent.

Rations on Gemini and the first Apollo spacecraft included products dehydrated through freeze drying and other methods. Some of these were compressed. A typical day's menu included approximately 50 percent rehydrated products, with the remainder being solid products rehydrated by saliva in the mouth. The solid products were eaten both during regular meals, during preparation of the products needing rehydration were being prepared, and as snacks between meals. The set of products for a typical menu for Gemini and Apollo crews during the first day of flight offers an example.

1) Meal "A"—applesauce, sugar frosted flakes, bacon squares, cinnamon toast, cocoa, orange drink (the bacon and toast were solids).

2) Meal "B"—beef with vegetables, spaghetti with meat sauce, cheese sandwich, apricot pudding, gingerbread (sandwich and gingerbread were solid, the rest had to be rehydrated).

3) Meal "C"— pea soup, tuna salad, cinnamon toast, fruit cake, pineapple-grapefruit drink (toast and cake were solid, the rest had to be rehydrated).

The total caloric value of the ration described was 2514 kcal. The net weight of the food was 580.6 g. There were four different menus with three to four meals per day. For the Gemini crews, the caloric value of the daily ration was set at 2500 kcal. The caloric value of the ration for the Apollo lunar landing crew was raised to 2800-3000 kcal per day.

On the Gemini spacecraft and the Apollo lunar module food products were rehydrated with water at a temperature of 21.1-26.7 °C; i.e., at room temperature. Rehydration took 10 min or less. The Apollo command module provided cold (7.2-12.8 °C) and hot (45.0-50.6 °C) water. The astronauts rated acceptability of the rehydrated food as higher than that of the solid products hydrated in the mouth, regardless of water temperature. The possibility of regulating water temperature raised the acceptability of the rehydrated food.

Since the rations for Gemini and Apollo used natural products and flight duration was limited to 14 days, multivitamins were not included, although, previously in the United States, it had been recommended that multivitamins be taken daily. In the opinion of Lachange,[25] it is necessary to supply spacecraft crews with vitamins, since the dynamics of nutritional status and individual needs for vitamins have not been studied adequately.

The dietary formula and the processes for preparing all forms of food for space flight are stipulated in the Flight Food Specification Document.[25] A number of works describe the technology of space food manufacture.[26,27]

As experience has been gleaned in supplying spacecraft crews with food during flight, it has become increasingly clear that to ensure the nutritional adequacy of rations we must first study the chemical composition of the food itself, as well as the dynamics of nutritional status of spacecraft crews in simulated conditions on the Earth and in actual flights.

Studies undertaken with this objective during flights of Gemini 5 and Gemini 7 on red blood cells marked with ^{14}C revealed a shortened life span for red blood cells in three of four astronauts.[28] This suggests the existence of a hemolytic state. On the last three Gemini flights, several astronauts displayed a decrease in the levels of vitamin E in plasma. This sparked scientists' interest in studying the role of vitamins and minerals in the diet of spacecraft crews.

Experience with previous space flights suggests that full consumption of products in rations is highly dependent on the sensory appeal of the food. Unfortunately, products used in flight were inferior in quality and taste to familiar "homemade" products. For this reason, the United States has devoted a great deal of attention to the taste and other sensory qualities of food for astronauts and has had some degree of success.[29] NASA has set general specifications for all food products that are stricter than those for commercial products[30] in order to ensure reliability and quality.

The United States has relied on general microbiological criteria used in sanitary practice and directed at detecting the most pathogenic food micro-organisms in conducting sanitary and bacteriological evaluations of astronaut rations.[31,32] The low level of moisture in dehydrated products and limits on the moisture content in ready-to-eat food guarantee minimal fungal contamination. Special attention has been given to methods of storing the remains of uneaten rehydrated food. On Gemini flights, 1-gram tablets of 8-hydro-oxinoinsulfate introduced into plastic pouches containing the uneaten portion proved to be adequately effective with respect to bacteriostatic action.

A great deal of attention was devoted to packaging rations. A day's ration of packaged food on Gemini weighed 725.6 g and was 2131 cm^3 in volume. When the daily caloric value was increased to 2800 kcal the ration weighed 850.5 g and had a volume of 2393 cm^3.

On the majority of flights, crews complied with mandated procedures for preparing and consuming food. The crews used individual containers, which made it easier to compute how much food was actually eaten by a given crewmember. The meal schedule was documented in a flight journal and communicated to Earth by radio. The quantity of uneaten food was subtracted to determine the total amount of food consumed.

The weight loss of the commander of Gemini 4 was 2.0 kg, and the weight loss of the pilot 3.9 kg. On Gemini 7, weight losses were 4.5 and 2.9 kg for the commander and pilot, respectively. The observed weight loss was evidently a consequence of inadequate consumption of food by the crews. During the flight of Gemini 5, food consumption was diminished, which was attributed to lack of appetite. Over the course of 8 days, the commander lost 3.3 kg and the pilot lost 3.9 kg.

Weight loss was observed in all United States and Soviet spacecraft crews on flights mentioned above. A number of authors believe that weight loss is not associated with flight duration or the amount of food consumed but is a consequence of diuresis and perspiration[33] resulting from the effects of weightlessness, especially during the initial period of the flight. However, without objective measurement of fluid balance and the amount of food consumed, this question is difficult to resolve. It has also been established that in-flight physical exercise and work in a pressure suit increase weight loss.

Attempts were made to assess the risk of nutritional inadequacy during flight by computing an indicator of food consumed and measuring the amount of released CO_2 adsorbed by lithium hydroxide in special canisters. When this method was used on Gemini 5, it was found that about one half of the astronaut's weight loss could be attributed to caloric deficit.

To prevent bone demineralization and support calcium balance, calcium lactate was added in fruit juice to the rations of certain crews. This made it possible to increase the amount of calcium ingested by Gemini 7 crews to the required level—approximately 950 mg/day.

The major components of the food supply system in the Apollo program were adopted as the basis for the feeding system for Skylab.[34]

Soyuz spacecraft did not have facilities for rehydrating food. Therefore rations consisted mainly of canned natural, rather than dehydrated, products of various consistencies (Fig. 1). Products with diminished levels of moisture were held to a minimum. The rations included products that had proved acceptable in previous flights: pureed soups, creamed cottage cheese, and drinks of cocoa and coffee in aluminum tubes, some of which could be heated in a special device (Fig. 2). Black currant juice, rich in vitamin C, stored in a special container was used. There was a large assortment of canned meats in metal cans. *Rossiyskiy* processed cheese was also packed in such cans. The rations also included various types of bread—*Stolovyy*, *Borodinskiy*, and *Rizhskiy*. Bread products were formed into small bite-size pieces and packed eight to a polyethylene film package. A packet of bread for a single meal weighed 50 g. Desserts included chocolate with a high melting point, honey cakes, fruit jellies, and prunes with nuts. All products in plastic pouches were divided into bite-size portions. Some of the products in the pouches were vacuum packed.

Daily rations for cosmonauts included two multivitamin tablets, called *Undevit* (A—3300 I.U., B_1—2.58 mg, B_2—2 mg, B_6—3 mg, B_{12}—12 mg, C—75 mg, E—10 mg, nicotinamide—20 mg, folic acid—0.5 mg, calcium pantothenate—3 mg, and rutin—10 mg).[35-37]

There were three variants of the daily rations, creating a 3-day menu cycle. An example of the daily ration is as follows:

1) Breakfast: ham (canned), *Borodinskiy* bread, chocolate candy with walnut praline, coffee with milk, and black currant juice.

2) Lunch: beef tongue (canned), *Rizhskiy* bread, and prunes with nuts.

3) Dinner: dried salted fish, borshcht, veal (canned), *Stolovyy* bread, pastry, and black currant juice.

4) Supper: creamed cottage cheese, candied fruit, and black currant juice.

The weight of a day's ration without the packaging was approximately 1460 g, with a caloric value of approximately 2800 kcal—139 g of protein, 88 g of fat, 345 g of carbohydrates, and 853-950 ml of water. The ration contained minerals in accordance with the general physiological nutritional norms adopted in the U.S.S.R. The caloric value of the ration was distributed as follows: breakfast—26 percent,

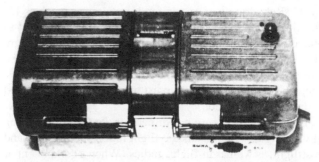

Fig. 1 Exterior view of the Soyuz food tube heater.

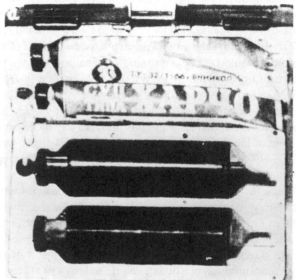

Fig. 2 Food tubes in the heater.

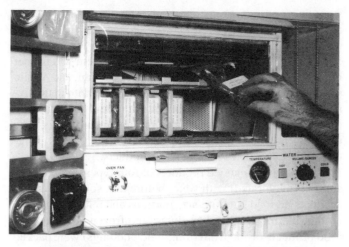

Fig. 3 Shuttle food system (NASA S82-26424).

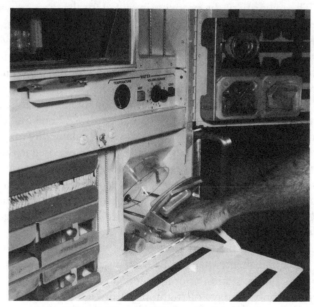

Fig. 4 Shuttle food rehydration device (NASA S82-26423).

lunch—21 percent, dinner—30 percent, and supper — 23 percent. In ground tests the assimilability of the nutrients was found to be 90 percent for protein, 97 percent for fats, 96 percent for carbohydrates, and 95 percent for calories. Cosmonauts flying on Soyuz rated the products in the rations as good.[35-40]

The rations on the U.S. Space Shuttles include thermostabilized, rehydratable, and partially dehydrated irradiated natural (fresh) products. The majority of products are packed in metal containers with nitrogen, and are similar in form to commercial products. The mean caloric value of a day's ration is approximately 3000 kcal, and the weight of the food before dehydration is 2.4 kg and after dehydration about 1.1 kg. Food is rehydrated with hot and cold water. The food values of the rations, on the whole, comply with the dietary recommendations of the Council on Food and Nutrition of the National Academy of Sciences (see Figs. 3 and 4).[41-43]

III. Food Supply System for Space Flights of Moderate Duration

Support of space flights of moderate duration (from 1 month to 1 year) required significant improvement of the previously developed and space-tested components of the onboard food supply system, as well as the introduction of new components. The most important task was improving the food value of the rations to support crew physiological needs on longer and more autonomous flights. It was important to expand the assortment of products and offer forms that would prevent the crews from growing tired of the food. Individual habits and preferences of the crewmembers had to be considered more carefully. It was essential to substantially increase the period over which the products retained their taste and other palatability factors, and to maintain the quality of the products in the rations. To make meals more pleasant, more foods had to be heated, the proportion of solid and dry products has to be decreased, and the resemblance of mealtime conditions and eating methods to those typical on Earth had to be increased. Meals had to become a source of enjoyment. Means of in-flight monitoring of crew food consumption and nutritional status also required further attention.

The U.S. Skylab crews remained in space for as long as 12 weeks. Skylab's onboard food supply system was further improved over the one used on Mercury, Gemini, and Apollo spacecraft and was significantly more appropriate to the living conditions on flights of moderate duration. A special 9.3-m^2 area in the cabin was set aside for leisure and meals. The menu cycle was lengthened to 6 days through use of a significantly expanded assortment of products.

The rations contained products of four types: those reconstituted (rehydrated) with water before use; solid dehydrated products divided into bite-size portions and rehydrated in the mouth; thermostabilized products; and frozen products. All food products (aside from drinks and puddings) were packed in aluminum cans. Drinks were packed in polyethylene accordion folded packages. The packaged products were stored in aluminum canisters.

The majority of the products intended for the three crews were stored onboard the station in 11 lockers at room temperature, in 5 lockers at a temperature of -18° C and below for deep frozen products, and in one refrigerator. The guaranteed shelf life of the products in the cabin of the station at room temperature (about 29 °C) was 2 years.

Unfortunately, during use of the station, the temperatures in the dining area periodically increased to 37.7 and 58 °C and, in the freezer to -8.3 °C. A study of the palatability of an analogous set of products stored on Earth and exposed to the same temperatures as those on the station showed decreased quality in 16 samples. Since altered storage conditions of products in flight may lead to loss of vitamins, it was decided to give members of the second and third crews vitamins before, during, and after flight.

The flight of the third Skylab crew was first planned for 56 days and then expanded to 84 days, but the rations remaining on the station after the second crew left were sufficient for only 69 days of flight, requiring the delivery of an additional 72 kg of products. However, specialists in nutrition managed to decrease this weight to 27 kg by using concentrates with increased caloric values of 3000 kcal/day. The assortment contained 70 different products. Daily rations were selected from these products, and menus were developed with consideration of the individual taste preferences of the crewmembers. This measure helped match the food to individual tastes, making it less likely that crewmembers would tire of their rations. The mean daily ration had a caloric value of approximately 3000 kcal and contained about 150 g of protein, 120 g of fat, 320 g of carbohydrates, 0.8 g of calcium, 2.2 g of phosphorus, 6.3 g of sodium, 4.3 g of potassium, and 0.32 g of magnesium. The weight of a day's ration was 1.9 kg, and the volume was 5.7 liters.[44] The food ration on Skylab was rather close in food value to that used on Salyut 6.[35,37,44]

Food was prepared and consumed at a special table, which contained heating trays and water guns for rehydrating the food and dispensing drinking water. The food was heated to 65 °C. Rehydration of certain foods required as much as 15-20 min, which meant that one of the crewmembers had to prepare the meal in advance. The products eaten hot were placed on the heating trays and the cold products in a chiller. After meals, the trays and table were cleaned with moist wipes. Utensils were cleaned with moist terry cloth towels soaked in disinfectant solution.

Balance studies were performed for the first time during Skylab flights. Astronauts ate flight rations during pre- and postflight, as well as in-flight studies. When a component of the ration could not be eaten, a system of rapid computation was used to prescribe dietary supplements of mineral tablets to compensate for the uneaten food. In their evening in-flight reports, the crew related what food had been consumed; the amounts of basic nutrients lacking were then computed rapidly on Earth, and the crew was instructed to take a certain quantity of tablets the next morning. The caloric value of the food consumed by the first crew per day pre- and in-flight was 2628 and 2509 kcal for the commander, 2822 and 2517 kcal for the co-pilot; and 2843 and 2593 kcal for the payload specialist. The actual calories consumed per day by the commander of the second crew, pre-, in-, and post-flight were 2732 ± 113, 2781 ± 259, and 2940 ± 149 kcal/day. This represents 40, 41, and 43 kcal/day per 1 kg body weight.

Mean weight loss in members of the first Skylab crew over the 28-day flight was 2.9 kg (3.9 percent); for the 59-day flight of the second crew, loss was 3.2 kg (4.6 percent). During the 84-day flight of the third crew, weight loss was diminished, equaling 1.1 kg (1.6 percent), as a result of the crew's consumption of a higher calorie ration—3000 kcal — and more physical training exercises. There is reason to believe that the third crew managed to maintain their preflight nutritional status.

The metabolic processes of Skylab crews were monitored pre- (on days 31, 27, and 21), in-, and postflight (on days 17, 18, and 18) for crews 1, 2, and 3, respectively. As had been the case for other flights, crewmembers experienced weight loss, accompanied by increased excretion of nitrogen, calcium, phosphorus, magnesium, and potassium.[35, 37,45,46]

Salyut 6 (September 29, 1977) utilized an improved food supply system, compared to those used on Vostok, Soyuz, Apollo-Soyuz, Gemini, and Salyuts 1 through 5. The system included rations; food storage containers; a dining table; an electric heater; utensils; devices for water regeneration, measurement, and dispensing of hot or cold water into the plastic pouches containing the rehydratable food; and receptacles for food scraps and discarded packaging. The cosmonauts cleaned their hands before eating, and utensils were cleaned using moist wipes with antimicrobial properties.[17,35,37,47-49]

The caloric value of the cosmonauts' rations was increased to 3150 kcal/day because of the expansion of the prescribed set of physical training exercises, which had proved effective in preventing the negative consequences of long-term hypokinesia and weightlessness. The rations, on the average, contained about 135 g of protein, 110 g of fats, 380 g of carbohydrates, 0.8 g of calcium, 1.7 g of phosphorus, 0.4 g of magnesium, 3.0 g of potassium, 4.5 g of sodium, and 50 mg of iron. On the flight of the first crew, cosmonauts took *Undevit* multivitamin tables (composition described above) twice a day. Starting with the flight of the second prime crew, *Aerovit* multivitamins (vitamin A—6600 I.U., B_1—2.58 mg, B_2—2 mg, B_6—10 mg, B_{12}—.025 mg, calcium pantothenate—10 mg, vitamin C—100 mg, vitamin E—20 mg, nicotinamide—15 mg, rutin—50 mg, and folic acid—0.5 mg) were used since they were more stable under storage. *Aerovit* had first been tested on Salyuts 3 and 5.

The mean weight of the daily ration was 1.7 kg, and its volume was 465 liters. The assortment of products and dishes was significantly expanded (from 44 on Salyut 4 to 70 on Salyut 6), which made it possible to switch from a 3-day to a 6-day menu cycle. On the whole, the new rations retained the traditional groupings of products: meats—25, dairy—5, bread—5, pastry—10, fruits and juices—12, hot drinks—3, and seasonings—2. There was a greater selection of heatable products and dishes in tubes, cans, and plastic wrap. A system for regenerating water from condensate of atmospheric moisture (SRV-12) made it possible to include a large number of freeze-dried entrees and drinks, which were reconstituted in their packages with hot water. The selection of fruit and vegetable juices reconstituted with cold water obtained from the water supply receptacles was increased. A total of 34 of the products could be heated. The crews responded favorably to this "innovation". Crewmembers noted that they did not grow as tired of the products, which retained their palatability for a longer period of time than on previous flights. The nutritional adequacy of the rations was initially determined under simulation conditions on the ground and, later, by evaluating parameters of cosmonaut nutritional status pre- and postflight, using data from clinical and physiological examinations postflight, and cosmonaut reports.[17,37,47-49]

Supplementary food products delivered to orbit by the Progress cargo vehicle and Soyuz and Soyuz-T transport spacecraft helped to solve the problem of feeding crews of Salyuts 6 and 7. The five prime crews of Salyut 6 were provided a rather wide selection of products and dishes (fresh vegetables and fruits, fruit and berry juices, seasoning, drinks, newly developed dehydrated and canned products), taking into account individual preferences. There was almost always a surplus of food products (flight rations plus supplementary products) onboard Salyut 6.

Despite this, of the 10 cosmonauts participating in the 5 prime crews, the majority—7 individuals—lost weight in amounts ranging from 1.8-6.4 kg, while the 3 others gained weight (0.2-3.5 kg) over the course of the flight. A number of authors explain changes in body weight by hypothesizing that individuals vary in their susceptibility to flight factors, in metabolism, and in the zeal with which they used prophylactic countermeasures. In particular, all members of the fourth prime crew, who strictly observed all prophylactic countermeasures and actively utilized such appetite enhancers as onion, garlic, and spices, gained weight. A study of parameters of nutritional status pre- and postflight did not reveal any significant changes in the cosmonauts.[37,48-52]

In general, the onboard food supply system for the long-term space station Salyut 7 (April 19, 1982) generally contained the same elements as that of Salyut 6, with the exception that, for the first time, there was a refrigerator for storage of fresh fruits and vegetables. A flight ration developed for the Salyut 7 crew was approximately the same in food value as that for Salyut 6 but consisted primarily (65 percent) of dehydrated products reconstituted with hot or cold water. This change was based on the experience of Salyut 6 crews, who received rations consisting of only 20 percent freeze-dried products, while the remaining 80 percent were primarily thermostabilized products. At the end of the second month of flight, the cosmonauts noted that they were growing tired of the sterilized products. The majority of dehydrated products included in the Salyut 7 ration had been tested in previous flights as supplementary products delivered to orbit by the transport vehicles. During the flights of the three Salyut 7 prime crews (211, 150, and 237 days in duration) all components of the food supply system functioned normally. The cosmonauts concluded that the rations helped them maintain a performance level adequate for completion of the flight program.[37,49,53]

A new menu-selection system for organizing flight rations was used for the first time on Salyut 7. In essence, this system involved packing the products in containers with other products of the same kind, rather than packaging a day's meals together. The new system facilitated tracking of the quantity of products used and allowed crewmembers to compose each meal on the basis of individual tastes. In practice, the crewmembers were frequently guided by their taste preferences, which did not always lead to a well-balanced menu with respect to food groups. Experience with the menu-selection system indicated that its success depended in many respects on preflight training of the crew in nutritional theory. The postflight nutritional status of the cosmonauts was, however, satisfactory.[49,53-55]

A record-setting space flight lasting 1 year was accomplished by a crew consisting of B.G. Titov and M.Kh. Manarov on the long-term space station complex Mir-Soyuz-TM-Kvant-Progress (December 21, 1987 to December 21, 1988). The onboard food supply system was, on the whole, analogous to that on Salyut 7. The rations consisted of 65 percent freeze-dried products that were reconstituted before use with hot or cold water, regenerated from humidity condensate, or brought from Earth. Since the products in standard flight rations are not recommended for storage for longer than 10 months, the Progress transport spacecraft delivered additional flight rations and drinking water requested by the crews, along with fresh apples, lemons, oranges, onions, garlic, cucumbers, honey, and other products with limited storage life. These measures substantially improved the crew's appetite and frame of mind.

On the whole, the cosmonauts evaluated the food supply system positively and willingly ate most of the products. No significant changes were noted in taste sensitivity, appetite, or digestive function.

After the 1-year flight, the commander lost 3.3 kg. During postflight clinical observation, his weight was observed to be 2.7 kg below baseline on day 4, and 0.5 kg below baseline on day 16. The flight engineer gained 2.1 kg. On day 16 postflight, his weight had returned to its preflight level. On the whole, over the 1-year flight, changes in weight were no greater than for shorter flights. With respect to anthropometric and biochemical parameters, no notable changes were found postflight. All this suggests that the rations used in flight, combined with the supplementary products regularly delivered to the station in orbit, proved adequate for the needs of the cosmonauts. The entire food supply system also proved efficient throughout the year.[56]

IV. Provision of Food for Long-Term Flights

There have not been any long-term space flights with durations greater than 1 year. In the future, plans call for the creation of a new generation of orbital stations, an expedition to Mars, and the establishment of planetary bases on the Moon and other celestial bodies of the solar system. All these and other permanently manned spacecraft require life support systems that are reliable and can function efficiently for several years. In particular, crews of these spacecraft and stations will need regular, well-balanced, and safe food to maintain their health and a high performance level throughout their missions.

Experience with previous space missions of up to 1 year suggests that, during space flight under relatively comfortable sanitary and hygienic conditions, the human body generally needs the same amounts of nutrients as on Earth. For this reason, the physiological nutritional norms for various demographic groups developed in the United States and the Russian Federation are acceptable for use in planning food supply systems for long-duration missions. Incidentally, within the limits of the stipulated age groups, these norms are valid for indefinite periods. Of course, during specific periods in flight, the amount of one or another nutrient needed and their optimal ratios in food may change, and this requires further study.

However, matters become more difficult when we turn to the issue of supplying space crews with high-quality, chemically well-balanced, and tasty food—a reliable source of the necessary quantity of energy and nutrients, especially essential nutrients. This is particularly true with respect to flights to other celestial bodies, when it becomes impossible to supplement onboard supplies with fresh products. Here, it seems promising to consider storing products in freezers and refrigerator chambers. However, refrigeration equipment has significant weight and volume and requires a significant expenditure of power, which is limited in flight. For this reason, as space flights become more autonomous so that onboard food supplies cannot be supplemented, the issue of guaranteed long-term storage of products in flight becomes more critical. Much work awaits us in this area.

The entire system of food preparation and consumption requires further improvement to make these processes more convenient, safer, easier, and less time-consuming. It is also necessary to improve the system of sanitary and antiepidemiological measures—those associated with the food supply technology, with the cosmonaut himself as a source of microbial contamination, and with prevention of contamination of the environment by food products.

Feeding ill crewmembers and dietary rehabilitation under conditions of altered physiological status and in emergency situations are other important topics.

The majority of authors writing today consider freeze-dried, vacuum-packed, and frozen products and dishes to be the most promising for use on long-term flights. Many countries are developing a wide assortment of such products, studying the best conditions for storing them (temperature and atmosphere, packaging, etc.), and evaluating their food value.[44,57-62] Development of food rations from freeze-dried products for long-term flights requires, first, the resolution of the following issues:

1) Is it possible to maintain good nutritional status on a diet based on dehydrated products and other preserved products over a long (2-3 year) period and evaluation of the nutritional acceptability of various degrees of rehydration?

2) What are the effects of long-term storage (2-4 year), with possible exposure to doses of cosmic radiation, on the food values and properties of dehydrated products?

3) What packaging is the most appropriate to storage conditions and safest from the standpoint of the products themselves, as well as the environment?

4) What types and assortments of dehydrated, frozen, irradiated, and other products are suitable with respect to physiological and hygienic parameters and palatability?

To solve some of these problems, the Russian Federation is conducting research studies continuing for as long as 1 year and using volunteers. The subjects consume a diet consisting totally of freeze-dried products under normal living conditions or in a sealed chamber (1 year). In three other experiments, subjects have received rations that were stored for 1-2 years with a portion irradiated by protons in a dose of 24,000 rad. The rations contain 3100-3200 kcal, 130-140 g of proteins, 96-125 g of fats, and 340-430 g of carbohydrates. Each subject takes a *Undevit* multivitamin tablet daily.[17]

All subjects undergo clinical medical monitoring. Parameters of protein, lipid, carbohydrate, vitamin, and mineral metabolism, the status of the gastrointestinal tract, the balance of a number of nutrients, and assimilation of the major nutrients are studied. Immune response and composition of intestinal microflora are also studied.[17]

The results of these studies support a conclusion that long-term (more than 1 year) human consumption of a diet consisting entirely of dehydrated products is possible, with adaptation requiring approximately 2 months.[17]

The results of consumption of dehydrated products after long-term storage and irradiation by protons were positive. The nutritional status of the subjects was evaluated as satisfactory, but at the same time it was deemed desirable for individuals on flights of as long as 2 years to take an *Undevit* multivitamin once a day, along with no less than 40 mg of vitamin E, 1 mg of vitamin A, and 0.5 g of calcium. These recommendations are based on results of measuring vitamins A and E in blood serum, and the discovery of symptoms of negative calcium balance.[17]

Nevertheless, as the durations of autonomous space flights increase beyond 2-3 years, the use of a food supply system based solely on supplies of food brought from Earth will become increasingly problematic. This raises the question of using various physicochemical and biological methods to extract nutrients from human wastes and by-products of various technological processes occurring in the onboard systems of the spacecraft. These issues have occupied researchers since the first short-term space flights.[63-65] Considering the aspects of the problem of providing food on long-term flights noted above, one may define the following possible basic types of system for feeding spacecraft crews.

1) Systems based exclusively on supplies of food brought from Earth. Considering the capabilities of modern food technology and the characteristics of the products and packaging that have been produced, an onboard food supply system of this type appears completely feasible for long-term flights with duration of 1, 2, and even 3 years. Thus, such a system is completely feasible for use on Mars flights. Of course, before such a system is approved for practical use in flight, considerable technological and design work and significant biomedical research will be needed to evaluate long-term storage of rations in simulated ground-based and flight conditions.

2) Mixed-type systems, in which space crews on long-term flights primarily use food supplies brought from Earth in the form of ready-to-eat products or preprocessed products requiring some additional culinary processing before use. As a supplementary source of nutrients, this system could use nutritive material obtained from processing crew wastes and by-products of technological processes of other spacecraft systems. For this purpose, the spacecraft must have special systems for obtaining this material from wastes through physicochemical and biological methods, and technological equipment for obtaining ready-to-eat food or individual nutrients from these nutritive materials, including those from nontraditional sources. The creation of reliable and relatively productive systems as components of onboard life support systems for transforming wastes into food products is still in the early stages. The task has proved to be more difficult than was initially thought. There has been some success in developing onboard greenhouses for growing algae. However, even here a great deal of additional work is needed, both in the technology for growing biomass and in the processing of this biomass into assimilable products. Use of the biomass in its raw form is limited in quantity by the biological, physiological, and psychological characteristics of humans. On flights lasting 1 to 2 years this issue is not critical but it would be very important to begin to test it.

3) Food supply systems primarily using food obtained from processing wastes, through the use of chemical, physical, and biological methods by onboard technological systems. Even for these systems to provide an adequate diet, certain essential nutrients would still have to be brought from Earth. These include vitamins, polyunsaturated fatty acids, amino acids, minerals, and spices and seasonings, which are too difficult to produce in the onboard systems of the spacecraft and of which relatively small amounts are required to meet physiological needs.

Under certain conditions, it would be possible to periodically supplement systems of the second or third type with additional supplies of food. At the present time, onboard food supplies to orbital stations are systematically supplemented, sometimes during crew exchange. Food products to meet the individual tastes of crewmembers have been delivered to space stations in orbit.[53,57,66]

However, creation of onboard food supply systems based on the use of food resources produced in flight as a result of waste processing remains an extremely complicated task. In the previous edition of "Foundations of Space Biology and Medicine," [2] the use of such food products in flight was considered in detail in Volume III, Chapter 2.

First, the chapter considered the use of physicochemical methods to produce food or rather individual nutrients: carbohydrates, glycerine, propylene glycol and ethyl alcohol, fats, and amino acids.[65,67-73] Unfortunately, today we can still only repeat the conclusion given there— that despite the importance of the problem, the results of numerous studies still concern only theoretical solutions of the problem and not concrete methods that can be applied in daily practice.

Next, the chapter considered the problem of obtaining food products as a result of biological production of food based on a partially or completely closed substance cycle. Such substance cycles occur naturally on the Earth. However, production of food products from wastes of crewmembers and the spacecraft biocomplex is evidently practical only for very long-term, completely autonomous flights or on long-duration stations.

The components of a recycling system on a spacecraft may be lower (one-celled algae) and higher autotrophic plants, lower heterotrophic organisms (yeasts, bacteria, and zooplankton), animal heterotrophic organisms (small animals and birds), humans; and a system of waste conversion.[63,65,74] Various combinations of biological and physicochemical methods for producing food are also possible. The previous edition of *Foundations of Space Biology and Medicine*[2] considered algae,[75-77] bacteria,[78,79] higher plants, [80,81] and fungi[80,82] in relative detail as potential sources of food in space.

Organisms capable of transforming human waste products into a nutritive biomass could theoretically also solve the problems of regenerating the cabin atmosphere and disposing of waste. In the opinion of certain researchers, autotrophic algae and bacteria are the most suitable organisms for a system of complete bioregeneration, considering the weight and volume required for this system. Higher plants may be grown hydroponically on large orbital and planetary stations, whereas animals may serve as an additional intermediate component of bioregeneration, requiring vegetable food.[76,81,83]

When the biomass obtained through regeneration of the atmosphere and wastes can supply a major portion of the diet, all that is required is to fine tune the system to match the elements of the bioregenerative system to the nutritional needs of the crewmembers. The food value of edible products obtained in a bioregenerative system are considered in detail in a special literature review.[84]

Bioregenerative systems for producing nutritive material must be supplemented with a technological system for processing them into products acceptable to cosmonauts in terms of taste and other aspects of palatability, as well as in terms of nutritive value.

There have certainly been some positive results toward solving the problem of bioregeneration of food. Work in this area is continuing; however, the successes are modest. Evidently, to create a reliable, complex, closed system for producing food in flight, especially ready-to-eat food and not just individual nutritive materials, an enormous amount of work still has to be done. Work in this area can be expected to intensify when space flights of 3 years and longer are scheduled, under which condition onboard systems based on food supplies would be seriously inferior to mixed or exclusively bioregenerative systems.

References

[1]Sisakyan, N.M., and Yazdovskiy, V.I., Eds. *The First Manned Space Flights*. Moscow, U.S.S.R. Academy of Sciences, 1962, pp. 37-39 (in Russian).

[2]Popov, I.G. Nutrition and water supply. In: Calvin, M., and Gazenko, O.G., Eds. *Foundations of Space Biology and Medicine*, Washington, D.C., NASA, 1975, vol. 3, chapter 2, pp. 35-69.

[3]Calloway, D.N., and Margen, S. *Clinical study of minimum protein and caloric requirements for man*. Annual Report, Grant NYR-050003-068, and Final Report, Contract NASA-3966, Washington, D.C., NASA Hq., 1966.

[4]Burnazyan, A.I.; Nefyodov, Yu.G.; and Parin, V.V., Eds. *Short Handbook on Space Biology and Medicine*, Moscow, Meditsina, 1967, pp. 314-315 (in Russian).

[5]Calloway, D.N. Nutritional aspects of all-purpose survival rations—A critical appraisal. *U.S. Armed Forces Medical Journal*, 1960, no. 11, pp. 403-417.

[6]Feeding man in space. *Canadian Food Industry*, 1961, vol. 32, no. 2, pp 22-27.

[7]Finkelstein, J.B. Nutrition research for space. *Journal of American Dietetic Association*, 1960, vol. 36, no. 4, pp. 313-317.

[8]Nanz, R.A. Food in flight. *Space World*, 1964, vol. A-3, pp. 12-14.

[9]Finkelstein, J.B. Progress in space feeding research. *Journal of American Dietetic Association*, 1962, vol. 40, no. 6,

pp. 529-531.

[10]Calloway, D.H. Nutritional aspects of astronautics. *Journal of American Dietetic Association*, 1964, vol. 44, no. 5, pp. 347-352.

[11]Klicka, M.V. Development of space foods. *Journal of American Dietetic Association,* 1964, vol. 44, pp. 358-361.

[12]Nanz, R.A.; Michel, E.L.; and Lachance, P.A. Evolution of a space feeding concept during the Mercury and Gemini space programs. *Food Technology,* 1967, no. 21, pp. 1596-1602.

[13]Sisakyan, N.M., and Yazdovskiy, V.I., Eds. *The First Multiman Space Flight*. Moscow, Nauka, 1964 (in Russian).

[14]Yazdovskiy, V.I., Ed. *The Second Multiman Space Flight*. Moscow, Nauka, 1965, pp. 22-27, 162-200 (in Russian).

[15]Popov, I.G. Some conclusions from the study of cosmonaut nutrition in space. In: Pokrovskiy, A.A, Ed. *Material From the XVIth Scientific Session of the Nutrition Institute of the U.S.S.R. Academy of Medicine*, Moscow, Meditsina, 1966, pp. 138–140 (in Russian).

[16]Kasyan, I.I.; Maksimov, D.G.; Popov, I.G.; Terentyev, D.G.; and Khagatuyants, L.S. Some results of medical studies of members of the Voskhod 2 crew. In: *Weightlessness,* Moscow, Meditsina, 1974, pp. 105-116 (in Russian).

[17]Bychkov, V.P. Feeding of spacecraft crews. In: Nefyodov, Yu.G., Ed. *Sanitary, Hygienic, and Physiological Aspects of Manned Spacecraft, Problems of Space Biology*, Moscow, Nauka, vol. 2, 1980, pp. 214-264 (in Russian).

[18]Dymza, N.A.; Stoewsand, G.S.; Donovan, P.; Barrett, F.F.; and Lachance, P.A. Development of nutrient defined formula diets for space. *Food Technology*, 1966, no. 20, pp. 109-112.

[19]National Academy of Sciences/National Research Council, Council on Food and Nutrition. Food and nutrition board recommended dietary allowances. Publication 1146 and previous editions, Washington, D.C., NAS-NRC, 1964.

[20]Sargent, F.J., and Johnson, R.E. The physiological basis for various constituents in survival rations, An integrative study of the all-purpose survival ration for temperate, cold, and hot weather. WADC 53-484, Part IV, Wright Patterson AFB, Ohio, USAF, 1957, pp. 53-484.

[21]Stone, S.E. Gemini flight food qualification testing requirements and problems. *Activities Report,* 1965, no. 17, pp. 34-43.

[22]Smith, K.J.; Speckmann, E.W.; Lachance, P.A.; and Dunco, D.P. Nutritional evaluation of a precooked dehydrated diet for possible use in aerospace systems. *Food Technology,* 1966, no. 20, pp. 101-105.

[23]Vanderveen, J.E.; Heidelbaugh, N.H.; and O'Hara, M.J. Study of man during a 56-day exposure to an oxygen helium atmosphere at 258 mm Hg total pressure. IXth Nutritional Evaluation of Feeding Bite-Size Foods, *Aerospace Medicine,* 1966, vol. 37, pp. 591-594.

[24]Welch, B.E. Dietary regimens in space cabin simulation studies. In: *Conference on Nutrition in Space and Related Waste Problems*, NASA SP-70, Washington, D.C., NASA Hq., 1964, pp. 181-187.

[25]Lachance, P.A. Gemini flight food specification document. CSD-G-079, Houston, NASA Manned Spacecraft Center, 1964.

[26]Hollender, H.A.; Klicka M.V.; and Lachance, P.A. Space feeding: Meeting the challenge. *Science Today*, 1968, vol. 13, no. 2.

[27]Klicka, M.V.; Hollender, H.A.; and Lachance, P.A. Food for astronauts. *Journal of American Dietetic Association*, 1967, no. 51, pp. 238-245.

[28]Fischer, C.L.; Johnson, P.C.; and Berry, C.A. Red blood mass and plasma volume changes in manned space flight. *Journal of American Medical Association*, 1967, vol. 200, pp. 579-583.

[29]Senter, R.J. Research on the acceptability of precooked dehydrated foods during confinement. AMRL-TD-63-9, Aerospace Medical Research Laboratories, Wright Patterson AFB, Ohio, USAF, 1963.

[30]National Aeronautics and Space Administration. *Inspection system provisions for suppliers of space materials, parts, components and services.* NPC-200-3, Washington, D.C., NASA Hq., 1962.

[31]U.S. General Services Administration. Clean room and work stations requirements, controlled environment. Federal standard 209, Washington, D.C., GSA, 1963.

[32]El-Risi, H.M. Microbiological requirements of space food prototypes. *Activities Report*, 1965, no. 17, pp. 374-380.

[33]Webb, P. Weight loss in man in space. *Science*, 1967, no. 155, pp. 558-559.

[34]U.S. Air Force. USAF Manned Orbiting Feeding System Assembly. Request for Proposal F-04695-67-R-0076, Washington, D.C., USAF, 1967.

[35]Burnazyan, A.I.; Nefyodov, Yu.G.; and Parin, V.V., Eds. *Short Handbook on Space Biology and Medicine.* Moscow, Meditsina, 1972, pp. 212-213, 233-235 (in Russian).

[36]Bychkov, V.P.; Chizhov, S.V.; Pak, Z.P.; Sitnikova, N.N.; and Koloskova, Yu.S. Onboard rations and water supply system. In: Gazenko, O.G.; Kakurin, L.I.; and Kuznetsov, A.G., Eds. *Space Flights on Soyuz Spacecraft*, Moscow, Nauka, 1976, chapter 4, pp. 65-89 (in Russian).

[37]Bychkov, V.P. Nutrition. In: Gazenko, O.G., Ed. *Space Biology and Medicine, A Manual*, Moscow, Nauka, 1987, pp. 108-115 (in Russian).

[38]Huber, C.S.; Heidelbaugh, N.D.; Smith, M.S.; and Klicka, M. Space foods. In: Birch, G.G.; Green, L.F.; and Plasket, L.G., Eds. *Health and Foods*, London, Applied Science, 1972, pp. 130-150.

[39]Roth, N.G., and Smith, M.S. Space food systems: Mercury through Apollo. *Advanced Space Science and Technology*, 1972, vol. 11, pp. 215-231.

[40]Vanderveen, J.E. Food, water and waste in space cabins. In: Armstrong, H.G., Ed. *Principles and Practice of Aviation Medicine*, 3rd Ed., Baltimore, Williams & Wilkins, 1952.

[41]Cooper, B.; Sams, P.; and Smith, M.A. *Space shuttle food supply system.* Preprints for 1975 annual scientific meeting of Aerospace Medical Association, San Francisco, Apr. 28-May 1, 1975.

[42]Smith, M.C.; Heidelbaugh, N.D.; Rambaut, P.C.; Rapp, R.M.; Wheeler, H.O.; Huber, C.S.; and Bourland, C.T. Apollo food technology. In: Johnston, R.S.; Lawrence, F.; Dietlein, M.D.; and Berry, C.A., Eds. *Biomedical Results of Apollo,* NASA SP-368, Washington, D.C., NASA Hq., 1975, pp. 437-468.

[43]Stadler, C.R.; Bourland, C.T.; Rapp, R.M.; and Sauer, R.L. Food system for Space Shuttle Columbia. *Journal of American Dietetic Association*, 1982, vol, 30, pp. 108-114.

[44]Rambaut, P.C., and Johnson, P.C. Nutrition. In: Nicogossian, A.E.; Huntoon, C.L.; and Pool, S.L., Eds. *Space Physiology and Medicine*, Second Edition, Philadelphia, Lea & Febiger, 1989, pp. 202-213.

[45]Leach, C.S., and Rambaut, P.C. Biochemical response of the Skylab crewmen. In: Johnston, R.S., and Dietlein, L.F., Ed. *Proceedings of the Skylab Life Science Symposium,* NASA TM X-58154, Houston, NASA Johnson Space Center, 1974, vol. 2, pp. 1-28.

[46]Rambaut, P.C.; Smith, M.C.; Leach, C.S.; Whedon, G.D.; and Reid, J. Nutrition and response to zero gravity. *Federation Proceedings*, 1977, vol. 36, pp. 1678-1682.

[47]Bychkov, V.P.; Guda, V.A.; Yefimov, V.P.; Kalandarov, S.; and Radchenko, N.D. Rations of Soyuz-9 crews. *Kosmicheskaya Biologiya i Aviakosmicheskaya Meditsina*, 1970, no. 6, pp. 59-60 (in Russian).

[48]Bychkov, V.P.; Kalandarov, S.; Markaryan, M.V.; Radchenko, N.D.; Stepchikov, K.A.; and Frumkin, M.L. Feeding the crewmembers of three Salyut-6 prime crews. *Kosmicheskaya Biologiya i Aviakosmicheskaya Meditsina*, 1981, no. 5, pp. 17-20 (in Russian).

[49]Burnazyan, A.I., and Gazenko, O.G., Eds. *Handbook on Space Biology and Medicine.* Moscow, Meditsina, 1984, pp. 195-199 (in Russian).

[50]Popov, I.G., and Latskevich, A.A. Concentration of free amino acids before and after a 175-day flight on Salyut-6. *Kosmicheskaya Biologiya i Aviakosmicheskaya Meditsina*, 1984, no. 2, pp. 26-33 (in Russian).

[51]Popov, I.G., and Latskevich, A.A. Certain characteristics of the levels of blood amino acids in cosmonauts completing a 185-day flight. *Kosmicheskaya Biologiya i Aviakosmicheskaya Meditsina*, 1983, no. 3, pp. 23-29 (in Russian).

[52]Ushakov, A.S.; Popova, I.A.; Goland-Ruvinova, L.G.; and Medkova, I.Ya. Biochemical description of neuro-endocrine reactions and metabolism. In: Gazenko, O.G., Ed. *Results of Medical Research Performed on the Salyut-6 - Soyuz Orbital Scientific Research Complex,* Moscow, Nauka, 1986, chapter 13, pp. 348-362 (in Russian).

[53]Bychkov, V.P.; Kalandarov, S.; Agureyev, A.N.; Popov, I.G.; Kochetkova, A.N.; and Ushakov, A.S. Feeding the crewmembers of the Salyut-7 orbital station. *Kosmicheskaya Biologiya i Aviakosmicheskaya Meditsina*, 1989, no. 4, pp. 9-14 (in Russian).

[54]Gazenko, O.G.; Grigoryev, A.I.; and Yegorov, A.D. Medical research program on long-term manned space flights on the Salyut-7- Soyuz orbital complex. *Kosmicheskaya*

Biologiya i Aviakosmicheskaya Meditsina, 1990, no. 2, pp. 9-15 (in Russian).

[55]Popov, I.G., and Latskevich, A.A. Amino acids in the blood of cosmonauts on flights varying in duration. In: Grigoryev, A.I., Ed. *Abstracts of Papers Presented at the IXth All-Union Conference*. Moscow-Kaluga, Institute of Biomedical Problems, pp. 544-545 (in Russian).

[56]Grigoryev, A. I.; Bugrov, S. A.; Bogomolov, V. V.; Yegorov, A. D.; Kozlovskaya, I. B.; Pestov, I. D.; Tarasov, I.K. Review of the major medical results of the 1-year flight on space station Mir. *Kosmicheskaya Biologiya i Aviakos-micheskaya Meditsina*, 1990, no. 5, pp. 3-10 (in Russian).

[57]Agureyev, A.N.; Bychkov, V.P.; Buneyeva, L.V.; Kalandarov, S.; and Sterlikova, N.P. Physiological/hygienic evaluation of the rations of the second prime crew of space station Mir. In: *Improvement of the Techniques, Technology, and Organization of Manufacture of Food Products and Rations*, Moscow, 1989, no. IV, pp. 299-302 (in Russian).

[58]Space Station Food Supply and Service System (FSSS). Technical Report, vol. 1, ZEMSCO-24210, 1987.

[59]Agureyev, A.N. Medical and technical aspects of nutrition in space flight. In: *Improvement of the Techniques, Technology, and Organization of Manufacture of Food Products and Rations*, Moscow, 1989, no. IV, pp. 290-294 (in Russian).

[60]Bourland, S.T. Designing a food system for Space Station Freedom. *Food Technology,* 1989, vol. 43, no. 2, pp. 76-82.

[61]Agureyev, A.N.; Gurova, L.A.; Karpova, O.K.; and Nedorubova, T.A. The problem of the scientific rationale for developing crew rations out of existing and future products. In: *Improvement of the Techniques, Technology, and Organization of Manufacture of Food Products and Rations*, Moscow, 1989, no. IV, pp. 262-266 (in Russian).

[62]Popov, I.G.; Bychkov, V.P.; and Korshunova, V.A. Issues of vitamin supplementation of the diet of cosmonauts on long-term flights. In: Grigoryev, A.I., Ed. *Space Biology and Aerospace Medicine. Abstracts of Papers Presented at the IXth All-Union Conference*, Moscow-Kaluga, Institute of Biomedical Problems, 1990, pp. 163-164 (in Russian).

[63]Nutrition for man in space. *Nutritional Review*, 1960, 18, no. 4, pp. 100–101.

[64]Ushakov, A.S., and Bychkov, V.P. Issues of nutrition in space flight conditions. In: *Problems of Space Biology, Volume 2*, Moscow, U.S.S.R. Academy of Sciences, 1962, pp. 48-53 (in Russian).

[65]Sisakyan, N.M.; Gazenko, O.G.; and Genin, A.M. Problems of space biology. In: Sisakyan, N.M., Ed. *Problems of Space Biology, Volume 1,* Moscow, U.S.S.R. Academy of Sciences, 1962, pp. 17-26 (in Russian).

[66]Bychkov, V.P.; Kalandarov, S.; Kochetkova, A.N.; Sedova, Ye.A.; and Ushakov, A.S. Feeding the crewmembers of three Salyut-7 orbital station prime crews. In: Gazenko, O.G., Ed. *Space Biology and Aerospace Medicine, Abstracts of Papers Presented at the VIIIth All-Union Conference,*

Moscow, Nauka, 1986, pp. 220-221 (in Russian).

[67]Fox, E.W. Prospectus for chemical synthesis of proteinaceous foodstuffs. In: *Closed Life-Support Systems,* NASA SP-134, Moffett Field, Calif., NASA Ames Research Center, 1967, pp. 189-200.

[68]Sinyak, Yu.Ye. On the possibility of physicochemical synthesis of carbohydrates in a spacecraft cabin. In: Sisakyan, N.M., and Yazdovskiy, V.I., Eds. *Problems of Space Biology, Volume 3*, Moscow, Nauka, 1964, pp. 401-410 (in Russian).

[69]Akerlof, G.C., and Mitchell, P.W. Study of the feasibility of the regeneration of carbohydrates in a closed circuit respiratory system. *Journal of Spacecraft and Rockets*, 1964, no. 1, p. 303.

[70]Budinikas, P., and Remus, G.A. Research and development study related to the synthesis of formaldehyde from CO_2 and H_2, NASA CR-7326, Washington, D.C., NASA Hq., 1968.

[71]Shapira, J. Design and evaluation of chemically synthesized food for long space missions. In: *The Closed Life-Support System,* NASA SP-134, Moffett Field, Calif., NASA Ames Research Center, 1967, p. 175-200.

[72]Shapira, J. Space feeding. Approaches to the chemical synthesis of food. *Cereal Science Today*, 1968, no. 13, p. 58.

[73]Ugolev, A.M.; Adamovich, B.A.; Krylov, O.V.; Sinyak, Yu.Ye.; Uspenskaya, V.A.; Ushakov, A.S.; and Shulgina, I.L Synthetic monosaccharides for human nutrition in space. In: *Abstracts of COSPAR Papers*, 1989, pp. 11-24.

[74]Genin, A.M., and Shepelev, Ye.Ya. Some problems and principles in forming a habitable environment based on the substance cycle. In: Proceedings of the XVth International Astronautics Congress, NASA TT-F-9131, Warsaw, Poland, 1964; Washington, D.C., NASA Hq., 1964 (in Russian).

[75]Powell, R.C.; Navels, E.M.; and McDowell, M.E. Algae feeding in humans. *Journal of Nutrition*, 1961, vol. 75, pp. 7-12.

[76]Casey, A.P., and Lubitz, J.A. Algae as food for space travel. *Food Technology,* 1963, no. 17, pp. 48-56.

[77]Kondratyev, Yu.I.; Bychkov, V.P.; Ushakov, A.S.; and Shepelev, Ye.Ya. Case study of the use of the biomass of one-celled algae for human nutrition. In: Chernigovskiy, V.N., Ed. *Job Performance. Issues of Habitability and Biotechnology. Problems of Space Biology, Volume 7*, Moscow, Nauka, 1967, pp. 364-370 (in Russian).

[78]Shapira, J., and Mandel, A.D. Nutritional evaluation of bacterial diets in growing rats. *Nature*, 1968, vol. 217, pp. 1061-1062.

[79]Waslien, C.J.; Calloway, D.H.; and Margen, S. Human tolerance to bacteria as food. *Nature*, 1969, vol. 221, pp. 84-85.

[80]Chuchkin, V.G.; Ushakov, A.S.; Rozhdestvenskiy, V.J.; Golovin, V.N.; Arbuzova, K.S.; Tsvetkova, G.V.; and Kostetskiy, A.V. Some aspects of utilization of higher plants as a nutrition source in space missions. In: Vishniac, W., and Favorite, F.G., Eds. *Life Sciences and Space Research VIII*, Proceedings of XIIth Plenary Meeting, COSPAR, Prague, Czechoslovakia, 1969; Amsterdam, North Holland, 1970, pp.

302-304.

[81]Boeing Co. Investigation of selected higher plants as gas exchange mechanisms for closed ecological systems. In: *Biologistics for Space Systems Symposium*, ARML-TDR062-127, Wright-Patterson AFB, Ohio, USAF, 1967.

[82]Cooke, G.D.; Beyers, R.J.; and Odum, E.P. The case for the multispecies ecological system with particular reference to succession and stability. In: *Bioregenerative Systems*, NASA SP-165, Washington, D.C., NASA Hq., 1968, pp. 129-139.

[83]National Academy of Science. Report of the Panel on Atmosphere Regeneration, Life Science Committee, Space Science Board, 1969, p. 88.

[84]Waslien, C.J. Impediments to the use of *Hydrogenomonas eutropha* as food for man. Doctoral dissertation, University of California, Berkeley, 1969, p. 173.

[85]Meleshko, G.I., and Shepelev, Ye.Ya. Biological life support systems. In: Gazenko, O.G., Ed. *Space Biology and Medicine: A Manual in Physiology*, Moscow, Nauka, 1987, chapter 4, pp. 123-146 (in Russian).

Chapter 12

Spaceflight Water Supply

Yu. Ye. Sinyak, V. B. Gaidadymov, V. M. Skuratov, R. L. Sauer, and R. W. Murray

I. General Issues

The importance of water for living creatures in general and humans in particular cannot be overestimated. The water contained in the human body (in the form of solutions and water-colloid complexes) is essential to virtually all metabolic processes and mechanisms for maintaining homeostasis. Moreover, water plays a major part in thermal regulation, especially at high ambient temperatures or when physiological heat production increases, for example, in strenuous exertion.

In the estimates of different authors, the body of an adult male is composed of 61–65 percent water.[1,2] Dehydration may have serious physiological effects. For example, water loss amounting to as little as 1 percent of body weight interferes with the functioning of various organs,[3] 10 percent loss causes serious problems, and a 20–22 percent loss is lethal.[1]

Dehydration could become a critical problem for humans in space. Numerous investigations have found that actual space flights and ground simulations alter fluid-electrolyte metabolism, reducing circulating blood volume and leading to loss of fluid and electrolytes.[4-6] A water loss of 3–5 percent in humans has been found to have serious deleterious effects on health status,[4] and this could have adverse consequences during re-entry and landing, when crewmembers undergo acceleration and are re-exposed to the Earth's gravity. For this reason, dehydration must not be allowed to occur on space flights. However, water stores substantially contribute to the launch weight of a spacecraft and must be held to a minimum. Thus, it is important to limit water consumption on the one hand and to develop efficient methods of water reclamation on the other.

A. Water Consumption Standards

The amount of water the human body needs to maintain a constant level of water balance varies as a function of environmental parameters, total heat production, and diet.

On the ground, water balance is achieved through consumption of about 2.2–2.8 liters per day by people doing light

physical work in a temperate climate.[1,7] Water losses in the course of a single day amount to 1.2–1.5 liters in urine, 400–700 mL in sweat, 350–400 mL in exhaled air, and 100–150 mL in feces. When the level of exertion and/or heat production increases, so does the amount of water lost through perspiration and insensible losses. Under such conditions, if water intake does not increase proportionally, urine concentration grows. The maximum possible urine concentration for healthy adults is 1400 mOsm/L, at which the minimum daily volume of excreted urine is 1.04 liters.[8] Physiologically, it is better to maintain a higher water intake than to allow a higher urine concentration.

In a temperate climate, water loss is counteracted by the consumption of drinking water (on the average, 1.5 liters) and dietary water (0.6–1.0 liter), and by water of metabolism (0.3.–0.4 liter). Given a normal diet, every 100 kcal of energy produced as a result of metabolism produces about 0.012 liter of water. At the same time, daily human fluid intake, even in a comfortable environment, may vary widely, ranging from 2–3.5 liters according to a number of authors.[9] Strenuous exertion in a high-temperature environment requires fluid intake of 6–6.5 liters per day; if solar radiation is intense, as in a desert, for example, 6–11 liters per day are required.[9,10]

Water requirements in space are affected by many factors associated with the microclimate and gravitational environment, physical activity, diet, physiological functions, etc. The issue of water consumption standards was considered intensively by researchers in the late 1960s and early 1970s, when space flights were of short duration and size and weight constraints on the spacecraft then used were of overriding importance. At that time, most authors agreed that, in space, water intake should equal 2.0–2.5 liters per crewmember per day.[10–14]

The development of water reclamation systems for use on spacecraft drastically altered the situation with regard to water intake standards. The first such water reclamation system was flown on the Salyut-4 station in 1974. Water reclamation systems transformed moisture-containing waste products (produced by humans, hardware, or biological systems) into potable water. In this situation, it seems more reasonable to speak not of standards for water intake, but rather of standards for water supply; i.e., the quantities of water that

The Russian portions of this chapter were translated by Galina Tverskaya and Lydia Stone.

Table 1 Daily water intake of Mir third and fourth prime crews

Mir crew	Water intake, L/man/day		
	Stored	Recycled	Total
Third	0.78	1.54	2.32
Fourth	0.45	1.75	2.20

must be produced by a water reclamation system over a 24-h period.

Experience with actual space flights has supported this approach. Table 1 cites water intake data for the third (V. Titov and M. Manarov) and the fourth (S. Krikalyov, A. Volkov, and V. Polyakov) Mir prime crews. The station carried two sources of water: stored water (Rodnik system) and water reclaimed from condensates of atmospheric moisture (SRV-K system).

B. Quality of Potable and Wash Water

Initially, in order to develop hygienic principles appropriate for use of water in space, all available data on the hygienic aspects of water supply were considered, but always from the perspective of the specific properties of the spacecraft environment, the sources of reclaimed water, and the conditions under which water production processes must operate in flight. However, the basic concept for space consumption remained unchanged from standards on the ground, i.e., that humans in space, like those on Earth, need water that is safe, meets physiological needs, and has acceptable aesthetic properties.

In the Soviet Union (currently Russian Federation) parameters that have been used as standards of water quality in space were taken from "USSR State Standards on Potable Water No. 2874" and "USSR State Standards on Sources of Centralized Water Supply, Procedures for Sampling and Quality Evaluation No. 2761-57," which were in force at that time.[15,16] Water quality control also involved selective measurement of various added preservatives and substances that could migrate into the water from storage containers. Since electrolytically introduced ionic silver had been selected as the preservative for water in the U.S.S.R., the flight-qualified water standards regulated silver levels. It should be mentioned here that standards regulating silver concentrations in stored and reclaimed water on spacecraft differ from those accepted in the United States or in the U.S.S.R. for potable water on the ground (0.05 mg/L).[15,26]

A distinguishing feature of the standards for quality of stores of potable water on spacecraft is that the water must comply with the requirements during two periods, i.e., preflight and during inflight storage.

The goal of developing efficient water supply systems using water reclaimed from human wastes and by-products of hardware and biological systems presented scientists and engineers with many new problems in hygiene, chemistry, engineering, and design.

Sanitary and hygienic studies targeted the composition of sources of reclaimed water[2,7,8,10]; changes occurring in them during the reclamation process[17-20]; efficiency of elimination of contaminants[2,21]; associated effectiveness in decreasing contaminants to toxicologically safe concentrations[2,22,23]; and a toxicological description of proposed water reclamation technologies.[2,24] On the basis of experimental data, "A List of Standards for Evaluating the Quality of Water Reclaimed by On Board Water Supply Systems" was compiled and approved by the U.S.S.R. Ministry of Health in 1967.

In the course of preparing this list and in the subsequent development of national standards (1967), several assumptions were made and these should be remembered when using these documents. First, the standards regulate the quality of water meant for consumption for a period no longer than 1/70–1/50 of the mean life span of man. This is the reason why some of the contaminant levels judged acceptable are higher than those pertaining to tap water.

Second, since it is forbidden to use any construction materials not explicitly approved by the U.S.S.R. Ministry of Health for use in the potable water supply systems, the number of toxic compounds for which standards are stipulated is significantly smaller than in the United States.

Third, since the nature and quantities of organic impurities in moisture-containing wastes are highly variable and may undergo chemical transformation during treatment of the water, reclaimed water quality is evaluated in an integral fashion, on the basis of chemical oxygen demand (COD) and/or total organic carbon.[25] When COD is used as the criterion, there are two standards: one for water reclaimed from a source free of toxic compounds and the other for water reclaimed from a product that does contain toxins.

Fourth, all standards set for quality of reclaimed water should be considered absolute only as applied to water produced by a system that has been meticulously designed, repeatedly tested, and already officially certified with respect to hygienic effectiveness. During the design, development, and testing of systems, compliance with these standards should be considered in relative terms; that is, they are used to evaluate the water supply system only for technological effectiveness. The final evaluation of these water reclamation systems must involve toxicological experiments on warm-blooded animals.

Table 2 presents standards regulating the quality of reclaimed water currently used in the United States[26] and in the Russian Federation.

C. In-Flight Monitoring of Water Quality

The conclusion that reclaimed water can safely be consumed by humans is based on a set of sanitary/hygienic studies utilizing chemical, toxicological, biological, and micro-

Table 2   United States and U.S.S.R. standards of the quality of reclaimed water[26]

Parameter	Standards			
	United States		Russia	
	Potable[26]	Hygiene[26]	Potable	Hygiene
pH value	6.0–8.0	5.0–8.0	6.0–9.5	4.5–9.5
Turbidity, no more than	1[b]	1[b]	1.5[a]	–
Color, true, no more than	15	15	20	–
Taste, rated, no higher than	2	–	2	–
Odor, rated, no higher than	3	3	2	3
Total hardness, mg-equiv/L, not over	–	–	7	7
Total number of solids, mg/L, no more than	100	500	–	–
Nitrogen as ammonia, mg/L, no more than	0.5	0.5	2	10
Calcium, mg/L, no more than	30	30	100	–
Magnesium, mg/L, no more than	50	50	50	–
Sulfate-ions, mg/L, no more than	250	250	500	–
Chlorine-ions, mg/L, no more than	200	200	350	350
Nitrogen in nitrates, mg/L, no more than	10	10	10	–
Total salt content (dry residue), mg/L, no less than	–	–	100	–
Silver, mg/L, no more than	0.05	0.05	0.5	2.0
Fluorine, mg/L, no more than	–	–	1.5	–
Arsenic, mg/L, no more than	0.01	0.01	–	–
Barium, mg/L, no more than	1.0	1.0	–	–
Cadmium, mg/L, no more than	0.005	0.005	–	–
Chromium, mg/L, no more than	0.05	0.05	–	–
Copper, mg/L, no more than	1.0	1.0	–	–
Iodine, mg/L, no more than	15.0	15.0	–	–
Iron, mg/L, no more than	0.3	0.3	0.3	–
Lead, mg/L, no more than	0.05	0.05	–	–
Manganese, mg/L, no more than	0.05	0.05	–	–
Mercury, mg/L, no more than	0.002	0.002	–	–
Nickel, mg/L, no more than	0.05	0.05	–	–
Selenium, mg/L, no more than	0.01	0.01	–	–
Zinc, mg/L, no more than	5.0	5.0	–	–
Sulfides, mg/L, no more than	0.05	0.05	–	–
COD, mg O_2/L, no more than	–	–	–	250
a) with no toxic substances in the source	–	–	100	–
b) with toxic substances in the source	–	–	50	–
Total organic carbon, mg/L, no more than	0.5	10	25	80
Organic acids, mg/L, no more than	0.5	0.5	–	–
Cyanides, mg/L, no more than	0.2	0.2	–	–
Phenols, mg/L, no more than	0.001	0.001	–	–
Halogen derivatives of hydrocarbons, mg/L, no more than	0.01	0.01	–	–
Alcohols, mg/L, no more than	0.5	0.5	–	–
Cations, mg/L, no more than	30	n/a	–	–
Radioactivity, pico-Curie/L	c	c	–	–
Microbiological parameter				
Maximum microbial count in 100 mL	1	1	–	–
Total bacterial count per 100 mL, no more than	1	1	10,000	100,000
Electric conductivity, x 10^{-4} S/cm, no more than				
a) purified water	–	–	1.5	1.4
b) conditioned water	–	–	1.5–7.5	–

[a] Rated against a turbidity standard of a suspension of kaolin in water, in mg/L.

[b] NTU or nephalometric turbidity unit.

[c] MCLs for radioactive constituents shall conform to Nuclear Regulatory Commission regulations.

Table 3 Standards for range of parameters of reclaimed water quality

Parameter, units	Potable water	Hygiene (wash) water
pH value, pH units	6.0–9.5	–
Total organic carbon, mg/L	0–25	0–80
Nitrogen as ammonia, mg/L	0–2.0	–
Ionic silver, mg/L	0.02–0.5	0.02–2.0
Microbial count, cells/mL	0–100	0–1000

biological methods and analyses of the technological effectiveness of water reclamation systems. Hygienic evaluation of the quality of water produced by a water reclamation system during the period of design, development, and operational life testing in ground-based experiments is based on criteria involving many chemical, physical, aesthetic, and biological parameters. The results of these experiments and tests are used to determine the operational lifetime of the entire water supply system and of its individual components and to specify the protocol for their use in space flight.

It should, however, be remembered that the operational lifetime of a system depends directly on the level of contaminants in the source used for water recovery, the nature and quantity of which, in turn, depend on a number of conditions and factors. Obviously, it is extremely difficult to simulate all these factors in ground-based tests. The feasible duration of a test and the amount of the water reclaimed in such cases cannot be compared with the continuous functioning of the water supply system in space; for example, the one on Mir, which was in continuous operation for 4 years and reclaimed 1500 kg of water during the flight of the third prime crew alone (366 days). In addition, it is virtually impossible to simulate, in these tests, all hypothetical situations that could affect the functioning of life support hardware, experimental equipment, or other units. This further decreases the cost effectiveness of these tests.

It is clear that, on long-duration space flights, in-flight measurements should be made of the physical, chemical, and bacteriological parameters of the potable water produced by the water reclamation system. It should be emphasized that high-quality water is one of the prerequisites for maintaining the health and performance of crewmembers exposed to the adverse effects of space. In future water supply systems involving continuous decontamination and conditioning, feedback from in-flight monitoring will ensure that the water produced meets physiological requirements.

The development of in-flight monitoring systems is complicated by the need to deal simultaneously with problems in hygiene, analytical chemistry, and precision engineering.

With respect to hygienic monitoring, size and weight constraints dictate that the minimum number of parameters must be used for water quality control. The only acceptable approach is to use integral parameters of water quality; in other words, parameters that provide information about the entire spectrum of potential contaminants.[27,29,30]

An automated system for in-flight monitoring of the quality of reclaimed water that was developed and tested by NASA in 1972 and 1973 can be considered a good prototype of such a system.[28] This system monitored ammonia and chlorine ions; pH; electrical conductivity; total, inorganic and organic carbon; and microbial contamination, including both total and viable cells. Except for the biosensor, the instrument was made from commercially available units, which were connected with tubes and pumps to operate automatically. A computer then analyzed the data obtained, initiated an alarm signal if any parameter exceeded the maximum allowable value, and activated a command to dump poor-quality water to a separate container.

In the U.S.S.R., a conductometric sensor, which signaled significant increases in level of contaminants, was added to the SRV-K water reclamation system in 1974.

In 1983, the U.S.S.R. Ministry of Health approved the "Provisional List of Parameters for Monitoring Water Quality." In contrast to the previously adopted documents, this list includes hygienic requirements not only for the water ultimately produced, but also for water quality at a number of intermediate stages of processing, making it possible to monitor individual components of the water reclamation system.[29] Two groups of parameters could thus be selected for monitoring purposes: parameters reflecting quality of water that had passed through the system as a whole; and parameters specific to each subsystem, i.e., parameters characterizing the performance of a given subsystem.[30] Table 3 presents standards for the in-flight-monitoring parameters of reclaimed water quality.

The NASA-developed instrument for monitoring the quality of reclaimed water mentioned above[28] employed a number of different procedures: potentiometric measurement of pH, ammonia and chlorine ions, conductometry, and high-temperature incineration followed by infrared detection of carbon dioxide to measure organic carbon.

The current Russian system for monitoring the quality of reclaimed water includes solid-state ion-selective electrodes for measuring ammonia and silver, potentiometric pH measurement, and potentiodynamic measurement of organic carbon. The last method was developed especially for this purpose.[31,32,146]

Conductivity has high potential as an integral parameter providing information about both organic and inorganic electrolytes in reclaimed water.[30,33,34] However, conductometry is nonspecific and, therefore, is best used in the segments of the system where ionized contaminants are most likely to occur.

D. Monitoring Microbial Contamination of Reclaimed Water

Microbiological safety is one of the most important quality requirements for potable water. This requirement cannot be overstated with regard to the quality of reclaimed water in space flight, in light of the increase in the "pathogenic potential" of microbes that takes place in the closed environments of spacecraft cabins.[35] In such environments, not only does the total level of microbial contamination increase, but also, and even more important, the proportion of pathogenic microbes with resistance to antibiotics increases.[36] Such microbial strains can spread among the crewmembers, causing a situation of "transient carriage" analogous to the spread of hospital infections.[37] In addition, alterations in the immune systems of crewmembers on long-term space flights occur in parallel to changes in the microbial status of the space environment.[38]

Current decontamination methods for reclaimed water include pasteurization and/or the addition of ionic silver.[2] These methods reduce microbial concentrations to levels compatible with applicable standards (see Table 2). However, the possibility of water becoming contaminated with environmental micro-organisms cannot be ruled out. This is especially true since the sources of water to be reclaimed are generally highly contaminated (the microbial count is 10^4 to 10^6 cells/mL, see Tables 6, 7, and 8), and there is a possibility of carry-over or bypass of the purification process. In addition, the interior surfaces of closed cabins, especially those made from nonmetallic materials, tend to become coated with a biofilm,[39] making it highly likely that the surfaces in contact with the water will become contaminated.

All of the above considerations emphasize the need for the microbiological monitoring of reclaimed water.

Before turning to the analysis of existing methods for evaluating the microbiological status of reclaimed water, the species composition of micro-organisms inhabiting the cabin, the human body, and reclaimed water in the spacecraft environment (see Table 4) should be discussed. A large number of proximate methods for microbiological monitoring of the environment have been developed recently. Of great interest are immunoserological methods, particularly those utilizing fluorescent antibodies.[49,50] These methods are very sensitive and highly specific; however, this, in itself, makes it difficult to use them to monitor the quality of reclaimed water, because its bacterial spectrum, as Table 4 shows, is extremely large and variable.

Another group of methods is based on the use of nutrient media labeled with radioactive isotopes of carbon (^{14}C), phosphorus (^{32}P), and sulfur.[51-53] These methods produce good results with a pure synchronized culture; however, their reproducibility is very low when naturally occurring water and other natural environments are analyzed. In addition, since

they require the use of radioactive isotopes and prolonged incubation, they are not suitable for use in space.

Methods based on bioluminescence, chemiluminescence, and fluorescence of different components of a bacterial cell are highly sensitive. These methods have been discussed by U.S. authors for use in detecting micro-organisms in reclaimed water. Levin recommended a method based on the measurement of adenosine triphosphate (ATP) by means of its bioluminescent reaction with luciferin-luciferase.[54]

The NASA-developed automated instrument mentioned above for monitoring the quality of reclaimed water[28] was equipped with a biosensor utilizing the chemiluminescent reaction of bacterial porphyrins with a luminol hydrogen peroxide mixture. Signals from incubated and nonincubated water samples were compared in order to distinguish between living and dead micro-organisms. Biosensor sensitivity was enhanced by concentrating micro-organisms on membrane filters. These procedures can detect as few as 10 microbial cells per milliliter, with a probability of 92 percent.

Other instruments using conductometry, potentiometry, and fluorescent microscopy have been designed.[55-57] However, the use of these methods presents a number of problems even on the ground; and the size, weight, and power requirements of the instruments needed to implement these methods preclude their use on spacecraft in the near future.

Another group of proximate methods uses biochemical indicators that can be dipped into the nutrient medium in which micro-organisms are cultivated.[58-60] These methods have adequate sensitivity and reproducibility, with response times between 2 and 6 h. The modification and refinement of these methods led to the development of very promising systems using paper indicator strips.[50,61] The same principle was used to develop a number of means for microbiological monitoring of reclaimed water.[62]

E. Sources of Water to be Reclaimed; Composition of Contaminants of Moisture-Containing Wastes

The following liquids are currently considered to be suitable sources of reclaimed water: humidity condensate, urine, wash water, fuel cell (electrochemical generator) by-products, and products of hydrogen peroxide decomposition. Sufficient quantities of these liquids are produced on spacecraft to meet the physiological and hygienic needs of crewmembers. For example, during Mir flights, the following quantities of liquids were produced per cosmonaut per day: 1.54–1.75 liters of humidity condensate, 1–1.5 liters of urine,[1-3] and 4.05 liters of wash water. In addition, 1-kW fuel cell produced 11 liters of water per day,[2] and the 0.8 kg oxygen obtained from hydrogen peroxide yielded 0.9 kg of water.[2]

The water vapor exuded and expired by the crewmembers forms humidity condensate in the cabin thermal regulation system. This condensate contains volatile organic and inorganic compounds. In addition to contaminants of anthropogenic origin, it also includes volatile compounds emitted from interior surfaces and products of biodegradation and pyroly-

Table 4 Generic composition of micro-organisms detected in different microbiocenoses of enclosed environments and space vehicles

Genus	Source (see reference list)									Current authors[b]
	(35)	(40.41)	(42,43,19)	(44)	(45)	(46)	(47)	(47)	(48)	
Achromobacter			W		BLSS					
Acinetobacter	SC	A, C, SC, SB	C, W, A			SB, SC	W	SC		WW-C, WW-D
Aeromonas	SC	SB, C	C, W			SB, SC	W			WW-C, WW-D
Alcaligenes										W
Arthrobacter		A, C, SC, SB	C, W							
Bacillus		SB				SB, SC			U	W
Citrobacter	SC	SB	C, W				W			W, WW-C, WW-D, U, WU, UC
Corynebacterium	SC	SB, A, C		SB	BLSS	SB, SC				
Enterobacter	SC	SC, C		SB		SB, SC		SB, SC		WW-C, C, WFC, FC, C, W
Enterococcus										WW-C, WW-D
Escherichia		SB, SC		SB[c]				SC	U	WW-C, WW-D
Flavobacterium					BLSS					
Herella			C, W	SB						
Klebsiella	SC	A, W, SB, SC		SB		SB, SC		SB		WW-C, WW-D, U, UC
Micrococcus	SC		C, W				W		U	
Moraxella	SC		C, W	SB		SB, SC	W			
Proteus		SB, SC		SB		SB, SC		SB, SC	U	WW-C, WW-D, W, WU, UC
Pseudomonas	SC	SB, SC, C	W	SB	BLSS	SB, SC			U	W, WW-C, WW-D, C,U, WU, UC, FC, WFC
Serrata				SB						
Staphylococcus	SC	SB, A, SC, C	C, W	SB		SB, SC	W	SB, SC	U	C, WW-C, WW-D, U, WU, UC
Streptococcus		C, SB	W					SB		WW-C, U, UC, WU
Yeast and mold fungi	SC	SC				SC		SC		

[a]Legend: atmosphere of the space cabin (A); biological life support system (BLSS); C, humidity condensate; fuel-cell by-products (FC); surface of the human body (SB); surface of the space cabin (SC); nonpreserved urine in storage (U); urine condensate (UC); water recovered from humidity condensate (W); water recovered from fuel-cell by-products (WFC); water recovered from urine (WU); contaminated wash water (WW-C); decontaminated wash water (WW-D).
[b]Obtained in collaboration with A.N. Viktorov, L.B. Zagibalova, K.V. Zarubina, and L.A. Vinogradova.
[c]Detected in the pharynx.

sis of polymers, paints, and varnishes. Various researchers have detected from 70–350 compounds in the humidity condensate of spacecraft cabins.[2,22,23,63]

Table 5 presents data on compounds detected in the humidity condensate of the Soviet space vehicles Vostok, Salyut, and Mir. The chemical composition of the condensates tends to vary quantitatively. Another feature is the presence of significant quantities of organic compounds, as revealed by chromatography and levels of COD, permanganate oxidizability, and total organic carbon. Of these contaminants, the most important are ethanol, acetic acid, ethylene glycol, and, occasionally, methanol. Inorganic compounds, with the excep-

Table 5 Physical properties, chemical composition and bacterial contamination of spacecraft cabin humidity condensate

Parameter, units	Space vehicles and mockups			
	Vostok[2]	Salyut mockup	Mir mockup	Mir station
COD, mg O_2/L	144–240	72–2880	150–375	437–1500
Permanganate oxidizability, mg O_2/L	25–30	19–81	33–81	–
Total organic carbon, mg/L	–	26–590	56–137	333–503
pH value, pH units	6.0–6.9	1.6–7.8	6.8–7.3	6.0–7.2
Specific electrical conductivity, x 10^4 S/cm	–	1.4–6.6	1.2–2.3	1.0–2.1
Transparency, cm	Turbid	10–20	30	–
Turbidity, mg/L	–	0.0–25	0–2	0.75–2
Odor, scored	3	1–4	5	4–5
Color (cobalt), deg	–	5–40	–	15
Total hardness mg-equiv/L	0.2–0.3	–	0.1–0.3	0.56
Nitrogen as ammonia, mg/L	70–160	15–275	17–33	13–32
Nitrogen as nitrates, mg/L	0.6–1.0	0.25–0.4	0	0.3
Nitrogen as nitrites, mg/L	–	0.9–1.15	0.04–0.25	0.03–0.0008
Chlorides, mg/L	3–22	1.9–50	0.8–2.8	2.55–3.69
Sulfates, mg/L	3–5	1–18	1–4	1–5
Calcium, mg/L	4–29	3.5–8.2	0.4–0.8	1.2–3.4
Magnesium, mg/L	–	0.2–4.8	0.1–0.8	–
Potassium, mg/L	–	0	0	–
Sodium, mg/L	–	0	0	–
Alcohols, mg/L	330–2500	–	–	–
Ethanol, mg/L	–	0.1–342	8–136	186–634
Methanol, mg/L	–	0.4–8.2	1.6–8.2	14.9–32.1
Propanol, mg/L	–	0.15–0.3	0	0
Butanol, mg/L	–	–	0–0.6	0–5.7
Isoamyl alcohol, mg/L	–	–	0	0–4
Ethylene glycol, mg/L	–	–	5.6–35	1.6–22.4
Organic acids:	15–27	–	–	–
Acetic, mg/L	–	0.8–98	17–48	0–47
Butyric, mg/L	–	0.1–1.2	0–1.6	1–13.7
Propionic, mg/L	–	0.01–1.1	0	0
Valeric, mg/L	–	–	0	1.1
Caproic, mg/L	–	0.15–18	0–3.8	0–19
Microbial contamination, x 10^3 cells/mL	–	2–800	2–380	0.06–4.5

tion of ammonia, are not present in significant amounts.

Humidity condensates tend to be highly contaminated by micro-organisms, probably because the latter form in the air conditioning system. Virtually all of the spacecraft cabin air circulates through this system, and the moisture condensed from the air is highly contaminated with environmental and human microflora. This process is markedly facilitated by microgravity. Table 4 presents a list of microbial genera occurring in humidity condensate.

Of all the sources of reclaimed water, urine is the most contaminated (see Table 6). Urine is a complex mixture of substances belonging to different chemical classes. Approximately 200 different compounds have been identified in urine.[64] The major organic substances are urea, uric acid, creatinine, amino acids, and lactic acid. The nitrogen in urea accounts for 85–89 percent of total urinary nitrogen, with other nitrogen-containing compounds, including ammonia salts, comprising the remaining 10–15 percent. Daily urine samples may contain as much as 16 grams of such salts as chlorides, sulfates, and phosphates and as much as 1.1–2.8 grams of amino acids. Volatile components of urine easily enter reclaimed water, making it unsuitable for drinking, with amines presenting the greatest danger. Moreover, alcohol, phenol, indole, furane, and pyrrole from urine may readily infiltrate the spacecraft cabin atmosphere. All these compounds are toxic and cannot be permitted in reclaimed water. Some of the salts in urine are in a supersaturated state.

Urine acts as a nutrient medium highly conducive to the growth and development of microorganisms, which may significantly alter its chemical composition and produce unde-

Table 6 Chemical composition of daily urine and condensate obtained during low-temperature evaporation in the water recovery system SRV-M

Chemical compounds and parameters, units	Urine[54]	Urine condensate[a]
Water, percent	95	99.9
Urea, mg/L	2000–35,000	0–17
Sodium chloride, mg/L	8000–10,000	1.2–2.8
Creatinine, mg/L	500–2400	–
Phosphates, mg/L	2000–13,000	–
Ammonia, mg/L	400–1200	0.5–2.5
Hippuric acid, mg/L	100–2500	–
Uric acid, mg/L	200–1200	–
Sodium, mg/L	4000–9000	–
Potassium, mg/L	2000–3300	–
Calcium, mg/L	200–970	1–2
Magnesium, mg/L	60–200	6–9
Sulfur as SO_4, mg/L	1800–3600	–
Inorganic sulfates, mg/L	1210–3030	0–30
Oxalic acid, mg/L	15–30	–
Nitrogen as amino acids, mg/L	180–530	–
Purine bases, mg/L	15–45	–
Phenols, mg/L	17–420	–
Volatile fatty acids, mg/L	≤ 60	–
Citric acid, mg/L	200–1000	–
Dry residue, mg/L	32–184	–
Nitrogen as nitrates, mg/L	–	0–0.2
Nitrogen as nitrites, mg/L	–	0.07
Iron, mg/L	–	1.9–32
Ethanol, mg/L	–	2.3–47
Methanol, mg/L	–	2.5–4.3
Acetic acid, mg/L	–	5.7–15.2
Acetaldehyde, mg/L	–	0–4.2
Acetone, mg/L	–	0–8.3
Total organic carbon, mg/L	11,800 ± 660[b]	10–78
COD, mg O_2/L	17,590 ± 1510[b]	70–100
Electric conductivity, x 10^{-4} S/cm	–	0.08–1.4
Odor, rated	–	5
Transparency, cm	–	30
pH value, pH units	–	3.7–6.4
Microbial contamination, 103 cells/mL	–	0.6–15

[a]Current authors' data.
[b]From Ref. 66.

sirable toxic substances. The main source of these substances is urea, which accounts for 25 grams of daily urine. Decomposition of this amount of urea through microbial action may produce as much as 14 g of ammonia. When untreated urine is stored under ambient conditions, the microbial count increases rapidly and may reach 10^{12} cells/mL. Microscopic fungi may also develop. Thus, if urine is to be used for water reclamation, it needs to be preserved to maintain chemical and microbiological stability.

Wash water recirculated after washing the face, hands, and body, as well as other sources of reclaimed water, contains many contaminants, mainly organic compounds, including detergents [for instance, katamin AB (alkyl dimethyl benzyl ammonium chloride) mixed with amine oxide, lactic acid, urea, and lipids]. Suspended substances are also present in substantial quantities. The main inorganic contaminant is sodium chloride. High microbial contamination is characteristic of wash water; thus, detergents should have disinfectant properties in order to stabilize the microbial level at (9-32) × 10^3 cells per milliliter. Table 7 lists the physical-chemical

Table 7 Physical-chemical parameters of wash water obtained on a mockup of Mir (data obtained in collaboration with A.A. Berlin)

Parameter values, units	Minimum–maximum
pH value, pH unit	6.5–8.1
Transparency, cm	0
Color, deg.	10–20
Odor, rated	0–5
Specific electrical conductivity, x 10^{-4} S/cm	2.2–6.0
Total hardness, mg-equiv/L	0.4–1.0
COD, mg O_2/L	1000–1750
Total organic carbon, mg/L	224–914
Urea, mg/L	62–166
Chlorides, mg/L	21–110
Detergent+disinfectant, mg/L (katamin AB+amine oxide)	120–340
Suspended substances, mg/L	750–1000
Sulfates, mg/L	28–31
Nitrogen as ammonia, mg/L	7–49
Nitrogen as nitrates, mg/L	0.25–0.31
Nitrogen as nitrites, mg/L	0.07–0.09
Microbial contamination, x 10^3 cells/mL	10–32

parameters of used wash water obtained in a mockup of Mir.

The least contaminated sources of reclaimed water are fuel cell by-products and water formed from the decomposition of hydrogen peroxide. The by-products of fuel cells (electrochemical generators) typically contain gaseous and dissolved hydrogen. At normal barometric pressure, hydrogen is biologically inactive; nevertheless, U.S. astronauts who drank water containing gaseous hydrogen complained of flatulence and bloating. The exact physical-chemical properties of by-products from fuel cells may vary as a function of fuel cell type. Table 8 presents data on the composition of by-products of electrochemical generators with different types of fuel cells.

II. Fill-and-Draw Water Supply Systems

The most reliable space flight water supply systems are those in which potable water is brought from the Earth (so-called "fill-and-draw" systems). Compliance with hygienic standards is assured by methods of preservation and/or by stabilization of the chemical and microbiological parameters of the water. Obviously, water that is to be preserved should start off by having acceptable aesthetic properties, as well as acceptable levels of chemical and biological toxins; and preservatives that are added should not negatively affect quality. The preservative should produce a sustained and reliable antimicrobial effect, stabilize taste and physical-chemical properties, be nontoxic to humans, not react with structural materials, and be compatible with the water supply system.[65]

Physical methods of water disinfection [e.g., heating (boiling or autoclaving), ultraviolet irradiation, ultrasonic and microwave treatments] are of limited utility for treating water stores because they do not produce a residual effect and thus cannot stabilize basic parameters of water quality or ensure bacteriological safety in the case of secondary contamination.[66] Nevertheless, in the Russian Federation, autoclaving is used to treat water in survival kits for use by cosmonauts who are forced to perform unscheduled landings in off-target area.[2] To exclude the possibility of contamination, this emergency water supply is never touched during flight, making autoclaving an acceptable method of water preservation.

Only chemical methods of decontamination have a residual effect, making them suitable to preserve water for use in space. Researchers have investigated such well-documented disin-

Table 8 Composition of fuel cell by-products

Parameter, units	Data of Chizhov and Sinyak[2]	Data of present authors	
		M ± m	(Min.–max.)
pH value, pH units	4.5–10.0	7.46 ± 0.53	(6.65–8.45)
COD, mg O_2/l	6.4–88	4.97 ± 1.73	(2.5–10)
Permanganate oxidizability, mg O_2/l	0.8–27	–	–
Total organic carbon, mg/L	–	1.06 ± 0.24	(1–2)
Nitrogen as ammonia, mg/L	0–0.52	0.08 ± 0.006	(0–0.18)
Nitrogen as nitrates, mg/L	0.12–0.25	0	
Nitrogen as nitrites, mg/L	0.007–0.025	0	
Calcium, mg/L	0	–	
Magnesium, mg/L	0–1.42	–	
Potassium, mg/L	0–117	0	
Sodium, mg/L	0–4.5	–	
Chlorides, mg/L	0–2.84	–	
Sulfates, mg/L	0	–	
Acetone, mg/L	0.5–1.0	0	
Methanol, mg/L	0.5–24	0	
Ethanol, mg/L	0.5–6.0	0	
Total hardness, mg-equiv/l	0	0.11 ± 0.07	(0–0.32)
Electrical conductivity, x 10^{-4} S/cm	–	3.47 ± 0.5	(0.4–17.9)
Microbial contamination, cells/mL	0–106	150 ± 10.6	(0–600)
Hydrogen: Gaseous, mL	–	232 ± 19.1	(5–700)
Dissolved, mL		12 ± 2.9	(6.2–15)

fectants as chlorine and its derivatives, ozone, iodine, heavy metals, and, in particular, silver and its derivatives. The investigators eventually had to reject most of the above disinfectants for a number of reasons. Chlorine must be used in doses so high (20–50 mg/L) that it affects the taste and odor of the water. Ozone does not produce a prolonged residual effect. The level of most heavy metals needed to kill bacteria is above the maximum permissible concentration with respect to toxicity.

Silver is a promising disinfectant. Bacterial loading studies of the bactericidal effects of various silver preparations have revealed high effectiveness. For example, 84–96 percent of E. *coli* cells died within 1 h, and 100 percent died within 6 h, after being added to water containing silver.

During the design and development of water supply systems, it was found that ionic silver tended to react with the materials used for the storage containers. In some cases, aluminum alloys were corroded, whereas, in others, silver was absorbed by the walls of the container.

Studies of samples of preserved water after prolonged storage, as well as after long-duration space flights, showed that silver levels diminished during storage and, at the termination of the storage period, had diminished from an initial level of 0.2 mg/L to 0.06–0.09 mg/L.[65]

The rate of silver absorption varies as a function of the ratio of the container surface area to volume; therefore, current Russian spacecraft water storage systems use spherical containers with volumes of up to 210 liters (the Rodnik system).[20]

The use of materials with minimum capacity to absorb ionic silver (Teflon® and similar materials, passivated stainless steel, and titanium) and water containers having optimal volume capacities, allows storage time to be extended to 2 years without the addition of more preservative.

American specialists followed another approach to water storage for space missions. On Apollo missions, sodium hypochlorite and monosodium phosphate were used to preserve stored water. The water system was regularly injected with ampoules containing sodium hypochlorite (5000 mg/L) and an aqueous solution (0.7 M) of sodium dehydrogen phosphate.[67] On the lunar module, water disinfection was achieved through the use of iodine (at a concentration of 10 mg/L).[2] Iodine is also used to preserve water on Space Shuttle flights. A packed bed of irradiated anion exchange resin provides iodine in quantities no less than 2.0 mg/L and no more than 4.0 mg/L at a flow rate of 12–60 lb/h flowing to the storage tanks. Such beds are also used at outlets to prevent back contamination.

III. Water Reclamation

A. Characteristics of Water Reclamation Systems

The weight of fill-and-draw water supply systems increases dramatically with mission duration, making them unfeasible for extended missions. Thus, water supply systems using water recycling or water reclamation had to be designed. Designers of such systems had to contend with the fact that, because of the lack of the liquid-gas interface in microgravity, extraction, rectification, and flotation processes cannot be used in space.

In light of the diversity and complexity of the chemical composition of human wastes, it is not possible to develop a water reclamation system that uses only a single method. Rather, the system should include a number of processes, as dictated by the chemical composition of the sources of reclaimed water and the type and amount of power available on the spacecraft.

It is very likely that it will not be possible to develop a single type of system that can be used in all situations. For example, a water supply system for a lunar spacecraft with fuel cells as components of the life support system would not be efficient on an extended mission space station; on such stations water should instead be reclaimed from human wastes and other moisture-containing by-products. On short-term flights, it would be difficult to use the radiation method, for example, since it requires that crewmembers be protected from ionizing radiation. At the same time, on extended flights on which power will be generated by nuclear reactors, the radiation method might be particularly cost effective.

When designing water reclamation technologies, it is important to consider how their behavior in microgravity differs from that on Earth. In the Earth's gravitational field, because of the difference in liquid and gas densities, the gas-liquid interface is stable; consequently, boiling, condensation, gas-liquid separation, and other processes occur normally. In microgravity, these mechanisms are disrupted. For example, in boiling, vapor bubbles do not separate and float to the surface but instead accumulate at the container wall, impeding heat transfer. In condensation, heat transfer is also impaired if special measures are not taken to remove the accumulating film of condensate. Thus, membranes, cyclonic separators, or centrifuges have to be used in microgravity to create artificial interfaces.

B. Design Principles for Water Reclamation Systems

The selection of water reclamation methods depends largely on the chemical and microbiological composition of waste products that serve as sources of reclaimed water. According to Kulskiy,[68] all contaminants in spacecraft wastes can be classified into six groups on the basis of particle size. Optimal methods can be identified for eliminating the contaminants in each group as a function of the type and amount of power available (thermal, electric, ionizing radiation, or solar radiation).

As a rule, a water reclamation system should include the following stages: 1) stabilization of physical-chemical and microbiological composition of waste products–decontamination and preservation; 2) removal of all impurities from the liquid media–filtration; 3) mineralization of resulting water using macro- and trace elements; 4) water preservation; and 5) water heating and/or cooling.

Stage 2 may include the process of transformation–oxidation of all organic components in the wastes and their subsequent demineralization.

These stages may be modified as a function of the use to which the reclaimed water is going be put. For example, stage 3 is unnecessary for wash water; stages 3 and 4 (mineralization and preservation) are unnecessary when reclaimed water is to be used for electrolytic generation of oxygen.

C. Pretreatment (Stabilization) of Wastes

Waste products used as sources for reclaimed water create a medium conducive to microbial proliferation. Microbial growth and development induce decomposition of organic and inorganic compounds, forming compounds of new classes, including ammonia, acetic and butyric acids, hydrogen sulfide, and others. In addition to their toxic effects on humans, these substances may degrade the hardware of the reclamation system. For example, urea transformation causes pH to shift toward alkaline values, causing sediments (e.g., calcium phosphate and magnesium hydroxides) to form and be deposited on membranes, tubes, valves, gas-liquid separators, sorption beds, and other elements of the reclamation system. Another consideration is the abundant offgassing of volatile compounds, which requires additional units for trapping and removal. Gaseous compounds, such as methane and nitrogen, can shield the surface of absorbers and intensify channel formation in the beds, thus reducing the dynamic capacity of ion-exchange resins and activated charcoals. Additionally, sediments and gaseous compounds may increase hydraulic resistance in the lines of the system and interfere with the functioning of the water pumps. For this reason, one of the stages of stabilization of moisture-containing human wastes is their decontamination and subsequent preservation.

It should be noted that moisture-containing wastes (even if they have been decontaminated) contain substances with unpleasant odors. It is thus desirable to bind volatile compounds to form thermally stable compounds or to expose them to partial transformation (oxidation) during the decontamination stage.

In summary, the stabilization unit should decontaminate and preserve wastes, as well as bind ammonia and other volatile compounds to form stable compounds. Methods of waste decontamination and preservation are described in detail in Chapter 13 of this volume.

D. Filtration (Removal of Suspended and Colloidal Impurities)

Virtually all moisture-containing wastes generated on manned space flights that are used as sources for water reclamation contain colloidal and suspended particles, as well as microbes. Removal of dispersed particles from these wastes typically precedes other stages of processing. Almost all processes used for this purpose on the ground can be used in space, with the exception of sedimentation and flotation, which will not work in microgravity. The most suitable process for waste clarification is filtration. Wastes are passed through porous partitions under the action of pressure gradients or centrifugal forces. Nonregenerable filters have been found to be more effective in extracting water from waste products.

Filter cartridges using filtration and precipitation have been employed successfully to clarify weakly contaminated wastes. The problem is that the process flow rate decreases rapidly for wastes that are strongly contaminated with suspended particles, demanding frequent replacement of filters.

Filters operating according to the bulk filtration principle are more suitable for strongly contaminated wastes. Such filters clarify by precipitating suspended particles in filter pores as a result of cohesion and adsorption. Normally, they consist of multiple layers made of different materials so that pores diminish in size from layer to layer; e.g., felt and nonwoven fabric, belting fabric, filter cardboard, and synthetic membranes. To clarify used bath and laundry water containing significant quantities of fats, the multilayer filters also include hydrophobic materials, such as wool.[69]

Waste clarification by filtration can be accelerated through contaminant coagulation. This method of clarification involves the agglomeration of colloidal and dispersed particles and neutralization of their Z-potential through adsorption of multicharged ions on their surface and coagulant hydrolysis. Coagulants containing multicharged cations (e.g., aluminum sulfate or iron compounds) are used to remove negatively charged colloidal particles. Activated silica is used for positively charged colloids. The process can be accelerated and the amount of coagulant needed can be reduced by using high-molecular-weight flocculants; e.g., polyacrylamide or quaternary ammonium bases of the B-2 or BA-3 type. The degree of coagulant hydrolysis depends on the pH value of the water being clarified and its buffer properties, which, in turn, are a function of its alkaline reserve. For example, the optimal pH range of hydrolysis is 4.95–5.4 for aluminum sulfate, 6.4–7.0 for sodium aluminate, and 9.0–10.5 for iron salts.

Organic flocculants can be used to clarify water with a low alkaline reserve and at a low temperature.

Filtering centrifuges equipped with an automatic precipitate discharge unit appear more promising for use in separating coagulated suspensions. However, methods to desiccate the sediments–either to extract more water or to preserve them for further storage–must be developed as well.

The efficacy of filtration can be increased, and the weight of water reclamation systems can be reduced, if electrocoagulation is used.[68,70] The advantages of this method are accelerated coagulation of dispersed contaminants through use of an electric field, independence of the process from the alkaline reserve of the wastes, and the low level of electrolyte contamination of the resulting water. When electrocoagulation is used to clarify water, the best results are obtained with aluminum electrodes having an electrical field intensity of 50–100 W/cm and a processing time of 6 min. This treatment provides a high level of clarification from suspended particles and detergent. Permanganate oxidizability of the filtrate does not exceed 50–90 mg O_2/L when either fat-based soaps or quaternary ammonia-based detergents are used. The use of electrocoagulation as part of a water supply system prevents the formation of gaseous by-products of electrolysis (primarily hydrogen), which constitute 3 percent of processed wastes by volume. This requires that cathode depolarization electrocoagulants be developed.

At the present time, the use of modern ultrafiltration hardware is being considered for clarification of moisture-containing wastes in future life-support systems.[71,72,147] The operational life of ultrafilters can be increased through the use of tangential-convective filtration and the method of wet oxidation to process concentrates. An advantage of this method is that it ensures that the water will be free of endotoxins. To achieve this goal, ultrafilters can also be used to follow sorption.

E. Removal of Soluble Contaminants from Moisture-Containing Wastes

1. Sorption

Sorption is widely used for decontaminating weakly contaminated waste products, such as humidity condensates. This method is cost effective; ensures 100 percent water extraction from wastes; and utilizes minimum power, which is required only to transport the wastes. The sorption method entails waste filtration through a series of beds of granular ion-exchange resins and molecular sorbents, which remove both electrolytes and molecular impurities. The most effective ion-exchange resins are synthetic cation- and anion-exchange resins, polymers that are not soluble in water, or organic solvents containing chemically active groups that participate in chemical exchange reactions with the ions of dissolved contaminants. To remove dissolved salts from water and ensure the necessary degree of purification, cation-exchange resins are used in acidic form and anion-exchange resins are used in basic form.

Typically, mixed beds of ion-exchange resins are used. However, in some cases, there are separate layers of cation- and anion-exchange resins. First, acids form through exchange on the cation-exchange resins. The specific acids generated depend on the anions that had been in the solution. Along with the solution, these enter the anion-exchange resin bed, where they are neutralized through anion exchange.

Ion-exchange processes occurring on mixed sorbent beds are not self-sustaining because of the depletion of ion-exchange resins, which must be either replaced or regenerated. In water supply systems, depleted sorption filters are usually replaced, since regeneration of the ion-exchange resin would complicate the system and diminish the amount of water extracted from waste products. In water supply systems, the sorption method is used to recover water from humidity condensates and used wash water. Cation-exchange resins of the polymerized type with highly acidic or alkaline functional groupings are used most frequently in water reclamation systems. Such ion-exchange resins have a high exchange capacity and satisfactory kinetic characteristics for sorption of ions with molecular weights to 300–350. They also meet radiation and mechanical stability requirements. Ionite consumption is mainly a function of the extent to which the waste is contaminated with ionic impurities. In humidity condensate, the level of such impurities is 3–4 kg/m^3, whereas they increase to 4–5 kg/m^3 when wash water is used.[71] For purposes of designing water reclamation systems, the performance characteristics of ion-exchange filters can be derived by computing ion exchange dynamics for various sorption isotherms and kinetic conditions.[73]

To decontaminate wastes containing molecular impurities, sorption systems use molecular sorbents and, especially, activated charcoals. Processes of waste decontamination using adsorption are very similar to ion-exchange processes. For this reason, the two process types are often combined in a single subassembly, in which electrolytes are first removed from wastes through ion exchange, and then are passed through adsorption filters for removal of organic molecular impurities. This sequence of operations is highly efficient and minimizes the consumption of materials.

Because of the type of contaminants in air moisture condensates, only small-pore activated charcoals are used to decontaminate them. Certain synthetic activated charcoals (PAU-SV, FAS) and granular charcoals (PC) are very efficient because they have high equilibrium constants for the low-molecular-weight, aliphatic, organic contaminants present in condensates.

To decontaminate wash water, activated charcoals with well-developed mesoporosity and microporosity (e.g., SKT-7C) are preferable. In ion-exchange resins, the dynamic capacity of sorbents is a function of contaminant levels in the wastes and is determined by the profile of their adsorption isotherms. The adsorption isotherms for most contaminants in weakly contaminated wastes are linear; i.e., the amount of contaminants adsorbed increases in proportion to concentration. For strongly contaminated wastes, adsorption can be described by Lengmuir's, Freindlich's, and other more complex isotherms.

There are no rigorous mathematical models of the dynamics of adsorption for moisture-containing wastes, although an attempt has been made to describe the dynamics of adsorption of binary mixtures.[74] In most cases, the sorption properties of multicomponent mixtures, such as actual waste products, can be approximated by a single hypothetical compound; and a mathematical model of sorption dynamics can be used to describe the process. An example of such an approach can be found in Zolotareva et al.,[75] in which mathematical modeling was employed to determine the optimal proportion of ion-exchange resins and adsorbents in a filter for air moisture condensate, with the operational lifetime of the water supply system used as the criterion for optimum performance.

The efficiency of sorbent systems for decontaminating wastes is not high because of the presence in the wastes of such organic compounds as low-molecular-weight alcohols, aldehydes, and urea. Decontamination of air moisture condensate requires amounts of sorbent equal to 3.0–4.0 percent of the volume of the processed decontaminated water. Wash water provides a slightly better ratio of 1.0 percent.

Greater efficiency can be attained with chemisorbents, such as activated charcoals impregnated with catalysts of dehydration of organic compounds. For example, nickel, platinum, and other metals of the platinum group act as efficient chemisorbents of most organic compounds. Chemisorption of alcohols, aldehydes, and organic acids are accompanied by dehydration.[76] Chemisorbents can sustain catalytic and electrocatalytic processes of oxidation of organic compounds with the involvement of absorbed oxygen.[77] The addition of catalysts of this kind to the sorption filters of waste decontamination systems may increase their capacity by several hundred percent, improve the quality of decontaminated water, and decrease the adjusted weight of the water supply system. The sorption method was used extensively in the first generation of water reclamation systems;[79–82,69] however, the adjusted weight of reclamation systems can be minimized only by using stationary decontamination processes.

2. Electrochemical Methods

One such stationary process is electrodialysis with ion-exchange membranes to remove electrolytes from wastes. This process involves treating wastes with direct or pulsating electrical current in a chamber bounded by selectively permeable cation-exchange and anion-exchange membranes. The current causes the impurities of the contaminant ions to migrate through the ion-exchange membranes toward the cathode and anode of the electrodialysis unit, removing them from the waste solution.

Electrodialysis is energy efficient and can readily be implemented in microgravity. The use of electrodialysis to decontaminate air moisture condensate was discussed by Armstrong[83] while Hansen and Berger[84] discussed its use for wash water decontamination and urine demineralization. These authors did not evaluate this method very highly because problems with use in a regenerative life support system and because it was used in combination with a relatively ineffective adsorption process for organic contaminants. Further studies demonstrated that electrodialysis units with ion-exchange fillers in desalinization chambers are well suited for use in decontaminating air moisture condensate. Glueckauf[85] showed that such systems can function like ion-exchange filters with continuous electrochemical regeneration. A maximum concentration technique proposed for decontamination of radioactive wastes[86] provided 98–99 percent water reclamation. In this case, power consumption was no more than several voltampere-hours per liter (VA-h/L).

Electrodialysis was investigated as a method of urine demineralization during the development of an electrochemical water reclamation system.[85,87,143] In this system, electrodialysis was employed to demineralize urine pretreated by electrodialysis for oxidation of organic contaminants. The method allowed extraction of approximately 90 percent of water from waste products, with power consumption of 25–35 VA-h/L. A prototype of the electrochemical water reclamation system was developed and successfully used in 30-day tests; however, a toxicological analysis of the reclaimed water detected the presence of oxidizing agents.

The combined use of electrochemical oxidation for organic contaminants and electrodialysis for deionization seems very promising for the design of a stationary system of water reclamation from condensates. A prototype was discussed in Putnam,[88] in which an attempt was made to implement both processes in one electrodialysis unit. However, it is more efficient to use a separate unit functioning as a short-circuited electrochemical cell to remove organic compounds.[89, 145]

In the design of electrochemical water reclamation systems, special attention must be given to the structuring of electrode processes specifically for use in microgravity and closed environments.[144] Gaseous by-products of electrode reactions in electrodialyzers are reclaimed through the use of the principle of a hydrogen electrodialyzer,[90] and solid ion-exchange electrolytes are reclaimed in combination with porous, catalytically active electrodes.[91]

3. Reverse Osmosis

Reverse osmosis, a universal method for removing organic and mineral contaminants from water, is one of the most promising methods for decontaminating wash water. Water is subjected to pressure exceeding osmotic pressure, which forces it through semipermeable membranes that are selectively permeable for water. Asymmetric membranes with 10-nm pores in the active layer are currently used most extensively. The permeability of asymmetric semipermeable membranes is optimal. Because of the simplicity of the hardware required, low power consumption, high selectivity with respect to most wash water contaminants, and a 95–97 percent water reclamation rate, this process is the most suitable one for decon-

taminating moisture-containing wastes when large quantities of water must be processed daily. The use of reverse osmosis has been investigated for wash water decontamination .[92–94] The best results have been obtained with polysulfonic and polyamide membranes. It has been noted that use of the nonionogenic surfactant, Triton X-100, makes it possible to maintain the selectivity of semipermeable membranes for a sustained period. It is recommended that reverse osmosis take place at high temperatures (50–75 °C) to diminish power consumption. Selectivity of 98–99 percent has been attained for inorganic compounds and 80 percent for organic compounds. This difference is mainly attributable to low selectivity for urea. The apparatus used has an effective membrane surface area of 0.3–0.38 m^2. The rate of water reclamation is 90–97.5 percent. Power consumption at a temperature of 53 °C is 10 VA-h/kg. Slightly poorer results are obtained when dynamic semipermeable membranes are used.

To ensure that the water processed through reverse osmosis is of adequate quality, the permeate should be exposed to additional sorption decontamination. To extend the performance of semipermeable membranes, reverse osmosis is usually combined with clarification processes; e.g., ultrafiltration.[95] The chief problem confronting designers of water systems using reverse osmosis is increasing the useful life of semipermeable membranes. If such systems are to become components of spacecraft life support systems, this parameter will have to be improved.

4. Distillation

Distillation is a universal method for purifying moisture-containing wastes. This method is suitable for reclaiming water from all sources except condensates, in which the major contaminants are volatile compounds. It is most efficient for water reclamation from urine. Since urine contains unstable organic compounds that disintegrate upon boiling (at normal barometric pressure) and strongly contaminate the condensate, distillation must take place at a temperature no greater than 65 °C. There are more than a dozen distillation technologies for recovering water from urine.[2,69,96,97,139] At present, the development of membrane distillation,[98,99] distillation with a thermal pump,[100,101] and distillation with catalytic oxidation in the vapor phase[13,26,102,103] are undergoing intensive study.

Methods of membrane evaporation with a diffusion gap and evaporation through hydrophobic porous membranes[99] are also under study. The major disadvantage of membrane methods is the high power expenditure (because of a relatively low coefficient of heat utilization) and the limited useful life of membranes (because of accumulation of deposits of organic and inorganic suspended particles on their surfaces). The useful life of semipermeable and porous membranes can be extended significantly by combining hydrophilic and hydrophobic membranes at the interface,[104] while their cost effectiveness can be increased by using a thermal pump of the refrigerant or thermoelectric type. This may help decrease power consumption to 300 VA-h/kg and extend the life of a distiller to tens of thousands of hours. The method of membrane distillation is the simplest and most reliable but requires greater quantities of expendables. Analyses of different variants of a spacecraft water supply system designed to function automatically for 500 days[105] showed that the method of membrane evaporation with vapor compression is the most suitable for reclaiming water from urine and other wastes. The most power-efficient methods of urine distillation are those utilizing heat produced by water vapor condensation.

Information about a new generation of water supply systems for a space station prototype can be found in Brose and Jackson.[106] In these systems, water is reclaimed from urine and concentrate in a reverse osmosis device through vapor compression. The reclamation device was manufactured and tested by the Hemtrick Co. It is a very sophisticated device with automated process control. Wastes are distilled in a rotating still at ambient temperature. Evaporation at subatmospheric pressure and vapor compression are provided by a vapor compressor located in the same device. Prolonged testing demonstrated that power consumption was 150 VA-h/kg with 90 percent of the water reclaimed.

In terms of performance, the use of a thermoelectric pump for reclaiming water from urine is similar to the vapor-compression method. The pump operates on the basis of the Peltier effect, the principle that a temperature rise or fall at the junction of two dissimilar metals carrying a small current will be proportional to the magnitude of the current. The heat of condensation is reclaimed by having this junction occur at the heat-transfer surface, separating the evaporator and condenser. Distillation providing phase separation in microgravity is performed in a rotating still. Extended tests of the system prototype showed that 90 percent of the water could be reclaimed at a power consumption of 250–300 VA-h/kg.

These distillation methods for recovering water from urine do not produce a condensate of adequate quality, since it typically still contains volatile organic and inorganic compounds. Sinyak and Chizhov have developed an oxidative-catalytic distillation method for contaminant oxidation in the vapor phase.[102,103] A water supply system using this method consumes minimum quantities of expendables. Water vapor and volatile compounds are passed through a heterogeneous catalyst layer (e.g., hopcalite), where they are oxidized at a temperature of 150 °C, to form carbon dioxide, nitrogen, sulfur dioxide, and water. In open-loop devices of this type, atmospheric oxygen is used as the oxidizer, while closed-loop devices use oxygen bound in the catalyst. In the latter case, the catalyst should be regenerated regularly.

The results of analyses of alternative processes for recovering urine from water[26] for use in an orbital space station water supply system[96] suggest that a distillation method involving catalytic oxidation of contaminants in the vapor phase is most suitable. This method has the lowest reduced weight, power consumption, and size because of the use of radioisotopic sources of thermal energy.[107,108]

5. Other Methods

In addition to the methods discussed, other procedures theoretically can be employed to recover water on spacecraft. However, for one reason or another, these procedures remain inadequately studied or are not being considered for incorporation in future reclamation systems. These include ozonization,[68] impulse processing,[70] catalytic oxidation in the presence of hydrogen peroxide,[109] radiation[110] and photochemical[2] oxidation, microbiological methods,[2,136] and others.

F. Artificial Mineralization of Reclaimed Water

Water reclaimed from moisture-containing wastes is virtually devoid of minerals and, thus, cannot be used for drinking on long-duration flights. Demineralized water does not taste very good, which decreases water consumption by crewmembers.[111] Some authors maintain that prolonged consumption of demineralized water may cause cardiovascular disorders.[112,113,142] In light of such adverse effects of microgravity as reduced water consumption and potential cardiovascular deconditioning, it becomes critically important to provide space crews with potable water containing a full complement of minerals.

The lowest acceptable level of total mineral concentration in reclaimed potable water is 100 mg/L total salts, with no less than 20 mg/L calcium, and no less than 10 mg/L magnesium.[114]

Demineralized reclaimed water can be enriched using reagent methods; i.e., solutions or tablets containing essential minerals can be added to the water,[115,116] or through dissolution of natural or artificial minerals.[117]

The reagent method of artificial mineralization of reclaimed water was tested in a year-long bioengineering study conducted in the U.S.S.R.[78] The method most suitable for artificial water mineralization in space flight depends on flight duration. For example, for flights no longer than 70 days, the addition of reagents seems to be justified;[118] whereas, for longer-duration flights, methods that do not require active participation by crewmembers are preferred. Shikina et al.[116] discussed various methods for artificial enrichment of reclaimed water that require dissolution of natural and artificial minerals. The major disadvantage of these methods is that it is very difficult to control salt concentrations in drinking water; thus, they can fluctuate to values outside the recommended range. A higher level of mineralization can be achieved if a mineral created by roasting dolomite at 700 °C is added to potable water.[119] However, this mineral, if allowed to remain in the water for a prolonged period, may increase its pH value to more than 9.0, requiring pH adjustment.

The recommended level of mineralization can be attained in reclaimed water through the use of plastic granules containing all physiologically important salts.[120] However, this method has the disadvantage of being nonstationary.

Another method of mineralization that can be employed to provide the recommended salt levels involves dissolving natural minerals in desalinated water that has been pretreated with carbon dioxide.[121] This method has been used extensively in preparing drinking water in arid zones. However, it cannot be readily incorporated in a life support system for use in microgravity. For this purpose, membrane methods of artificial mineralization based on dialysis and electrodialysis are under development.[84,85,122] The electrodialysis method appears attractive for use on spacecraft because salt concentrations may be adjusted by varying the current density. A disadvantage of the method is that it involves osmotic transfer of the solvent to the concentrate, necessitating the development of compensatory measures for use when there are pauses in the operation of the water supply system.

IV. Water Reclamation Systems

The multiple sources of water in the life support system of manned spacecraft complicate consideration of different design concepts for water supply systems. Water from different sources can be processed in separate systems and/or mixed together and processed in a single system. The former approach makes it possible to gradually increase the closure of the water reclamation process, as is currently being done on space station Mir. The overall design concept for such systems involves modular design of different units and their maximum standardization.

Each water reclamation subsystem is associated with one or more devices in which moisture-containing waste products are collected. For example, the subsystem for reclaiming water from air moisture condensate is associated with a cooling/drying component, which controls the temperature and humidity of the spacecraft cabin and collects air moisture condensate. The subsystem for water reclamation from wash water is associated with shower and wash-basin facilities, whereas the subsystem for recovering water from urine is connected with the commode.

The subsystem for recovering water from air moisture condensate[71] using the sorption method of decontamination includes the following processes. The air moisture condensate that builds up in the cooling/drying component is pumped out to the condensate separator, where it is separated from the gaseous phase. The separated condensate is collected in the interior of a bellows pump and periodically fed to the decontamination subassembly, which contains a series of beds of ion-exchange resins and activated charcoal. To prevent microbial proliferation on the sorbents, small quantities of bactericidal sorbents containing silver or iodine are sometimes added to the first and last beds.[123]

Decontaminated condensate is fed to the conductivity sensor, where its ionic strength is measured and then, depending on the measured value, is passed either to the water conditioning subassembly or to the reprocessing water container. The water is conditioned by enriching the demineralized water with calcium, magnesium, potassium, sodium, bicarbonates, and trace elements (fluorine and iodine), as well as oligodynamic quantities of silver or milligram doses of acti-

vated iodine. Reclaimed water that meets the requirements for reclaimed potable water[124] is transported to the potable water container, from which it is dispensed to the crew through a dispensing and heating subassembly, where it is pasteurized and, if necessary, cooled. The subsystem for recovering water from air moisture condensate can also be used for final decontamination of this condensate and of by-products of carbon dioxide hydration forming in the Sabatier or Bosch reactors.[26,125]

Early design configurations for water reclamation systems involved reclamation of potable water from urine.[2,69,78] Today, because of psychological considerations, it is considered preferable to use the water reclaimed from urine in the oxygen supply system. One of the modifications of the subsystem for recovering water from urine through membrane evaporation includes urine collection and separation from carrier air and preservation by the addition of chemicals, distillation at normal barometric pressure through a polymer membrane surface, final purification, and disinfection of the condensate.[71] This design is highly reliable, since it contains no very complicated devices and since the phase interface is created by a polymer membrane. Sometimes the diffusion gap is maintained by a slightly positive pressure, dispensing with the need for a bellows pump. Reliable performance of the system depends on use of the appropriate type and quantity of preservative, which can inhibit bacterial hydrolysis of urea and also bind volatile compounds, e.g., ammonia. Membrane distillers have the disadvantage that their performance declines during long use, requiring regular replacement. The performance of membrane distillers can be improved significantly by the use of hydrophobic membranes.[104] Water reclamation by membrane distillers is as high as 80–90 percent.

The reclamation of water from spent wash water has been emphasized because the relative amount of water used by a crew for personal hygiene is very high. On interplanetary flights, systems based on filtration, (e.g., clarification by ultrafiltration, reverse osmosis to remove dissolved contaminants, and sorption for final decontamination) are the most efficient.[95,126] On long-term orbital flights, where expendables can be resupplied, processes based on clarification using filter cartridges and final decontamination by sorption are more cost effective.[127]

One variant of the design configuration for recovering water from wash water includes the following stages: water from the shower is separated in a centrifugal or cyclonic separator and fed to the waste storage subassembly, then it passes through a preliminary filter into a pump and then into an ultrafiltration device for clarification. A high-pressure pump moves the clarified wastes into a reverse osmosis device. The permeate undergoes final decontamination through sorption and is disinfected by ionic silver or ultraviolet irradiation. The concentrate from the reverse osmosis device undergoes further concentration, along with urine, by distillation. According to different authors, water reclamation from hygiene water varies from 90–97.5 percent.

Water reclamation systems in which there are separate sub-

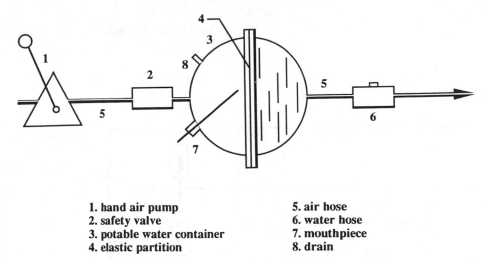

1. hand air pump
2. safety valve
3. potable water container
4. elastic partition

5. air hose
6. water hose
7. mouthpiece
8. drain

Fig. 1 Flow chart for a spacecraft water supply system using water stores.

systems for each water source seem to be preferable from the standpoint of low launch weight, but they are too complicated as a result of the presence of a large number of components, and their maintenance and servicing are time-consuming. According to Hall et al.,[96] maintenance work performed on the life support system by the crew costs about 35,000 U.S. dollars per hour, increasing the cost of life support. An alternative approach to water supply system design, involving the reclamation of water from a mixture of waste products, including solid wastes, has been considered. An integrated system of waste processing utilizing radioisotopic thermal elements (RITE), can treat a mixture of urine, feces, wash water, air moisture condensate, packaging material, food debris, and garbage.[108] Such systems are discussed in greater detail in Chapter 13 of the current volume.

V. Water Supply Systems on Manned Spacecraft

The Vostok and Voskhod spacecraft used stored water supplies.[128] Water tanks were made of polymer films and other elastic materials housed in metal containers (see Fig. 1). Potable water was preserved using silver compounds or ionic silver at a concentration of 0.1 mg/L. The outlet nozzle was filled with silver-impregnated, activated charcoal to enhance the reliability of water disinfection and deodorization. A cosmonaut could obtain water simply by sucking on the nozzle. The water supply subsystem, as well as other Voskhod life support subsystems, was designed to sustain one cosmonaut on a 12-day flight. The amount of water provided, including dietary water, was 2.2 kg/day.[128]

The Soyuz water supply system also used stored water preserved with ionic silver. The major component of the system was a tank consisting of two hemispheres separated by a polymer membrane. Water sufficient to fill the entire tank was pumped into one of the hemispheres, stretching the membrane to the container wall. When water was needed, a cosmonaut would use a hand pump to create air pressure on the membrane. Then he pushed a button valve on the nozzle to

dispense water. Air pressure in the device was controlled by a valve.

Most of the water for the Apollo water supply system was produced by fuel-cell cryogenic hydrogen and oxygen (Fig. 2). This water was used for drinking and food rehydration. Air moisture condensate was used for thermal regulation. A small store of water was brought from the Earth.

The Apollo command and lunar modules were each equipped with their own water supply systems,[67] which differed in design. In the command module, potable water was supplied by a system utilizing fuel-cell water, whereas water stores were used in the lunar module, which had no fuel cells (see Fig. 3).

Water from fuel cells located in the service module entered the command module through a water pipe. Before it reached the command module, it was cooled to 24 °C and its pressure was decreased from 4.2–1.7 atm. On Apollo 1 through 11, a hydrophobic-hydrophilic filter that separated gas from liquid was used. A special hydrogen separation device was used on Apollo 12 and subsequent flights. This device consisted of a silver-palladium tube, through which hydrogen was diffused from the water and vented overboard.

Water was dispensed into a container, where it was stored and used for food preparation. Potable water was supplemented with sodium hypochlorite, which helped to maintain its aesthetic, physical-chemical, and bacteriological parameters.

In the lunar module, potable water was stored in three containers. On the lunar surface, the astronauts used water from the main 181-liter container located in the lunar lander. During ascent from the Moon's surface and during docking with the command module, they used water stored in two 18-liter containers. The space between the walls of the container and the water membrane was filled with nitrogen at a pressure of 3.2 atm. Water was preserved with iodine. Seven days prior to launch, a solution of iodine at a concentration of 30 mg/L was added to the system. After a 1-h soak, the system was filled with deionized water containing 10 mg/L of iodine and

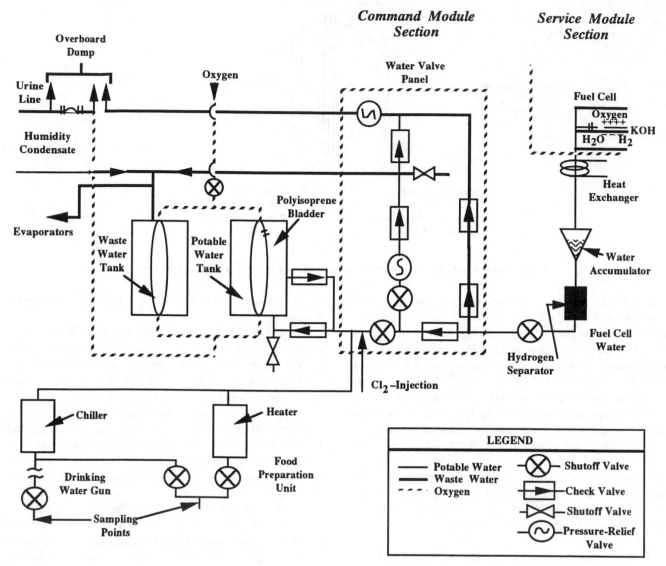

Fig. 2 Apollo Command Module water supply system.[67]

this water was actually consumed by astronauts.

The water supply system for the Space Shuttle[129] is, in many respects, similar to that of Apollo with fuel cell water as the primary water source. The maximum production rate was 11.34 kg/h when the three fuel cells were under maximum power demand. The fuel cells produce a hydrogen-enriched water, which is passed through a matrix of silver-palladium tubes to remove 95 percent of the hydrogen. The excess hydrogen is vented overboard, and the potable water is fed into storage tanks.

Water storage consists of four stainless steel tanks.[130] Each has a usable capacity of 74 kg and weighs 17.9 kg dry.[131] The potable water is routed from the potable water tank to the galley system, which is in the cabin middeck (working) area. The galley has a dispenser for drinking water and water to mix with rehydratable food. The system provides chilled water at 7–10 °C or water heated to a selected level as high as 49 °C, all at a maximum flow rate of 27 kg/h.

The water management system is serviced on the ground

before each mission. The water supplied by the ground support equipment is deionized and iodinated. New and refurbished systems are treated with concentrated iodine solutions of 25–50 mg/L of water. The solution is drained after a 3–4 h soak and refilled with water containing about 6 mg iodine per liter of water. For normal ground servicing of the water supply system, treatment is with deionized water with sampling before iodine addition. After this initial sampling, a solution containing iodine at levels of 5.0–10.0 mg/L water is injected. Dilutions by residual water results in an iodine concentration of 3–5 ppm.

In-flight iodination is achieved by passing the water through a packed bed of iodinated anion-exchange resin. The concentration of iodine is maintained at a level of 2.0–4.0 mg/L. Tests of the effectiveness of this method have found elevated microbial counts in only 46 of 853 water samples.

On Skylab flights, the water supply system utilized stores of deionized water. The system provided all the water used by the crew for drinking, food rehydration, washing, house-

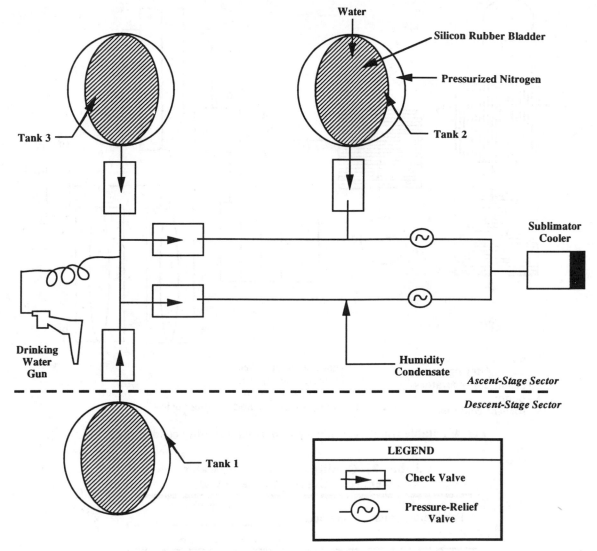

Fig. 3 Apollo Lunar Module water supply systems.[67]

keeping, and waste management.[132–135] The total amount of stored water was approximately 3000 kg. This water was stored in 10 stainless steel tanks, each with a capacity of 268 kg, which were located in the front portion of the orbital workshop module of the station along its interior perimeter.

Each container was equipped with a bellows membrane, through which water was forced from the container under pressure of gaseous nitrogen. To prevent water freezing on unmanned flights, each container was provided with an electric heater. Water was stored at a controlled temperature not above 13 °C. Cold water for drinking and cooking was maintained at 7 °C and was dispensed in 14.8-cm^3 portions by means of a valve. Hot water for cooking was heated to 65 °C and was dispensed in portions of 29.6–177.4 cm^3. Wash water was maintained at 52 °C.

Water use by the crew, consisting of three astronauts, included 10.9 kg/day for drinking and cooking and 3.2 kg/day for personal hygiene and housekeeping. During the three Skylab flights, the crews consumed 1812 kg of water.

The water supply system included water storage tanks, devices for microbial monitoring, and devices for water distribution and dispensing.

Waterlines containing cold and hot water for beverages, drinking water, and to reconstitute dehydrated food were placed under the dining table, which accommodated three crewmembers. At each seat was a nozzle that delivered drinking water. In the center of the dining table, there was a valve for water delivery for rehydrating food. Dehydrated food items were stored in plastic bags, into which cold or hot water could be injected. After water injection, the bags were shaken to prepare beverages, which the astronauts drank through the same opening used to input the water.

Water was piped to the table from the tanks through rigid pipes or flexible tubes. There was a separate line with a heater to the commode, which delivered 50 mL of water at a time, and another line to the washing facility.

Skylab also carried water supplies for the water-cooled extravehicular activity space suits. In addition, water was pro-

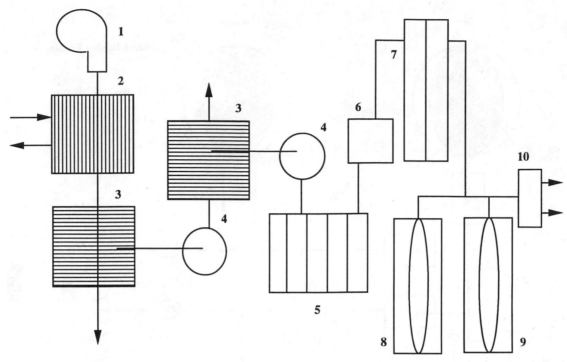

1 - fan
2 - cooling-drying unit
3 - gas-liquid separators
4 - pump
5 - sorbent columns

6 - conductometric sensor
7 - mineralization unit
8,9 - potable water tank
10 - water dispenser and heating device

Fig. 4 Potable water recycling system using humidity condensate.

**Table 9   Quality of recovered water
after five flights on Salyut-6**

Parameter, units	Standard	Flight				
		1	2	3	4	5
pH, pH units	6.5–9.6	7.5	7.0	7.8	7.5	7.1
Transparency, cm	30	30	30	30	30	30
Odor, rated	2	0	1	0	0	0
Taste, rated	2	0	1	0	0	0
Total hardness, mg-equiv/L	7	1.6	2.1	5.2	2.8	1.6
Nitrogen, as ammonia, mg/L	2.0	0.2	0.3	0.4	0.2	0.2
Bichromate oxidizability, mg O_2/L	100	30	21	22	25	30

vided for use in the event of a fire.

In addition to the main water tanks, the station also carried a special container with water to be used in various experimental studies. There was a portable container holding 12 kg of water for contingency situations.

Emphasis was placed on the level of microbial contami-

nation of water supplies, which were preserved by means of iodine. Before launch, iodine was added to every container in concentrations of 12 mg/L. Iodine concentration was measured regularly during water sampling. Since the iodine concentration diminished as the flight continued, additional amounts were administered to bring it up to the requisite levels.

The water supply for the Salyut station (beginning with Salyut-4) included both stored water supplies and water reclaimed from air moisture condensate.[20,136,137] Stored water was preserved using ionic silver at a concentration of 0.2 mg/L. The Rodnik system was used starting with the fourth expedition on Salyut-6. This system could be used repeatedly by replenishment from water tanks delivered by cargo vehicles. The Rodnik system accommodated the delivery, storage, transfer, and distribution of about 410 liters of potable water.

The configuration of the system for recovering water from air moisture condensate (SRV-K) included gas-liquid phase separation, water decontamination, enrichment with minerals, preservation with ionic silver, and heating. Reclamation was based on sorption with ion-exchange resins (cationites and anionites) and activated charcoal. The former were used to remove ionized compounds, and the latter removed organic (nonelectrolyte) compounds (Fig. 4).

The water reclamation system provided cosmonauts with cold and hot (to 80 °C) water, which they used to prepare hot drinks; e.g., tea, coffee, or fruit juices. Reclaimed water was used, also, to rehydrate freeze-dried foodstuffs. Some of the hot water was used for personal hygiene.

At the end of each flight, reclaimed water samples were delivered to a laboratory on the ground for analysis. Table 9 presents data obtained from the measurement of water reclaimed by the SRV-K system.

Salyut-6 crewmembers rated the taste and odor of stored water supplies, as well as water reclaimed by the SRV-K system, as good. It should be emphasized that cosmonauts seemed to prefer hot water from the reclamation system to the stored cold water. Beginning with the second expedition, average consumption of hot water in the form of tea, coffee, and juices was 1.50, 1.22, 1.14, and 1.04 L/man/day compared to cold water consumption, which was 0.63, 0.57, 0.66, and 0.61 L/man/day, for crews 2–5, respectively.

The operation of the SRV-K water reclamation system confirmed the efficiency of using water reclamation systems on spacecraft. Use of these systems make possible large decreases in the launch weight of life support systems and the amount of cargo that must be delivered to orbital stations from Earth.

The water supply system for Mir flights provides both stored water supplies and reclaimed water. Water stored in the Rodnik system is dispensed by a special pump and a water container. Water is reclaimed from air moisture condensate, urine, and spent wash water. Water is reclaimed from air moisture condensate by a sorption system resembling the one used on the Salyut stations. Water is extracted from urine by membrane, low-temperature evaporation, and subsequent condensation and sorption. The resultant condensate (distilled water) is used to generate oxygen in an electrolysis system. If necessary, water reclaimed from urine, after mineralization and preservation, can be consumed by cosmonauts. However, for psychological reasons, cosmonauts obtain the water they need from the Rodnik system.

In the future, when a carbon dioxide hydration system becomes operational, the water it generates will undergo sorption so it can be used by the crew. Sorption processes, in which a mixture of katamin AB and amine oxide has been used as a detergent and disinfectant, are used to recover water from wash water.

During Mir flights, water reclamation from water containing human wastes (wash water, urine, and perspiration) was accomplished for the first time in space.

As soon as a biological component is incorporated into the life support system, the water supply system will reclaim water from condensates produced by algal reactors and greenhouses, since all wastes will probably be transformed by bioengineering systems.[138]

Water supply systems for Space Station will probably also include reclamation of water from all moisture-containing wastes.[140,141] Potable water will be reclaimed from air moisture condensate. Plans call for urine and used wash water to be reclaimed to obtain wash water. Feces is not a suitable source of water because its moisture content is low and difficult to extract. The final selection of a process to be used for the reclamation system has not yet occurred.

The design of water supply systems for flights to Mars will depend on the design of life support systems and propulsion systems selected for the spacecraft. In any event, any system selected will have to meet the requirements of maximum reliability and high closure of water reclamation for extended missions.

References

[1]Babskiy, Ye.B.; Zubkov, A.A.; Kositskiy, G.I.; and Khodorov, V.I. *Human Physiology.* Moscow, Meditsina, 1966, pp. 236–240 (in Russian).

[2]Chizhov, S.V., and Sinyak, Yu.Ye. *Water Supply of Space Crews. Problems of Space Biology, Volume 24,* Moscow, Nauka, 1973, p. 268 (in Russian).

[3]Genitsinskiy, A.G. *Physiological Mechanisms of Fluid-Electrolyte Balance.* Moscow, U.S.S.R. Academy of Sciences, 1963 (in Russian).

[4]Balakhovskiy, N.S. Metabolic processes in real space flights and prolonged hypokinesia studies. Abstract of dissertation for degree of Doctor of Medical Sciences, Moscow, 1974, p. 6 (in Russian).

[5]Grigoryev, A.I.; Kozyrevskaya, G.I.; Natochin, Yu.V.; Tigranyan, R.A.; Balakhovskiy, I.S.; Belyakova, N.I.; Kalita, N.F.; Dlusskaya, I.G.; and Koselev, R.K. Metabolic and endocrine processes. In: *Space Flights on Soyuz Spacecraft: Biomedical Investigations,* Moscow, Nauka, 1976, pp. 266–303 (in Russian).

[6]Grigoryev, A.I.; Ushakov, A.S.; Popova, I.A.; et al. *Fluid-electrolyte Metabolism and Renal Function.* Moscow, Nauka, 1986, pp. 145–159, 328–333 (in Russian).

[7]Calloway, D.H., and Pace, N. Life support requirements of astronautics. Part 1, Basic Data. *Environmental Biology and Medicine,* 1971, vol. 1, pp. 165–202.

[8]Calloway, D.H. Basic data for planning life support systems. In: Calvin, M., and Gazenko, O. G., Eds. *Foundations of Space Biology and Medicine*, Washington, D.C., NASA Hq., 1975, vol. III, pp 3–21.

[9]Kerpel-Fronius, E. *Pathology and Clinical Medicine.* Moscow, Budapest-Inostrannaya Literatura, 1964, pp. 24–86 (translated into Russian).

[10]Voronin, G.I., and Polivoda, A.I. *Life Support of Space Crews.* Moscow, Mashinostroyeniye, 1967, p. 212 (in Russian).

[11]Sisakyan, N.M.; Gazenko, O.G.; and Genin, A.M. Problems of space biology. In: Sisakyan, N.M., and Yazdovskiy, V.I., Eds. *Problems of Space Biology, Vol. 1,* Moscow, U.S.S.R. Academy of Sciences, 1962, pp. 17–26 (in Russian).

[12]Chizhov, S.V. Nutrition and water supply. In: Yazdovskiy, V. I., Ed. *Space Biology and Medicine. Biomedical Problems of Space Flight*s, Moscow, Nauka, 1966, p. 317 (in Russian).

[13]Bambenek, R.A., and Zeff, I.D. Life support system design maintainability. *Space Aeronautics*, 1962, vol. 37, no. 1, pp. 54–59.

[14]Bambenek, R.A., and Zeff, I.D. Developmental status of advanced life support systems. Preprint 2107-61, American Rocket Society, 1961.

[15]U.S.S.R. State Standards. *Potable Water*, GOST 2874–83, Moscow, Izdatelstvo Standartov, 1983 (in Russian).

[16]U.S.S.R. State Standards. *Sources of centralized water supply for drinking and housekeeping. Procedures for water sampling and quality evaluation*, GOST 2761-57, Moscow, Izdatelstvo Standartov, 1954 (in Russian).

[17]Dmitriyev, M.T.; Malyshev, A.G.; and Rastyannikov, Ye.G. Specific organic compounds in waste products. *Kosmicheskaya Biologiya i Aviakosmicheskaya Meditsina*, 1987, no. 4, pp. 50–56 (in Russian).

[18]Chizhov, S.V.; Omelyanets, N.I.; Vladavets, V.V.; Kalina, G.P.; Sinyak, Yu.V.; Korchak, G.I.; Vinogradova, L.S.; Shikina, M.I.; Shmargun, L.M.; and Kolesina, N.B. Microorganisms in water recovered from air moisture condensate in an enclosed environment. *Kosmicheskaya Biologiya i Aviakosmicheskaya Meditsina*, 1979, no. 2, pp. 52–57 (in Russian).

[19]Shikina, M.I.; Vinogradova, L.A.; and Kolesina, N.V. Microorganisms in potable water recovered from air moisture condensate in an enclosed environment. *Kosmicheskaya Biologiya i Aviakosmicheskaya Meditsina*, 1988, no. 2, pp. 53–56 (in Russian).

[20]Pak, Z.P.; Sinyak, Yu.Ye.; and Chizhov, S.V. Water supply. In: Gurovskiy, N.N., Ed. *Medical Results of Salyut-6-Soyuz Flights*, Moscow, Nauka, 1986, pp. 50–52 (in Russian).

[21]Putnam, D.F. Wash water reclamation technology for advanced spacecraft. American Society of Mechanical Engineers (ASME) Paper 77 ENAs-50, 1977, p. 9.

[22]Putnam, D.F., and Wells, G.W. Water recovery for spacecraft application. In: *Proceedings of XXIVth International Aeronautical Federation (IAF) Congress*, Baku, U.S.S.R., 1973, pp. 45–55.

[23]Slonim, A.R.; Rotz, A.I.; Herald, A.B.; and London, S.A. Potable water standards for aerospace systems. *Aerospace Medicine*, 1967, vol. 37, no. 9, pp. 789–799.

[24]Pak, Z.P.; Lobacheva, G.V.; Spiryayeva M.M.; Bekhumova, Yu.Ye.; Korotkova, T.P.; Petina, V.P.; and Yevdokimova, Ye.S. Toxicological-hygienic aspects of improving final purification of water recovered from urine. *Kosmicheskaya Biologiya i Aviakosmicheskaya Meditsina*, 1981, no. 6, p. 51–57 (in Russian).

[25]Skuratov, V.M.; Gaydadymov, V.V.; and Chizhov, S.V. Evaluation of recovered water quality for total organic carbon. *Kosmicheskaya Biologiya i Aviakosmicheskaya Meditsina*, 1976, no. 6, pp. 66–70 (in Russian).

[26]*Space Station Program Definition and Requirements.* JSC 30000, Section 3, Revision J, Houston, NASA Johnson Space Center, 1991.

[27]Skuratov, V.M.; Gaydadymov, V.B.; and Chizhov, S.V. Hygienic principles of operational monitoring of the quality of recovered water in space flight. *Kosmicheskaya Biologiya i Aviakosmicheskaya Meditsina*, 1981, no. 6, pp. 48–51 (in Russian).

[28]Misselhorn, I.E.; Hartung, W.H.; Witz, S.W.; and Sanders, C.A. *An automated instrument for monitoring the quality of recovered water.* ASME Paper AV 73-11, 1973.

[29]Skuratov, V.M. Operational monitoring of the quality of recovered water in space flight. In: *Abstracts from 22nd Meeting Intercosmos Working Group on Space Biology and Medicine*, Varna, Bulgaria, 1989, p. 225 (in Russian).

[30]Skuratov, V.M.; Sinyak, Yu.Ye.; Pak, Z.P.; et al. Problem of increasing the hygienic reliability of regenerative systems of water supply based on monitoring the quality of recovered water. In: O.G. Gazenko, Ed. *Abstracts of Papers Delivered at the 8th National Conference on Space Biology and Aerospace Medicine*, Moscow/Kaluga, 1986, p. 238 (in Russian).

[31]Vasilyev, Yu.B.; Gaydadymov, V.B.; Gromyko, V.A.; et al. Potentiometric method for measuring organic compounds. U.S.S.R. Author's Certificate no. 573745, Class G 01, no. 27/48, 1974 (in Russian).

[32]Vasilyev, Yu.B.; Gaydadymov, V.B.; Skuratov, V.M.; Gromyko V.A.; et al. Method for measuring organic contaminants in water. U.S.S.R. Author's Certificate no. 750364, Class G 01, no. 27/48, 1980 (in Russian).

[33]Skuratov, V.N. Use of conductometry for monitoring the quality of recovered water. In: Kakurin, L.I., Ed. *Important Problems of Space Biology and Medicine*, Moscow, Institute of Biomedical Problems, 1977, Volume 1, Conference Abstracts, pp. 34–35 (in Russian).

[34]Idzikovskiy, A.I.; Latyshenko, K.P.; and Skuratov, V.M. Mathematical modeling of conductometric instruments for monitoring the quality of recovered water in a closed ecological system. In: *Abstracts of Papers Delivered at the National Conference on Modeling Systems of Automated Design,* 1989, Tambov, pp. 124–125 (in Russian).

[35]Viktorov, A.N., and Novikova, N.D. Microbial development on construction materials used in a manned enclosed

environment. *Kosmicheskaya Biologiya i Aviakosmicheskaya Meditsina*, 1985, no. 2, pp. 66–69 (in Russian).

[36]Zaloguyev, S.N.; Viktorov, A.N.; Shilov, V.M.; et al. Ecological aspects of microbial development in space cabins. In: O.G. Gazenko, Ed. *Abstracts of Papers Delivered at 8th National Conference on Space Biology and Aerospace Medicine,* Moscow/Kaluga, Institute of Biomedical Problems, 1986, pp. 233–234 (in Russian).

[37]Viktorov, A.N. Medical relevance of the formation of the ecological system "man-microorganisms" in manned enclosures. In: Gazenko, O.G., Ed. *Abstracts of Papers Delivered at 8th National Conference on Space Biology and Aerospace Medicine,* Moscow-Kaluga, Institute of Biomedical Problems, 1986, pp. 221–222 (in Russian).

[38]Konstantinova, I.V. Immunological investigations. In: Gurovskiy, N.N., Ed. *Medical Results of Salyut-6-Soyuz Flights,* Moscow, Nauka, 1986, pp. 114–123 (in Russian).

[39]Novikova, N.D.; Orlova, M.N.; and Dyachenko, M.B. On the problem of biostability of construction materials for manned enclosures. In: Gazenko, O.G., Ed. *Abstracts of Papers Delivered at 8th National Conference on Space Biology and Aerospace Medicine,* Moscow-Kaluga, Institute of Biomedical Problems, 1986, pp. 245–246 (in Russian).

[40]Startseva, N.D. Gram-negative bacteria on man's skin in normal and enclosed environments. In: Kakurin, L.I., Ed. *Important Problems of Space Biology and Medicine*, Moscow, Institute of Biomedical Problems, 1977, Volume 1, Conference Abstracts, pp. 214–215 (in Russian).

[41]Startseva, N.D. Gram-negative bacteria as potential pathogens in manned space vehicles. Abstract of dissertation, Moscow, 1975 (in Russian).

[42]Shikina, M.I.; Vinogradova, L.A.; and Kolesina, N.B. Study of metabolism in microbial cells of water-containing waste products and recovered water in an enclosure. In: *Important Problems of Space Biology and Medicine,* Moscow, Institute of Biomedical Problems, 1980, pp. 152–153 (in Russian).

[43]Shikina, M.I.; Kolesina, N.B.; and Vinogradova, L.A. On the study of microflora of recovered water in an enclosure. In: Islinskiy, A.Yu., Ed. *Papers Presented at the 15th Gagarin Lecture Series,* Moscow, U.S.S.R. Academy of Sciences, 1985, p. 78 (in Russian).

[44]Berry, C.A. Medical care of space crews. In: Calvin, M., and Gazenko, O.G., Eds. *Foundations of Space Biology and Medicine,* Washington, D.C., NASA Hq., 1975, vol. III, pp. 345–372.

[45]Kondratyeva, E.M. Composition and dynamics of the bacteriocenosis associated with algae in a man-rated biological life support system. *Kosmicheskaya Biologiya i Aviakosmicheskaya Meditsina,* 1985, no. 2, pp. 69–74 (in Russian).

[46]Zaloguyev, S.N.; Viktorov, A.N.; Gorshkov, V.P.; and Novikova, N.D. Sanitary-microbiological characterization of the environment. In: Gurovskiy, N.N., Ed. *Medical Results of Salyut-6-Soyuz Flights*, Moscow, Nauka, 1986, pp. 43–46 (in Russian).

[47]Zaloguyev, S.N.; Viktorov, A.N.; Shilov, V.M.; Gorshkov, V.P.; Zarubin, M.M.; Shinkareva, M.M.; and Norkina, T.Yu. Results of microbiological examinations performed during Salyut-6 flights. *Kosmicheskaya Biologiya i Aviakosmicheskaya Meditsina,* 1985, no. 2, pp. 64–66 (in Russian).

[48]Lebedeva, T.Ye.; Yakimova, I.V.; Nazarov, N.M.; and Chizhov S.V. The role of microflora of a manned enclosure during the formation of urine ammonia. In: *Important Problems of Space Biology,* Moscow, Institute of Biomedical Problems, 1980, pp. 15–158 (in Russian).

[49]Meyssel, M.N. Fluorescent microscopy and cytochemistry in general microbiology. *Uspekhi Mikrobiologii,* 1971, vol. 7, pp. 3–32 (in Russian).

[50]Nikitin, V.M. *Handbook of Methods for Biochemical Identification of Microbes.* Kishinev, Kartya Moldavenske, 1986, p. 296 (in Russian).

[51]Korsh, L.Ye.; Zheverzheyeva, V.F.; and Nikiforova, Ye.P. Specificity of the radioisotope method for rapid identification of *E. coli* in C-14 water. In: *Papers Presented at a Conference on Research Results,* Moscow, Sysin Research Institute, 1968, pp. 34–36 (in Russian).

[52]Alekseyeva, M.M., and Khudarov, G.D. Comparative evaluation of methods for detecting P-32 labeled tuberculosis mycobacteria on various surfaces. In: *Proceedings of the Central Research Institute on Disinfection*, Moscow, 1961, no. 14, pp. 37–86 (in Russian).

[53]Sedova, T.S., and Grechko, V.V. Use of radioactive sulfur to prepare labeled bacteria. *Zhurnal Mikrobiologii, Epidemiologii i Immunobiologii,* 1960, no. 3, pp. 31–35 (in Russian).

[54]Levin, G.V. Rapid detection of microorganisms in aerospace water systems. *Aerospace Medicine,* 1968, vol. 38, no. 1, pp. 14–16.

[55]Geating, I.A., and Rubek, F.P. *Bacterial sensor for reprocessed water. Microbiology research, design, and fabrication.* AMRL-TR-68-173, Wright-Patterson AFB, Ohio, U.S. Air Force, 1969.

[56]Wilkins, J.R., and Grana, D.C. Apparatus and process for microbial detection and enumeration. *Scientific and Technical Aerospace Reports*, 1981, vol. 19, no. 20, p. 2811.

[57]Pierson, L.D., and Brown, H.D. Inflight microbial analysis technology. SAE Technical Paper no. 871493, *Papers presented at the 17th Intersociety Conference on Environmental Systems*, Seattle, 1987, pp. 1–3.

[58]Korn, M.Ya., and Kushnarev, V.M. The effect of various tetrazolium salts on bacterial proliferation. *Mikrobiologiya*, 1965, no. 3, pp. 469–472 (in Russian).

[59]Test for measuring microorganisms in blood. U.S. Patent, Class 195-103 5M (C 12 K 1/04), no. 4026767.

[60]Microbial medium containing a fluorescent growth indicator. U.S. Patent, Class 195–100 (C 12 K 1/06, 1/10), no. 4049499.

[61]Nikitin, V.M., and Polugard, S.V. *Rapid Methods for Microbial Detection Using Enzymes.* Kishinev, Shtintza, 1979, p. 350 (in Russian).

[62]Skuratov, V.M.; Georgitsa, F.I.; Nikitin, V.M.; et al. Microbiological monitoring of recovered water. In: *Abstracts of Papers Presented at the 22nd Meetings of Intercosmos Working Group on Space Biology and Medicine*, Varna, Bulgaria, 1989, p. 225 (in Russian).

[63]Clemedson, G.M. Toxicological aspects of the sealed cabin atmosphere of space vehicles. *Astronautics*, 1959, vol. 1, no. 4, pp. 133–158.

[64]Tolkachevskaya, N.F. *Chemical Composition of Blood, Secreta, Excreta, and Fluids in the Normal Man*. Moscow, Medgiz, 1940, pp. 53–54 (in Russian).

[65]Chizhov, S.V.; Pak, Z.P.; Sitnikova, N.N.; Koloskova, Yu.S. Water supply system. In: Gazenko, O.G.; Kakurin, L.I.; and Kuznetsov, A.G., Eds. *Space Flights on Soyuz Spacecraft*, Moscow, Nauka, 1976, pp. 79–88 (in Russian).

[66]Skuratov, V.M. Content of organic carbon as an index of the quality of recovered water. *Important Problems of Space Biology*. Moscow, IMBP, 1975, pp. 204–206 (in Russian).

[67]Sauer, R.L., and Calley, D.J. Potable water supply. In: Johnston, R.S.; Dietlein, L.F.; and Berry, C.A. Biomedical Results of Apollo, NASA SP-368, Washington, D.C., NASA Hq., 1975, pp. 226–233, pp. 485–516.

[68]Kulskiy, L.A. *Theoretical Foundations and Technology of Water Treatment*. Kiev, Naukova Dumka, 1983, pp. 44–48 (in Russian).

[69]Allen, G.E.; Bonura, M.S.; Thomas, E.C.; and Putnam, D.F. *Integrated temperature control, humidity control and water recovery subsystem of a 90-day space station simulator test*. ASME Paper 1970. Av./Spt-18, 1970, p. 5.

[70]Rukobratskiy, N.I. Study of water regeneration by electric effects. Abstract of dissertation for degree of Candidate in Technological Sciences, Leningrad, 1979 (in Russian).

[71]Chizhov, S.V.; Adamovich, B.A.; Sinyak, Yu.E.; et al. Advanced methods of recovery for space life support systems. In: Napolitano, L.G., Ed. *Astronautical Research. Proceedings of the 22nd Congress of the International Astronautical Federation, Brussels, Belgium 1971*, Dordrecht-Boston, Reidel, 1973, pp. 163–169.

[72]Verostko, C. E.; Price, D. F.; Garcia, R.; et al. *Test results of a shower water recovery system*. Society of Automotive Engineers (SAE) Technical Paper No. 871512, 1987, p. 13.

[73]Senyavin, M.M.; Rubinshteyn, R.N.; Venetsianov, Ye.V.; et al. *Fundamentals of Calculation and Optimization of Ion-Exchange Processes*. Moscow, Nauka, 1972, p. 172 (in Russian).

[74]Koganovskiy, M.A.; Klimenko, N.A.; Levchenko, T.M.; Marutovskiy, R.M.; and Roda, I.G. *Purification and Use of Sewage Water for Industrial Supply*. Moscow, Khimiya, 1977, p. 288 (in Russian).

[75]Zolotareva, E.L.; Kolosova, G.M.; Gaydadymov, V.B.; Argin, M.A.; and Komarova, I.V. Selection of optimal ratios of sorbents for condensate decontamination. *Khimiya i Technologiya Vody*, 1982, vol. 4, no. 3, pp. 260–263 (in Russian).

[76]Bagotskiy, V.S., Ed. *Electrocatalysis*. Moscow, Nauka, 1980, p. 272 (in Russian).

[77]Podlovchenko, V.I., and Korchinskiy, G.A. On the interaction of methanol and ethanol with oxygen adsorbed on a platinized platinum electrode. *Vestnik Moskovskogo Universiteta*, 1970, no. 3, p. 310 (in Russian).

[78]Burnazyan, A.I.; Parin, V.V.; Nefyodov, Yu.G.; Adamovich B.A.; Maksimovich, S.B.; Goldshvend. B.L.; Samsonov, N.N; and Kirikov, G.N. Year-long bioengineering experiment in a ground-based complex of life support systems. *Kosmicheskaya Biologiya i Aviakosmicheskaya Meditsina*, 1969, vol. 3, no. 1, pp. 9–19.

[79]Jackson, J.K.; Putnam, D.F.; and Thomas, E.C. *Evaluation of closed-cycle life support system during a 60-day manned test*. SAE Technical Paper No. 68-0341, 1968.

[80]Malin, R.L. Facilities and support systems for a 90-day test of a regenerative life support system. Paper presented at *Space Simulation Processes Symposium*, New York, Washington, D.C., 1972, pp. 69–72.

[81]Pearson, A.O., and Jackson, J.K. Summary of a 90-day manned test of a regenerative life support system. *Astronautical Research, 1971*, Dordrecht-Boston, Reidel, 1973, pp. 149–162.

[82]Secord, T.C., and Bonura M.S. Life support system data: sixty-two days of testing in a manned space laboratory simulator. *Journal of Spacecraft and Rockets*, 1966, vol. 3, no. 3, pp. 1527–1533.

[83]Armstrong, R.C. Life support system for space flights of extended time periods. NASA CR-614, Washington, D.C., NASA Hq., 1964, p. 115.

[84]Hansen, C.D., and Berger, C. *Water reclamation from urine by electrodialysis*. ASME Paper 65-Av-16, 1965, p. 11.

[85]Glueckauf, E. Electrode ionization by ion-exchange bed. *British Chemical Engineering*, 1959, no. 12, p. 137.

[86]Walters, W.R.; Weiser, D.W.; and Marec, L.J. Concentration of radioactive aqueous wastes. *Industrial Engineering and Chemistry*, 1955, vol. 47, no. 1, p. 61.

[87]Putnam, D.F., and Vaughan, R.L. *Water reclamation from urine by electrolysis-electrodialysis*. ASME Paper 71-Av-11, 1971, p. 9.

[88]Putnam, D.F. *Chemical aspects of urine distillation*. ASME Paper no. Av–24, 1985, p. 13.

[89]Rosener, A.A.; Parker, D.M.; and Narris, S.C. *Space shower habitability technology*. AIAA Paper no. 71-Av-26, 1971.

[90]Justi, E., and Winzel, A. *Fuel Cells-Kalte Verbrennung*, Steiner, Wiesbaden, 1962, pp. 110–141.

[91]Podshivalov, S.A.; Ivanov, E.I.; Muratov, A.I.; Zakiyev, A.L.; and Moskalev, V.L. *Power Units on Space Vehicles*. Moscow, Energoizdat, 1981, p. 223 (in Russian).

[92]Ray, R.J.; Babcock, W.C.; Barss, R.P.; Andrews, T.A.; and La Chepella, E.D. A novel reverse-osmosis wash water recycle system for manned space station. SAE Technical Paper no. 840933, 1984, pp. 1–9.

[93]Slavin, T.J.; Peters, H.H.; and Cao, T.Q. Shower water recovery by reverse osmosis. SAE Technical Paper no.

871511, 1987, p. 10.

[94]Swamikanni, X.X.; Kulnarri, S.; Funk, E.W.; and Madson, B.B. Recovery of Space Station hygiene water by membrane technology. SAE Technical Paper, no. 881032, 1988, p. 9.

[95]Starikov, Ye.N., and Volgin, V.D. On the repeated use of wash water reclaimed by reverse osmosis in space life support systems. In: *Important Problems of Space Biology and Medicine*, Moscow, Institute of Biomedical Problems, 1980, pp. 165–168 (in Russian).

[96]Hall, J.B.; Pickett, S.J.; and Sage, K.H. Manned space station environmental control and life support system computer-aided technology assessment program. SAE Technical Paper, no. 840957, 1984.

[97]Secord, T., and Ingelfinger, A. Life support for a large space station. *Astronautics and Aeronautics*, 1970, no. 2, pp. 56–64.

[98]Blecher, W.A. Development of a prototype vapor diffusion water reclamation system. ASME Paper 71-Av-31, 1971.

[99]Ripperger, S. Transmembrane distillation. *PT/Process Technology*, 1986, vol. 41, no. 8, pp. 50–53.

[100]Hickman, C.D. Centrifugal boiler compression still. *Industrial Engineering and Chemistry*, 1957, vol. 49, no. 7, p. 84.

[101]Trusch, R.B. Thermoelectric integrated membrane evaporation system. U.S. Patent no. 4316774, B 01 D 3/10, 1982.

[102]Sinyak, Yu.Ye. Processes of deep catalytic oxidation in space life support systems. In: *Problems of Kinetics and Catalysis,* Moscow, Nauka, 1981, vol. 18, pp. 185–196 (in Russian).

[103]Sinyak, Yu.Ye., and Chizhov, S.V. Water reclamation in a space cabin. In: Sisakyan, N.M., and Yazdovskiy, V.I., Eds. *Problems of Space Biology, Volume 3*, Moscow, Nauka, 1964, pp. 104–112 (in Russian).

[104]Volgin, V.D.; Starikov E.N.; Sinyak Yu.Ye.; and Chizhov S.V. Method for water desalination. U.S.S.R. Author's Certificate. no. 1126307, B 01 D 13/00, 1984 (in Russian).

[105]Dooling, D. Closed loop life support systems. *Space Flights*, 1972, vol. 4, no. 4, pp. 134–139.

[106]Brose, H.F., and Jackson, J.K. *Experience and trends in life support systems for near-Earth applications.* AIAA Paper no. 827, 1971, 11 pp.

[107]Serebryakov, V.N. *Foundations of the design of space life support systems.* Moscow, Mashinostroyeniye, 1983, p. 160 (in Russian).

[108]Murray, R.W.; Shivers, R.W.; Ingelfinger, A.L.; and Metzger, C.A. *Integrated waste management-water system using radioisotopes for thermal energy.* ASME Paper, 71-Av-1, 1971, p. 9.

[109]Vasilenko, I.I.; Shevel, N.M.; and Sinyak, Yu.Ye. Gas-liquid oxidation of acetone by hydrogen peroxide on oxide catalysts. *Kosmicheskaya Biologiya i Aviakosmicheskaya Meditsina*, 1988, no. 1, pp. 78–81 (in Russian).

[110]Dolin, P.I.; Shubin, V.N.; and Brusentseva, S.A. *Radiation Decontamination of Water.* Moscow, Nauka, 1973,

p. 152 (in Russian).

[111]Suckling, E.W. *The examination of water and water supplies.* London, Churchill, 1944, p. 849.

[112]Ananyev, N.I. The effect of potable water trace elements on the cardiovascular system. *Gigiyena i Sanitaria*, 1961, no. 14, pp. 37–86.

[113]Winton, E., and McCabe, L. Health and mineralization of water. *Journal of the American Water Works Association*, 1970, no. 1, pp. 7–11.

[114]Novikov, Yu.V.; Plitman, S.I.; Levin, V.I.; and Petrov, Yu.A. Hygienic standards for minimum levels of magnesium in potable water. *Gigiyena i Sanitaria*, 1983, no. 9, pp. 7–11.

[115]Paley, P.N.; Novikov, Yu.P.; and Elpiner, L.I. Facilities for mineralization of desalinated water. In: Elpiner, L.I., Ed. *Water Supply of Deep Sea Fishing Vessels*, Moscow, Pishchevaya Promyshlenost, 1977, p. 171 (in Russian).

[116]Shikina, M.I., and Chizhov, S.V. Artificial mineralization of recovered water in space flight. *Kosmicheskaya Biologiya i Aviakosmicheskaya Meditsina*, 1971, no. 2, pp. 28–31 (in Russian).

[117]Shikina, M.I.; Aladinskaya, T.I.; Volkova, L.N.; and Dupik, Z.A. Artificial mineralization of desalted potable water using salts in tablet and powder form. *Kosmicheskaya Biologiya i Aviakosmicheskaya Meditsina*, 1989, no. 4, p. 74 (in Russian).

[118]Yegorov, A.I. *Preparation of Artificial Potable Water.* Moscow, Stroyizdat, 1988, p. 112 (in Russian).

[119]Zabarillo, L.B.; Zhumanov, O.; Shabolovskaya, G.K.; et al. Control of trace elements in water. *Khimiya i Technologiya Vody*, 1985, vol. 7, no. 3, pp. 65–67 (in Russian).

[120]Sokolova, O.A.; Saldadze, G.K.; Medvedev, I.N.; et al. Plastic granules for water treatment. *Khimiya i Technologiya Vody*, 1985, vol. 7, no. 3, pp. 65–67 (in Russian).

[121]Ipatov, P.F.; Smirnov, V.A.; Vilkova, P.I.; and Abramova, V.S. Processes of distillate enrichment with calcium hydrocarbonate and a technology of preparing desalinated potable water. In: Yegorov, A.I., Ed. *Water Desalination and Use for Industrial Purposes*, Moscow, VNII Vodgeo, 1982, pp. 13–15 (in Russian).

[122]Yakubov, H.G. On the hygienic evaluation of a method of electrodialytic mineralization of desalinated water. *Gigiyena i Sanitariya*, 1987, pp. 68–69 (In Russian).

[123]Shaydarova, V.V.; Salikova, M.I.; Ballod, A.A.; Nolde, T.V.; and Lugovaya, L. Water Disinfection by silver-plated sorbents. In: *Proceedings of Third Conference of Young Researchers*, Moscow, Institute of Biomedical Problems, 1969, p. 189 (in Russian).

[124]U.S. National Academy of Sciences. Water quality standards for the long-duration manned space mission. Report of the Ad Hoc Committee of the Space Science Board, Washington, D.C., 1967.

[125]Ohya, Haruhiko and Oguchi, Mitzio. Utilization of membranes for water recycle systems. SAE Technical Paper no. 851394, 1985, p. 7.

[126]Gaydadymov, V.B.; Prishchep A.G.; Zarubina K.V.; et

al. Sorption method of water regeneration for personal hygiene procedures. *Kosmicheskaya Biologiya i Aviakosmicheskaya Meditsina*, 1976, no. 1, pp. 73–75 (in Russian).

[127]Putnam, D.F. Wash water reclamation technology for advanced spacecraft. ASME Paper 77, ENAs-50, 1977, p. 9.

[128]Adamovich, B. A. Life support systems for short- and medium-term space flights. In: Calvin, M., and Gazenko, O. G., Eds. *Foundations of Space Biology and Medicine*, Washington, D.C., NASA Hq., 1975, vol. III, pp. 227–246.

[129]Sauer, R.L. The Potable Water STS-1 Medical Report. NASA Technical Memorandum 58240, Houston, NASA Johnson Space Center, Oct. 1981.

[130]Feindler, Claus. Development of a bladderless tank for Space Shuttle. In: *Proceedings of Space Shuttle Technology Conferences, Volume II, Biotechnology*, TR-114, Fla., NASA John F. Kennedy Space Center, 1971.

[131]Rockwell International. Potable Water Servicing Fill System, Model S70-0537, P/N GW70-680537. STS-83-0434, *Space Shuttle Tech Manual WPA001-2*, Downey, Calif., North American Space Operations, 1983.

[132]Belew, L.F.; Stuhlinger, E.; and George, C. *Skylab Guidebook*. Huntsville, Ala., NASA Marshall Space Flight Center, 1978.

[133]Hopson, G.D. et al. MSFC Skylab thermal and environmental control system mission evaluation. TMX-64822, NASA, 1974, p. 488.

[134]Stokes, J.W. An evaluation of Skylab habitability hardware. The Skylab Results. *Advances In the Astronautical Sciences*, 31, Pt. 1, CAAS-74-135, San Diego, Calif., American Astronautical Society, 1975, pp. 349–366.

[135]Summerlin, L.B. *Skylab Classroom in Space*. Washington, D.C., NASA Hq., 1977.

[136]Sinyak, Yu.Ye. Water supply. In: Gazenko, O.G., Ed. *Space Biology and Medicine*, Moscow, Nauka, 1987, p. 155 (in Russian).

[137]Kryuchkov, B.I.; Kutepov, A.; and Frolov, I. Salyut-6 life support system. *Aviatsiya i Kosmonavtika*, 1978, no. 12, pp. 34–35 (in Russian).

[138]Shepelev, Ye.Ya. Biological life support systems. In: Calvin, M., and Gazenko, O.G., Eds. *Foundations of Space Biology and Medicine*, Washington, D.C., NASA Hq., 1975, vol. III, pp. 274–311.

[139]Putnam, D.F. Chemical aspects of urine distillation. ASME Paper NAv-24, 1985, p. 13.

[140]Janik, D. S.; Crump, W. J.; Macler, B. A.; Wydeveen,T.; and Sauer, R. L. Problems in water recycling for Space Station Freedom and long-duration life support. SAE Technical Paper no. 891539, *Proceedings of 19th Intersociety Conference on Environmental Systems*, San Diego, Calif., 1989.

[141]Janik, D.S.; Sauer, R.L.; Pierson, D.L.; and Thorstenson, Y.R. Quality requirements for reclaimed/recycled water. NASA TM 58279, Houston, NASA Johnson Space Center, Mar. 1987.

[142]Voynar, A.O. *The Biological Role of Microorganisms in Animals and Humans*. Moscow, Vyschaya Shkola, 1960, p. 544 (in Russian).

[143]Gaydadymov, V.B.; Gromyko, V.A.; Sinyak, Yu.Ye.; et al. Study of water reclamation from urine by the electrochemical method. In: *Abstracts of Papers Presented at the 24th IAF Congress*, Baku, U.S.S.R., Oct. 1973, pp. 176–178. (In Russian.).

[144]Gaydadymov, V.B., and Sinyak, Yu.Ye. Electrochemical and electrocatalytic methods of water recovery for life support systems and environmental chemistry. In: *Abstracts of Papers Presented at National Conference on Electrochemistry and Environmental Protection*, Irkutsk, 1984, p. 8 (in Russian).

[145]Grebenyuk, V.D.; Sobolevskaya, T.T.; Zhiginas, L.H.; Novikov, V.M.; Bobe, L.S.; and Amiragov, M.S. Decontamination of aqueous solutions containing organic and mineral compounds by electrodialysis. *Khimiya i Technologiya Vody*, 1983, vol. 5, no. 6, pp. 532–536. (In Russian).

[146]Serebryakov, I.V.; Gromyko, V.A.; Levina, G.D.; Sinyak, Yu.Ye.; Gaydadymov, V.B.; Vasilyev, Yu.B.; and Chizhov, S.V. Automatic instrument for evaluating the quality and origin of organic contaminants in water. In: *Aviation and Space Lectures 1979-1980. Systems for Life Support and Safety of Manned Flights*, Moscow, U.S.S.R. Academ of Sciences, 1983, p. 214 (in Russian).

[147]Reuder, J.L.; Turner, L.D.; and Humphries, W.K. Preliminary design of the space station environmental control and life support system. SAE Technical Paper no. 881021, 1988, p. 10.

Chapter 13

Waste Disposal and Management Systems

V. V. Popov and N. M. Nazarov

I. Introduction

The generation of wastes in spacecraft cabins poses the risk of contamination of the environment by noxious and toxic gases, as well as by microbes. The wastes presenting the greatest risk—urine, feces, and food scraps—should be collected individually and contained as they are formed.

Once they are collected and contained, waste products provide an environment conducive to the development of microbes, leading to offgassing, and creating the potential for spread beyond the confines of the waste storage receptacles. Thus, waste receptacles must be designed so that they can be easily and reliably mounted, removed, transported, and depressurized for disposing of wastes overboard. In addition, effective and safe preserving agents must be used.

As crew size and mission durations increase, it may become more cost effective to transform wastes into substances that are more compact and suitable for long-term storage or that can be productively utilized in other life support subsystems, rather than simply storing and disposing of them.

II. Qualitative and Quantitative Description of Wastes

The waste products produced in spacecraft include the following:

1) Liquid and solid human wastes (e.g., urine, feces, hair, nails, and vomitus);

2) Housekeeping wastes (e.g., food scraps, used cleaning products, discarded clothing, and trash);

3) Wastes produced by life support subsystems (e.g., byproducts of the water reclamation subsystem, the nonrecyclable biomass of lower and higher plants, used nutrient media, and nonregenerable absorbents, filters, and similar materials); and

4) Wastes produced by spacecraft systems (reagents, films, and paper, as well as worn out or damaged materials or equipment).

U.S. authors have cited 1500 types of waste products from 220 sources.[1] A number of researchers have computed the total amount of waste produced per day by one crewmember or an entire crew. However, the values computed, especially with regard to wastes produced by spacecraft systems and trash, vary significantly as a function of flight mission, living conditions, and other factors and should not be taken as absolute. It should be noted that, according to U.S. data,[2] although feces is the most unpleasant waste product, it comprises only 10 percent of the total amount of solid wastes produced. Food scraps and food packaging comprise about 50 percent. Wastes produced by sanitation measures and personal hygiene (wipes, towels, swabs, hair, and wastes produced by medical and housekeeping procedures) account for about 10 percent. Discarded clothing, paper, fragments of recording tape, photographic film, etc., comprise approximately 25 percent.

Volatile substances released by urine, feces, and food scraps are the most significant potential contaminants of cabin air (and of reclaimed water, if it is used). Gas chromatography used in combination with mass spectrometry has detected approximately 300 such compounds, 40 of which have been identified.[3] These include ketones, alcohols, lactones, terpenes, furanes, dimethyl sulfones, pyrroles, and allyl isocyonate. It has been found that diet has virtually no effect on the composition of volatile human metabolites, the predominant components of which are ammonia and amines. Ketones are another group of volatile metabolites. Ketones are resistant to oxidants but are transformed into secondary alcohols in the presence of strong reducing agents. The ketone acetone readily reduces to form isopropanol, which is a more toxic compound. Other volatile metabolites include certain organic acids, primarily of the fatty acid series, as well as propanol and isobutyl alcohol, which oxidize in the presence of oxidants to form aldehydes and then carboxylic acids. Other gaseous substances emitted by waste products include phenol and other cyclic unsaturated hydrocarbons with narcotic properties.

Thus, the large number of volatile and toxic substances that waste products can release into a spacecraft cabin atmosphere presents a serious hazard and makes air regeneration and water reclamation difficult. In addition, microbial action, especially biodegradation and fermentation, on stored wastes may lead to the formation of additional volatile and toxic gases.

Human wastes generally contain *E. coli*, diphtheroid mi-

This chapter was translated from Russian by Galina Tverskaya and Lydia Razran Stone. Nigel J.C. Packham provided technical editing of the translation.

crobes, *Streptococci, Staphylococci,* and *Micrococci.*[4] In healthy individuals, urine always contains nine bacterial species: hemolytic *Streptococci, E. coli, Str. faecalis, St. aureus, Pr. mirabilis, Klebsiella, Pseudomonas, Str. epidermidis,* and *Pr. rettgeri.* Micro-organisms forming in a number of different environments, including wastes, can contaminate the air of enclosed cabin environments. The following microbes have been detected in the humidity condensates from the air of enclosed environments: *E. coli, Staphylococcus albus, Pseudomonas alcaligens, Aeromonas, Citrobacter, Streptococcus faecalis,* and *Bacillus subtilis.*[5] During long-term storage, the number of microbial species found in wastes decreases and, by the end of the first month, *Pseudomonas* cultures become prevalent.

The biochemical processes through which microbes can transform waste products are quite diverse. For example, they decompose urea into ammonia and carbon dioxide and proteins into hydrogen sulfide or indole, and they ferment carbohydrates.

Data on the chemical and microbiological composition of wastes suggest that measures should be taken to protect enclosed environments from chemical and microbiological contamination. Theoretical calculations for the design of waste management subsystems on future space missions, especially flights to Mars, are typically based on parameters such as the average production of waste products per day per person or for an entire crew, projected waste generation during an entire flight, and water content (the latter is usually used to compute water balance). Table 1 cites estimates of waste streams taken from the literature.[2,6-8] The differences in values obtained for the same parameters can be attributed to differences in the way data were collected or differences in the approach to waste management design.

The present authors agree completely with Rasmussen et al.,[9] who argue that the management of various types of waste is a potentially critical problem for long-duration flights and that there must be regular reviews of mission plans and programs to fill in the gaps and make corrections in waste inventories. The waste management problem may become critical when waste products produced by servicing operations (e.g., fragments of wire insulation, grease residue, and broken electronic components) increase.

Thus, unless appropriate measures have not been worked out for dealing with them, the formation and accumulation of waste products on a spacecraft may have two types of adverse effects, the potential hazard of crew contact with toxic gases and microbes, and the potential hazard of the spacecraft becoming "cluttered" with waste products produced by experiments and servicing operations.

These problems can be dealt with using the following approaches: 1) improving existing means for collecting, storing, and disposing of wastes through compacting and use of preserving agents, and 2) developing waste processing technologies to improve conditions of waste storage and disposal, to extract water from wastes, and to recycle wastes in closed life support systems.

Table 1   Estimates of Wastes Streams (g r a m s / m a n / d a y)

Type of waste	Source of data	Total	Water content
Urine	6	1270–2110	–
	7	1550	1485
	8	1630	1570
Feces	6	96–132	75–111
	7	161	120
	8	150	114
Food scraps	7	93	59
	8	45–170	–
Trash	6	810–1620	≤1088
	7	902	81
Food packaging	2	536	
Wash water	2	160	
Wastes from experiments and maintenance	2	820	

III. Waste Collection and Storage on Spacecraft

Starting with the Vostok program, early Soviet waste systems involved progressively more sophisticated use of pneumatic principles (entrained air streams) to separate wastes from the body and direct them into a containment system; both solid and liquid wastes could be collected simultaneously but were stored in separate containers. Early U.S. spacecraft utilized "personal" collection systems, which had to be affixed to the body. Procedures for using these devices were time-consuming and unpleasant. On Apollo, urine was vented and feces were collected in bags, mixed with bactericide, and stored. Skylab stations were equipped with devices for separate collection of urine, feces, and housekeeping wastes. The urine collector used in the Skylab program was equipped with a blower, generating air flow at a speed of 0.3 m^3/min, to carry the liquid into bags. The subsystem also included a liquid/gas separator, a urine container, urine sample vials, and a cooling surface containing the coolant used in the thermal regulation subsystem. Urine was fed into a container and was transferred to the oxygen tank of the Saturn rocket, where all waste products were stored. A blower was also used to collect feces in plastic bags, which were then sealed and stored in containers. In both devices, the air stream passed through filters to remove trace contaminants and bacteria. On Soviet Salyut stations, feces were collected in a bag and then stored in sealed metal containers, which were ejected to space about once a week. The urine collector was separate from the main commode. On Mir, urine and feces are collected in the same commode and urine is recovered after passing through an air/liquid separator. On the U.S. Shuttle Orbiter, feces are col-

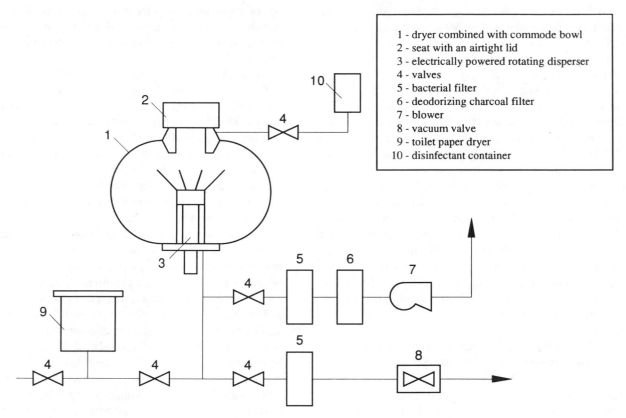

Fig. 1 Flow chart of a feces vacuum dryer.

1 - dryer combined with commode bowl
2 - seat with an airtight lid
3 - electrically powered rotating disperser
4 - valves
5 - bacterial filter
6 - deodorizing charcoal filter
7 - blower
8 - vacuum valve
9 - toilet paper dryer
10 - disinfectant container

lected in the commode storage container, vacuum dried, and held. Urine is sent to a waste water tank, which is vented when full.

There is no question that these devices need considerable improvement, particularly 1) to eliminate unpleasant odors and 2) to provide more efficient use of container capacity. Vacuum methods of waste processing, particularly for feces, are to be recommended for these purposes. Wastes may be vacuum dried by exposure to space, inhibiting microbial proliferation and significantly decreasing the rate of degradation of organic compounds. Through the use of this method, waste products can be desiccated to a residual humidity level of 3–10 percent in approximately 24 h without additional heating. However, the method requires the use of a relatively large number of disposable containers or storage tank liners (an amount equal to 10 percent of the initial weight of the wastes being processed); in addition, some cabin air is lost.

A vacuum drying waste management subsystem manufactured by General Electric Company, along with other life support subsystems, was subjected to a 90-day test in a McDonnell Douglas space station simulator. Four subjects participated in the test.[10] The waste management subsystems consisted of a fecal processor; a urine collector; devices for packaging, transporting, and storing wastes; a toilet paper dryer; and a device for dumping liquid wastes overboard. A diagram of the feces vacuum dryer is shown in Fig. 1. The fecal processor includes a commode bowl, a spherical commode chamber, and a rotating disperser (slinger). It is is

equipped with a bacterial filter for the vacuum dryer, a blower, and bacterial and deodorant filters for the air blower used for feces. The processor is designed for use in microgravity with feces directed into the collector by means of air flow. Disinfectants can be added. The test demonstrated that one device can function effectively for 180–200 eliminations. Storage and collection of other waste products (toilet paper, filter materials, various wipes, packaging foils, and bags) required a 166-liter aluminum container, five 12-liter boxes, 42 containers for wet and 41 containers for dry food wastes. The test demonstrated the need for further research on disinfectants, bacterial monitoring, and the selection of adequate storage containers.

The vacuum processing subsystem has the capability to collect, desiccate, sterilize, compact, and store different wastes (urine, feces, and others) from six crewmembers until the wastes can be returned to Earth on a cargo spacecraft.[2] The air stream velocity in the feces collection unit is 0.566 m^3/min, and the air passes through a 0.08-μm mesh filter. The time needed to dry feces from one elimination to 10 percent humidity is 2–6 h (without additional heating), and the loss of air for one use is 57 liters. The air stream velocity in the urine collector is 0.283m^3/min of air, and 0.263 kg of water are used for each flush. The processing subassembly can accommodate 6.8 kg/day and a volume of 28 liters per day of wastes (in uncompacted form). It consists of a drying chamber, a compactor, and a storage container. The drying temperature is $121\,^\circ$C, and the drying time is 4 h. The dried wastes are compacted once a week at a pressure of 5 atm, reducing their bulk by a factor of 4. Dried, compacted wastes are automatically fed into the storage container. The authors believe that a technology using both vacuum drying and heating has advantages in terms of rate of processing.

Waste storage containers should obviously be light, strong, and leak proof. Of concern are volatile compounds offgassed by wastes. It has been asserted that "under ideal conditions, 1 gram of waste products may produce as much as 0.3 m^3 of gas."[11] This is, indeed, a real danger, particularly when different wastes are stored together, facilitating intensive microbial proliferation. However, when feces and food scraps are stored together in a pressurized container, a pressure increase is noted only during the first 7–10 days. Subsequently, pressure decreases, often to below ambient pressure. This is due primarily to the uptake of oxygen from the air in contact with organic wastes. Pressure increases or decreases may jeopardize waste containment, which can be guaranteed only when chemical or physical methods of preservation are used for decontamination purposes.

IV. Methods of Waste Preservation and Decontamination of Sanitary Facilities

The fact that a number of different types of microbes proliferate in moisture-containing waste products dictates the use of disinfectants with sporicidal, fungicidal, and bactericidal effects, which are also able to stabilize labile chemical components.

The biological decomposition of wastes can be slowed by freezing and storing at a temperature of -10 °C, but the wastes must remain frozen throughout the storage period and then must be thawed before water extraction can occur. Wet heat sterilization requires exposure to steam at a minimum temperature of 121 °C for 15 min, whereas dry heat sterilization requires a minimum of 160 °C and exposure of 60 min.

Organic wastes can be stabilized by desiccation because microbes cannot grow without moisture. Desiccation may be achieved through exposure to the vacuum of space, but this method poses the risk of cabin depressurization. The incineration of organic compounds to form water and carbon dioxide is an effective method of waste disposal. However, the amount of oxygen consumed and carbon dioxide, nitrogen and sulfur oxides, and other contaminants produced may challenge the air purification and regeneration subsystem.

Mention should be made of the use of microwaves as a physical method of decontaminating moisture-containing wastes. The microwave method has been demonstrated to decrease the number of *Ps. aeruginosa* cells, starting at a temperature as low as 56–58 °C. As temperature is increased beyond this point, level of disinfection increases as well.[12]

Physical methods of waste processing also include ultraviolet irradiation, ultrasonic treatment, and exposure to ionizing radiation. However, these methods are not very effective; they are energy inefficient, and the last method requires bulky shielding from ionizing radiation. These physical methods of decontamination have in common the disadvantage that they do not have a residual effect; and, consequently, processed wastes are subject to recontamination with microbes.[13,14]

While biological oxidation of water-containing wastes can, in theory, be performed in space, this method is not cost effective. Biological mineralization can prove cost effective only in a closed bioregenerative life support system.

Chemical methods should be considered the methods of choice for decontaminating wastes for prolonged storage. The major advantage of such methods is that they have a residual effect; i.e., they destroy microbes that enter the medium after it has been treated. Moreover, chemical processing of moisture-containing wastes can be used to modify their chemical composition and stabilize labile components. Chemical treatment of wastes can readily be combined with water reclamation procedures to improve water quality. Chemical methods of decontamination include chlorination, ozonation, and the use of preparations such as silver, iodine, hydrogen peroxide, and bromine. When chemical methods of decontamination are developed, it is important to consider the chemical composition of the waste products, their projected storage time, and the water reclamation techniques that will be used. This is necessary because certain chemical compounds in the wastes inhibit decontamination capacity. It has been demonstrated that some detergents and pesticides reduce the decontaminating capacity of chloride-containing substances.[15] Even chlorination of water can be accompanied by the formation of carcinogenic and toxic compounds.[16]

The use of electrochemical methods to decontaminate moisture-containing human wastes through exposure to electrical current to produce sodium hypochlorite is of potential practical interest. Electrochemical treatment of urine produces mono- and di-chloramines, which bind ammonia, producing a prolonged bactericidal effect.[17] The efficacy of sterilization with sodium hypochlorite can be enhanced by the addition of sodium phosphate. It has been found that water can be decontaminated through use of sodium hypochlorite isolated from solutions of table salt, sea water, or mineralized ground water.[18,19] Electrochemical treatment of moisture-containing human wastes appears to be an attractive technique for use in space, since it does not require toxic chemicals and can be automated readily. Its major disadvantage is the instability of sodium hypochlorite.

Some authors recommend the use of silver salts, cuprous bromide, copper sulfate, iodine, or surfactants as preservatives for urine.[20,21] Waste collectors can be disinfected using "vescodim" (a mixture of iodine and surfactants).[11]

Cuprous bromide is an optimal preserving agent with respect to decontamination efficacy and cost and can also reduce the production of ammonia and nitrogen oxides.[22] This compound, in a concentration of 5–8 grams per 100 grams of waste, can be effectively used in storing both urine and feces; however, it should be distributed uniformly throughout the waste mass, which requires a special mixer. If such a mixer is used, the preserving effect lasts for at least 1 year.

However, not all the compounds recommended can be used in a medium containing a mixture of a number of contaminants of organic and mineral origin. For example, silver salts can easily interact with sodium chloride and precipitate in urine, diminishing their effectiveness. Properties of phenol-containing preserving agents (benzyl phenyl, benzyl chlorophenyl, phenyl trichloroacetate, hexachlorophene, resorcin, and paranitrophenol) have also been investigated. These compounds, when added to urine at a concentration of 1 percent, have kept it from rotting for as long as 100 days.[23] However, some of these compounds are volatile and may contaminate reclaimed water or the spacecraft cabin atmosphere. Investigations of the effects of paranitrophenol on the gaseous compounds emitted by stored urine showed that the amount of ammonia, aliphatic amines, acetone, organic acids, and nitrogen oxides diminished, whereas the total quantity of organic compounds measured in terms of total carbon and carbon dioxide remained unchanged.

Urine and other moisture-containing wastes can be preserved with quaternary ammonium compounds such as alkyl dimethyl benzyl ammonium chloride (cipheral, roccal, ketavlon), in which alkyl radicals contain different numbers of carbon atoms (from 8 to 10). These compounds belong to the class of cation-active compounds, i.e., the organic portion of the molecule has a positive charge. These compounds are of low toxicity for warm-blooded animals and have detergent and bactericidal properties. Soviet chemists have synthesized a homolog of alkyl dimethyl benzyl ammonium chloride (catamine) and cation-active preparations of pyridine compounds (catapines).[24,25]

A mixture of sulfuric acid, chromium oxide, and copper sulfate has been recommended to decontaminate physical-chemical subsystems recovering water from urine.[26,27] This preparation is highly effective as a disinfectant and stabilizes labile ammonium salts. However, its use requires stringent safety measures because of its high reactivity.

Wash water can be decontaminated with the iodine sorption method, utilizing sorption and desorption.[28] When water is passed through an iodine-saturated anion-exchange resin, aqueous solutions of hypoiodite and hydrogen iodide are formed, undergo a series of reversible and irreversible transformations, and are ultimately converted into molecular iodine and hypoiodous acid.[29]

Experience with space flight has shown that some crewmembers experience space motion sickness symptoms, one of which is vomiting. Vomitus forms a rich nutrient substrate for microbes. It does not remain in its original form for long, and its fermentation is accompanied by the emission of various gaseous compounds. This presents the danger of rupture of the vomitus collectors and emission of their contents into the cabin atmosphere. Vomitus can be preserved by drying in the vacuum of space.[30] However, chemical treatment is an even simpler method for preserving vomitus in space. Food preservatives can be used for this purpose.

On the whole, chemical methods that utilize decontaminating and preserving agents selected specifically to treat dif-ferent types of waste should be considered as one of the most promising ways to further improve waste management subsystems. Chemical methods can be particularly effective when combined with physical techniques. In the future, when waste storage is replaced by waste recycling, chemical methods will be used in waste collection and initial processing devices to prevent the decomposition of unstable compounds and the uncontrolled growth of microbes.

V. Procedures for Eliminating Wastes in Space

Over time, the development of waste management technologies has tended to move from storage of wastes to waste processing using vacuum, chemical, or thermal methods. The use of a bioregenerative controlled ecological life support system (CELSS), which includes plants, has made it practical to use still another method—biological mineralization. The concept underlying the use of this method was advanced in the late 1960s[8,31-33] and remains essentially unchanged today.

The selection of a method of disposing of or dumping wastes should be based on a number of factors, the most significant of which are 1) access to cargo spacecraft and number of crewmembers, 2) possibility of dumping waste containers into space, 3) risk of depressurization and effects on the spacecraft exterior of venting gases in space, and 4) possibility of utilizing waste products in life support systems or as rocket propellant.

Theoretical design work to determine an appropriate profile for the life support system in general and a waste management subsystem in particular has encompassed the following options: biological mineralization, radioactive irradiation, freezing, use of preserving agents, vacuum and thermal-vacuum drying, pyrolysis and subsequent combustion of the vapor-gas mixture, wet oxidation, and use of wastes as a shield against cosmic rays or as rocket propellant.

Waste collection, transportation, and accumulation and the addition of preservatives, storage, and disposal are operations that generally do not involve changes in the state of aggregation of the wastes; i.e., they do not involve waste processing or destruction. Vacuum drying entails a decrease in the mass of wastes, which, stretching the point somewhat, can be classified as a form of elimination. However, it should be remembered that the water vapor and volatile substances released into space may condense on exterior surfaces, antennas, and optical instruments, requiring preventive measures. In principle, there are two ways to eliminate wastes through utilizing them as rocket propellants: by heating the vapor-gas mixture in electrothermal engines,[34,35] or by creating a propellant that is a composite of solid and liquid components.[36]

In the first instance, the vapor-gas mixture can be produced by pyrolysis or waste combustion. In the second case, proposals include a propellant called MONEX made from human wastes (5–65 percent); metallic additives, specifically, powdered aluminum (10–40 percent); and inorganic oxidizers, primarily ammonium nitrite (5–50 percent). Sixty-day tests established that the specific impulse of the propellants in the effective range is about 250 s. This approach to waste processing meets environmental standards, provides partial or total waste disposal, complies with the requirement that space not be polluted (through high-temperature sterilization), and saves on weight (since smaller amounts of propellant stores are needed).

Further developments in this direction were described by Grishin,[37] who compared electrothermal engines utilizing life support system wastes (carbon dioxide, methane, water vapor, urine, and concentrated urine) to two-component liquid propellant rockets using a standard propellant and discussed the potential of their joint use. It would be practical to utilize first methane and then carbon dioxide and concentrated urine. Joint use of the two systems would reduce total weight by 20.7 percent (through saving propellant), energy consumption by 1.3 percent, and heat production by 8.6 percent. Although implementing this approach would present some technical difficulties, it would certainly merit further study in developing a manned Mars mission.

Of great interest is thermal processing of waste products, which involves partial or complete elimination of the wastes themselves and the recycling of water and other substances in the life support system. Thermal methods, although they may differ in hardware and design, are basically similar in the nature of their effects on the processed material. The solid residue left after thermal processing of wastes is more suitable for prolonged storage than that produced by vacuum drying. The condensate produced by catalytic or high-temperature oxidation of the vapor-gas mixture contains only insignificant amounts of organic substances and is suitable for preparation of potable or wash water. The various methods (thermal drying, pyrolysis, and incineration) differ primarily with respect to the completeness of combustion and oxygen uptake, the amount of water and carbon dioxide extracted, the methods of heat addition and removal, and the convenience of subsequent handling of the solid residue.

Thermal drying at 120–130 °C not only decontaminates wastes but also provides relatively complete water extraction. Final oxidation of volatile substances requires approximately 2 grams of oxygen per 100 grams of dry weight. This method is expedient if heat is being produced by other technological processes and, particularly, if water contained in plants and algae has to be returned for recycling in the life support system.

Pyrolysis at 250–300 °C helps accelerate waste processing and reduces, by a factor of 1.5, the amount of solid residue that must be stored. However, this process requires more oxygen than thermal drying and, even more important, more power and better thermal insulation of hardware. Under certain conditions, the solid residue can be used as a sorbent for trapping acidic gases (nitrogen and sulfur oxides).

Power constraints make incineration preferable to drying or pyrolysis. In theory, the heat production capacity of human wastes should be sufficient to sustain stable combustion even when humidity exceeds 90 percent. In practice, complete oxidation of wastes requires that an oxidizing agent be delivered to the thermal processing area beginning at the ignition point (400–450 °C) and continuing throughout the process of incineration (650–700 °C). Complete incineration has the following advantages over thermal drying and pyrolysis: solid residue (ashes) can be handled easily and is of minimum weight and volume; chemical energy (heat of combustion) can, in principle, be utilized; and wastes are almost completely recovered (except for 40–60 percent of ashes, which weigh 1–2 percent of the initial weight of waste products). The major disadvantage is the need for significant quantities of oxygen.

In view of the fact that, on future manned missions, microbial contamination of wastes will present a significant danger and water recovery will be an important benefit, some authors propose the use of high-temperature (650 °C) technological processes.[38] These produce a sterile condensate that is acceptable as a source of reclaimed potable water. These processes can be implemented by utilizing heat produced by radioisotopic elements, which are more reliable than other sources. General Electric Company has designed, developed, and tested a system (which is actually a modified, improved vacuum dryer) containing an electric heater that simulates heat produced by a radioisotopic source. A diagram of the system is shown in Fig. 2.

This system's efficiency was tested in a life support situation involving four individuals for 180 days. All waste products (urine, feces, atmospheric humidity condensate, wash water, food scraps, packages, wipes, and paper) were collected in an evaporator, from which a vapor-gas mixture was transported to three parallel catalytic cartridges and then to a condenser. During this process, the solid dried residue was fed by a metering screw into an incineration chamber, where it underwent thermal decomposition and oxidation; and the resultant gas was dumped overboard. The gaseous compounds from the condenser, also, were vented into a vacuum, while carrier air underwent sterilization. The high-temperature subassembly, which contained a heater, cartridges, an incineration chamber, and a sterilizer, was vacuum insulated in a titanium housing. A table cites the results of analyzing condensate measurements from 10 trials, in which the concentrations of contaminants in the water were below standard limits. The water recovery coefficient was 98.2 percent. The temperature of 650 ± 10 °C was maintained by a 400-W heater. These results confirm the utility of combining water recovery and waste processing subsystems based on incineration.

Another author[39] describes an incinerator that uses heat from a ^{238}Ru source and is designed to operate for a period of 6 months to 3 years. This incinerator, which weighs 340 kg and requires 1270 W, extracts water from solid and liquid wastes and reduces their bulk by a factor of approximately 100. A detailed description of this technology can be found in Jakut,[40] which cites equipment used, power requirements, and formulas for estimating the cost effectiveness of system components.

The efficiency of incineration, which can be applied to

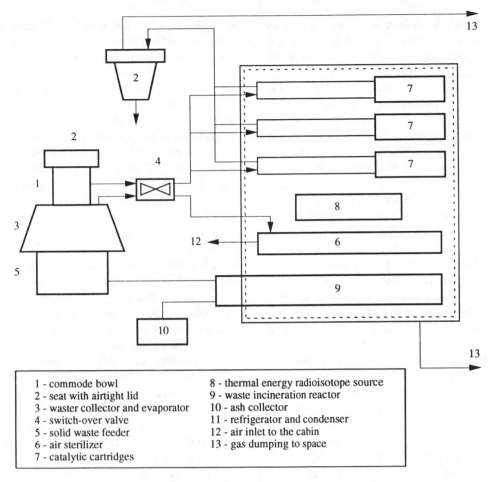

1 - commode bowl
2 - seat with airtight lid
3 - waster collector and evaporator
4 - switch-over valve
5 - solid waste feeder
6 - air sterilizer
7 - catalytic cartridges
8 - thermal energy radioisotope source
9 - waste incineration reactor
10 - ash collector
11 - refrigerator and condenser
12 - air inlet to the cabin
13 - gas dumping to space

Fig. 2 Flow chart of a waste incineration unit.

virtually any type of waste product, depends on whether the process is continuous; whether materials differing in their moisture content, chemical parameters, and rheological properties are used; whether heat sources are efficient; and whether the condensate produced will be used for water recovery.

One promising technology for the future involves using microwaves for heating. This technique has the following important advantages: 1) heat can be applied almost instantaneously and in controlled amounts to the material being processed (minimizing heat loss); and 2) microwave sources may already be present on the spacecraft for heating food, sterilizing water and medical instruments, etc. Its disadvantages are the low efficiency of commercial devices; the bulkiness and low reliability of converters (magnetrons); and the complexity of design, development, and adjustment of microwave heaters. It appears, however, that these problems will be resolved in the future.

These considerations were taken into account in the development of an apparatus for thermal processing of human wastes and wastes of a biological system, using cycles of drying, pyrolysis, and incineration.[41,42] The use of an afterburner permits not only final oxidation of the resultant vapor-gas mixture but also provides a constant loading level, which protects the microwave source.

The method of wet oxidation of waste products is of inter-est for space vehicles that have bioregenerative life support systems. This technology has recently been used extensively, particularly in sewage treatment. With respect to the waste products under discussion here, the best results were obtained when the autoclaving chamber functioned cyclically at a temperature of 250–300 °C and at a pressure of 2–5 MPa at the beginning and 13–17 MPa at the end of the process.[42] After the process was complete, the gases obtained (nitrogen, carbon dioxide, residual oxygen, and traces of carbon monoxide, methane, and other trace contaminants) were cleaner than those produced by other thermal methods. The liquid phase contained up to 90 percent of the original mineral salts in forms assimilable by autotrophic organisms. The recovery coefficients for the major biogenic elements were: K and Na, 80 percent; P, 45 percent; Ca, 80 percent; Mg, 40 percent; S, 25 percent; Fe, 60 percent; Al, 40 percent; Si, 30 percent; and total N, 75 percent. Although these values vary slightly as a function of the type of waste, overall, the recovery coefficient is higher than that for other thermal processing technologies. The recovered solution can be enriched and then used for plant cultivation.

Wet oxidation can be used to process virtually all waste products and, thus, may be used on future missions of more than 1 year in duration, with a crew of at least six.[43] The most important units required for this subsystem are a crusher, a heat exchanger, and a phase separator. A technology such as this processes the entire waste stream into 0.2 percent ashes, 91 percent pure sterile saltwater for further treatment in the water recovery subsystem, and 8 percent carbon dioxide.

A further improvement of this technology utilizes supercritical water oxidation for human waste processing.[44] A prototype includes two reactors: one for waste oxidation (urine, flush water, feces, wipes, trash, and wash water) and the other for oxidation of the gaseous products of waste decomposition (similar to the afterburner used in thermal treatment). In addition, the system includes a heat exchanger, which heats the water-oxidizer mixture to supercritical temperatures (above 374 °C), high- and low-pressure evaporators, pumps for wastes and water, compressors for the oxidizing agent and fuel, a water tank, and gas and water analyzers.

This system functioned cyclically. Feces mixed with urine and hydrogen were fed in batches into the waste oxidation reactor. The oxidizer, mixed with water heated to a supercritical temperature, was fed into the reactor simultaneously with the wastes. In the reactor, wastes underwent oxidation, and the temperature rose to 600 °C. The residue remained in the reactor, whereas the vapor-gas mixture was transported to the second reactor for final oxidation. Hydrogen was also fed into the second reactor to maintain chemical reactions. Results of this test suggested that this technology can be used in space.

In addition to thermal methods of waste processing, biological life support systems can also use methods of biological mineralization analogous to natural processes on the Earth. However, as early as 1964, it was demonstrated that biological mineralization would require bulky and heavy equipment and would have power requirements similar to those of other systems.[45] It was found that only 40 percent of organic substances could be processed biologically; thus, physical-chemical methods of waste recovery and annihilation would also be required. This conclusion, which, as a first approximation, was correct, neglected to consider the potential use of the products of biological processing for plant cultivation.

Special studies have evaluated different methods of waste management by measuring the biological activity in the resultant condensate and mineralized solution. These studies demonstrated that mineralized wheat straw, after hydroaerobic degradation, exerts a stimulating and protective effect on plant growth and development.[46] It has been proposed, also, that anaerobic processes occur in addition to aerobic ones.[47] The use of natural soils for plant cultivation has been recommended for future large space stations,[48] and this is related to the issue of biological mineralization.

The investigation of waste degradation on solid substrates is of theoretical and practical interest. Here, natural mechanisms responsible for the degradation, transformation, and synthesis of organic compounds can occur, ensuring continuous renewal of all the properties and functions of the soil. As a result, mineral nutrients are transformed into elements utilizable by plants. Newly formed humus substances foster

maintenance and renewal of the soil structure, which determines its water and air budget and provides the plants and soil biocenoses with biologically active substances.

Experimental studies were performed to investigate these issues. They demonstrated that the preliminary microbiological degradation of waste products in fermenters, combined with the subsequent addition of liquid and solid products of degradation to the plant substrate, supported high productivity in the biomass for a number of years without substrate replacement.[49] There was virtually total utilization of the substances added (and, consequently, total elimination of organic wastes), since the substrate itself did not increase or decrease in volume.

In summary, there are a number of different technologies for waste management and disposal available today. However, ironically, in actual space programs, because of serious technical, financial, and logistics problems, only a small portion of such technological capabilities are utilized. Thus, for example, no modern spacecraft has facilities for treatment and recovery of solid wastes, and Mir alone has a subsystem for recovering water from urine. The Salyut and Mir stations have a subsystem for collecting, containing, preserving, and disposing of wastes from the inhabited modules of the station. Food wastes, personal hygiene products, housekeeping refuse, and pouches containing feces are collected in metal containers and ejected into space through a special hatch or packed in bilayer bags, which the cosmonauts load into the crew cabin of the transport or cargo vehicles. After the transport or cargo ship separate from the station, the crew cabin and its contents burn up upon entry into the atmosphere.

On the U.S. Space Station, plans call for feces to be collected in a bag and then compacted for biodegradation. Urine will be sent to a vapor compression distillation system to be recovered as potable water. There is no question that we must advance from this type of waste disposal to subsystems for treating and recovering wastes. Appropriate waste treatment and recovery technologies have been developed; what is required now is that efforts be directed at their practical implementation and utilization.

References

[1]*Housekeeping Concepts for Manned Space Systems.* Data Book, vol. 3, Waste Control Search/Report Computer Program, NASA CR-115038, Washington, D.C., NASA Hq., 1971.

[2]Antell, R.W., et al. *Modular Space Station Phase B, Extension Preliminary System Design.* Vol. 4, Subsystem Analysis; Part III, Environmental Control Life Support Subsystem, NASA CR-115408, Washington, D.C., NASA Hq., 1972, pp. 3.1-3–3.1-163.

[3]Zlatkis, A., and Liebich, A.M. Profile of volatile metabolites in human urine. *Clinical Chemistry*, 1971, vol. 17, pp. 592–594.

[4]Kaplan, A.Ye. Methods of bacteriological analysis of urine in massive bacteriuria. *Laboratornoye Delo*, 1977, No.

1, pp. 46–49 (in Russian).

[5]Guskova, Ye.I.; Kuznetsova, L.A.; Shikina, M.I.; and Kolesina, N.B. Preservation of atmospheric moisture condensate in space flight. In: Kakurin, L.I., Ed. *Abstracts of Papers Presented at a Conference on Current Problems of Space Biology and Medicine*, Moscow, Institute of Biomedical Problems, 1977, p. 8 (in Russian).

[6]Wydeven, T., and Golub, M.A. Generation rates and chemical compositions of waste streams in a typical crew space habitat. Moffett Field, Calif., NASA Ames Research Center.

[7]Cullingford, H.S., and Novara, M. Conceptual design of a piloted Mars sprint life support system. SAE Technical Paper, Series 1988, No. 881059, pp. 1–10.

[8]Laubach, G.E., and Schaedle, G.C. An introduction to the waste management problem for large space stations. ASME Paper, 1970, NAV/SPT-24, p. 8.

[9]Rasmussen, D.N., et al. OSSA space station waste inventory. SAE Technical Paper Series, 17th Intersociety Conference on Environmental Systems, Seattle, Wash., July 13–15, 1987, pp. 1–6.

[10]Shook, R.E., and Wells, G.W. Waste management for the 90-day space station simulator test. ASME Paper, 1971, NAV-7, p. 12.

[11]Jones, W.L., and Pecoraro, J.N. Isolation and removal of waste products. Unpublished manuscript, 1970.

[12]Sobolevskiy, V.G.; Viktorov, A.N.; Klimarev, S.I.; and Grishayenkov, B.G. On the potential use of SHF energy for water disinfection in deep-sea diving facilities. In: *Abstracts of Papers Presented at the All-Union Conference on Space Biology and Aerospace Medicine,* Moscow-Kaluga, U.S.S.R. Academy of Sciences, 1990, p. 493 (in Russian).

[13]Vashkov, V.I. *Antimicrobial Drugs and Disinfection Procedures for Infectious Diseases.* Moscow, Meditsina, 1977, pp. 5–8 (in Russian).

[14]Dolivo-Dobrovolskiy, L.B., and Kuznetsov, S.I. Bactericidal effects of ultrasonic oscillations in water. *Gigiyena i Sanitariya*, 1943, pp. 1–8 (in Russian).

[15]Shtannikov, Ye.V., and Ilyin, I.Ye. Hygienic evaluation of the barrier role of water pipe purification facilities in relation to surfactants and products of their transformation. *Gigiyena i Sanitariya*, 1979, no. 1 (in Russian).

[16]Ilyin, I.Ye. Study of the toxicity of products of transformation of surfactants formed during water chlorination. *Gigiyena i Sanitariya*, 1980, no. 2, pp. 11–14 (in Russian).

[17]Gaydadymov, V.B. Water recovery from urine by electrochemical oxidation and electrodialysis. In: *Life Support and Safety Systems for Flight Vehicles*, Moscow, Nauka, 1983, p. 181 (in Russian).

[18]Sergunina, P.A. Sanitary studies of decontamination of potable water and housekeeping sewage by sodium chloride products. Abstract of dissertation for degree of Doctor of Biological Sciences, Moscow, 1969, pp. 24 (in Russian).

[19]Sokolova, N.F. Water decontamination by sodium chloride electrolysis products. In: *Proceedings of National Conference on Disinfection and Sterilization*, Moscow, 1969, pp. 29–31 (in Russian).

[20]Rogatina, L.N. Development of fecal preserving agents for space flights. In: Chernigovskiy, V.N., Ed. *Work Performance, Issues of Habitability and Biotechnology. Problems of Space Biology, Volume 7,* Moscow, Nauka, 1967, pp. 415–428 (in Russian).

[21]Borshchenko, V.V.; Prishchep, A.G.; Zarubina, K.V.; and Shumilina, G.A. Development of urine preserving agents for prolonged space flights. In: *Abstracts of Papers Presented at IVth National. Conference on Space Biology and Aerospace Medicine*, Moscow, Kaluga, U.S.S.R. Academy of Sciences, 1972, vol. 1, pp. 175–178 (in Russian).

[22]Kustov, V.V.; Mikhaylov, V.I.; Poddubnaya, L.T.; and Rogatina, L.N. Toxic gaseous compounds released during urine storage. In: Chernigovskiy, V.N., Ed. *Work Performance, Issues of Habitability and Biotechnology. Problems of Space Biology, Volume 7,* Moscow, Nauka, 1967, pp. 432–435 (in Russian).

[23]Borshchenko, V.V.; Vashkov, V.I.; and Rogatina, L.N. Study of urine preservation methods as related to space flight. In: Chernigovskiy, V.N., Ed. *Medical and Biological Problems of Manned Space Flight. Problems of Space Biology, Volume 16,* Moscow, Nauka, 1971, pp. 249–253 (in Russian).

[24]Vashkov, V.I. Methods for reducing microbial concentrations in small closed areas used for long-term manned experiments. In: Chernigovskiy, V.N., Ed. *Work Performance, Issues of Habitability and Biotechnology. Problems of Space Biology, Volume 7,* Moscow, Nauka, 1967, pp. 408–412 (in Russian).

[25]Skala, L.Z. Antimicrobial properties of iodides and their use for skin and hand disinfection. Abstract of doctoral dissertation in biological sciences, Moscow, 1968 (in Russian).

[26]Putnam, D.F. Chemical aspects of urine distillation. *Papers of American Society of Mechanical Engineering*, 1965, No. 2465, AV-24, p. 13.

[27]Putnam, D.F., and Wells, G. Water recovery for space flight. In: *Proceedings of the XXIII International Astronautics Congress*, Baku, IAF, Oct. 1973.

[28]Tolstykh, I.M.; Smirnov, D.V.; Sitnikova, N.N.; and Ovechkina, E.I. Decontamination of wash water by the iodine absorption method. In: *Abstracts of Papers Presented at the All-Union Conference on Space Biology and Aerospace Medicine*, Moscow, Kaluga, U.S.S.R. Academy of Sciences, U.S.S.R. Ministry of Health, 1990, p. 503 (in Russian).

[29]Mokhnach, V.O. *Theoretical Foundations of the Biological Effect of Haloid Compounds.* Moscow - Leningrad, 1968 (in Russian).

[30]Goldblith, S.A., and Wick, E.L. Analysis of human fecal components and study of methods for their recovery in space systems. ASD-TR 61419, Wright-Patterson AFB, Ohio, Aerospace Medical Laboratory, 1961.

[31]Shepelev, Ye.Ya. Spacecraft life support systems based on biological recycling. In: Yazdovskiy, V.I., Ed. *Space Biology and Medicine, Biomedical Problems of Space Flights,* Moscow, Nauka, 1966, pp. 330–362 (in Russian).

[32]Yazdovskiy, V.I.; Agre, A.L.; Gusarov, B.G.; Sinyak,

Yu.Ye.; Chizhov, S.V.; and Tsitovich, S.I. Transformation of human and biological wastes through recycling in small enclosed areas. In: *Proceedings of XVIIth International Astronautical Congress,* Madrid, International Astronautics Federation, 1966 (in Russian).

[33]United Aircraft Corporation. Trade-off study and conceptual design of regenerative advanced integrated life support systems (AILSS). NASA CR-1458, Washington, D.C., NASA Hq., 1968.

[34]Bliss, T.R., et al. Biowaste resistojet system definition for the NASA Space Station. AIAA Paper no. 1132, 1970, p. 13.

[35]Greco, R.V., et al. *Development of a biowaste resistojet propulsion system: propellant management and control subsystem.* AIAA Paper 448, 1972, p. 19.

[36]U.S. Patent No. 3773574, NKI 149-22, 1967.

[37]Grishin, S.D. Optimization of life support systems for flying vehicles based on waste utilization in the propulsion system. *Aviation and Cosmonautics Lectures (1979–1980),* Section on Life Support Systems and Flight Vehicle Safety, Moscow, 1983, pp. 52–57 (in Russian).

[38]Murray, R.W.; Shivers, R.W.; Ingelfinger, A.L.; and Metzger, C.A. Integrated waste management-water system using radioisotopes for thermal energy, ASME Paper 71-Av-1, 1971, p. 8.

[39]Wastes to water. *Spaceflight,* 1972, vol. 14, no. 10, p. 380.

[40]Jakut, M.M. Cost analysis of water recovery systems, NASA CR-124098, Washington, D.C., NASA Hq., 1972.

[41]U.S.S.R. Patent No. 473880b, MKI G 23, 1972 (in Russian).

[42]Guryeva, T.S.; Dagayeva, L.V.; Zablotskiy, L.L.; and Sinyak, G.S. Problems of human waste management and utilization in life support systems. In: *Vth Tsiolkovskiy Lectures,* Kaluga, U.S.S.R. Academy of Sciences, 1971, pp. 124–131 (in Russian).

[43]Jagow, R.B. Development of a spacecraft wet oxidation waste processing system. ASME Paper NAV-2, 1972, p. 11.

[44]Hong, G.T.; Fowler, P.K.; Killilea, W.R.; and Swallow, K.C. *Supercritical water oxidation: treatment of human waste and system configuration trade-off study.* SAE Technical Paper Series, paper presented at *17th Intersociety Conf. on Environmental Systems,* Seattle, Wash., July 13–15, 1987, No. 871444, pp. 1–5.

[45]Drake, G.L. Integration and mechanics of waste collection and processing. Paper in: *Proceedings of Conference on Nutrition in Space and Related Waste Problems,* Tampa, Fla., 1964, Washington, D.C., NASA Hq., pp. 265–271.

[46]Deshevaya, Ye.A.; Kryuchkova, I.V.; Shaydorov, Yu.I.; and Popov, V.V. Study of wheat straw degradation in an artificial environment. *Kosmicheskaya Biologiya i Aviakosmicheskaya Meditsina,* 1983, no. 1, pp. 75–78 (in Russian).

[47]Modell, M., and Spurlock, T. Closed ecological life support systems for long-duration manned missions. In: *Proceedings of 9th Intersociety Conference on Environmental Systems,* July 16–19, 1979, San Francisco.

[48]Smith, W.L., and Brose, H.I. *Habitability support systems—a new reality.* AIAA Paper 78-1668, 1980.

[49]Shepelev, Ye.Ya.; Shaydorov, Yu.I.; and Popov, V.V. Processing of plant waste on a solid substrate for a biological life support system. *Kosmicheskaya Biologiya i Aviakosmicheskaya Meditsina,* 1983, no. 6, pp. 74–76 (in Russian).

Chapter 14

Individual Systems for Crewmember Life Support and Extravehicular Activity

James W. McBarron II, Charles E. Whitsett, Guy I. Severin, and Isaak P. Abramov

In Chapter 7, Volume III, of the first edition of *Foundations of Space Biology and Medicine,* Walton Jones presented detailed information on individual life support systems (LSSs) used by the United States and Soviet Union through 1975. Since 1975, extravehicular activity (EVA) life support, pressure suit, and propulsion/maneuvering technologies have advanced to support the requirements of the U.S. Space Shuttle and the U.S.S.R. Salyut and Mir orbital stations.

In the current chapter, we present information on the individual intravehicular activity (IVA) and EVA life support and manned maneuvering systems currently in use by the United States and Russia. Rather than emphasize development history, this chapter begins with an introduction to terminology, followed by a brief discussion of the essential philosophy used to develop these systems, and continues by focusing in more detail on engineering design. At the end of this chapter, Tables 1 through 7 provide information on the design and performance characteristics of U.S. and Soviet (Russian) individual EVA LSSs, space suits, and manned maneuvering units (MMUs), along with a summary of EVA statistics, systems, and accomplishments.

I. Terminology

It is easy to become confused by the multitude of names for hardware performing similar functions. The names of the hardware tend to change with the program (i.e., Apollo to Skylab to Shuttle, Mir to Buran) and with time, in general, as a result of upgrades resulting from lessons learned. This is true of both the U.S. and Soviet (Russian) space programs. A chapter such as this, which describes the efforts of both space programs faces twice the usual confusion. To aid the

reader, the following nomenclature is used consistently in this chapter:

1) "Space suit" always denotes one subsystem (i.e., the anthropomorphic enclosure) of an individual LSS.

2) The term "individual LSS" describes the entire system needed to provide life support to a crewmember in an environment that would not otherwise support life. The word "individual" is used to distinguish this system from the vehicle or spacecraft LSS. The term "individual LSS" encompasses two major classes of system differing with respect to the primary use of each system.

3) A system that provides individual life support *inside* a vehicle or base will be called an "individual IVA LSS" or "IVA system" for simplification when there is no risk of confusion with the vehicular LSS.

4) A system used *outside* a vehicle or base will be called an "individual EVA LSS" or an "EVA system."

This terminology is meant to describe systems and not individual subsystems. An entire system is described as being IVA or EVA, although certain systems can be used under both conditions.

In the popular literature, the term "space suit" tends to be used to describe an entire system, whereas the engineering community makes a distinction between the space suit (as the anthropomorphic shell) and the entire system, which always includes some form of LSS. The entire EVA system consists of the space suit and the LSS [called, in the United States, an extravehicular mobility unit (EMU) and, in Russia, a space suit or EVA semirigid suit with a built-in LSS]. The terminology selected here runs the risk of creating a problem opposite to the one just described. It is possible the term "individual LSS" will be misunderstood to refer to a part of the system (i.e., only the mechanical and electrical components that comprise the life support subsystem). We hope that our definition of terms will prevent this from happening.

II. Individual Life Support System Design Philosophy

In both the U.S. and U.S.S.R. space programs, the individual LSS was developed for 1) IVA, to provide life support and work capability in the event of cabin pressure loss or atmospheric contamination; and 2) EVA, allowing a human

The Russian coauthors are grateful to V.I. Svertshek and A.Yu. Stoklitskiy for consultation and to V.A. Frolov for help in the preparation of this chapter. The U.S. coauthors are grateful to Michael Rouen for recommendations regarding content organization, Natalie Karakulko for the translation from Russian to English, Patricia F. Kanz for manuscript editing, and Robert Herman for identification of figures. All the authors are grateful for the helpful technical coordination support provided by Dr. Ingemar Skoog, Dornier GmbH.

We sadly note the deaths of Charles E. Whitsett and Natalie Karakulko, which occurred during the preparation of this chapter for publication.

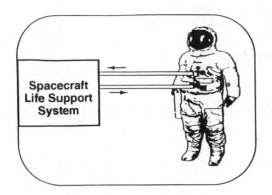

CLOSED VENTILATION LOOP

- Metabolic rate limited by available gas cooling
- Used by USSR Shuttle Buran
- Used by U.S. Mercury, Gemini, and Apollo Command Module Spacecraft

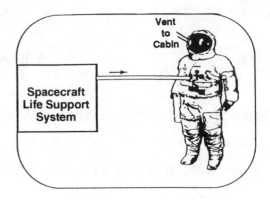

OPEN VENTILATION LOOP

- High potential oxygen expenditure during cabin depressurization
- Metabolic rate limited by available gas cooling
- Used by USSR Vostok, Voskhod, Soyuz, Soyuz-T, and Soyuz-TM Project Spacecraft
- Used by U.S. Shuttle Orbiter

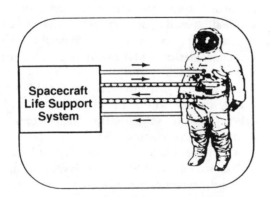

CLOSED VENTILATION AND WATER COOLING LOOPS

- Higher metabolic rate accommodated by both gas and water cooling
- Used in U.S. Apollo Lunar Module

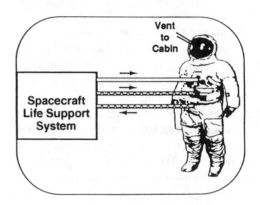

OPEN VENTILATION AND CLOSED WATER COOLING LOOPS

- High oxygen expendables use during cabin depressurization
- Not known to have been used

Fig. 1   Intravehicular individual life support systems.

to perform useful work and exploration tasks in the vacuum of space either in orbit or on a planetary surface.

In the design of both the IVA and individual EVA LSSs, basic factors such as the following must be considered:

1) major physiological and hygienic conditions needed to sustain life;

2) human capabilities (strength, dexterity, and vision) required to perform necessary tasks;

3) dangerous or hazardous environments (e.g., thermal extremes, vacuum, radiation, micrometeorites, space debris, and atomic oxygen);

4) amount of physical exertion (energy consumption) required of the crewmember to accomplish the mission;

5) spacecraft support capabilities affecting servicing and recharge between sorties;

6) crewmember safety and reliability;

7) provisions for accommodating failures and emergencies;

8) system constraints, as dictated by interactions with the vehicle, station, or base from which the individual LSS operates; and

9) mission and program requirements affecting equipment life, maintainability, sortie duration, and frequency.

The possible interactions of individual LSSs with the parent vehicle LSS are schematically summarized in Fig. 1 for the individual IVA LSS and in Fig. 2 for the individual EVA LSS. These schematics pertain to interactions during normal use of the systems; for example, for EVA, during operations outside the spacecraft. Different conditions could apply during emergencies or backup situations. Recharges of self-contained EVA LSS and airlock operations are not covered in these figures.

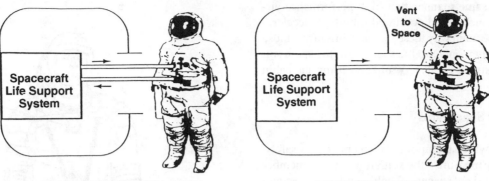

CLOSED VENTILATION LOOP

- Metabolic rate limited by available gas cooling
- Used for Gemini and Apollo Command Module Spacecraft EVA

OPEN VENTILATION LOOP

- High potential oxygen expenditure during EVA
- Used for Voskhod-2 EVA (Emergency Oxygen Umbilical)

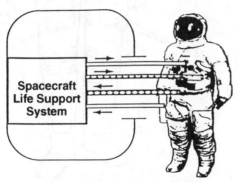

CLOSED VENTILATION AND WATER COOLING LOOPS

- Used for Apollo Lunar Module "Standup" EVA

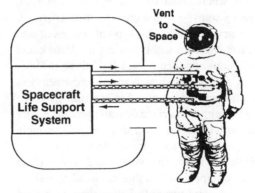

OPEN VENTILATION AND CLOSED WATER COOLING LOOPS

- Higher metabolic rate accommodated by both gas and water cooling
- Used for U.S. Skylab Space Station EVA

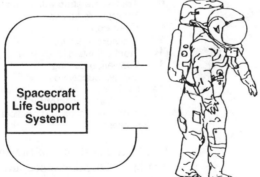

SELF-CONTAINED LIFE SUPPORT

- Used for emergency escape for U.S. Space Shuttle Orbiter
- Used for Apollo Lunar Surface and Shuttle Orbiter Spacecraft EVA
- Used for USSR Salyut and MIR Space Stations and Soyuz-4/5
- Planned use for USSR Shuttle Buran and U.S. Space Station Freedom

Fig. 2 Extravehicular individual life support systems.

A number of possible combinations have been implemented in actual flight systems. The proper selection of a schematic arrangement depends on the factors listed above.

III. Intravehicular Life Support Systems

The IVA LSS is used to provide life support in the event of vehicle failure. The system design is strongly driven by the interfaces with the vehicle and the kind of contingency for which protection is being provided. Both the U.S. and Russian (continuing the Soviet) programs have used the space suit subsystem of their early systems in both the IVA and EVA modes. As the programs matured, both countries moved away from this dual use and now have systems specifically designed for IVA use. The IVA systems of both programs use space suits that are similar to high-performance aircraft pressure suits, because the latter are designed to provide protection for similar problems, such as loss of cabin pressure. In addition, both systems may incorporate "g-suit" provisions to prevent pooling of blood in the lower body during return from orbit, in the same manner that high-performance aircraft suits prevent such blood pooling during high-acceleration maneuvers. The main way these systems differ from those used in aviation is that, onboard the spacecraft, the space suit worn in the pressurized cabin is ventilated using the cabin atmosphere.

A. Intravehicular Space Suits

The IVA suit provides an important element of crew safety. Unlike other safety measures, the suit allows a crewmember to stay in a depressurized spacecraft cabin under any vacuum conditions for a virtually unlimited period, dependent only upon available cabin LSS supplies. In addition, it can be used if the onboard spacecraft LSS fails, if the cabin atmospheric system malfunctions, when smoke and toxic gases are present, and during emergency transfer of the crew to another area of the vehicle or to a rescue vehicle. This type of space suit was first used to ensure cosmonaut safety during the Vostok and Project Mercury missions conducted from 1961 through 1963.

The IVA suit may also be designed to sustain crewmembers during launch or after orbital reentry for ejection from the spacecraft followed by either a surface or water landing. Other measures, such as inflatable flotation devices and portable radio station and signaling devices, are added to ensure crew safety after landing. In 1965, the Voskhod 2 and Project Gemini 4 IVA suits—equipped with a thermal insulating shell, helmet visor light filter, and portable LSS—were also used for EVA.

The multipurpose use of the IVA suits led to changes in their specifications, resulting in decreased reliability for EVA and unnecessary complexity for IVA. Therefore, both Russia and the United States implemented the use of two different types of space suit on Soyuz-Salyut, Soyuz-TM-Mir, and Space Shuttle spacecraft. A highly reliable reusable semi-rigid suit (using a hard upper torso) with a built-in (Russian) or integrated (U.S.) LSS was designed for EVA. This system is used pressurized almost exclusively and has a number of features that are not needed for IVA space suits. A lightweight, "soft-type" space suit was designed and custom made for each crewmember to wear during hazardous flight phases (launch, orbital insertion, orbital operations, reentry, and landing).

A space suit is worn during these hazardous flight phases under the assumption that rapid depressurization of the crew cabin may occur in two ways: accidentally, as the result of a mechanical problem; or deliberately, to evacuate the cabin atmosphere in the event of a fire. In all other cases, cabin depressurization is most likely to be slow and may, for example, be caused by depressurization at vehicle joints or from vehicular micrometeorite damage. If, at such time, crewmembers are not wearing space suits, or it is important to allow the cabin pressure to decrease to the lowest acceptable level, the crew must have sufficient time to don and pressurize the suits or to move to a safe area in the vehicle.

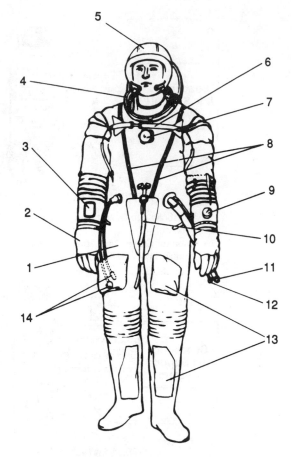

1	Shell of suit
2	Glove
3	Mirror
4	Helmet connector
5	Headset cap
6	Transverse strap with a spring hook
7	Pressure regulator
8	Front zippers
9	Pressure indicator
10	Front adjusting torso strap
11	Ventilation ducting
12	Oxygen supply hose
13	Pockets
14	Electrical connector for communications and medical sensors

Fig. 3   General view of the Soyuz-TM intravehicular space suit.

B. Soyuz-TM Spacecraft IVA Space Suit

A major feature of the IVA suit used in Soyuz vehicles is a "soft" nondetachable helmet with a folding manually closed visor (Fig. 3). The suit ensures the necessary compatibility with the shock-absorbing seat during acceleration (Fig. 4) and consists of a multilayer suit, individual built-in helmet, soft shoes, and quick-don gloves. It is designed for a comfortable sitting posture. In weightlessness, cosmonauts can don the suit in about 5 min.

The space suit shell is composed of restraint and pressure (inner) layers. The pressure layer is made of rubberized ny-

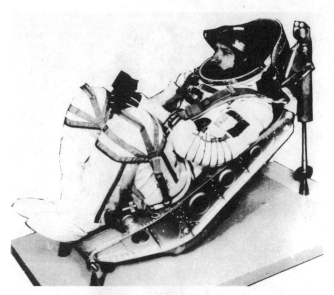

Fig. 4 Cosmonaut's posture in the Soyuz-TM shock absorbing seat.

lon and rubberized knitwear (part of the helmet and components of articulation joints). The suit is donned through a front opening tunnel made of pressure bladder material, which, when rolled and tied, is sealed. Adequate seal for pressurization is ensured by the use of two zippers and lacings located below the waistline. To provide mobility, the shell is outfitted with sealed wrist bearings, attachable gloves, and soft fabric joints for shoulder, elbow, and knee articulation. The adjustable strap at the front, as well as straps for adjusting arm and leg assemblies, is designed to keep suit size unaltered under excessive pressurization and to provide customized fit for each cosmonaut.

Air supplied to the suit from the onboard system (Fig. 5) in the pressurized cabin is fed through an external umbilical, then through separate ducts to the helmet, arms, and feet. In the event of cabin depressurization to 533.3 hPa (7.73 psia), an electropneumatic valve is activated by the vehicle automatic control unit, and oxygen is fed to the helmet from the onboard supply at a flow rate of 1.5 kg/h (3.3 lb/h).

When the cabin is depressurized, the suit is pressurized

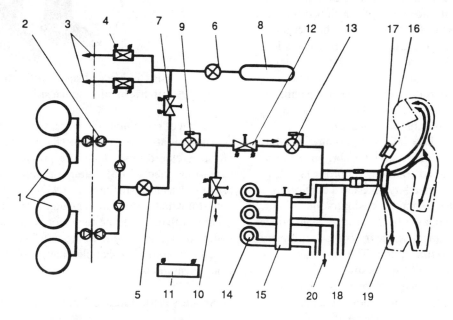

1	Primary oxygen supply located in a separable section of the space vehicle
2	Check valves (6 locations)
3	Jettisoning gas before landing
4	Electropneumatic valves
5,6	Manual valves
7,10,12	Controlled electropneumatic valves (7 is activated during separation of descent vehicle, 12 operates with loss of cabin pressure, 10 is used to compensate for a cabin leak)
8	Oxygen supply in the descent vehicle
9,13	Pressure regulator (first and second stages)
11	Automatic assembly with pressure relay
14	Fans
15	Distributive unit
16	Pressure suit
17	Pressure regulator of pressure suit
18	Group input of hoses
19	Distribution of ventilation
20	Ventilation and oxygen supply distribution to second and third pressure suits

Fig. 5 Diagram of the spacecraft life support system for the Soyuz TM space vehicle intravehicular spacesuit.

automatically by activating a pressure regulator, which maintains either one of two selected absolute pressure modes: 410.6 hPa or 262.6 hPa (5.95 psia or 3.81 psia). The pressure regulator is also used as a relief valve, which opens at a pressure of 466 hPa (6.76 psia) and as a suction valve supplying air from the atmosphere (in the event of ventilation or oxygen supply failure) at ambient pressure close to that on Earth (when the helmet is closed).

C. IVA Space Suit Designed for Buran

An IVA space suit and a closed-loop spacecraft LSS was designed for long-term survival in the event of cabin depressurization in the Buran. The space suit was designed to 1) be compatible with an ejection seat, 2) give maximum convenience and comfort with the suit at ventilation pressure level, 3) be easily donned and pressurized within 5–7 min, 4) minimize constraint on the cosmonaut's movements when worn in a pressurized cabin, 5) enable maximum ergonomic capabilities under peak work demands at nominal operational pressure, and 6) have fewer sizes while providing individual fit.

Like the Soyuz IVA suit, the space suit designed for the Shuttle Buran (Fig. 6) was to be "soft" with a helmet integrated into the upper torso, featuring the following major units: a pressure retention shell, an internal ventilation system, gloves, an external umbilical, a pressure regulator, a breathing valve, and a headset cap. A flotation device and a built-in parachute harness were to be included. The suit was to be donned over a special undergarment and a g-suit.

The shell was to contain three layers: a pressure restraint layer constructed using a "super modular" fabric made of a rigidly bonded polymer thread (durable fireproof layer), a pressure bladder layer (rubberized nylon), and a comfort lining. The lining was intended to make it easier to don the suit and to protect the rubberized layer from damage. Ventilation ducting and heat-resistant panels (made of woolen knitwear) were to be laced to the internal lining. The suit was to be donned similarly to the Soyuz TM space suit.

In contrast to the IVA suit designed for Soyuz, the parachute system of the Buran IVA suit incorporated a modified, mass-produced parachute harness. The shape of the suit shell and the availability of front and back torso straps for adjusting a cosmonaut's posture ensured compatibility with the ejection seat. The suit was to be manufactured in several sizes or custom made for each cosmonaut. Special pressure restraint strap adjusters were to be used to fit the suit for height. In the pressurized cabin, oxygen supply, thermal conditioning, and removal of carbon dioxide, moisture, and contaminants were controlled by an independent unit that would ventilate the suit with cabin atmosphere and then discharge back into the cabin.

In the event of cabin depressurization, the unit (Fig. 7) would automatically switch to a closed-loop mode, which would automatically purge the system and the suit with oxygen to change suit internal atmospheric composition. Once the process was completed, oxygen gas usage would become

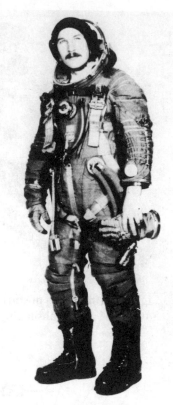

Fig. 6 View of the Shuttle Buran intravehicular space suit.

a function of consumption by cosmonauts and suit leakage.

The crew also would have had the capacity to switch manually to a closed-loop mode in a pressurized crew cabin in case of an onboard LSS failure or smoke in the cabin. Suit pressure was to be maintained by an onboard leakage compensator with the pressure regulator in the suit functioning as a safety valve. The same regulator would allow the cosmonaut to decrease pressure in the suit. The system was also to contain equipment to handle emergencies should any LSS component fail.

D. Space Shuttle Launch/Entry Suit (LES)

Starting in September 1988 (flight of STS-26), a suit that combined features of high-altitude flight suits and anti-g suits was used to protect crewmembers in emergencies on takeoff and landing (Figs. 8 and 9). The LES design is an integral part of the Crew Escape System, which allows airborne escape from the Shuttle in a situation where the craft is operational but unable to reach a landing field. The system also enhances the crewmember's ability to safely escape from a disabled Shuttle on the launch pad or elsewhere on the ground.

The environments of the upper atmosphere and space are hostile. One threat to a crewmember's safety during exposure to the upper atmosphere is the near vacuum pressure. Because of the danger of a sudden failure in cabin pressure and consequent explosive decompression at extreme altitudes, a counterpressure garment was developed and incorporated

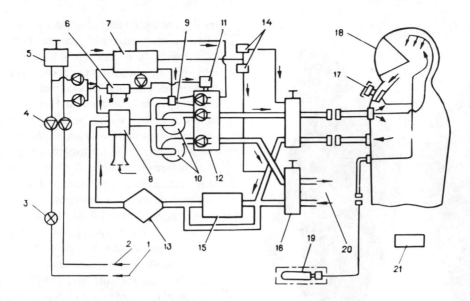

1,2 From standby and primary oxygen supply
3 Standby oxygen valve
4 Check valve
5 Remote manual control
6 Electropneumatic valve
7 Oxygen automatic unit
8 Pneumatic valve
9 Ejector
10 Primary and standby fans
11 Automatic purging unit
12 Valve unit
13 Cooling and drying unit

14 Compensators for pressure suit pressure drop
15 Carbon dioxide and impurities absorption unit
16 Valve to control ventilation and to isolate the suit from the system
17 Pressure regulator of pressure suit
18 Pressure suit
19 Unit for supplying oxygen after ejection
20 To second pressure suit
21 Pressure relay unit

Fig. 7 Diagram of spacecraft life support system for Buran IVA suit.

in the LES to provide high-altitude protection. The garment applies a direct mechanical counterpressure through a series of bladders positioned over the body.

The LES consists of a helmet and a counterpressure/ antiexposure suit integrated into one unit (Fig. 10). The unit provides the necessary protection to sustain the crewmember at or below 30,480 m (100,000 ft) altitude for approximately 40 min. The LES also includes a personal parachute assembly consisting of a parachute harness and parachute pack. An emergency oxygen system is attached to the crewmember by the harness assembly and provides 100 percent oxygen upon demand. The system can be used at any time during high-altitude bailout or ground egress and will provide a minimum of 10 min of oxygen at an average consumption rate of 37 liters (1.3 ft^3) per minute at sea level. Each of the system's two cylinders has a capacity of 0.98 liters (60 in^3) and is pressurized to 20.7 MPa (3000 psia) with 100 percent oxygen. High-pressure reducers mounted on top of the cylinders reduce the pressure from 20.7 MPa to 0.48 MPa (3000 to 70 psia). To activate the system, the crewmember pulls a "green apple" to allow the oxygen to flow to a suit-mounted breath-

ing regulator.

The parachute pack has an automatic opener, a pilot chute, a drogue chute, a main canopy, a personal life raft, a sea dye marker, and an emergency locator beacon, as shown in Fig. 11. When packed, the parachute pack measures 63.5 cm (25 inches) high, 43.2 cm (17 inches) wide, and 10.2 cm (4 inches) thick. This allows the parachute pack to replace previously used orbiter seat back cushions. The automatic opener is an aneroid sensing element preset for activation at 4267 meters (14000 feet) altitude. The drogue chute is employed to place the crewmember in a preferred feet-down orientation. The drogue chute controls the descent to 4267 meters (14,000 feet) and is extracted by a spring-loaded pilot chute. The main canopy is a modified 7.9-meter (26-foot) conical NB-6 U.S. Navy parachute.

The parachute harness has an automatic saltwater-initiated, parachute riser release system (SEAWARS) to protect the user from wind drag. The harness provides interfaces for the emergency oxygen system, escape pole lanyard, personal lowering device, personal flotation device, and a supply of drinking water.

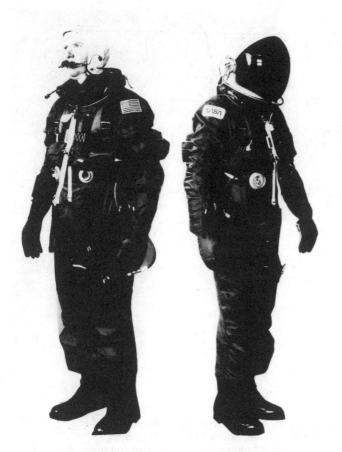

Fig. 8   View of the Space Shuttle launch/entry suit.

The personal flotation device is located on the harness and has automatic water-initiated inflation. The flotation device keeps an unconscious crewmember's head out of the water.

The personal life raft is a modified LRU-18 personal life raft and is located at the bottom of the parachute pack. The life raft provides the crewmember a comfortable, stable, highly visible, and sheltered platform for surviving the hazards of the sea. The raft is partially inflated automatically by water activation of the first CO2 cylinder. The floating crewmember can easily board the raft in its partially inflated condition by pushing one side into the water and sliding aboard. Once inside the raft, the crewmember can fully inflate it by manually activating a second CO_2 cylinder. Water in the raft can be removed using the bailing bag or hand pump assembly tethered to the raft. The high freeboard of the raft provides shelter, and an attached canopy affords additional protection from the weather.

Between the crewmember's back and the parachute pack is a 2-liter (67.63 oz) supply of drinking water. The water is contained in 16 packets distributed over the back surface area of the harness assembly.

The LES helmet is a dome-type full-pressure helmet consisting of a fiberglass shell fitted with a large movable visor and a connecting ring incorporating a bearing. The helmet is supported entirely about the shoulders by an adjustable formed wire support system, which allows complete freedom of head movement within the helmet. A lightweight "skull cap" communications carrier with integral buffet protection pads is worn inside the helmet. Thus, the nonconformal helmet system virtually eliminates headboard weight and stress caused by head movements. This helmet also includes an independently operated sunshade and an antisuffocation valve. To minimize helmet visor fogging, inflowing oxygen is directed by a spray bar and flows across the inside surface of the visor. Additionally, an antifogging compound is applied to the visor before every flight. The helmet pressure control system is referenced to suit pressure and delivers 100 percent oxygen on demand to maintain positive breathing pressure of approximately 2.5 hPa (1.0 in of H2O) above suit pressure while connected to the normal orbiter oxygen supply or the emergency oxygen system. Suit pressure is controlled by an aneroid-operated suit pressure controller designed to maintain a minimum suit pressure of 193 hPa (2.80 psia) absolute. A functional diagram of the LES is shown in Fig. 12.

Mobility of the LES is enhanced by minimizing bladder coverage over the joints of the body, leaving the joints relatively free of the restricting counterpressure and using link net restraint material at the neck and shoulder areas of the unit. The lower extremity bladder system is capable of independently providing protection against blood pooling caused by gravity during the reentry phase. The lightweight emergency pressure suit allows a crewmember to survive extremely low barometric pressures until reaching an optimum altitude for bailing out of the Shuttle.

To protect the crewmember from extreme cold and the hazards of a hostile environment, the "open areas" of the suit (areas not covered by pressure bladders) are sealed with a Gortex® material, thus making the garment a full-body dry suit, which provides cold atmosphere [-12.2 °C (10 °F)] ambient and cold water [7.2 °C (45 °F)] protection by ensuring that body heat loss is no greater than 0.14 °C (32.25 °F) per hour while in the life raft.

A helmet retention assembly (HRA) was developed to provide a way to use only the helmet while on orbit. Because the helmet retention system and pressure controls are suit mounted, the full-pressure helmet could not otherwise have been worn independently. The HRA provides for helmet retention and oxygen breathing without using the counterpressure/antiexposure suit, allowing the crewmembers to don the helmet for EVA prebreathe or on-orbit emergency operations (when it is necessary to breathe 100 percent orbiter-supplied oxygen).

Because the suit is a multilayered garment and may be worn for long periods of time, it can become uncomfortable from heat buildup. To overcome the heat buildup and provide thermal regulation during launch and reentry, a personal suit ventilation system is provided for each crewmember. It consists of a small centrifugal blower and a 28-V brushless DC motor operating from orbiter power. The unit fits into a 12.7-cm (5-in) square container, which is mounted to each crew seat. The system ventilates the suit with ambient cabin air at 169.9–283.2 liters (6–10 ft^3) per min.

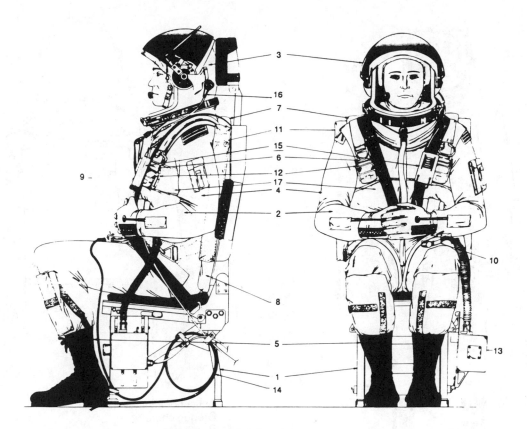

1	Mission specialist seat
2	Crewmember
3	Helmet
4	Antiexposure/counterpressure garment
5	Boots
6	Parachute harness
7	Parachute pack
8	Life raft with sea dye marker
9	Suit-mounted O_2 manifold
10	Anti-G suit controller
11	Emergency O_2 supply
12	Seawars
13	Ventilation fan
14	Orbiter O_2 line
15	Headset interface unit
16	Communication line to headset interface unit
17	Flotation device

Fig. 9   View of the Space Shuttle launch/entry suit.

IV. Extravehicular Life Support Systems

EVA LSSs are used to provide protection from the vacuum and thermal conditions of Earth orbit and lunar and planetary environments. Unlike individual IVA LSSs, EVA systems are designed for extended-duration missions to accomplish a given objective (e.g., study of planetary surface geology or orbital station repairs or maintenance). Because these systems are to be used for 6- to 8-hr work periods, pressurized mobility and dexterity are key design drivers. This contrasts to IVA systems where unpressurized mobility and longer term comfort drives design since pressurized operation is of limited duration in confined spaces (i.e., in a spacecraft couch).

EVA systems may require significant separation distances from the vehicle LSS, which requires the design of the individual LSS to provide for autonomy from the vehicle LSS, except for recharge. Both the U.S. and Russian space programs have matured to designs of individual EVA LSSs that are self-contained and dedicated for EVA use.

The EVA LSS designs implemented by both the U.S.S.R. (now Russian) and U.S. space programs have maintained an anthropomorphic space suit shape with a portable LSS mounted primarily on the back and controls and displays mounted on the front. Both programs have arrived at semi-rigid designs for the space suit as well. In a semirigid design, part of the suit is a rigid structure and part is a soft

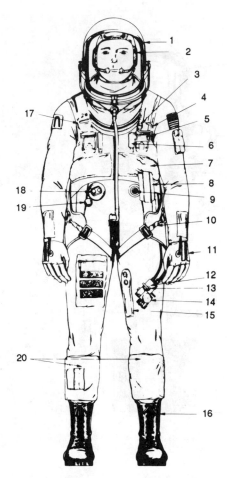

1   Helmet
2   Communications carrier (comm cap)
3   Parachute arming lanyard (red apple)
4   Rip cord handle (D-ring)
5   Upper parachute attach fittings (frost
     fittings)
6   Sea water activation release system
     (seawars)
7   Life preserver unit (LPU)
8   Carabiner
9   Suit ventilator valve
10   Lower parachute attach fittings (ejector snaps)
11   Suit gloves
12   Suit oxygen manifold
13   Suit oxygen on/off valve
14   G-suit controller valve
15   Shroud cutter
16   Boots
17   Pole lanyard attach ring (harness ring)
18   Suit controller valve
19   Emergency O_2 system activation
     lanyard (green apple)
20   Survival gear
     • survival radio
     • signal mirror
     • chem lights
     • pen gun flare kit
     • smoke flare
     • motion sickness pills

**Fig. 10 General view of the Shuttle
orbiter launch/entry suit.**

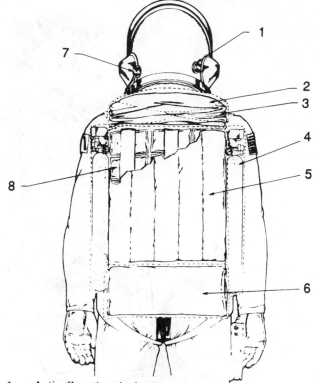

1   Antisuffocation device
2   Drogue chute
3   Pilot chute
4   Emergency oxygen system
5   Parachute pack   • automatic opener
                       • main canopy
                       • locator beacon
6   Life raft (LRU-18) • sea dye marker
7   Radio communication line (to headset interface unit)
8   Emergency water supply

**Fig. 11 Shuttle orbiter launch/
entry suit parachute pack.**

structure. Both the U.S. and Russian designs incorporate hard upper torsos and helmets and soft lower torsos, legs, boots, arms, and gloves. While retaining these features, designers from the different programs have arrived at different entry methods.

A. Salyut, Mir, and Buran EVA Suits

As early as the 1960s, Soviet scientists developed the concept of a semirigid space suit for potential use on lunar missions and EVA. The semirigid design used for orbital stations Salyut and Mir was optimal for meeting U.S.S.R. EVA requirements.

First worn by G. Grechko and Y. Romanenko in 1977, the semirigid suit included a suit pressurized shell and portable life support system (PLSS) (Fig. 13). The main feature of this suit is the hard metallic torso with an integral nondetachable helmet. The lower torso and arm assemblies were made of soft elastic materials. The cosmonaut could step into the suit through its rear hatch (Fig. 14). The main

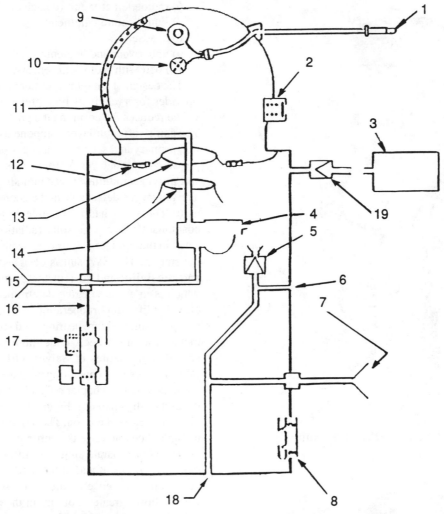

1	Radio communications electrical cable	11	Oxygen delivery spray bar
2	Antisuffocation valve	12	Exhalation valve (2 ea)
3	Gloves	13	Breathing compartment neck seal
4	Breathing regulator	14	Inner blade neck seal
5	Helmet vent check valve	15	Oxygen supply inlet
6	Arm openings	16	Coverall gas container
7	Ventilation gas inlet	17	Pressure controller (dual system)
8	Relief valve	18	Leg openings
9	Earphone (2 ea)	19	Glove inflation valve
10	Microphone (2 ea)		

Fig. 12 Diagram of the Shuttle Orbiter launch/entry space suit.

portion of the PLSS was mounted on the inside of the rear door, and controls and indicators were mounted on the front of the rigid torso of the EVA system.

The semirigid structure offered important advantages over other existing designs, namely:

1) small dimensions of the pressurized torso;

2) simplicity of operation and high safety and reliability resulting from elimination of external lines connecting the PLSS with the suit (PLSS in pressurized portion of suit);

3) the ability to use a single-size space suit for cosmonauts of different sizes; and

4) the simplicity of replacing components and conducting repairs, because of easily accessible locations of major LSS

units inside a pressurized suit.

The design for "ingressing" the suit has proved to be extremely effective; a trained cosmonaut can don and pressurize the suit unassisted in 2–3 min.

The EVA suit used on Salyut and Mir includes the following major components:.

1) rigid upper part of the suit with helmet and control panels;

2) hatch to the suit containing autonomous LSS;

3) soft lower part of the suit shell, including the lower torso and boots;

4) soft arms with gloves;

5) vacuum-shield thermal insulation suit;

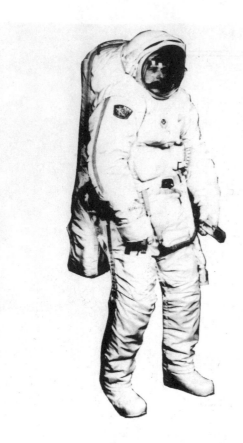

Fig. 13 Mir Orlan DMA EVA suit.

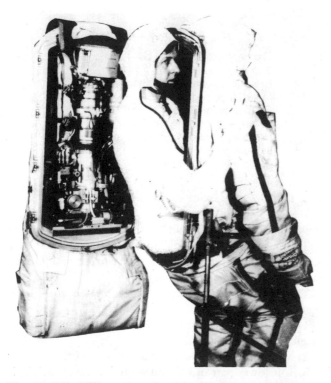

Fig. 14 Mir EVA space suit with an open entry door.

6) radiotelemetry unit (detachable);

7) liquid cooling garment;

8) headset;

9) underwear and hygienic shield; and

10) belt with biological sensors.

The design of the semirigid suit used on Mir (Orlan-DMA) provides for a relatively high pressure of 400 hPa (5.8 psia), which reduces the cosmonaut's prebreathe time before EVA. The suit's soft multilayer components include a comfort lining, primary and secondary airtight pressure bladders, and a pressure restraint layer. A protective shell worn over the space suit provides multilayer, vacuum-shield, thermal insulation. The gloves are detachable and custom made for each cosmonaut. The visor has a movable light filter to protect the cosmonaut's face from solar radiation. The main frame located in the rigid torso is used to secure the EVA suit onboard the station. The EVA suit is designed to ensure high safety and reliability and sustain the cosmonaut's performance, which is to a great degree determined by suit mobility and effective life support operation.

Space suit pressure bearings and soft joints enable the cosmonauts to move freely under high pressure. Table 2 shows articulation features of Salyut (Orlan-D) and Mir (Orlan-DMA) EVA suits at operating pressures of 400 hPa (5.8 psia). (Note that, in this chapter only, all of the tables are located at the end of the chapter.) Figure 15 diagrams cosmonaut mobility and range of motion. The mobility parameters presented in Table 2 characterize the entire multilayer assembly rather than that of a separate joint. The difference between the joints in the Orlan-D suit and in the modified DMA suit is the reduced circumference of the space suit shell's lower torso, which allows greater mobility in the airlock and easier passage through the hatch. (The space suit's mobility in the leg area is decreased, but the cosmonaut's work capacity in weightlessness is not impeded.)

The use of the space suit by a wider range of on-orbit based cosmonauts necessitated an increase in the diameter of the arm and glove-connector assembly, thus reducing the articulation of the elbow joint. The length of the elastic shell for the limb and the lower torso is adjusted on orbit by the cosmonaut. The suit components that can be damaged and cause depressurization are backed up: double visors and two pressure bladders are used in soft suit elements, with the secondary pressure bladder being activated automatically if the primary one fails. During normal operation of the space suit, the secondary bladder is not pressurized, since the intrashell space is joined with the inner part of the suit through ports, which are closed by aneroid valves (when the primary shell is depressurized). Connectors and movable joints of the suit (suit entry hatch and shoulder pressure bearing) are double-sealed (Fig. 16). Component joints, metal welded seams, and other critical spots on the suit are additionally protected with sealing fabric or rubber glue-on patches. In addition, the design of the suit allows for the replacement of damaged or worn-out soft portions (arm and leg assemblies) onboard the orbital station. Arm assemblies are replaced where they are

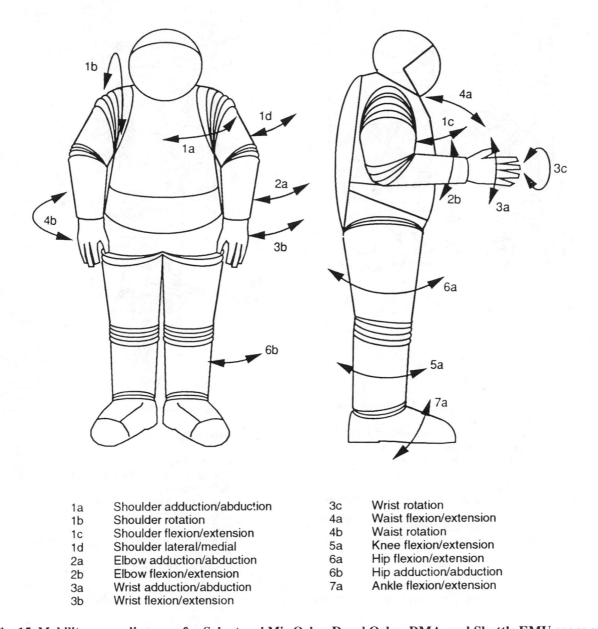

1a	Shoulder adduction/abduction	3c	Wrist rotation
1b	Shoulder rotation	4a	Waist flexion/extension
1c	Shoulder flexion/extension	4b	Waist rotation
1d	Shoulder lateral/medial	5a	Knee flexion/extension
2a	Elbow adduction/abduction	6a	Hip flexion/extension
2b	Elbow flexion/extension	6b	Hip adduction/abduction
3a	Wrist adduction/abduction	7a	Ankle flexion/extension
3b	Wrist flexion/extension		

Fig. 15 Mobility range diagrams for Salyut and Mir Orlan-D and Orlan-DMA, and Shuttle EMU space suits.

joined at the pressure bearing, leg assemblies at the joint with the rigid upper torso. This feature contributes to the on-orbit life of the suit and simplifies tailoring of fit for each cosmonaut.

Gloves are the most vulnerable suit component. The problem of suit depressurization caused by glove damage has been addressed by introducing pressure-sealing arm cuffs, which are activated if glove pressure drops. The 15 min of pressurization provided allow the cosmonaut time to return to the station.

The outer insulation layer of the EVA suit is designed to minimize heat exchange with the space environment. The thermal protection shell consists of five layers of aluminized Mylar® film insulated from each other by a mesh layer and an outer material made of phenilon (a woven Nomex® fiber fabric) having the following characteristics: solar absorptiv-

ity $\alpha_s = 0.38$, emissivity $\varepsilon = 0.9$. The maximum calculated heat loss from the thermal protection shell is no more than 139.5 W (476.2 Btu/h), whereas the heat gain is less than 93 W (317.4 Btu/h). The protection layers of the EVA suit help to prevent it from depressurizing from penetration by space particles.

B. EVA Portable Life Support System for Salyut, Mir, and Buran

A closed-loop PLSS provides the required microclimate inside the Russian EVA suits (Fig. 17). The PLSS features an oxygen supply unit with a pressure regulator; a ventilation and atmosphere regulation unit; a system of thermal regulation; and power equipment, controls, and monitoring devices.

Under normal conditions, the oxygen system provides a

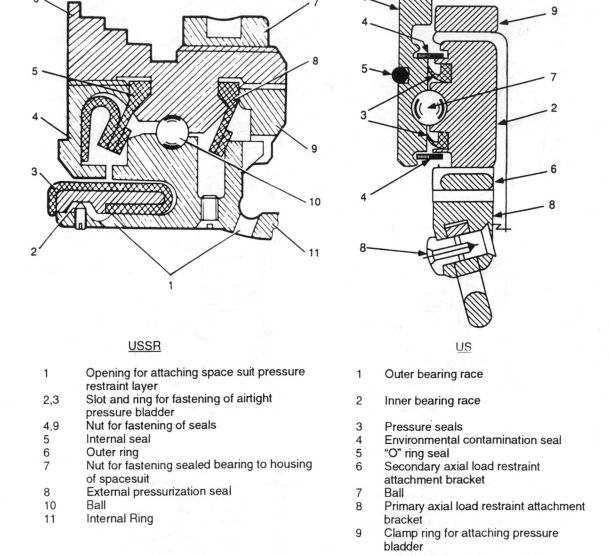

<table>
<tr><td colspan="2"><u>USSR</u></td></tr>
<tr><td>1</td><td>Opening for attaching space suit pressure restraint layer</td></tr>
<tr><td>2,3</td><td>Slot and ring for fastening of airtight pressure bladder</td></tr>
<tr><td>4,9</td><td>Nut for fastening of seals</td></tr>
<tr><td>5</td><td>Internal seal</td></tr>
<tr><td>6</td><td>Outer ring</td></tr>
<tr><td>7</td><td>Nut for fastening sealed bearing to housing of spacesuit</td></tr>
<tr><td>8</td><td>External pressurization seal</td></tr>
<tr><td>10</td><td>Ball</td></tr>
<tr><td>11</td><td>Internal Ring</td></tr>
</table>

<table>
<tr><td colspan="2"><u>US</u></td></tr>
<tr><td>1</td><td>Outer bearing race</td></tr>
<tr><td>2</td><td>Inner bearing race</td></tr>
<tr><td>3</td><td>Pressure seals</td></tr>
<tr><td>4</td><td>Environmental contamination seal</td></tr>
<tr><td>5</td><td>"O" ring seal</td></tr>
<tr><td>6</td><td>Secondary axial load restraint attachment bracket</td></tr>
<tr><td>7</td><td>Ball</td></tr>
<tr><td>8</td><td>Primary axial load restraint attachment bracket</td></tr>
<tr><td>9</td><td>Clamp ring for attaching pressure bladder</td></tr>
</table>

Fig. 16 Cross section of space suit shoulder pressure bearings and seals.

crewmember oxygen for breathing, using two redundant oxygen pressure regulators having pressure control settings at 392 hPa and 265 hPa (5.7 psia and 3.8 psia). These regulators provide oxygen, as needed; i.e., proportionally to a pressure drop inside the suit. The supply of oxygen to a crewmember can be initiated manually using the ejector built into the ventilation assembly and located on the helmet's gas inflow duct. The ejector can be used to 1) maintain EVA suit pressure during depressurization, 2) provide closed-loop air circulation if both ventilators or the power supply fails, 3) sustain an acceptable level of CO_2 in the helmet if a CO_2 control cartridge fails, by purging the suit with pure oxygen at a flow rate of 1 kg/h (2.2 lb/h), and 4)improve thermal conditions if the thermal regulating system fails.

Additionally, a separate oxygen system is available for the Orlan-DM and DMA designs. This system can be used during the nominal situations and the contingencies listed above, allowing continuous oxygen flow into the individual LSS.

The cosmonaut manually activates the emergency oxygen supply from a backup system. If the pressure of the individual LSS drops below 220 hPa (3.2 psia), the emergency oxygen supply is automatically activated by pressure regulators and supplies a maximum of 3 kg/h (6.6 lb/h) operating together with an emergency supply activated manually.

Internal ventilation is necessary to maintain the gaseous atmosphere composition of the space suit within acceptable limits. The gas flow removes some human metabolic products (carbon dioxide, contaminants, humidity) and, partially, heat. To support closed-loop ventilation, a sealed electric motor drives a centrifugal fan. The system has two fans: primary and secondary. If the primary fan does not operate, the secondary fan turns on automatically. In special cases, the design provides for simultaneous use of two fans. The increase in the gas flow rate can compensate for a malfunction in the water cooling system or reduce helmet fogging potential during work in the shade.

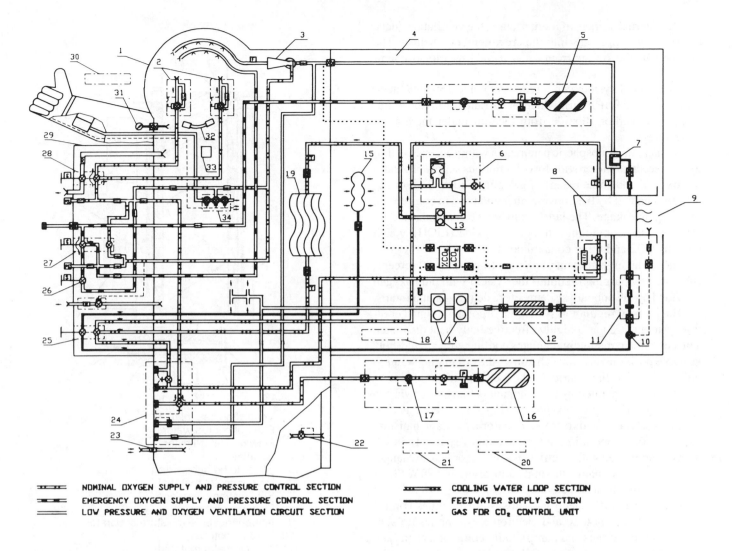

NOMINAL OXYGEN SUPPLY AND PRESSURE CONTROL SECTION
EMERGENCY OXYGEN SUPPLY AND PRESSURE CONTROL SECTION
LOW PRESSURE AND OXYGEN VENTILATION CIRCUIT SECTION

COOLING WATER LOOP SECTION
FEEDWATER SUPPLY SECTION
GAS FOR CO_2 CONTROL UNIT

1 Pressure suit
2 Pressure regulators in pressure suit
3 Ejector
4 Internal cavity of back part of suit
5 Standby oxygen reserve tank
6 Hydro accumulator with gas bubble separator
7 Moisture separator
8 Heat exchanger
9 Vapor venting into vacuum of space
10 Regulator
11 Flow rate filter-limiter
12 CO_2 absorption cartridge
13 Water pump
14 Primary and standby fans
15 Water supply tank
16 Primary oxygen supply tank
17 Regulator
18 Electroautomatic monitoring units control
   and medical equipment
19 Liquid cooling suit
20 Self-contained electrical power supply

21 Radiotelemetry system and antenna feeder unit
22 Valve to activate standby airtight pressure bladder
23 Relief valve
24 Communications connector
25 Water temperature control valve and water supply
   switch to the heat exchanger
26 Standby oxygen reserve supply handle
27 Actuator for switching on ejector and emergency
   oxygen supply
28 Pressure conditions mode switch
29 Pneumohydraulic systems control panel
30 Electrical control and monitoring panel
31 Pressure gauge for control of pressure in suit
32 Medical sensors belt
33 Radio communication headset

In case EMU and Orbital Station
communication is maintained through
as EVA umbilical, numbers 20 and 21
may not be engaged.

Fig. 17 Diagram of Orbital Station Mir EMU life support system.

The internal surface of a suit secures the ventilation ducts. These ducts supply gas into the crewmember's helmet. The gas reenters the system from the arm and lower torso assemblies.

The level of system ventilation is equal to 150 ± 25 liters/min (5.30 ± 0.9 ft^3/min), which is sufficient to remove humidity and carbon dioxide from the suit under the highest work rates.

To maintain atmospheric parameters within acceptable limits, it is necessary to provide for a continuous supply of breathing oxygen and some means of gas purification. The former is both breathed by the crewmember and used to compensate for oxygen leakage. The latter includes the contaminant control cartridge containing lithium hydroxide (LiOH), which absorbs CO2 and other contaminants.

The initial high content of oxygen (more than 90 percent) is created by purging (venting) the system with pure oxygen provided by the onboard system before denitrogenation starts.

The thermal regulation system incorporates a liquid cooling system (LCS) as a highly effective body heat dissipater. The cosmonaut manually regulates cooling with a "cold-hot" variable position valve, which allows the circulating water to either bypass or flow through a heat exchanger.

Moisture generated by a cosmonaut is transported via circulating gas to the heat exchanger (Fig. 18) where it is condensed and channeled to the sublimator by a static moisture separator for evaporation in the vacuum of space. The LCS garment combined with an efficient sublimator/heat exchanger ensures the cosmonaut's thermal equilibrium to 698 W (2381 Btu/h) during physical activity.

The space suit's electrical subsystem includes control panel, electrical motors, and electronic assemblies (to support operation of fans and pump), radio communications and telemetric devices, sensors and regulators, power supply, cables, etc. The design provides a choice of two sources of power supply. The first option (Orlan-D and -DM) takes advantage of the orbital station's electrical power. The electricity reaches the cosmonaut through a 25-m (82-ft) umbilical cable, which also supports radio communications and transmission of the telemetry data. Orlan-DMA allows a cosmonaut to conduct autonomous operations. Here, the cosmonaut is provided an independent power supply and radiotelemetry and antenna units. Table 3 cites the parameters of the independent power supply unit.

The communication system of the space suit includes the headset, antenna-feeder, and transceivers located in the self-contained life support assembly. The system provides two-way semiduplex radio communication between two EVA crewmembers and with the radio station onboard the orbital station, which has communication capability to Earth.

The transceiver houses two units—primary and backup. The electric power supply to the radio station and activation of the backup unit are controlled from the suit control panel. Transceivers are activated either by voice or a "push-to-talk" switch.

The headset contains two earphones, two microphones,

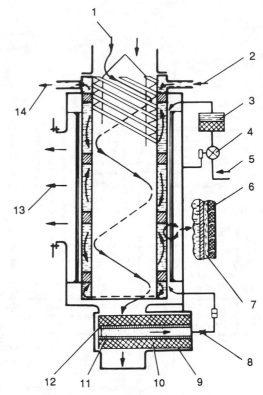

1   Ventilation gas inlet
2   Entry of cooled water
3   Flow rate filter-limiter
4   Regulator
5   Water to be sublimated
6   Porous metal material
7   Sublimation clearance
8   Flow rate orifice
9   Interchangeable moisture separator
10 Porous material
11 Porous metal material
12 Wick material
13 Exit of vapor into vacuum
14 Exit of cooled water

Fig. 18 Diagram of Mir EVA suit sublimator/heat exchanger with a moisture separator.

and an amplifier.

The operation of the individual LSS is monitored by a set of sensors and caution and warning (C&W) units, with telemetry transmitted to Earth; major parameters are also displayed on the suit display.

In addition to the controls of the electrical subsystem, various switches control pneumatic and hydraulic subsystems. Some of these switches perform multiple functions. For example, one can be used either as a sublimator ON switch or as a switch to control heat removal. Similarly, another can be used either to activate an emergency oxygen supply or as an ejector ON switch.

The display module shows the oxygen pressure in the actuated primary or secondary tank, voltage, and C&W signals. C&W signals indicate low pressure in space suit and oxygen tanks, drop of ventilation flow, and ON position of the injector switch. The design provides redundant output of these signals to helmet-mounted light-emitting diode (LED) displays.

The telemetry parameters include the gas pressures, temperature of liquid cooling and ventilation gas, ventilation flow, content of CO_2 inside the suit, and C&W signals. The telemetry system transmits (downloads) this data to the control center on the ground.

C. Operational Modifications of U.S.S.R. Suits

A number of modifications have been made to the semirigid suit during the period of its use on Salyut and Mir. On Salyut, the Orlan-DM space suit assembly was connected with the onboard systems by an umbilical containing power supply, radio communication lines, and lines for transmitting telemetric data on suit performance and cosmonaut medical status. This configuration ensured high reliability of electric and radio equipment. Additionally, the umbilical served as another tether in case the cosmonaut accidentally broke away from the station. Connection with the spacecraft through an umbilical is acceptable during work on the orbital station in the vicinity of the airlock.

For Mir, the suit underwent major modifications. Its period of operation was increased to 6 h, and several basic design changes were made. In contrast to the Salyut space suit, the Mir suit (Orlan-DMA) can operate without being connected by the umbilical to onboard systems. This major difference was achieved by adding a special portable unit containing a power supply and radiotelemetric and antenna feeder units. The antenna is an integral part of the suit's outer protection layer. The modified suit also has sealing cuffs to back up the gloves and a capability for replacement of arm and leg assemblies.

A number of other suit components have also been modified (e.g., increased water tank volume of simpler design, new components for better suit compatibility with a manned maneuvering unit).

It was planned to use an Orlan-DMA suit (the type used on Mir) for the Shuttle Buran. This suit was to be compatible with Buran's operational requirements, including short-term orbital exposure.

The location of major PLSS assemblies in the pack and the fact that they share a pressurized area with a suit provides a number of advantages in terms of torso dimensions, safety, and reliability. Connections between internal units, as well as between the PLSS and other EVA suit units, are simpler; the number of units exposed to the vacuum is smaller; thermal conditions are more favorable; and units are easily detachable. A major disadvantage of the airtight pack is that some of its assemblies operate in an almost pure oxygen environment. To alleviate associated risks, special fire safety measures are provided. In addition to the measures and designs described, high safety and reliability of an EVA suit and PLSS are achieved by including redundant basic life support subsystems and components.

The pressure layer, elements of the oxygen supply system, ventilation fan, radio communications system, electrical wiring, space suit and system pressurizing components have redundant backups. A fully self-contained emergency oxygen supply system is available and capable of compensating (for up to 25 min) for excessive leaks from the suit and backing up ventilation and thermal regulation systems (including cases of electrical power failure).

To increase the safety and reliability of the EVA suit, certain easily replaceable components (having a limited service life) must be changed and major suit systems must be routinely maintained and tested before each EVA. The replaceable components include the main oxygen tank, carbon dioxide absorbing cartridge, moisture separator, water flow rate limiter to the heat exchanger, and space suit gloves.

D. U.S. Shuttle Extravehicular Mobility Unit Space Suit

The original design of the Space Shuttle included a "shirtsleeve" cabin environment, which precluded the need for all crewmembers to wear an IVA space suit to protect against loss of cabin pressure. This approach permitted the space suit and LSS to be integrated into an EMU optimized solely for EVA.

The Shuttle EMU was first used during the STS-6 mission, when EVA was performed by Astronauts S. Musgrave and D. Peterson in 1983. This EMU included a suit with a "hard" fiberglass upper torso; "soft" arms; gloves; lower torso; legs and boots; and a detachable, bubble-shaped helmet. The PLSS was mounted to the back of the hard upper torso with manual controls and displays mounted on the front (Figs. 19 and 20). The astronauts donned the lower torso first and then donned the upper torso through a waist entry opening. This arrangement had the following features:

1) conformal fit of the hard upper torso;

2) increased safety and reliability, since all ventilation loop gas and cooling water plumbing between the suit and PLSS are internal;

3) a minimum number of upper torso sizes required to provide excellent suit fit;

4) maintenance access to almost all active PLSS components without disassembly of the PLSS from the hard upper torso;

5) minimum front-to-back dimension required to access the flight deck through the orbiter inner deck access hatch openings; and

6) minimum spacecraft airlock volume necessary for stowage and EMU donning.

This design for ingressing the suit has proved to be effective. Donning time and difficulty are minimal for trained astronauts.

The Shuttle EMU space suit assembly has the following features:

1) hard upper torso and arms—the portion of the pressure suit above the waist, excluding the gloves and helmet;

2) lower torso assembly—the portion of the pressure suit

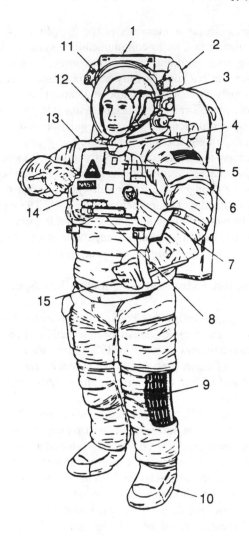

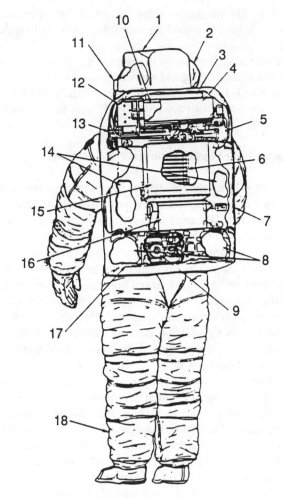

1 TV Camera
2 EV lights
3 Radio communications headset
4 Insuit drink bag
5 Connection for service and cooling
   umbilical
6 MMU mount
7 Temperature control valve
8 O_2 control actuator
9 Liquid cooling and ventilation garment
10 Boots
11 Extravehicular visor assembly
12 Helmet
13 Hard upper torso
14 Display and control module
15 Gloves

Fig. 19 Shuttle EMU components (front).

1 TV Camera
2 EV lights
3 Antenna
4 Muffler
5 Fan/separator/pump/motor assembly
6 H_2O tank
7 Primary life support subsystem
8 Secondary O_2 tanks
9 O_2 regulators
10 Radio
11 EV lights
12 Caution and warning computer
13 Sublimator
14 Primary O_2 tasks
15 CO_2/contaminant control cartridge
16 Battery
17 Secondary oxygen supply
18 Lower torso assembly

Fig. 20 Shuttle EMU components (back).

below the hard upper torso including the waist, legs, and boots;

3) helmet/visor assembly—the portion of the pressure suit providing pressure protection for the head; visibility; and impact, light glare, and thermal protection;

4) communications carrier assembly—a cap worn under the pressure suit helmet to position and hold redundant earphones and microphones;

5) liquid cooling and vent garment (LCVG)—a garment worn under the space suit with attached tubes to provide circulation of cooling water and suction return of gas ventilation flow at the arms and feet;

6) disposable absorption collection trunk—a device to collect and retain the female crewmember's urine;

7) urine collection device—a device to collect and retain

the male crewmember's urine; and

8) operational bioinstrumentation system—instrumentation to monitor the crewmember's heart rate during EVA.

1. Mobility Features

The purpose of a pressurized suit is to maintain the crewmember at a safe pressure while providing the necessary range of body motions and dexterity for useful work with minimal energy expenditure and fatigue.

Most approaches to suit joint design for two-axis motion (i.e., flexion/extension or adduction/abduction) have been "soft" fabric, flat-pattern constructed joints (Fig. 21).

Flat-pattern "soft joints" have been selected over "hard joints" because they can be overflexed without bruising the crewmember. These joints have no "hard" limits in range. Flat-pattern "soft joints" also were selected over other hybrid joint types (such as rolling convoluted and toroidal types) because they are lighter, smaller, less expensive to manufacture, and collapsible, requiring less stowage volume.

Axial restraint webbing carries longitudinal suit structural loads and prevents axial growth of the joint under pressure. When the joint is bent or flexed, restraint lines follow the angle of the joint, allowing inside fabric elements to be compressed while outside fabric elements extend. This maintains the joint at nearly constant volume, minimizing the work to compress the gas within the joint while bending. This also provides a neutral range of stability while bent; i.e., once bent, the joint stays in the desired position with minimal application of force.

The Shuttle EMU suit design emphasizes upper body mobility; leg mobility is less important, since the legs serve mainly to locate and hold the body in a comfortable position for working and for crewmember restraint while positioned in EVA foot restraints.

Tactility is the ability to feel forces and shapes through the suit and is primarily essential in the gloves. The most desirable features of gloves are snug fit without pressure points or discomfort and low-torque finger, thumb, and wrist joints to allow long periods of work with minimum hand fatigue. Gloves are made in standard sizes and are custom made to individual astronaut hands when standard sizes are not adequate.

2. Redundancy Features

Two sets of axial structural load restraint webbing and attachment brackets are provided for each limb (one primary set and one secondary set). One set consists of two webbings located on each side of the limbs.

Pressure bearings at the shoulders, upper arms, gloves, and waist are designed to include dual seals for pressure retention. Provisions allow each seal to be leak-checked on the ground during preflight checkout. A diagram of the Shuttle EMU suit shoulder pressure bearing is shown in Fig. 16.

The Shuttle EMU design includes a thermal and microme-

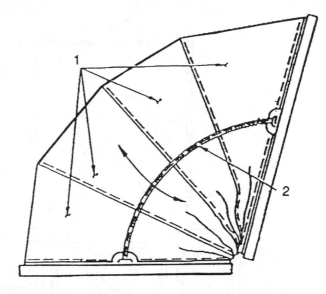

Developed flat pattern sections are gore-shaped

1 Flexible, flat pattern sections
2 Neutral axis restraint

Fig. 21 Shuttle EMU suit "soft" flat-pattern joint.

teoroid garment (TMG), which provides protection from spaceborne particles and a thermal environment temperature range between 113 and -118 °C (235 and -180 °F). The TMG is constructed of seven layers of coated and uncoated fabrics. Between the outer and inner layers are five plies of aluminized Mylar® film. The outermost ply is a woven fabric blend of Gortex®, Teflon®, Kevlar®, and Nomex® fibers. The fabric exhibits the following characteristics: solar absorptivity $\alpha_s = 0.18$, emissivity $\varepsilon = 0.84$. The maximum calculated heat loss from the TMG in a typical cold orbital environment is no greater than 130 W (444 Btu/h). Similarly, the maximum heat gain in a typical hot orbital environment is 88 W (300 Btu/h). The innermost TMG material layer is a neoprene-coated ripstop nylon fabric. The energy-absorbing characteristics of this layer, together with other TMG material layers, prevent micrometeorites from penetrating the suit pressure bladder.

E. U.S. Shuttle EMU Portable Life Support System

The PLSS is a closed-loop assembly that, under nominal conditions, supplies the crewmember oxygen for breathing, ventilation, and pressurization and water for cooling. This system is shown in Fig. 22. In conjunction with a space suit, it provides the following functions to support EVA:

1) maintains necessary suit pressure;

2) provides breathable oxygen supply;

3) removes CO_2, trace contaminants, and odor;

4) controls humidity;

5) provides adequate thermal regulation, removing both metabolic and equipment heat;

6) provides adequate gas ventilation flow to remove ex-

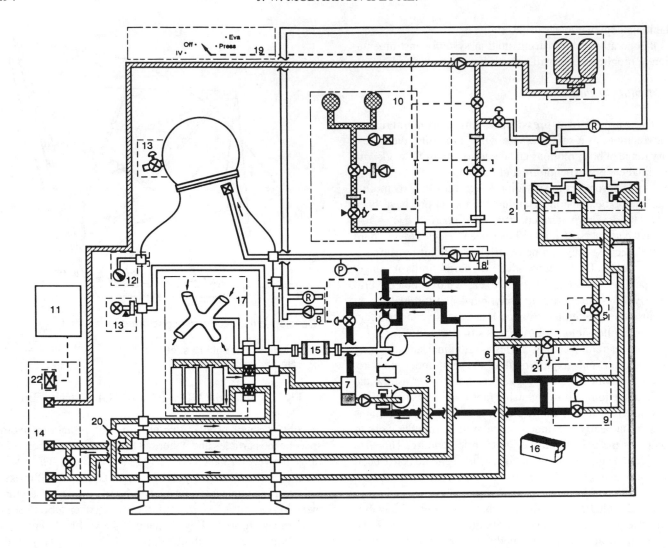

Oxygen Ventilating Circuit
Feedwater Curcuit
Liquid Transport Circuit
Condensate Circuit
Primary Oxygen Circuit
Secondary Oxygen Curcuit

1   Primary oxygen supply
2   Primary pressure control module
3   Fan/water pump/water separator assembly
4   Water storage tanks
5   Feedwater regulator
6   Sublimator/heat exchanger
7   Gas trap
8   Suit positive and negative pressure relief valves
9   Water controls
10   Emergency oxygen supply system
11   Electrical controls and display

12   Suit pressure gauge
13   Redundant gas purge valves
14   Common multiple connector
15   Contaminant control cartridge
16   Battery
17   Liquid cooling ventilation garment
18   Vent flow sensor
19   Four-position oxygen control
20   Cooling control valve
21   Feedwater valve
22   Power and communications connector

Fig. 22   Diagram of Shuttle EMU portable life support system.

pired CO_2 from the helmet;

7) provides an electrical power source; and

8) provides system control, monitoring, warnings, and communications.

Design considerations for selection of the normal operating pressure include

1) decompression sickness (bends) prevention, which depends upon the starting pressure of the spacecraft cabin and the final total suit pressure;

2) maximum suit mobility, especially glove dexterity, which requires suit pressure to be kept to a minimum;

3) minimum suit pressure requiring 100 percent oxygen gas concentration (minimum dilutant gas). Normoxic oxygen level established minimum nominal suit pressure at 255 hPa (3.7 psia) partial pressure of O_2 for 100 percent O_2; and

4) oxygen toxicity levels set maximum suit pressure for 100 percent oxygen gas composition; i.e., 413 hPa (6.0 psia) for continuous exposure or 689 hPa (10 psia) for up to 18-h exposure every 120 h.

The normal suit pressure is set at 297 hPa (4.3 psia). The primary oxygen regulator overrides the secondary regulator during normal operation, since it is preset to operate at a higher pressure than the secondary regulator.

The operating bands of both regulators are separated by 34.5 hPa (0.5 psia) minimum so that pressure-monitoring instruments, with error bands, can determine (unambiguously) which regulator is controlling suit pressure. The primary oxygen regulator band is 297 ± 7 hPa (4.3 ± 0.1 psia) over a flow range of 0.009–0.150 kg/h (0.02–0.33 lb/h) oxygen and a supply pressure range of 0.45–7.24 MPa (65–1050 psia).

An emergency backup system is required to provide minimum suit pressure, helmet CO_2 removal, ventilation flow, and some body cooling. This secondary backup system is a purge flow system. The secondary O_2 regulator band is centered on 238 hPa (3.45 psia) and maintains suit pressure at 230–269 hPa (3.34–3.90 psia). The system will automatically activate in the event of pressure falling to the secondary oxygen regulation level.

The primary oxygen supply contains 0.54 kg (1.2 lb) of usable oxygen stored at 6.2 ± 0.3 MPa (900 ± 50 psia). The system is rechargeable from the orbiter oxygen supply system. The emergency oxygen supply is sized to maintain the suit at the emergency pressure over the flow range of 0–2.4 kg/h (0–5.26 lb/h) O_2 and a supply pressure range of 2.5–51.0 MPa (365–7400 psia). It supplies about 30 min of emergency oxygen at a flow rate of approximately 2.3 kg/h (5 lb/h) or 1 h of oxygen at 1.1 kg/h (2.5 lb/h), depending on which of two available purge orifices is manually selected by the EVA astronaut. The emergency oxygen supply contains 1.2 kg (2.6 lb) of oxygen and is not rechargeable by the orbiter.

An important function of the LSS is the removal of expired CO_2 from the suit environment. Studies have shown that even moderate increases in the CO_2 level in the bloodstream cause varying physiological reactions, ranging from increased heart and respiration rates, mental depression, headaches, dizziness, and nausea (at lower concentrations), to

mental stupor and finally unconsciousness (at higher concentrations). Both concentration level and duration of exposure are factors in determining the allowable maximum limits of CO_2 under normal conditions. Because of hardware and software monitoring capabilities, NASA medical personnel have set the helmet allowable limits for U.S. space-flight conditions at 20 hPa (15 mm Hg). A lag time exists and a warning is given to the crewmember when 10.7 hPa (8.0 mm Hg) is detected.

The production of CO_2 depends on two major independent factors: metabolic rate and respiration quotient (RQ). The RQ is the ratio between O_2 intake and CO_2 production and is largely a factor of diet. A diet high in carbohydrates yields a higher RQ value and results in a higher CO_2 production rate for a given activity. On the other hand, a high fat diet results in higher oxygen consumption (lower RQ) for a given activity and, thus, a lower CO_2 production rate. Figure 23 shows the relationship between O_2 consumption and CO_2 generation as a function of metabolic rate and RQ.

The U.S. EMU suit uses LiOH for CO_2 control. LiOH was chosen because of its high CO_2 absorption capacity and its relatively low weight and volume. LiOH, as a CO_2 absorbent, has the following properties:

Chemical formula: LiOH
Molecular weight: 23.95
Density of crystals: 2.54 g/cm^3 (0.092 lb/in^3)
Bulk density of granular LiOH: 0.401–0.448 g/cm^3 (0.015–0.016 lb/in^3)
Theoretical CO_2 absorption capacity: 0.917 kg CO_2 /kg LiOH (0.917 lb CO_2/lb LiOH)
Water of reaction: 0.409 kg H_2O/kg CO_2 (0.409 lb H_2O/lb CO_2)

The U.S. EMU PLSS contaminant control cartridge is designed to remove CO_2, trace gases, and control particulates. In addition to an activated charcoal bed for odor and trace gas control and a particulate filter for removing small contaminants, the cartridge contains 1.1 kg (2.43 lb) of LiOH. This amount of LiOH allows the LSS to maintain CO_2 levels in the suit helmet at or below 10.1 hPa (7.6 mm Hg) for a minimum of 7 h at normal mission conditions, with an average activity level of 293 W (1000 Btu/h) and an RQ equal to 0.90.

To maintain astronaut comfort and prevent fogging of the suit helmet, the PLSS must have some means of removing excess moisture from the ventilation loop. Moisture is present because of normal evaporation from the skin surface and through the lungs and respiratory tract.

The U.S. EMU PLSS uses a sublimator to condense the water vapor out of the vent loop. Ventilation flow is cooled under normal conditions from 39.4 °C to 13.9 °C (103 °C to 57 °F). As the water vapor is condensed in the sublimator, it is carried along the walls into a "slurper" hole array. The slurper moves the condensate along to a rotary water separator, where centrifugal force is used to generate sufficient pres-

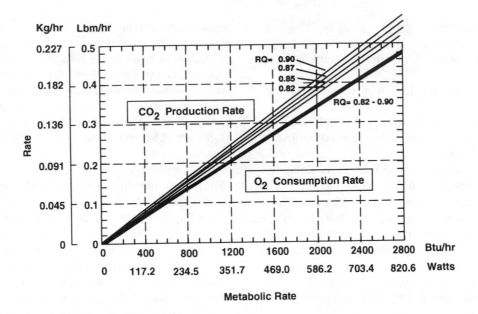

Fig. 23 Diagram of oxygen consumption and CO₂ production as function of metabolic rate and respiration quotient.

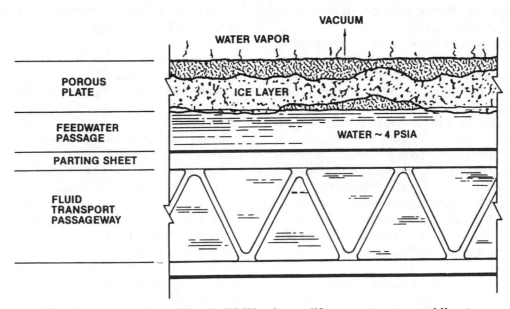

Fig. 24 Cross section of Shuttle EMU primary life support system sublimator.

sure to return the condensate to the water storage system and allow it to be used in the cooling control system as an expendable.

Another design concern for a closed-loop subsystem such as the PLSS is the removal of internal body heat. As stated previously, the technology selected for any system of the EMU is closely linked to the spacecraft being used and how readily it can support the requirements of that technology approach. In the U.S. Space Shuttle Program, the vehicle's abundant water resource lends itself to a cooling system design that uses expendable water as the heat dissipation medium. The heart of the Shuttle EMU cooling system is an onboard heat exchanger called a sublimator, which uses the phase change characteristics of water under vacuum or near vacuum condi-

tions (Fig. 24). The rest of the cooling system involves water storage capability to provide the water to feed the sublimator and its associated plumbing and valving. Additionally, a separate plumbing arrangement is required to route the water from the crewmember, where it picks up the generated heat, to the sublimator and back to the crewmember. The sublimator contains an ice layer encapsulated in a metal mesh structure known as a porous plate.

The circulation loop must contain a pump to provide water flow, and the crewmember must be able to regulate temperature as cooling needs dictate. In the Shuttle EMU, the heat acquisition plumbing is found in an LCVG, which is form-fitting to the crewmember and allows for circulation of 108.9 kg (240 lb) of water per hour around the body. This water is circulated by a pump, which is magnetically coupled to the shaft of the EMU's ventilation fan and routes the water to the cooling control valve. This valve is a diverter type and allows the crewmember to optimize cooling by selecting how much of the water that circulates over the body will be routed through and cooled by the sublimator. The cooling control valve has continuous control, which allows a range from 0.9 to 108.9 kg/hr (2 to 240 lb/hr) of water to be sent to the sublimator for heat rejection. Comfort with liquid cooling is best achieved by controlling coolant temperature rather than varying flow rate through the LCVG. Manually adjusted fluid bypass of the sublimator varies coolant temperature over 7.2–27.2 °C (45–82 °F), a range that was previously derived through tests with many suit subjects over a wide range of metabolic loads. Varying water loop temperature is superior to varying flow rate, since the former approach could expose a crewmember to a low flow rate of very cold water at approximately 0 °C (32 °F).

Since a vacuum environment is required for this cooling system, thermal regulation while connected to the orbiter during prebreathe operations uses an onboard heat exchanger that cools EMU circulating water and is connected to the EMU by an umbilical.

The metabolic load design baseline used for the Shuttle EMU is 293 W (1000 Btu/h) nominal, with peak loads up to 469 W (1600 Btu/h) for 1 h and 586 W (2000 Btu/h) for 15 min.

The method for controlling the CO_2 level in the oral/nasal area and preventing helmet visor fogging involves directing low dew point ventilation flow over the crewmember's head and down over the face. This entrains exhaled breath and sweeps it downward into the torso area of the suit, where it is returned to the LSS for cooling, dehumidification, and CO_2 removal.

A gas flow rate of 169.9 liters/min (6 ft^3/min) across the oral/nasal passages is required to control CO_2 level in the helmet. Higher gas flows consume excessive battery power and increase noise, which can interfere with audio communication.

An antifog compound consisting of a detergent-like wetting agent is applied over the visor inner surface of the helmet interior before each EVA to help control visor fogging.

Electric power is provided by a silver oxide/zinc battery, which internally supplies all power. The battery provides 16.8 V and contains 26.6 Ah of energy when fully charged. The battery is rechargeable by the orbiter in about 19 h.

The monitoring system consists of instrumentation and a microprocessor, which monitors and displays system and consumable status. The monitoring system generates an alert or warning message to the crewmember as needed, which is announced by a tone over the communication system and presented on the chest-mounted liquid crystal display. The display is backlit and provides sufficient contrast to be readable in either direct sunlight or darkness.

Controls are provided for the pressure regulators, thermal control system, fan, power, monitoring system, and communi-cation system. All controls are located on the chest-mounted display and controls module.

Full duplex communications are provided between each EVA crewmember and the orbiter by the communication system. The system also provides continuous medical electro-cardiographic monitoring of the EVA crewmembers. The radio consists of two amplitude modulation (AM) transmitters and three AM receivers operating in the ultra-high frequency. The system provides backup simplex modes of operation. EMU system performance data are provided on a time-share basis with the electrocardiogram information, with updates every 2 min.

The LSS is designed to be fail-safe. The PLSS has no redundancy. If the ventilation, CO_2 removal, or cooling system fails and the crewmember activates a purge valve, or if the suit develops a leak up to a rate of 2.3 kg/h (5 lb/h) of O2, the secondary oxygen pack (SOP) takes over automatically. The diagram of the EMU LSS is shown in Fig. 22. The SOP provides 30 min of oxygen in an open-loop purge mode, which is sufficient to control the helmet CO_2 level, provide limited cooling, and allow the astronaut to terminate the EVA in an orderly fashion and return to the vehicle airlock. CO_2 levels in the helmet are allowed to reach 20 hPa (15 mm Hg) during an emergency.

F. Safety and Reliability of an Individual Life Support System Designed for EVA

Longer space flights, more elaborate EVA tasks, and the need for reusability place stringent requirements on the reliability and operating life of an EVA suit. The main emphasis is on crewmember safety, which includes preventing (or at least reducing to a reasonable level) harmful effects caused by failure of EVA suit components.

Emergencies can occur when a space suit shell or an LSS component is damaged during work or as a result of equipment failure, such as malfunction of the valves, or non-airtight joints, a leaking seal, or a break in electrical circuits. Emergencies also can be caused by a number of other EVA conditions, such as failure to return to the cabin or airlock on schedule, crewmember fatigue, or human performance error. Knowledge of the period during which a crewmember would be able to rescue himself after various types of system failure is critical in evaluating system failure effects and improving safety and reliability. This period is called time to unconsciousness, i.e., time elapsed from equipment failure to crewmember unconsciousness. Analyses have shown that a crewmember's safety in an EVA suit depends primarily on its capacity to maintain pressurization within acceptable limits and on fail-safe operation of the oxygen supply and atmosphere-maintaining units supplying adequate gas composition.

The following major reliability factors are considered when designing an individual LSS:

1) No catastrophic effects may be caused by failure of any one element. Depressurization (to an intolerable level), explosion, or fire must be completely ruled out by an appropri-

ate layout and design and high-quality construction of components. Given these conditions, the probability of two or more similar failures in one subsystem is considered highly unlikely.

2) A contingency system must be built into the LSS to ensure that an EVA crewmember can survive until return to the vehicle or transfer to a rescue vehicle.

3) A critical subsystem or unit with high failure probability normally should have a redundant system.

4) With components used many times, crewmembers must be able to perform preventive maintenance of systems, troubleshoot problems, and replace components as necessary while in flight.

5) Because of the suit's oxygen-rich atmosphere, particular attention must be paid to fire prevention safety measures.

6) Control functions should be reasonably divided between automatic and manual (to decrease the workload on crewmembers, particularly under stress).

7) The control system must give the crewmember ample C&W information in case of emergency.

8) Failure of certain secondary units should not compel immediate work stoppage by a crewmember.

9) Emergency provisions to maintain suit pressure at a level necessary to support life must be automatically activated.

System reliability during performance under excessive pressure is also ensured by its predetermined safety margin and proof pressure testing.

The Russian safety margin for operating pressure is as follows:

1) For pressurized suit shell and pressurized volumes (oxygen tanks, etc.), ≥ 3.0.

2) For the other elements in the unit, ≥ 2.0 (relative to the applied loads).

3) For electrical components operating in an almost pure oxygen atmosphere, ≥ 4.0 (ratio of current level causing short circuit or materials ignition to operating nominal current level).

These were the primary factors used in the selection of the configuration and design of the space suit assembly for EVA on Salyut and Mir.

The U.S. safety margin for EMU operating pressure is as follows:

1) For pressurized suit shell fabric elements, ≥ 2.0 over normal operating pressure; included are both pressure-induced and measured crewmember-induced manloads into the suit pressure shell structure.

2) For metallic parts and other elements in the unit, ≥ 1.5 for material yield and ≥ 2.0 for material ultimate.

3) For electrical components operating in an almost pure oxygen atmosphere, electrical current is limited to prevent ignition of materials under worst case conditions of short-circuit current and the environment. Energy storage or conversion devices capable of providing a short-circuit current and discharge rate sufficient to ignite materials are not allowed inside the suit environment unless adequate electrical current limiting is provided.

G. Future Development Trends

Space research and continuing orbital operations pose new EVA challenges—mainly, to improve space suit and LSSs so work in space will be more efficient. The issues include improving performance (primarily crewmember mobility), eliminating or reducing prebreathe time, increasing the operating life of subsystems and components, lowering the weight of expendable consumables that must be transported into orbit, increasing the use of microprocessors to monitor and control EVA suit systems, and decreasing the operating costs in flight and on the ground.

EVA efficiency may be increased through the use of robotic manipulators and the development of special tools and equipment that more fully consider human ergonomics in a space suit.

V. Manned Maneuvering Units

This section provides a definition of the manned maneuvering unit (MMU) and the history of its development in the U.S. and the U.S.S.R. Next, we describe MMU designs for the reusable spacecraft Space Shuttle and the Mir orbital station. In conclusion, we discuss some design issues related to MMU operations for future space missions.

The MMU is a self-contained propulsive system. It expands the operating range of EVA by allowing crewmembers to maneuver in open space, i.e., to fly around the spacecraft or to nearby free-flying objects. Without an MMU, EVA maneuvers require the crewmember to use restraint cables (safety tethers) and external handrails or foot restraints located on the surface of the spacecraft.

A. Historical Background

The U.S. Air Force was the first to conduct serious long-term research on mobility in weightlessness. Since its start in the 1950s, this research included studies, designs, models and prototypes. As a result of these efforts, the first backpack MMU was developed and used onboard the Gemini 9 spacecraft (Fig. 25).

The first MMU used in space was the handheld unit operated by astronaut Edward White during the Gemini 4 mission in June of 1965 (Fig. 26). Both of the Gemini MMUs had serious design flaws—no lateral control, and the handheld unit could not be easily aligned with the pilot's center of gravity.

During 1973–1974, the flight of the zero-gravity laboratory of the Skylab orbital station made possible the evaluation of three MMU designs. The first design—"Jet Shoes"—involved attaching jets under the astronaut's feet and required that he pedal to operate them (Fig. 27). The second design was an upgrade of the Gemini handheld approach. The third design embodied the principle of a fixed-position, multiple-thruster backpack (Figs. 28 and 29). The second and third designs were incorporated into one experiment, lasting 14 h,

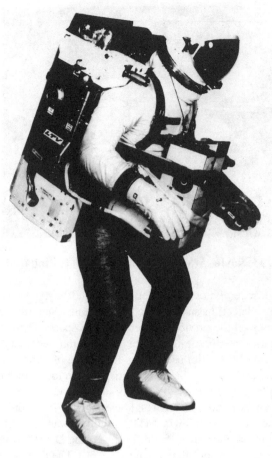

Fig. 25 Gemini manned maneuvering unit.

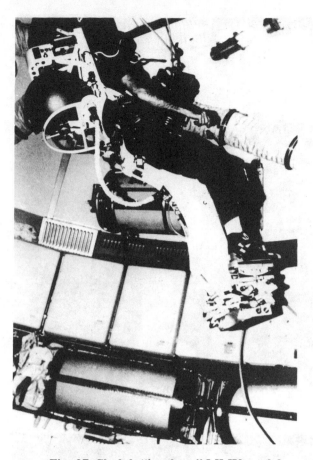

Fig. 27 Skylab "jet shoes" MMU model.

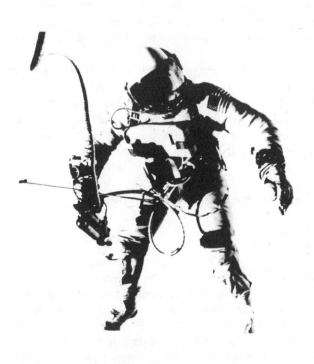

Fig. 26 Gemini handheld maneuvering unit.

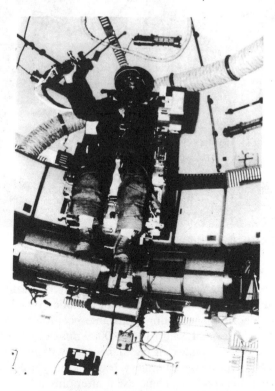

Fig. 28 Skylab handheld maneuvering unit.

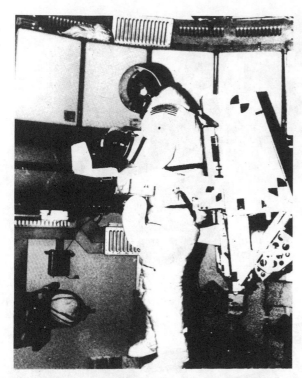

Fig. 29 Skylab experimental MMU.

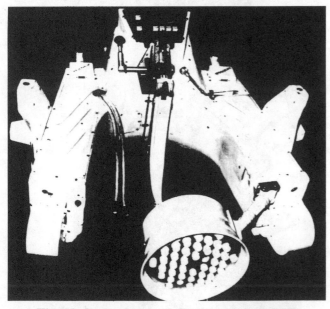

Fig. 30 General view of the first Soviet MMU.

during which 5 astronauts conducted 14 tests, proving that the backpack design had the best flight and control qualities. This unit had three different modes of attitude control and provided precise maneuvering and stable positioning capabilities [±0 0.03 m (±1.18 in) and ±0.0009 m/s (±0.04 in/s)]. It could perform complex zigzag maneuvers without touching any object inside the laboratory. It was so easy to operate that the mission specialist could use it after only a few minutes of on-orbit training. Demonstrated functional tasks in-

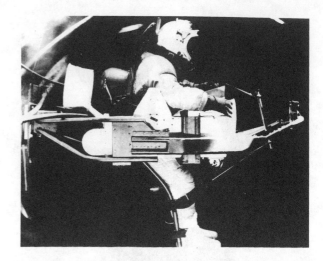

Fig. 31 Soviet MMU and space suit on testing unit.

cluded rescue of a crewmember and a failed MMU, transfer of cargo, detection and capture of a spinning satellite, and operations on the service platform in open space. These experiments gave the designers the information necessary to prepare the MMUs for use during the Shuttle missions.

In the early 1960s, Soviet scientists began to explore the same subject—to provide the means and methods for maneuvering under conditions of weightlessness. In 1968, the development of the first Soviet MMU prototype was completed. Enclasping a cosmonaut from the front, the U-shaped unit combined two propulsion systems (Fig. 30). The first system had two blocks of rocket microengines with each block containing 42 engines. Using a single-shot approach, this gunpowder-based system enabled linear movement of a cosmonaut in the forward or backward direction. The second system had 14 thrusters and control capacity with 6 degrees-of-freedom, enabling it to perform translation and rotation maneuvers.

After the completion of dynamic tests (Fig. 31), this unit was ready for use in open space. Because the progress of the MMU development was ahead of other developments (e.g., functional tasks to perform in open space and appropriate equipment of the spacecraft), this work was temporarily stopped. Eventually, Mir missions led to the renewal of the MMU work.

B. Space Shuttle Manned Maneuvering Unit

1. Development

April 1975 marked the formal beginning of a new U.S. MMU project. The purpose of this project was to accelerate the transition from the Skylab experiments to the Space Shuttle operational environment. Actual work on this project started 4-1/2 years later (in September 1979) after a sufficient level of funding was reached. Figure 32 depicts the main phases of these efforts. The project team reevaluated, redesigned, and retested all major MMU components: hand controllers, elec-

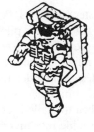

Skylab M509 Experiment Results
- Flown by 5 pilots for 14 hours
- Demonstrated MMU capability
  - Precise control
  - Intricate trajectories
  - EVA type tasks
- Established design criteria for shuttle MMU

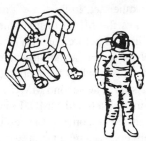

Development Activity
- New technology
- Conceptual design
- Interface definition
- Breadboard components and mockups
- Man-machine evaluation

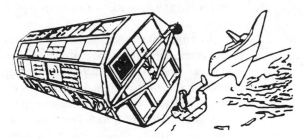

Space Shuttle Support
- Extends EVA capability
- Reach appendages outside bay
- Servicing or repair
- Remove protective covers
- Free-flying payloads
  - Docking not required
  - Min. contamination/perturbation
- Orbiter or payload contingencies
- Crew rescue operations

Fig. 32 Main phases of Shuttle MMU development.

tronic control circuitry, thrusters, regulators, and valves. The objective was to evaluate various operational parameters, such as the unit's reachability, visibility, and usability. Wearing space suits, test personnel conducted evaluations in laboratory conditions and simulated weightlessness. Also, there was progress in designing interfaces with the spacecraft and the Individual EVA LSS.

These extensive efforts led to modifications of the Skylab unit aimed at improving the MMU's maneuverability and usability. The first modification related to the overuse of propellant by the space attitude control system. Mechanically, an astronaut dressed in a space suit represents a flexible system. To compensate for frequent changes in the astronaut's center of gravity, the MMU thrusters were active all the time. A special control law that ignored high attitude rates while resisting small attitude rotations with a low duty cycle solved the problem. This modification introduced the automatic attitude hold (AAH) mode, which, functioning automatically, maintains the MMU in an inertial attitude during flight by using thrusters to counteract induced rotations as sensed by rate gyros. When a pushbutton switch at the top of the rotational hand controller (RHC) handle is depressed, the MMU is activated in the AAH mode. Once activated, it maintains a stable attitude within a displacement dead band of ±1.25° and a drift rate of approximately ±0.01° per second. The AAH is disabled independently in the pitch, roll, or yaw axis when the pilot initiates a manual rotational command by deflecting

the RHC handgrip for that particular axis. These independent inhibits may occur in any combination or sequence. The control techniques above are intuitively simple, require minimum effort to learn, and provide maneuvering flexibility during operation.

The second modification dealt with the human factors aspect of the RHC. Typically, the spacecraft rotation is proportional to the deflection of the RHC handgrip. It is similar to the relation between the speed of a car and the extent of pressure on the car's accelerator pedal. Dressed in a pressurized space suit, the MMU pilot experienced fatigue of the arms and forearms because of the extended duration of the command. For example, it took 36 s to make a 180° turn, given angular rotation of 5° per second. After extensive testing of the several models, it was established that the fingertip controller design was the simplest and required the least effort to control. Using the space suit under excessive pressure, it required a force of less than 8.9 N (2 lbf) to advance fingertips over a distance less than 0.6 cm (0.24 in).

2. Description

The Space Shuttle MMU (Fig. 33) is a self-contained propulsive backpack that allows the EVA astronaut to reach areas beyond the confines of the Shuttle. Its modular design allows it to be stored in the payload bay area. The flight support station (FSS) is the servicing and mounting interface struc-

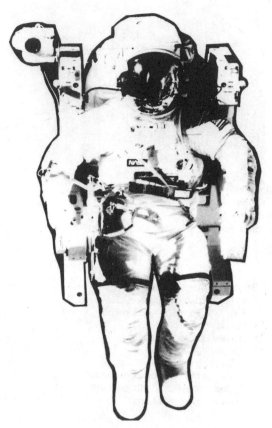

Fig. 33 Shuttle EMU/MMU.

ture between the MMU and the Shuttle. It has all the necessary hardware for storing, donning, doffing, and servicing; e.g., handrails, release levers, foot restraint, quick-disconnect hoses, and valves for propellant refueling. At this station, the MMU can be readily recharged, donned, doffed, and stowed by one crewmember.

To perform the desired maneuver, the astronaut uses hand controllers located at the ends of two control arms. These controllers allow the pilot to input commands to the control electronics assembly, which activates the appropriate thrusters. The left-hand translational hand controller (THC) handles three-degree-of-freedom translation inputs, e.g., forward/back, left/right, and up/down. The right-hand RHC handles three-degree-of-freedom rotational inputs, e.g., ± roll, ± pitch, and ± yaw. The rotational inputs are: rotate left/right (roll), shift up/down (pitch), and turn left/right (yaw).

In the event of a thruster malfunction, the rotation of the THC grip isolates the propellant tanks. If AAH mode is required, then a pushbutton switch located at the top of the RHC handle can be used as described above. To select another control mode (normal or proximity operations such as "axis inhibit" and "satellite stabilize") or to enable/disable gyro power, the appropriate left-hand switches are activated. The two right-hand switches allow the pilot to select active control and propulsion subsystems.

In addition to visual observation of velocity and its position in space, the pilot can monitor the thruster fire commands by looking at the thruster cue lights. Periodically turning the head to the left and to the right, the pilot can also check pressure of the remaining propellant (gaseous nitrogen, GN2).

To provide higher reliability and relatively lower weight and cost, the MMU design includes redundant sets of components, which operate simultaneously (Figs. 34 and 35). If a malfunction occurs, then the failed set is shut down and the MMU continues to provide maneuvering capabilities using the other set. In this case, cross-feed of the propellant tanks allows the MMU to maintain the same maneuvering capabilities as before but with a 50 percent loss of translation acceleration. For an additional redundancy, two MMUs are usually flown when their operations are required on a Shuttle mission. The second MMU can be used to retrieve an astronaut with a failed MMU. Finally, if both MMUs fail, then the Shuttle can come to the rescue by performing retrieval maneuvers. As a result, a crewmember can safely work near the spacecraft at a distance of 137.16 m (450 ft) without a safety tether.

As a miniature spacecraft, the MMU has all the traditional subsystems: propulsion, power, control, thermal control, structures, and mechanisms. Each set of the propulsion subsystem has four three-thruster triad assemblies to provide a motion in space. Each of the 24 corner-mounted thrusters delivers 7.56 N (1.70 lbf) of thrust. Two fuel tanks store the propellant, GN2. At a maximum nominal recharge pressure of 20.7 MPa (3000 psia), each tank has a capacity of 5.9 kg (13.0 lb) of propellant. Given a load of 199.58 kg (440.0 lb) for the astronaut and EMU, the MMU's maximum delta velocity is 20.12 m/s (66 ft/s). However, the lack of a C&W subsystem leads to larger fuel margins, reducing the effective delta velocity to 13.72 m/s (45.0 ft/s). The control electronics assembly activates the appropriate thrusters. It contains gyros, control logic, thruster select logic relays, and valve drive amplifiers required for stabilization and maneuvering control of the MMU. Gyro circuitry provides attitude and rate information.

Structurally, the MMU has mechanisms for folding and adjustment. The latter allows adjustment for different sizes of astronauts: from 5th percentile to 95th percentile pilots. The white color of the MMU's thermal coating keeps the temperature of its components below their upper limit of 65.7 °C (150.3 °F). To maintain the temperature of the critical components above their lower limit, the MMU employs electric heaters. The 154.22-kg (340-lb) MMU aircraft-type structure consists of an aluminum framework. In extended "flight" configuration, its approximate dimensions are 127 cm (50 in) high × 86 cm (33.9 in) wide × 122 cm (48.0 in) deep.

Before an MMU is launched on a repeat mission for a maximum of 6 h of EVA, its two batteries and two propellant tanks require complete recharging and refueling. To satisfy this requirement, the 113.4-kg (250-lb) FSS provides access to the GN2 resources of the host spacecraft. During refueling, the usual pressure of the propellant is approximately 15.2 MPa (2200 psia). For the purpose of temperature control, the spacecraft monitors all MMU/FSS temperature sensor data

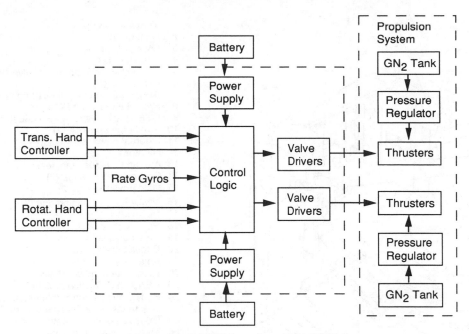

Fig. 34 Shuttle MMU functional block diagram.

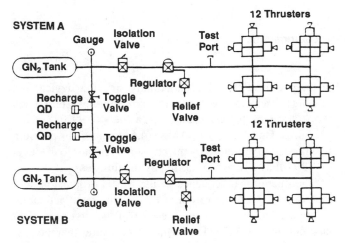

Fig. 35 Shuttle MMU propulsion subsystem schematic.

and supplies power to electric heaters. Table 5 lists the key features of the Space Shuttle MMU and Fig. 36 identifies MMU components.

C. Orbital Station Mir Manned Maneuvering Unit

The Mir MMU is a backpack mobility unit that enclasps the cosmonaut from the back (Fig. 37). Unlike the Shuttle MMU, the Mir MMU is attached in front of the space suit using a rigid frame belt. Mounted on two MMU hinges, the frame belt (Fig. 38) contains various attachment devices: a central latch, two side pins, an assembly to attach telescopic control arms, and additional side rests to increase the rigidity of the attachment. Two control panels with hand controllers are located at the ends of two control arms (Fig. 39). The left-hand and right-hand controllers (respectively) handle trans-

lation and rotation inputs. When stowed or when engaged in work on the exterior surface of a spacecraft, the control arms are retracted into "transport" position. For maneuvering, the arms are released and rotated to their "working" position. The length of the arms can be adjusted to accommodate the reach of the cosmonaut.

The assembly for attachment to the station is located at the center of the frame belt. In addition to the capability of being attached to the station, this assembly can be used to hold various objects during EVA. The frame belt (Fig. 38) has two segments of unequal length that fasten together with the lateral latch. When unlatched, the backpack and the shorter segment of the belt can be rotated on hinges relative to the longer segment. The EVA cosmonaut can attach the space suit to the central latch and the lateral pin located on the longer segment of the frame belt, without assistance or special tools. After the backpack is rotated back to its initial position and the lateral latch is closed, the cosmonaut-to-MMU attachment becomes rigid and secure.

The Mir MMU has the same main subsystems as the spacecraft: power, propulsion, control, telemetry, etc. Figure 40 shows a schematic diagram of the unit.

The MMU power subsystem supplies electrical power to the other subsystems of the unit. It includes two silver zinc batteries (primary and backup), a power distribution system, and circuitry protection blocks. If the space suit's power supply fails, then the MMU supplies electrical power to the suit as well. The parameters of the subsystem are as follows: 27 V (7 V/-4 V), 18.0 Ah (primary battery) and 8.5 Ah (spare battery) of power.

The MMU propulsion subsystem consists of two identical units. Each propulsion unit includes a propellant tank with a valve; a check valve; an electrical isolation valve; a pressure regulator valve; 16 thrusters (with thrust of 5.0 N each),

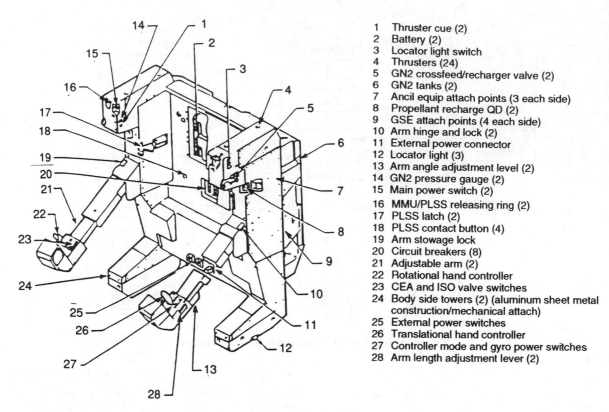

1	Thruster cue (2)
2	Battery (2)
3	Locator light switch
4	Thrusters (24)
5	GN2 crossfeed/recharger valve (2)
6	GN2 tanks (2)
7	Ancil equip attach points (3 each side)
8	Propellant recharge QD (2)
9	GSE attach points (4 each side)
10	Arm hinge and lock (2)
11	External power connector
12	Locator light (3)
13	Arm angle adjustment level (2)
14	GN2 pressure gauge (2)
15	Main power switch (2)
16	MMU/PLSS releasing ring (2)
17	PLSS latch (2)
18	PLSS contact button (4)
19	Arm stowage lock
20	Circuit breakers (8)
21	Adjustable arm (2)
22	Rotational hand controller
23	CEA and ISO valve switches
24	Body side towers (2) (aluminum sheet metal construction/mechanical attach)
25	External power switches
26	Translational hand controller
27	Controller mode and gyro power switches
28	Arm length adjustment lever (2)

Fig. 36 Shuttle MMU components.

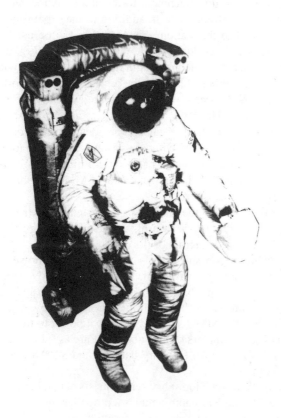

Fig. 37 Mir MMU for EVA operations.

postregulator safety valve; and, finally, signaling devices and sensors to measure pressure in the tank and subsystem. Each propellant tank has a capacity of 28 liters (0.99 ft^3) of air, pressurized to a level of 32.0 MPa (4.641 psia). This pressure is subsequently reduced by the pressure regulator to the level of 1.25 MPa (181 psia) required by the thruster.

The operational sequence of the MMU propulsion subsystem requires deactivation of the first unit and activation of the second unit after the pressure in the first propellant tank falls to 11.0 MPa (1595 psia). This ensures that the cosmonaut can return to the spacecraft from the maximum operating range of the MMU. A unit is activated from the control panel by triggering the opening of the electric isolation valve. A cross-feed valve interconnects and isolates both sets. When opened, the valve connects the fuel tank of the failed unit (failure of pressure regulator, thrusters, etc.) to the working unit.

The 32 thrusters are grouped into 4 blocks of 8, and these blocks are positioned to 1) cause the resultant translational thrust to go through the system's (MMU-suited cosmonaut's) center of gravity and 2) allow each rotation to be effected by a pair of forces that are in a plane perpendicular to the coordinate axis of rotation. This arrangement minimizes rotational disturbances during translational maneuvers and minimizes translational disturbances during rotations.

The MMU control subsystem provides for input of commands necessary to activate thrusters in different modes of maneuvering: translations, rotations, and AAH. It includes

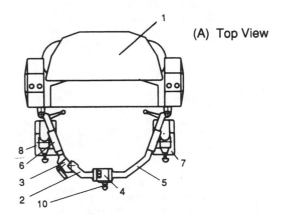

(A) Top View

(B) Waist Frame Open

A	Top view
B	View with the waist frame open
1	MMU rear section
2	Waist frame
3	Lateral latch
4	Central latch
5,6	Left and right segments of the waist
7,8	Control panels with hand controllers
9	Pin for EMU attachment
10	MMU attachment point

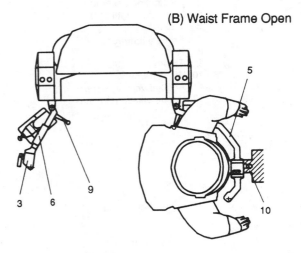

Fig. 38 Diagram of Mir MMU-cosmonaut attachment.

two identical units, each of which consists of a gyroscopic sensor of angular velocities, control electronics assembly (CEA), and static DC/AC converter to supply electric power for the gyromotors of the angular velocity sensors. Located between the propellant tanks, a pressurized chassis encloses all CEA, gyro, and converter assemblies.

To perform a maneuver, the cosmonaut uses the THCs and RHCs on the control panels. The design of the control subsystem provides for semiautomatic control, AAH, and direct control modes. The semiautomatic mode allows the pilot to select the economy or accelerated (thrust augmentation) operating regime. In the economy regime, a singular pressing of the THC handgrip causes the CEA to activate the appropriate thrusters for 1 s. Pressing the RHC handgrip leads to continuous rotation of the unit with the angular rate of 3° per

second until the pilot releases the RHC handgrip in a neutral position. In the accelerated (thrust augmentation) regime, these parameters are equal to 4 s and 8° per second. Which regime is selected is a function of the type of operation and the distance from the object. Usually, the pilot selects the economy regime during proximity operations (including hovering near the exterior of the spacecraft); larger distances require the accelerated regime.

To aid the pilot in controlling the unit, the design includes the AAH mode, which maintains the MMU in a given inertial attitude within a precision (displacement dead band) of ± 2°. By pressing a zero-reset pushbutton on the control panel, the pilot sets an initial inertial attitude. To change the attitude, the pilot performs the necessary rotation by deflecting the RHC handgrip. Upon release of the handgrip, the subsystem maintains the new inertial attitude.

The direct control mode allows the pilot to select the duration of thruster firing and rotational rate, which could be helpful during the servicing of a rotating object. In this mode, a special timing device interprets the control commands by activating the thruster for a specific duration. A single pressing of the handgrip fires the thruster for 2 s (THC grip) for translational movement or for 0.2 s for rotational movement (RHC grip). Other translational/rotational rates require multiple presses of the handgrip.

The MMU communications subsystem performs radiotelemetry and audio functions. The radiotelemetry equipment collects sensor-generated measurements of the 100 MMU operational parameters and, after processing, transmits them to the spacecraft, which downloads the telemetry data to the ground. This approach allows ground control to monitor the MMU operations during its operation in open space. Audio data on the subsystem states are broadcast to the interphone headset of the space suit.

The navigation (locator) lights provide visual aid to the spacecraft observer in locating the MMU. The headlight provides worksite lighting in shaded parts of the spacecraft orbit. To maintain the appropriate interior thermal environment, all the MMU subsystems are installed inside and shielded with vacuum seal insulation. Table 5 lists the key features of the Mir station MMU.

All MMU subsystems have high reliability. For safety reasons, all main subsystems (power, propulsion, and radiotelemetry) are backed up. This allows the pilot to return safely to the spacecraft with no external aid if a single subsystem fails.

The MMU control subsystem sends separate command signals from the hand controllers through each of the two semiautomatic mode control circuits and direct mode control circuits. Cross-connected with both propulsion units, the command signals from each control circuit are sent to both simultaneously. As this takes place, the cosmonaut-selected propulsion unit engages (fires) its thrusters.

The frame belt has quick-disconnect mechanical and electric joints to effect the prompt release of the cosmonaut from the unit in an emergency (e.g., failure of the lateral and cen-

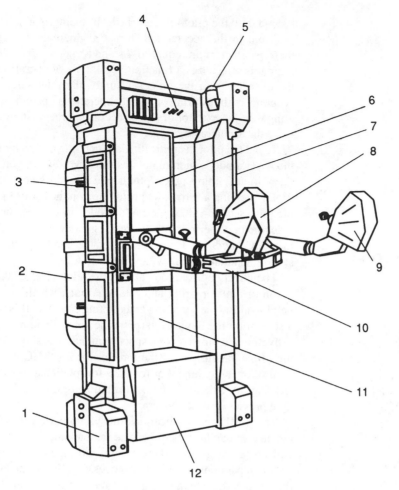

Fig. 39 Mir MMU components.

1   Sets of thrusters (4)
2   Gas pressure vessel (2)
3   Secondary battery
4   Distribution assembly
5   Navigation lights (4)
6   CEA 12
7   Primary battery
8   RHC
9   THC
10 Waist frame
11 Angular velocity sensor unit
12 Pneumatic components

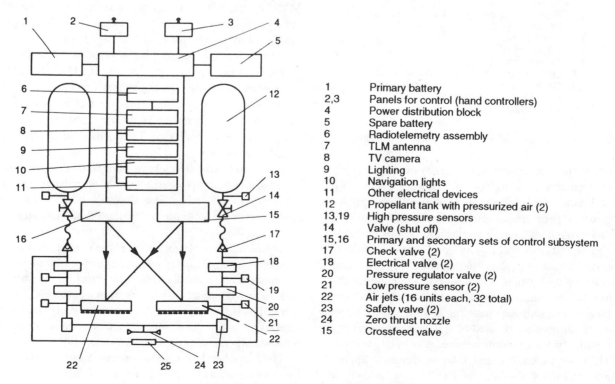

Fig. 40 Block diagram of Mir MMU.

1   Primary battery
2,3   Panels for control (hand controllers)
4   Power distribution block
5   Spare battery
6   Radiotelemetry assembly
7   TLM antenna
8   TV camera
9   Lighting
10   Navigation lights
11   Other electrical devices
12   Propellant tank with pressurized air (2)
13,19   High pressure sensors
14   Valve (shut off)
15,16   Primary and secondary sets of control subsystem
17   Check valve (2)
18   Electrical valve (2)
20   Pressure regulator valve (2)
21   Low pressure sensor (2)
22   Air jets (16 units each, 32 total)
23   Safety valve (2)
24   Zero thrust nozzle
15   Crossfeed valve

tral latches of the frame belt).

In the propulsion subsystem, the safety output valve has a zero thrust nozzle, which reduces the resultant thrust of air outflow and force impact on the cosmonaut to zero. In the case of a malfunction (e.g., breakdown of the regulator diaphragm), the same line is used to jettison air flow.

To increase the reliability of data communications, the MMU and space suit telemetry subsystems transmit (simultaneously) a composite set of MMU-space suit telemetry data.

D. Summary of Flight Experience

The Shuttle MMU has been used by six astronauts during nine open-space EVA sorties. The cumulative total of these MMU operations is equal to 10 h 22 min (Table 6).

In February 1984, astronaut Bruce McCandless was the first MMU pilot during the STS 41-B mission. He and his fellow astronaut, Robert Stewart, conducted thorough engineering tests of the unit. The operating range of the first flight without use of a safety tether was 96.93 m (320 ft). In addition, the possibility of a load transfer was tested.

The next flight, STS 41-C, refined the operations of inspecting the rotating object, docking, and load transfer. Dur-

ing the STS 51-A mission, the astronauts captured two communications satellites. Using the AAH mode, the astronauts quickly stopped rotation of the 3000-kg (1365-lb) satellite and positioned it for capture by the spacecraft's manipulator arm. After retrieval and secure placement in the payload cargo bay of the Shuttle, the satellites were returned to Earth for repair.

In February 1990, Soviet Cosmonauts A.A. Serebrov and A.S. Viktorenko conducted tests of the Mir MMU. To provide additional safety in unforeseen contingencies (the Mir cannot perform the complete set of retrieval maneuvers necessary to rescue a cosmonaut), the aerial MMU tests included a safety winch with a high-strength synthetic lifeline connecting the MMU pilot with the spacecraft. During its operations, the lifeline tracking system minimized lifeline tension, virtually excluding the effects of flight dynamics on the cosmonaut. Following the cosmonaut's egress from the airlock, the safety winch was attached to the frame belt of the cosmonaut. The maximum operating range of the space flight (measured by the released length of the lifeline) was equal to 45 m (147.6 ft).

The cosmonauts rated the unit's technical and human engineering characteristics highly. They confirmed that the

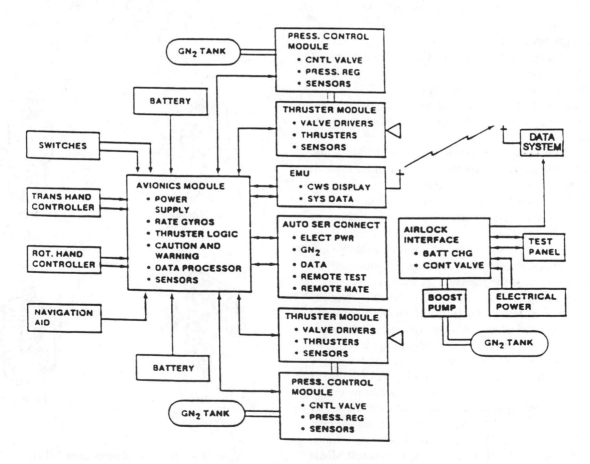

Fig. 41 Functional block diagram of an advanced MMU model.

MMU can be used during assembly, rescue, maintenance, research, and other operations in open space at a distance from the base spacecraft.

E. Future Directions of MMU Development and Application

Future orbital stations (like the U.S. Space Station) will provide an MMU that can be used to perform the following tasks:
1) Rescue operations
    – Rescue of a crewmember outside the spacecraft
    – Emergency passage in open space from a spacecraft in distress to another spacecraft
    – Retrieval of valuable equipment
    – Retrieval of a second failed MMU
2) Transport operations
    – Equipment transfer to a manipulator-unreachable zone
    – Rapid transfer of an astronaut from a remote position to the airlock (in medical emergencies)
3) Inspection operations
    – Inspection of space objects
    – External control of the station's operations and its structural connectivity (with the potential to intervene, if necessary)
    – Inspection of otherwise inaccessible places on the space station
4) Assembly operations
    – Assembly (support, alignment and connection) of large structures
    – Backup of a failed manipulator
    – Replacement or repair of elements in otherwise inaccessible places or on the surface of other space objects.

All operations noted above increase flight efficiency and reduce station maintenance expenses, because of the reduced redundancy requirements of some of the station's components.

The existing Shuttle MMU must be modified to satisfy enhanced operational requirements for speed, duration of flight, versatility, duration of checkout, service, training, and extended total duration of on-orbit operations. Table 5 compares enhanced and existing characteristics. Functionally, it is necessary to increase the sizes and pressures of the propellant tanks; to install an expert subsystem assembly, navigation subsystem, and remote control; to provide for on-orbit checkout, service, and repair; and to design a possibile means of piloting by either an astronaut or a robot. Figure 41 shows the functional diagram of an advanced MMU model.

The data in Table 5 show a threefold increase of the effective delta velocity of the advanced versus current model. In addition to the larger capacity of the fuel tanks and the higher pressure of refueling, it is also important to increase the efficient use of the propellant. Because of checkout requirements, potential failures, and inaccurate gauges, the current MMU model can use only two-thirds of the total propellant. The

new requirement for reduced fuel consumption will be satisfied by the expert subsystem of the advanced MMU model.

The expert subsystem will provide continuous monitoring of system parameters, fault detection and isolation of the failed subsystems, monitoring of the state and consumption rate of the expendables, directional analysis, data storage, C&W, signaling, and display of information. The MMU operational data could be output to the helmet-based display of the space suit. The display data would combine the MMU and space suit data for subsequent transmission to the spacecraft. If the space suit has an audio control subsystem, then it could be used by the expert system and as a regime of MMU control.

The versatility of future flights could be significantly increased if some MMU control parameters could be reprogrammed; e.g., a displacement dead band of AAH mode, thruster select logic, thrust levels, and compensation for a new center of gravity during load transfer. For each planned activity, a threshold of each expendable item could be

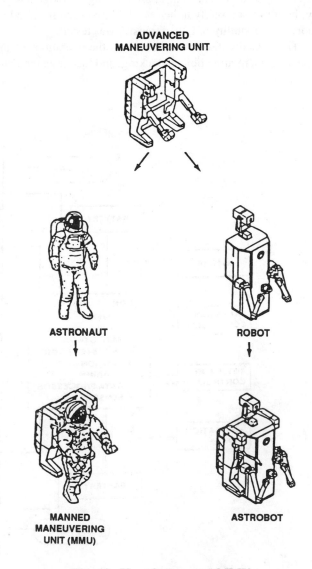

Fig. 42 Use of advanced MMU model as a transport device.

precalculated. Reacting to a threshold violation, an autonomous fault detection, isolation, and recovery (FDIR) function of the expert subsystem will decrease duration of training and preflight onboard checkout. It will allow the EVA crewmember to don and egress in less than 1 min, compared to the current duration of 20 min.

The possibility of a robotic EVA in open space is an additional advantage of the expert subsystem. In this regime, instead of the space suit, a robot would be attached to the MMU and left in a "ready-to-fly" position, while the flight crew would remain inside the spacecraft (Fig. 42). An optical device for data transmission and an electrical interface unit would connect the two systems. If a new task for a robot should arise, the MMU/robot system would be checked out and prepared to execute the task. Sending maneuvering commands directly to the expert subsystem could free the robot's hands for carrying loads. Later modifications could transform a robot into a more autonomous assistant (and, subsequently, an apprentice). In this regime, the EVA crewmember would issue audio commands to the robot to pick up a tool, hold a light, or help during assembly operations. If a task should require human participation, then a crewmember would doff the robot, place it on a stand, and don the MMU.

A laser and radio-frequency radar will supply navigational data to the expert subsystem. The expert subsystem will process these data and output the results to the helmet-based display of the space suit.

On-orbit service and repair will be another operational feature of the advanced model. Because of the high cost of a spacecraft mission, the advanced MMU will have to remain in operational condition for 1 year until its return to Earth for tuning and upgrade.

Other structural modifications of the current model will involve improving the connection with the space suit, improving hardware and procedures to free the pilot's hands for work, and simplifying preflight MMU preparations (change and recharging/refueling of the expendables, etc.).

If the spacecraft has no mechanism for MMU retrieval or to ensure against inability of the crewmember to operate the primary system, it may be necessary to use a backup MMU or provide some means to automatically return the crewmember to the spacecraft.

Recommended Reading

Abramov, I. P.; Severin, G.I.; Stoklitskiy, A.Y.; and Sharipov, P.H. *EMU and Systems for EVA.* Moscow, Mashinnostroyenie, 1984, pp. 8–21, 189–192, 207–211 (in Russian).

Balinskas, R.; McBarron, J.W. II; and Spampinato, P.M. Shuttle Extravehicular Mobility Unit operational enhancements. Society of Automotive Engineers (SAE) Technical Paper 901317, delivered at the 20th Intersociety Conference on Environmental Systems, July 9–20, 1990, Williamsburg, Va.

Compton, W.D., and Benson, C.D. *Living and Working in Space: A History of Skylab.* NASA SP-4208, Washington, D.C., NASA Hq., 1983.

Correale, J. V. Evolution of the Shuttle Extravehicular Mobility Unit. American Society of Mechanical Engineers (ASME) Publication 79-ENAs-24, 1979.

Grimwood, J. M.; Hacker, B.C.; and Vorzimmer, P. J. *Project Gemini Technology and Operations — A Chronology.* NASA SP-4002, Washington, D.C., NASA Hq., 1969, p. 270.

Jones, W.L. Individual life-support systems outside a spacecraft cabin, space suits and capsules. In: Calvin, M., and Gazenko, O.G., Eds. *Foundations of Space Biology and Medicine,* Volume III, Washington, D.C., NASA Hq., 1975, pp. 193–226.

Lutz, C.C.; Stutesman, H.L.; Carson, M.A.; and McBarron, J.W. II. Apollo experience report—Development of the Extravehicular Mobility Unit. NASA TND-8093, Washington, D.C., NASA Hq., 1975, p. 6.

Machell, R.M., Ed. *Summary of Gemini Extravehicular Activity.* NASA SP-149, Washington, D.C., NASA Hq., 1967.

McBarron, J.W. II. U.S. and Soviet EVA operation. Presentation for the 18th Intersociety Conference on Environmental Systems, July 1988.

McBarron, J.W. II. U.S. Prebreathe protocol. Proceedings of the 9th International Academy of Astronautics Man-in-Space Symposium, Cologne, Germany, 1991.

McBarron, J.W. II. Past, present and future: The U.S. EVA program. Proceedings of the 9th International Academy of Astronautics Man-in-Space Symposium, Cologne, Germany, 1991.

McBarron, J.W. II; Abramov, I.P.; and Wilde, R.C. Extravehicular individual life support: A comparison of American and Russian Systems. SAE Technical Paper 932223, 23rd International Conference on Environmental Systems, Colorado Springs, 1993.

McBarron, J.W. II; Balinkskas, R.; and Spampinato, P.M. Shuttle Extravehicular Mobility Unit operational enhancements. SAE Technical Paper 901317, 20th Intersociety Conference on Environmental Systems, Williamsburg, Va., 1990.

McBarron, J.W. II; Lutz, G.C.; Statesman, H.L.; and Carson, M.A. Apollo experience report—Development of the Extravehicular Mobility Unit. NASA TND-8093, Houston, NASA Johnson Space Center, 1975.

McBarron, J. W. II, and McMann, H.J. Challenges in the development of the Shuttle Extravehicular Mobility Unit. In: *Proceedings, Space Shuttle Technical Conference,* Houston, NASA Conference Publication 2342, Part 2, NASA Johnson Space Center, 1985, pp. 435–449.

National Aeronautics and Space Administration. Advancing automation and robotics technology for the Space Station and for the U.S. economy. NASA TM 87566, I-7, Washington, D.C., NASA Hq., 1985.

National Aeronautics and Space Administration. *Gemini Summary Conference, February 1–2, 1967.* NASA SP-138, Houston, NASA Manned Spacecraft Center, 1967.

National Aeronautics and Space Administration. Control law

for astronaut stabilization (CLAS). Invention Disclosure MSC-16917, Houston, NASA Johnson Space Center, 12, 1977.

National Aeronautics and Space Administration. Skylab Mission Report—First Visit. JSC-08414, Houston, NASA Johnson Space Center, 1973.

National Aeronautics and Space Administration. Skylab Mission Report—Second Visit. JSC-08662, Houston, NASA Johnson Space Center, 1974.

National Aeronautics and Space Administration. Skylab Mission Report—Third Visit. JSC-08963, Houston, NASA Johnson Space Center, 1974.

National Aeronautics and Space Administration. Apollo Program Summary Report. JSC-09463, Houston, NASA Johnson Space Center, 1975.

National Aeronautics and Space Administration. Apollo 9 mission report. MSC-PA-R-69-2, Houston, NASA Manned Spacecraft Center, 1969.

National Aeronautics and Space Administration. Apollo 11 mission report. MSC-00171, Houston, NASA Manned Spacecraft Center, 1969.

National Aeronautics and Space Administration. Apollo 12 mission report. MSC-01855, Houston, NASA Manned Spacecraft Center, 1970.

National Aeronautics and Space Administration. Apollo 14 mission report. MSC-04122, Houston, NASA Manned Spacecraft Center, 1971.

National Aeronautics and Space Administration. Apollo 15 mission report. MSC-05161, Houston, NASA Manned Spacecraft Center, 1971.

National Aeronautics and Space Administration. Apollo 16 mission report. MSC-07230, Houston, NASA Manned Spacecraft Center, 1972.

National Aeronautics and Space Administration. Apollo 17 mission report. MSC-07904, Houston, NASA Manned Spacecraft Center, 1973.

National Aeronautics and Space Administration. Operational data book, vol. I. MMU-SE-17-73, Rev. C, Houston, NASA Johnson Space Center, 1985.

National Aeronautics and Space Administration. Shuttle flight data and in-flight anomaly list, STS-1 through STS-50, and STS-52 through STS-56. JSC-19413, Rev. T, Houston, NASA Johnson Space Center, 1993.

Newkirk, R.W.; Ertel, I.D.; and Brooks, C.G. *Skylab —A Chronology.* NASA SP-4011, Washington, D.C., NASA Hq., 1977, p. 363.

Parker, J. Jr., and West, V.R. *Bioastronautics Data Book..* NASA SP-3006, Washington, D.C., NASA Hq., 1973, pp. 48, 811, 813.

Severin, G.I.; Abramov, I.P.; and Svertshek, V.I. Problems of employing rescue equipment in manned spacecraft. IAA-87-576, paper delivered at the 38th International Astronautical Federation (IAF) Congress, England, 1987, pp. 1–7.

Severin, G.I.; Abramov, I.P.; and Svertshek, V.I. EMU and safety problems. IAF-88-515, paper delivered at the 39th IAF Congress, India, 1988, pp. 1–17.

Severin, G.I.; Abramov, I.P.; and Svertshek, V.I. EMU, its basic concepts and designs. European Space Agency (ESA) SP-280, paper delivered at ESA Workshop on Crew Safety and Rescue, Le Bourget, Noordwijk, 13–17.

Severin, G. I.; Svertshek, V.I.; Abramov, I.P.; and Frolov, V.A. EMU used by cosmonauts to build and maintain orbital stations, Means of increasing the EMU's operational efficiency. IAF-90-075, paper delivered at 41st IAF Congress, Dresden, East Germany, 1990, pp. 1–9.

Severin, G.I.; Abramov, I.P.; Sverschek, V.I.; and Stoklitskiy, A.Yu. Development of space suits. In: *Gagarin Scientific Lectures on Aeronautics and Aviation, 1990 and 1991.* Moscow, Nauka, 1991, pp. 12–28 (in Russian).

Whitsett, C.E., and McCandless B. II. Skylab experiment M509, Astronaut Maneuvering Unit orbital test results and future applications. In: *The Skylab Results: Advances in the Astronautical Sciences,* Vol. 31, Part 1, The American Astronautical Society, Tarzana, Calif., 1975.

Whitsett, C.E.; Rodriguez, M.; and Rogers, L.J.A. Recent Shuttle EVA operations and experience. SAE Technical Paper 851328, presented at 15th Intersociety Conference on Environmental Systems, San Francisco, July 15–17, 1985.

Whitsett, C. E. Role of the Manned Maneuvering Unit for the Space Station. SAE Technical Paper 861012, presented at the 16th Intersociety Conference on Environmental Systems, San Diego, Calif., July 14–16, 1986.

Table 1 Space suit design characteristics

Characteristic	Intravehicular			Extravehicular	
	U.S. Shuttle LES	Soviet Soyuz TM	Soviet Shuttle Buran	U.S. Shuttle EMU	Soviet Salyut and Mir Stations
Spacecraft module pressure, hPa (psia)	1013 (14.7)	1013 (14.7)	1013 (14.7)	1013 (14.7)	1013 (14.7)
Normal suit operating pressure, hPa (psia)	207 (3.0)	410 (5.9)	431 (6.3)	296 (4.3)	392 (5.7)
Secondary operating pressure, hPa (psia)	None	265 (3.8)[a]	265 (3.8) and 220 (3.2)[a]	227–269 (3.3–3.9)	265 (3.8) and 220 (3.2)[a]
Prebreathe time period	None	None	None	Footnote b	30 min
Leakage rate allowable, sccm (in³/min)	≤4400 (269)	≤1000 (61)	≤660 (40)	≤50 (3)	≤330 (20)
Weight, charged, kg (lb)	10.4 (23)	10 (22)	≤17 (37)	120 (264)	≤105 (231) for Orlan-DMA with battery power ≤88 (194) for Orlan-DMA with umbilical power and for Salyut
Crewperson size accommodated, cm (in)					
• Height	155–188 (61–74)	161–185[c] (63–73)	161–185[c] (63–73)	155–188 (61–74)	161–185[d] (63–73)
• Chest	81–109 (32–43)	96–108[c] (38–43)	96–108[c] (38–43)	81–109 (32–43)	96–108[d] (38–43)
• Arm span	155–196 (61–77)	Footnote e	Footnote e	155–196 (61–77)	Footnote e
• Leg length	69–91 (27–36)	72–91 (28–36)	72–91 (28–36)	69–91 (27–36)	72–91 (28–36)
Suit mobility—joint types and bearing locations					
• Shoulder and upper arm	Soft joint	Soft joint with 2 degrees of freedom (DOFs)	Similar to Soyuz TM	Combination of soft joint with pivoting gimbal with pressure bearing	Combination of soft joint with pressure bearing
• Elbow	Soft joint	Soft joint with 1 DOF	Soft joint with 2 DOFs	Soft joint with 1 DOF and pressure bearing	Similar to Buran
• Wrist	Soft joint	Combination of pressure bearing and soft joint with 1 DOF	Combination of pressure bearing and soft joint with 2 DOFs	Combination of pressure bearing and soft joint with gimbal ring with 2 DOFs	Similar to Buran
• Waist	Soft joint	None	None	Soft joint with pressure bearing	None
• Hip	Soft joint	None	Soft joint with 1 DOF	Soft joint with multi-DOFs	Similar to Buran

Table 1 Space suit design characteristics (continued)

Characteristic	Intravehicular			Extravehicular	
	U.S. Shuttle LES	Soviet Soyuz TM	Soviet Shuttle Buran	U.S. Shuttle EMU	Soviet Salyut and Mir Stations
Suit mobility (cont'd)					
• Knee	Soft joint	Soft joint with 1 DOF	Similar to Soyuz TM	Soft joint with 1 DOF	Similar to Soyuz TM
• Ankle	Soft joint	None	None	Soft joint with 2 DOFs	Soft joint with 1 DOF
Operational life	6.5 yr[f]	4 yr[f]	4 yr[f]	8 yr: nonmetallic materials; 15 yr: metallic materials	4 yr[g] (limited by nonmetallic materials)
Mission EVAs	None	None	None	3-6: Shuttle orbiter; 24: Space Station	10 (15–20 with replacement of space suit "soft" parts)

[a] 265 hPa (3.8 psia) for work regime of short duration; 220 hPa (3.2 psia) pressure for automatic emergency oxygen supply
[b] U.S.Shuttle EMU Prebreathe Protocol:
1. In cabin
   • Prebreathe O_2 for 1 h at 1013 hPa (14.7 psia) cabin pressure.
   • Depress cabin to 703 hPa (10.2 psia) for 12 to 24 h.
   • Prebreathe O_2 for 40 min in suit at 703 hPa (10.2 psia).
   • Depress airlock.
2. In suit
   • Prebreathe O_2 for 4 1/2 h in suit at 1013 hPa (14.7 psia)
   • Depress airlock
[c] Other sizes require special order.
[d] Provided with one size of the space suit type.
[e] Parameter not determined.
[f] Another use is possible after inspection.
[g] With routine use and replacement of consumable components.

Table 2 Mobility parameters of EVA space suit joints

Joint component and type mobility movement[a]	Maximum flexure angle, degrees			Operating angle of flexing, degrees			Magnitude of flexing moment at operating angle, N·m (lb·ft)		
	U.S. Shuttle EMU	Soviet Orlan DMA	Soviet Orlan D	U.S. Shuttle EMU	Soviet Orlan DMA	Soviet Orlan D	U.S. Shuttle EMU	Soviet Orlan DMA	Soviet Orlan D
Shoulder									
1a — abduction/adduction	97	90	90	70	60	60	16.2 (11.9)	5.0 (3.7)	5.0 (3.7)
1b — rotation (x-z plane)	102	--	--	102	--	--	1.7 (1.3)	--	--
1c — flexion/extension	117	180	180	70	180	180	1.4 (1.0)	1.5 (1.1)	1.5 (1.1)
1d — lateral/medial	84	--	--	34	--	--	3.7 (2.7)	--	--
Elbow									
2a — abduction/adduction[b]	132	25	--	80	25	--	3.4 (2.5)	21.0 (15.4)	--
2b — flexion/extension	132	120	120	100	60	60	5.7 (4.2)	2.8 (2.1)	2.6 (1.9)
Wrist									
3a — abduction/adduction	85	75	70	70	75	70	2.7 (2.0)	2.2 (1.6)	2.6 (1.9)
3b — flexion/extension	140	110	95	120	110	95	4.4 (3.2)	1.0 (0.7)	2.6 (1.9)
3c — rotation	243	180	180	180	180	180	0.2 (0.2)	0.7 (0.5)	0.7 (0.5)
Waist									
4a — flexion/extension	85	20	40	60	20	20	7.7 (5.7)	8.5 (6.3)	4.0 (2.9)
4b — rotation	104	--	--	150	--	--	4.3 (3.2)	--	--
Knee									
5a — flexion/extension[c]	77	110	120	60	60	60	4.2 (3.1)	6.0 (4.4)	4.8 (3.5)
Hip									
6a — flexion/extension	50	20	40	40	20	20	28.1 (20.7)	8.5 (6.3)	4.0 (2.9)
6b — adduction/abduction	11	--	--	10	--	--	38.1 (28.0)	--	--

Table 2 Mobility parameters of EVA space suit joints (continued)

Joint component and type mobility movement[a]	Maximum flexure angle, degrees			Operating angle of flexing, degrees			Magnitude of flexing moment at operating angle, N·m (lb·ft)		
	U.S. Shuttle	Soviet Orlan		U.S. Shuttle	Soviet Orlan		U.S. Shuttle	Soviet Orlan	
	EMU	DMA	D	EMU	DMA	D	EMU	DMA	D
Ankle 7a — flexion/extension	+30/-26	±30	±30	±15	±15	±15	2.2 (1.6)	1.8 (1.3)	4.8 (3.5)

Glove fingers grasp capability	U.S. Shuttle EMU: • Ability to hold tools and handholds for 5 min. • Maintain 69 hPa (1.0 psia) grasp of objects with surface temperature between -118 °C (-180 °F) and 112 °C (+235 °F) for 30 s. Orlan-D/DMA: Ability to hold a 4.5-cm (1.8-in) diameter rod for 5 min.

[a] The references throughout this table refer specifically to the designators on the mobility diagram, Fig. 17.

[b] Elbow adduction/abduction is accommodated by the flexion/extension joint after the arm bearing is rotated to align the suit elbow perpendicular with the adduction/abduction plane.

[c] Knee mobility data recorded from standing position.

Table 3 Individual EVA Life Support System design characteristics

Characteristic	U.S. Shuttle EMU	Soviet Salyut Orlan-D	Soviet Mir Orlan DMA
EVA duration without expendable recharge or replacement, h	7	5	6
Mission EVA's capability with expendables recharge	3-6: orbiter 24: Space Station	10	Replaced after every EVA
CO_2 control method and maximum limits allowed, hPa (mm Hg)	Absorption by LiOH 20(15)	Absorption by LiOH 21(16)	Absorption by LiOH 21(16)
Oxygen flow rate into helmet/suit		0 - 3.2 (0.1) by regulator	Same as Orlan-D
• Nominal L/min (ft³/min)	1.4 - 7.1 (0.05 - 0.2) through regulator	12.5 (0.44) by injector	
• Emergency supply on L/min (ft³/min)	1.4 - 96.3 (0.05 - 3.4)	25 (0.88) when manually activating emergency supply 38 (1.34) when suit pressure drops below 220 hPa (3.2 psia) and emergency supply is activated	
Temperature control method	Gas flow Liquid cooling regulated manually	Gas flow Liquid cooling regulated manually	Same as Orlan-D
Total metabolic capacity, W (Btu/h)	293 (1000) average 117 and 469 (400 and 1600) for 1 h 586 (2000) for 15 min	349 (1190) average 698 (2380) short term	
Ambient thermal load, W (Btu/h)	-134 to 181 (-455 to 619)		
Ventilation gas flow, L/min (ft³/mn)	170 (6.0)	150 ± 25 (±0.9)	150 (5.3)
Water cooling fluid flow rate L/min (lb/in)	1.8 (4.0)	1.5-3.0 (3.3-6.6)	1.5-3.0 (3.3-6.6)
Humidity control method	Condensation with condensate removal into sublimator for evaporation into vacuum	Condensation with condensate removal into sublimator for evaporation into vacuum	Same as Orlan-D

Table 3   Individual EVA Life Support System design characteristics (continued)

Characteristic	U.S. Shuttle EMU	Soviet Salyut Orlan-D	Soviet Mir Orlan DMA
Oxygen supply	Gaseous O_2 supplied as function of suit pressure	Gaseous O_2 supplied as function of suit pressure; supplied continually through ejector and in emergency directly into helmet	Same as Orlan-D
Storage pressure			
• Primary supply	6.2 MPa (900 psia)	41.2 MPa (5975 psia)	Same as Orlan-D
Quantity	0.6 kg (1.3 lb)	1.0 kg (2.2 lb)	
• Secondary supply	41.3 MPa (5990 psia)	41.2 MPa (5975 psia)	
Quantity	1.2 kg (2.6 lb)	1.0 kg (2.2 lb)	
Power supply methods	Portable or onboard	Onboard	Portable or onboard
Source type, EVA	AgZn battery	Umbilical	AgZn battery
Voltage	16.5	27	27
Total Watts capacity	405 W/h, 26.6 Ah	≤32 W	42 W, 19 Ah
Recharge or regeneration capabilities	Recharged with 4.08 kg (9.0 lb) H_2O for cooling	Recharged with 2.9 kg (6.4 lb) H_2O for cooling	Recharged with 3.6 kg (7.9 lb) H_2O for cooling
	Battery recharged or replaced after each EVA sortie; wet life 135 days, and 8 discharge/recharge cycles	Not applicable	Battery replaced after each EVA sortie; Wet life 180 days max
	Primary O_2 tank only recharged	Primary and secondary O_2 tanks replaced	Primary and secondary O_2 tanks replaced
	CO_2 absorption cartridge replaced	CO_2 absorption cartridge replaced	CO_2 absorption cartridge replaced
Instrumentation sensors and warning parameters provided	Total 16	Total 14	Total 22
• Pressure	8	3	3
• Temperature	1	4	4
• Electrical	4	3	5
• Discrete	3	4	10

Table 4 Individual EVA life support system dimensions

Feature or characteristic, units	U.S. Shuttle EMU (Maximum size)	Soviet Mir Orlan DMA (Maximum size)	Remarks
1, cm (in)	192 (75.6)	189 (74.4)	
2, cm (in)	85 (33.5)	80 (31.5)	Hands down
3, cm (in)	66 (26)	68 (26.8)	Hands pressed
4, cm (in)	51 (20.1)	53 (20.9)	
5, cm (in)	81 (31.9)	119 (46.9)	
6, cm (in)	58 (22.8)	48 (18.9)	
7, cm (in)	18 (7.1)	19 (7.5)	
SS pressure when measuring, hPa (psi)	296 (4.3)	400 (5.8)	Normal operating pressure
Packed volume, m^3 (ft^3)	0.48 (16.95)	0.37 (13.07)	
Weight, fully charged, kg (lb)	123 (272)	105 (232)	Without airlock equipment
Hatch diameter, m (in)	0.9 (35.4)	0.8 (31.5)	

Table 5 Comparison of MMU models

Characteristic	Space Shuttle	Mir	Advanced
Self-contained propulsive backpack	Yes	Yes	Yes
Modular design, onboard storage (prior to EVA)	Yes	Yes	Yes
Capability to pass through airlock hatches	Yes	Yes	Yes
Operated by one person, does not require extra help	Yes	Yes	Yes
Noncontaminating gaseous propellant	Yes	Yes	Yes
Manual translation and rotational control, automatic attitude hold (AAH) mode	Yes	Yes	Yes
Additional safety measures	Retrieval by Orbiter	Ensured by winch	Ensured by second MMU
Mechanical interface for attaching additional equipment	Yes	Yes	Yes
EVA time spent for donning, checkout, doffing and service, min	45	30	2
Duration of EVA operations outside spacecraft, h	6	6	8
Effective delta velocity, m/s (ft/s)	13.7 (45)	25 (82)	40 (130)
Recharge pressure, MPa (kpsi)	15 (2.2)	32 (4.6)	31 (4.5)
Operating range, m (ft)	137.2 (450)	60 (197)	1000 (3200)
Weight, kg (lb)	154 (340)	218 (481)	204 (450)
Weight of flight support station (FSS), kg (lb)	113 (250)	Not required	23 (50)
Caution and warning and signaling	No	Yes	Yes
Flight telemetry data	No	Yes	Yes
Self-test and FDIR	No	No	Yes
Remote control, checkout, and service	No	Yes	Yes
Reprogramming of control parameters and constraint on orbit	No	No	Yes
Repair and service on orbit	No	Yes	Yes
Total duration of orbital use	3 weeks	3 years	1 year
Robotic operations	No	No	Yes
Frequency of EVA flights	2/year	10/year	24/year
Total impulse, N/s (lb/s)	4670 (1050)	12,000 (2697)	13,500 (3035)
Number of jets	24	32	24
Thrust per jet, N (lb)	7.6 (1.7)	5.0 (1.1)	8.9 (2)
Displacement deadband in AAH mod	±1.25°	±2.0°	±2.0°

Table 6 Statistics of U.S. and U.S.S.R. MMU flight experience

Mission	Name of pilot	Flight date	Duration of flight, hr:min	Operating range, m	Delta velocity,[a] m/s
41-B Shuttle	B. McCandless	2/07/84	01:22	96.93	15.84
41-B Shuttle	R. Stewart	2/07/84	01:09	91.60	12.80
41-B Shuttle	B. McCandless	2/09/84	00:47	18.30[a]	17.05
41-B Shuttle	R. Stewart	2/09/84	00:44	18.30[a]	12.20
41-B Shuttle	B. McCandless	2/09/84	01:08	18.30[a]	11.67
41-C Shuttle	G. Nelson	4/08/84	00:42	41.60[a]	12.50
41-C Shuttle	J. Van Hoften	4/11/84	00:28	15.24[b]	15.24
51-A Shuttle	J. Allen	11/12/84	02:22	30.48[a]	11.88
51-A Shuttle	D. Gardner	11/14/84	01:40	30.48[a]	12.80
		U.S. Total	10:22		
Mir	A. A. Serebrov	2/01/90	00:40	33.00	15.50
Mir	A. S. Viktorenko	2/05/90	00:93	45.00	21.00
		U.S.S.R. Total	01:33		

[a] Calculated.

[b] In payload cargo bay, calculated.

Table 7   Summary of EVA statistics, systems, and accomplishments

Mission	Astronaut/ cosmonaut[a]	EVA date	Space suit and life support system	EVA duration, hr:min[b]	Significant accomplishments/comments
Voskhod 2	A. A. Leonov	3/18/65	Berkut, LSS KP-55, emergency oxygen and electrical umbilical	0:12	First human EVA; assessment of human EVA capabilities; pressure airlock used for first time.
Gemini 4	E. White (J. McDivitt)	6/3/65	G-4C and oxygen, electrical umbilical/ ventilation control module (VCM)	0:36	First U.S. EVA; first use of a handheld propulsion unit and tether for evaluation of body attitude and position control.
Gemini 9-A	E. Cernan (T. Stafford)	6/5/66	G-4C and oxygen, electrical umbilical/ environmental control life support system (ECLSS)	2:07	"Standup" EVA from spacecraft hatch opening initially to acclimate crewman to conditions. Astronaut maneuvering unit (AMU) evaluation not completed. High workloads exceeded capacity of ECLSS, resulting in helmet visor fogging and reduced visibility. High workloads caused by difficulty of maintaining necessary body position and restraint relative to workstation.
Gemini 10	M. Collins (J. Young)	7/19/66	G-4C and spacecraft LSS umbilicals	0:50	Standup EVA; ultraviolet (UV) photos of star fields taken. First EVA retrieval of an experiment (micrometeorite collection package from Agena target vehicle).
		7/20/66	G-4C and oxygen, electrical umbilical/ECLSS	0:39	First free-space transfer (used handheld propulsion unit). EVA ended early due to unrelated spacecraft problem.
Gemini 11	D. Gordon (P. Conrad)	9/13/66	G-4C and oxygen, umbilical/ECLSS	0:33	EVA traverse and attachment of tether from the Agena target vehicle to Gemini spacecraft docking bar demonstrated. EVA ended early due to crewman fatigue.
		9/14/66	G-4C and spacecraft LSS umbilicals	2:10	"Standup" EVA from spacecraft hatch opening for Agena target vehicle tether operations support.
Gemini 12	E. Aldrin (J. Lovell)	11/12/66	G-4C and spacecraft LSS umbilicals	2:29	"Standup" EVA from spacecraft hatch opening to acclimatize crewman to EVA conditions.
		11/13/66	G-4C and oxygen, electrical umbilical/ ECLSS	2:06	Successfully accomplished all representative EVA work tasks including Agena target vehicle 30.5 m (100 ft) tether attachment, UV stellar photography, and evaluation of various restraint systems including a waist tether and positive positioning "Dutch Shoe" restraints at spacecraft adapter.
		11/14/66	G-4C and spacecraft LSS umbilical	0:55	Second "standup" EVA from spacecraft hatch opening.
Soyuz 5 Soyuz 4	A.S. Yeliseyev E. V. Khrunov	1/16/69	Yastreb, LSS RVR-1P, electrical umbilical	0:37	Crew moved from one spacecraft to another in space for the first time.

Table 7 Summary of EVA statistics, systems, and accomplishments (continued)

Mission	Astronaut/cosmonaut[a]	EVA date	Space suit and life support system	EVA duration, hr:min[b]	Significant accomplishments/comments
Apollo 9	D. Scott	3/6/69	A-7L and command module (CM) environ-mental control system (ECS) umbilicals	0:47	Command module pilot performed "standup" EVA out of CM hatch. Retrieved thermal experiment samples and performed photography.
	R. Schweickart (J. McDivitt)		A-7L and -6 PLSS	1:01	Lunar module pilot egressed LM side hatch and demonstrated extravehicular transfer using handrails. Demonstration of PLSS recharge performed after EVA completed.
Apollo 11	N. Armstrong E. Aldrin	7/20/69	A-7L and -6 PLSS	2:32	First manned excursion on the lunar surface at landing site in Sea of Tranquillity. Crewmen collected 21 kg (46.3 lb) of material during 60 m (197 ft) surface traverse.
Apollo 12	C. Conrad A. Bean	11/19/69	A-7L and -6 PLSS	3:56 3:49	Second manned excursion on lunar surface at landing site in Ocean of Storms. Crewmen collected 34.3 kg (75.6 lb) of lunar material and returned parts from Surveyor 3 during two EVAs.
Apollo 14	A. Shepard E. Mitchell	2/5/71	A-7L and -6 PLSS/ buddy secondary life support system (BSLSS)	4:48 4:35	Third manned excursion on lunar surface at landing site in Fra Mauro area. Crewmen collected 42.8 kg (94.4 lb) of lunar material during two EVAs. Crewmen traversed ~1.5 km (0.9 mile) from LM.
Apollo 15	D. Scott	7/30/71	A-7LB and LM ECS oxygen umbilical	0:33	"Standup" EVA (through LM to CM hatch) for lunar surface observations and photographs.
	J. Irwin D. Scott	7/31/71 8/1/71 8/2/71	A-7LB and -7 PLSS	6:33 7:12 4:50	Fourth manned excursion on lunar surface in Hadley Apennine region. First use of Lunar Rover. Crewmen collected 76.7 kg (169 lb) of lunar material during three EVAs.
	A. Worden (D. Scott) (J. Irwin)	8/5/71	A-7L CMP and CM ECS oxygen umbilical	0:39	First transearth EVA performed for retrieval of experimental photographic film package during flight back to Earth.
Apollo 16	C. Duke J. Young	4/21/72 4/22/72 4/23/72	A-7LB and -7 PLSS	7:11 7:23 5:40	Fifth manned excursion on lunar surface in Descartes area. Crewmen collected 94.3 kg (208 lb) of lunar material during three EVAs.
	K. Mattingly (C. Duke) (J. Young)	4/25/72	A-7L CMP and CM ECS oxygen umbilical	1:24	Second transearth EVA for retrieval of experimental photographic film package and microbial response experiment.

Table 7 Summary of EVA statistics, systems, and accomplishments (continued)

Mission	Astronaut/cosmonaut[a]	EVA date	Space suit and life support system	EVA duration, hr:min[b]	Significant accomplishments/comments
Apollo 17	H. Schmitt E. Cernan	12/11/72 12/12/72 12/13/72	A-7LB and -7 PLSS	7:12 7:37 7:15	Sixth manned excursion on lunar surface in Taurus-Littrow area. Crewmen collected 110.4 kg (243 lb) of lunar material during three EVAs. Lunar Rover allowed crewmen to travel ~7 8 km (4.9 miles) from LM. Eight explosive charges placed on lunar surface to be activated later for a seismographic experiment.
	R. Evans (M. Schmitt) (E. Cernan)	12/17/72	A-7LB, CMP and CM ECS oxygen umbilical	1:06	Third transearth EVA performed during flight back to Earth.
Skylab 2	P.J. Weitz (C. Conrad) (J. Kerwin)	5/25/73	A-7LB, CMP and CM ECS oxygen umbilical	0:37	"Standup" EVA through CM hatch in unsuccessful attempt to free jammed orbital workshop solar panel.
	C. Conrad J. Kerwin	6/7/736	A-7LB EV and umbilical/astronaut ECS life support assembly (ALSA)	3:30	First EVA from orbital workshop airlock. Deployed jammed solar panel restoring power to workshop.
	C. Conrad P.J. Weitz	6/19/73	A-7LB EV and umbilical/ALSA	1:44	Recovered film from Apollo telescope mount camera and repaired stuck power module electric relay by striking battery housing with a hammer.
Skylab 3	O. Garriott J. Lousma	8/6/73	A-7LB EV and umbilical/ALSA	6:29	Constructed and deployed twin-pole thermal shield which reduced interior temperature to nominal level, loaded ATM camera with film, and inspected several malfunctioning items.
	O. Garriott J. Lousma	8/24/73	A-7LB EV and umbilical/ALSA	4:30	Installed backup package of six rate gyros on docking adapter adding back gyro system and redundancy, and exchanged ATM film.
	A. Bean O. Garriott	9/22/73	A-7LB EV and umbilical/ALSA	2:41	Recovered film from ATM camera.
Skylab 4	E. G. Gibson W. R. Pogue	11/22/73	A-7LB EV and umbilical/ALSA	6:34	Photographed contamination surrounding the workshop, reloaded ATM cameras with film, and repaired inoperative microwave sensor antenna restoring more than half of its function.
	G.P. Carr W.R. Pogue	12/25/73	A-7LB EV and umbilical/ALSA	6:54	Photographed comet Kohoutek, reloaded ATM cameras, pinned open a malfunctioning UV spectroheliograph aperture door, installed electronographic camera, and used screwdriver to pry open jammed filter wheel in X-ray telescope.
	G.P. Carr E.G. Gibson	12/29/73	A-7LB EV and umbilical/ALSA	3:29	Observed and photographed comet Kohoutek, and retrieved experimental materials samples.
	G.P. Carr E.G. Gibson	2/3/74	A-7LB EV and umbilical/ALSA	5:19	Recovered film from ATM camera and retrieved particle collection experiments.

Table 7 Summary of EVA statistics, systems, and accomplishments (continued)

Mission	Astronaut/cosmonaut[a]	EVA date	Space suit and life support system	EVA duration, hr:min[b]	Significant accomplishments/comments
Salyut 6 Orbital Station (OS)	Yu.V.. Romanenko G.M. Grechko	12/20/77	Orlan-D	1:28	Inspected OS docking unit outer surface (Romanenko stayed in depressurized airlock); semirigid space suit design used for first time.
Salyut 6	V. V. Kovalyonok A. S.Ivanchenkov	7/29/78	Orlan-D	2:06	Retrieved samples exposed to outer space and installed new samples.
Salyut 6	V. A. Lyakhov V. V. Ryumin	8/15/79	Orlan-D	1:23	Unplanned EVA with translation to the end of OS to dislodge a jammed radio telescope antenna. Dismantled research equipment.
Salyut 7	A. N. Berezovoy V. V. Lebedev	7/30/82	Orlan-D	2:33	Dismantled and partially replaced samples and research equipment. Performed engineering checks to evaluate different types of mechanical joints.
STS-6	S. Musgrave D. Peterson	4/7/83	Shuttle EMU	3:59	First Shuttle Program EVA performed to verify contingency procedures and evaluate EMU performance.
Salyut 7	V. A. Lyakhov A.P. Alexandrov	11/1/83	Orlan-D	2:50	Mounted an additional solar cell panel. Repaired EVA suit pressure shell on board the station.
		11/3/83	Orlan-D	2:55	Mounted a second additional solar cell panel.
STS-41B	B. McCandless R. Stewart	2/7/84	Shuttle EMU	5:35	First use of MMU.
		2/9/84	Shuttle EMU	6:02	Continued MMU evaluations.
STS-41C	G. Nelson J. Van Hoften	4/8/84	Shuttle EMU	2:59	First use of EVA for retrieval, repair and deployment of solar maximum satellite (SMS).
		4/11/84	Shuttle EMU	7:07	Replaced SMS modular attitude control system and performed MMU evaluation. MMU capture unsuccessful due to unexpected spacecraft protuberance.
Salyut 7	L. D. Kizim V. A. Solovyov	4/23/84	Orlan-D	4:15	Installed ramp and other equipment and prepared work station for repair of hydraulic subsystem of the integrated propulsion system (IPS).
		4/26/84	Orlan-D	5:00	Repaired IPS hydraulics.
		4/29/84	Orlan-D	2:45	Continued IPS repairs.
		5/4/84	Orlan-D	2:45	Continued IPS repairs.
		5/19/84	Orlan-D	3:05	Installed additional solar cell panels.
Salyut 7	V.A.Dzhanibekov S. E. Savitskaya	7/25/84	Orlan-D	3:35	First U.S.S.R. woman to perform EVA. Demonstrated work with manual welding tool. Retrieved samples located on station's external surface.

Table 7 Summary of EVA statistics, systems, and accomplishments (continued)

Mission	Astronaut/cosmonaut[a]	EVA date	Space suit and life support system	EVA duration, hr:min[b]	Significant accomplishments/comments
Salyut 7	L. D. Kizim V. A. Solovyov	8/8/84	Orlan-D	5:00	Flattened hydraulic duct work at rear of station's assembly module. Dismantled solar cell component for return to Earth. Orlan-D water pump failed. Performed work with two ventilation fans working simultaneously (while the liquid cooling system was not functioning).
STS-41G	K. Sullivan D. Leetsma	10/11/84	Shuttle EMU	3:29	First U.S. woman to perform EVA. Transferred hydrazine fuel using orbital refueling system ball valve repair kit. Unscheduled EVA task performed to lock gimbals on Ku-band antenna.
STS-51A	J. Allen D. Gardner	11/12/84	Shuttle EMU	6:13	Retrieved and berthed Palapa B2 satellite which, when launched in February 1984, failed to obtain proper orbit after motors misfired. MMU was used to capture and de-spin satellite.
		11/14/84	Shuttle EMU	6:01	Retrieved and berthed Westar VI satellite. Astronaut Allen held and maneuvered satellite while standing on end of the remote manipulator system (RMS) arm. MMU was used to capture and de-spin satellite.
STS-51D	J. Hoffman D. Griggs	4/16/85	Shuttle EMU	3:10	First unscheduled EVA to attach special in-flight fabricated fly-swatter-like device to orbiter RMS arm which was used the next day in an attempt to activate payload time sequencer on Syncom satellite. Payload sequencer did not activate after it was snagged by RMS arm.
Salyut 7	V.A. Dzhanibekov V. P. Savinykh	8/2/85	Orlan-DM	5:00	Installed additional solar panels on third solar cell; modified suit used for EVA.
STS-51I	J. Van Hoften W. Fisher	8/31/85	Shuttle EMU	7:20	Syncom IV-3 satellite captured and attached to RMS.
		9/1/85	Shuttle EMU	4:31	Repaired Syncom IV-3 and manually redeployed the satellite.
STS-61B	J. Ross S. Spring	11/29/85	Shuttle EMU	5:34	Performed Experimental Assembly of Structures in EVA/Assembly Concept for Construction of Erectable Space Structures (EASE/ACCESS) demonstrations and simulated heat pipe manipulation. First flight with EMU Real Time Data System.
		12/1/85	Shuttle EMU	6:46	Performed additional EASE/ACCESS demonstrations and heat pipe manipulations. Deployed small tracking test satellite.

Table 7 Summary of EVA statistics, systems, and accomplishments (continued)

Mission	Astronaut/cosmonaut[a]	EVA date	Space suit and life support system	EVA duration, hr:min[b]	Significant accomplishments/comments
Salyut 7	L.D. Kizim V.A. Solovyov	5/28/86	Orlan-DM	3:50	Tested methods for installing large structures using hinged lattice truss.
		5/31/86	Orlan-DM	5:00	Continued testing methods for installing large structures.
Mir	Yu.V. Romanenko A. I. Laveykin	4/11/87	Orlan-DM	3:40	Unscheduled EVA to remove a foreign object interfering with docking Kvant with the station.
		6/12/87	Orlan-DM	1:53	Mounted solar cell on truss structure and two sections of photoelectric transducers.
		6/16/87	Orlan-DM	3:15	Completed installation of solar cell and unfolding the truss. Installed test samples.
Mir	V. G. Titov M. K. Manarov	2/26/88	Orlan-DM	4:25	Mounted an experimental solar cell, installed test samples.
		6/30/88	Orlan-DM	5:10	Replaced sensor unit on Kvant module X-ray telescope. Work was not completed because of breakdown of device for dislodging the sensor unit.
		10/20/88	Orlan-DMA	4:12	Completed replacing the sensor on the Kvant module X-ray telescope. First phase of evaluation of modified EMU using OS power cable.
Mir	A. A. Volkov J.L. Chretien	12/9/88	Orlan-DMA	6:00	Conducted experiments with the Soviet-French program Aragats. Mounted and deployed a truss structure, mounted a panel with test samples to study space exposure effect on different materials.
Mir	A. S. Viktorenko A. A. Serebrov	1/8/90	Orlan-DMA	2:56	Mounted two star-navigation sensors to raise accuracy of the navigation and guidance system of the station.
		1/11/90	Orlan-DMA	2:54	Mounted scientific equipment on Kvant module. Retrieved samples, prepared transfer to house module Kristall.
Mir	A. S. Viktorenko A. A. Serebrov	1/26/90	Orlan-DMA	3:02	First egress from Kvant 2 airlock. Tested modified self-contained EMUs; installed additional equipment on the module. First EVA without power umbilical.
		2/1/90	Orlan-DMA	4:59	First Soviet test of an MMU, with Serebrov moving from the station as far as 33 m.
		2/5/90	Orlan-DMA	3:45	Cosmonaut Viktorenko performed additional detailed testing of the MMU.
Mir	A.Ya. Solovyov A. N. Balandin	7/17/90	Orlan-DMA	7:00	Inspected and repaired Soyuz TM damaged thermal insulation. After return to airlock, hatch failed to close completely.
					Kvant 2 instrumentation module depressurized to let cosmonauts enter station.

Table 7 Summary of EVA statistics, systems, and accomplishments (continued)

Mission	Astronaut/ cosmonaut[a]	EVA date	Space suit and life support system	EVA duration, hr:min[b]	Significant accomplishments/comments
Mir	A.Ya. Solovyov A. N. Balandin	7/26/90	Orlan-DMA	3:31	Dismantled equipment on Kvant 2 module exterior, inspected damaged hatch, closed it; sealed and pressurized module.
Mir	G.M. Manakov G.M. Strekalov	10/30/90	Orlan-DMA	2:45	Attempted hatch repair using special hardware. Troubleshooting revealed need to replace one of hatch axis support brackets.
Mir	V.M.Afanasyev M.K. Manarov	1/7/91	Orlan-DMA	5:18	Repaired Kvant 2 module hatch and replaced bracket and bearing. Disassembled instruments, took out solar battery truss to be installed.
		1/23/91		5:33	Installed 14 m (46 ft) boom on station core.
		1/26/91		6:20	Lifted solar battery trusses by the boom from egress hatch and installed on Kvant module.
STS-37	J. Ross J. Apt	4/7/91	Shuttle EMU	4:31	Performed unscheduled EVA to manually deploy jammed Gamma Ray Observatory (GRO) antenna necessary for GRO deployment.
		4/8/91	Shuttle EMU	5:58	Performed evaluation of prototype Space Station translation equipment and methods, and conducted tests to measure loads induced by crewman during performance of typical EVA tasks.
Mir	V.M.Afanasyev M. K. Manarov	4/25/91	Orlan-DMA	3:34	Conducted experiment to test construction techniques for assembly of large structures in space. Inspected damaged antenna located on the end plane of Kvant module which contributed to Progress M7 supply ship docking problems.
Mir	A. P.Artsebarskiy S.K. Krikalev	6/24/91	Orlan-DMA	4:58	Repaired damaged antenna at the edge of Kvant module.
		6/28/91	Orlan-DMA	3:25	Installed research equipment; prepared a derrick.
		7/15/91	Orlan-DMA	5:56	Prepared the work station (based on the Kvant module) for the Sofor experiment designed to develop new methods ofassembling large structures in space, using thermal mechanical connections.
		7/19/91	Orlan-DMA	5:28	Installed the work platform and berth, and assembled the Sofor truss structure.
		7/23/91	Orlan-DMA	5:42	Continued assembling the Sofor truss structure.
		7/27/91	Orlan-DMA	6:49	Completed Sofor experiment. Assembled and mounted 14 m (46 ft) truss.

Table 7 Summary of EVA statistics, systems, and accomplishments (continued)

Mission	Astronaut/ cosmonaut[a]	EVA date	Space suit and life support system	EVA duration, hr:min[b]	Significant accomplishments/comments
Mir	A.A. Volkov S.M. Krikalev	2/20/92	Orlan-DMA	4:13	Installed scientific equipment on Kvant module, collected samples from experimental solar panel. Due to malfunctioning of space suit cooling garment, commander had to be connected to the airlock cooling system for the better portion of the work period.
STS-49	P.J. Thuot R.J. Hieb	5/10/92	Shuttle EMU	3:53	Attempts to manually attach a capture bar to Intelsat VI-F3 satellite unsuccessful. Capture bar attachment was necessary to provide mechanical interface for satellite grapple by orbiter RMS end effector.
	P.J. Thuot R.J. Hieb	5/11/92	Shuttle EMU	5:38	Additional attempts to manually attach capture bar to satellite unsuccessful. Installed new payload bay video camera to replace unit that failed to operate previous day.
	P.J. Thuot R.J. Hieb T.D. Akers	5/13/92	Shuttle EMU	8:30	First 3-man EVA team; performed manual satellite grapple using "real-time" mission-developed procedure; successfully attached capture bar to Intelsat VI-F3 satellite; and performed scheduled EVA to check out and attach propulsion motor to satellite in support of satellite redeployment to correct operational orbit.
	K.C. Thornton T.D. Akers	5/14/92	Shuttle EMU	7:47	Performed Assembly of Station by EVA Methods (ASEM) experiment; evaluated Multi-Purpose Experiment Support Structure (MPESS) attachment and handheld crew propulsion device (CPD). Unscheduled EVA task to manually restow orbiter Ku-band antenna.
Mir	A. S. Viktorenko A. Yu. Kaleri	7/08/92	Orlan-DMA	2:03	Installed vacuum lines on station surface for operation of gyrodines on Kvant 2 module.
Mir	A.Ya. Solovyov S.V. Avdeyev	9/03/92	Orlan-DMA	3:56	Performed preparatory work for the reinstallation of a movable propulsion system (MPS) for space station complex.
		9/07/92	Orlan-DMA	5:08	Installed a cable on Sofor truss for the MPS and mated connectors to Kvant module.
		9/11/92	Orlan-DMA	5:44	Mated MPS with Sofor truss and activated it.
		9/15/92	Orlan-DMA	3:33	Dismantled Kristall, module antenna, and scientific equipment.

Table 7 Summary of EVA statistics, systems, and accomplishments (continued)

Mission	Astronaut/cosmonaut[a]	EVA date	Space suit and life support system	EVA duration, hr:min[b]	Significant accomplishments/comments
STS-54	G.J. Harbaugh M. Runco, Jr.	1/17/93	Shuttle EMU	4:32	Conducted EVA environment adaptation and EVA tasks evaluation including work site restraint methods, translation with tools, equipment, and a simulated large orbital replacement unit.
Mir	G.M. Manakov A.F. Politshuk	4/19/93	Orlan-DMA	5:25	Removed and transferred a solar array electric drive from the Kristall module and installed it on the Kvant module.
		6/18/93	Orlan-DMA	4:33	Removed and transferred the second solar array electric drive from the Kristall module and installed it on the Kvant module.
STS-57	D. Low J Wisoff	6/25/93	Shuttle EMU	5:47	Performed contingency EVA task to latch and lock European Retrievable Carrier (EURECA) spacecraft antennas. Also conducted EVA task evaluation, including: simulated ORU mass handling and manipulations; and ability to align a large mass precisely.
STS-51	C. Weitz J. Newman	9/16/93	Shuttle EMU	7:08	Conducted EVA environment adaptation and EVA task evaluations, including: encumbered/unencumbered cargo bay translations; work site restraint ingress/egress; EVA tools and tethers testing.
Mir	V.V. Tsibliyev A.A. Serebrov	9/16/93	Orlan-DMA	4:18	Installed RAPAN experimental truss with scientific equipment on the Kvant module, removed metallic and nonmetallic material samples; and installed specimens of composite materials on truss.
		9/2093	Orlan-DMA	3:13	Installed a platform with scientific equipment on the RAPAN truss.
		9/28/93	Orlan-DMA	1:51	Dissembled panel from cosmic ray experiment and installed new scientific cassette with samples of construction materials.
		10/22/93	Orlan-DMA	0:38	Installed new equipment unit for measuring micrometeorite streams, visually inspected and took video of individual components of station looking for metal corrosion and changes in coloration.
		10/29/93	Orlan-DMA	4:12	Visually inspected elements status of external station surface and performed set of preventive maintenance operations.

Table 7   Summary of EVA statistics, systems, and accomplishments (continued)

Mission	Astronaut/ cosmonaut[a]	EVA date	Space suit and life support system	EVA duration, hr:min[b]	Significant accomplishments/comments
STS-61	J. Hoffman S. Musgrave	12/4 and 12/5/93	Shuttle EMU	7:57	Performed Hubble Space Telescope (HST) repair tasks: rate sensing gyroscope units #2 and #3 replacement; electronic control unit #1 and #3 replacement; fuse plugs replacement; and solar array carrier preparation for next EVA.
	K. Thornton T. Akers	12/5 and 12/6/93	Shuttle EMU	6:37	Performed HST twin solar arrays replacement. One of two arrays was jettisoned in space.
	J. Hoffman S. Musgrave	12/6 and 12/7/93	Shuttle EMU	6:49	Performed HST repairs: wide-field planetary camera replacement; and magnetic servicing system #1 and #2.
STS-61	K. Thornton T. Akers	12/7 and 12/8/93	Shuttle EMU	6:58	Performed HST repairs: high speed photometer replacement; corrective optics space telescope axial replacement; and D-224 computer coprocessor replacement.
	J. Hoffman S. Musgrave	12/8 and 12/9/93	Shuttle EMU	7:23	Performed HST repairs: Goddard high resolution spectrograph cable replacement; solar array drive electronics replacement; and improved thermal insulation over the magnetometers.

[a] Astronauts exposed to vacuum conditions within the spacecraft during EVA are shown within ( ).

[b] Gemini 4 through 12, Apollo 11, and for all Soviet spacecraft and orbital stations, EVA duration based on time from spacecraft hatch opening to hatch closure

Apollo 12 EVA duration based on time from spacecraft egress to ingress.

Apollo 14 through Apollo 17 EVA duration based on time spacecraft cabin pressure was less than 3.0 psia.

Shuttle STS-6 through STS-54 EVA duration based on time that spacecraft airlock pressure was at 0 psia.

Chapter 15

Physical-Chemical Life Support Systems

William R. Humphries, Panchalam K. Seshan, and Peggy L. Evanich

Physical-chemical life support systems can be either open, nonregenerative systems or closed, regenerative systems. Open, nonregenerative systems are those in which both the materials essential to sustain human life and the reagents for treatment and contaminant removal are provided as expendable supplies. Such systems are most suited for short-duration missions. In contrast, closed, regenerative systems employ selected chemical processes for recovery of air and water from waste products and for regeneration of contaminant removal adsorbents and other reagents required for future long-duration missions. Food supplies are provided as expendables for both open and closed physical-chemical life support systems. As the duration of human space missions increases and as missions focus on the exploration of environments far from Earth so as to make resupply prohibitive, regenerative physical-chemical life support systems will become increasingly mandatory. For support of such remote, long-duration missions, many attributes, such as reliability, maintainability, and controllability, must become inherent in the life support system design to prevent undue safety hazards to the crew, to maximize crew productivity, and to enhance crew psychological well-being.

I. History and Evolution of Life Support Capability in Spacecraft*

A. Overview

With the evolution of human space flight has come a wealth of knowledge on supporting human life in the hostile environment of outer space. Each successive manned space program has built and improved upon the last, learning from the successes and failures experienced on each mission. As crew size and mission duration and complexity have increased, the spacecraft Environmental Control and Life Support System (ECLSS) has been adapted and improved based on lessons learned from the past.

On early space flights carrying animals, life support systems used stored consumables and simple open-loop systems. On early Soviet flights potassium superoxide (KO_2) was used as an oxygen source and as a carbon dioxide adsorber. The first higher-order living creature placed in Earth orbit was a female mixed-breed dog named Layka, launched on Sputnik II by the Soviet Union on November 3, 1957. Layka's open-loop life support system was a hermetically sealed, air-conditioned compartment complete with food and water. A typical U.S. design was that used to sustain a monkey named Gordo, who rode a ballistic path through space in the nose cone of a Jupiter missile in December 1958. Carbon dioxide was absorbed by pellets of baralyme, and the breathing gas was compressed oxygen from a cylinder. Temperature control was partially achieved by insulating layers of metal foil and fiberglass, and water vapor was absorbed by a porous material. The waste management system consisted of a diaper on the monkey. Gordo was provided neither food nor water.[1]

Support of human life in space was the next ECLSS goal. Life support systems have succeeded in supporting human life on the Moon and for mission durations over a year. The design of ECLSSs for future manned missions must begin with a knowledge of past designs. This knowledge should come from the manned space programs of both the United States and the Soviet Union. Both countries have been pursuing the manned exploration of space for more than 30 years, resulting in a considerable experience base.

A summary of the ECLSS on U.S. manned spacecraft is presented in Table 1 for Mercury, Gemini, Apollo, Skylab, Spacelab, Space Shuttle, and Space Station. A summary of the ECLSS on Soviet spacecraft is presented in Table 2 for Vostok, Voskhod, Soyuz, Salyut, and Mir.

B. ECLSS Design History on U.S. Spacecraft

Manned space flight in the United States began with Alan Shepard's 15-min suborbital flight aboard the Freedom 7 Mercury-Redstone 3 spacecraft on May 5, 1961. Thirty years later the United States is planning to launch a space station designed to remain in orbit for 30 years. U.S. ECLSS design

The authors express sincere appreciation for the contributions of James L. Reuter and Richard G. Schunk (NASA Marshall Space Flight Center, U.S.A.); Bryce L. Diamont (McDonnell-Douglas Space Systems Company, U.S.A.); Joseph F. Ferrall, Naresh K. Rohatgi, Ph.D., and Darrell L. Jan, Ph.D. (Jet Propulsion Laboratory, U.S.A.); and Edwin L. Force, Ph.D. (NASA Ames Research Center, U.S.A.).

*Section 1 of this chapter is adapted from Ref. 41, and used with permission of the Society of Automotive Engineers, Inc., 1990.

Table 1a - ECLSS on U.S. Spacecraft (Modified from Ref. 41 with permission of Society of Automotive Engineers, © 1990)

Subsystem	Mercury	Gemini	Apollo CM	Apollo LM	Skylab	Orbiter	Spacelab	Space Station
Atmosphere Revitalization								
CO_2 Removal	Two LiOH canisters operated in parallel, with airflow through only one. After the first canister was spent, airflow was diverted through the second, and the spent one was replaced.	Similar to Mercury design	Similar to Mercury design	Similar to Mercury design	Two canister molecular sieve. Each regenerative canister contained Zeolite 5A. CO_2 was vacuum desorbed to space.	Similar to Mercury design	Similar to Mercury design. Eight canisters included on each mission.	Four-bed molecular sieve. Includes two regenerative desiccant beds to remove water and two regenerative Zeolite 5A molecular sieve beds. CO_2 heat and pressure desorbed to an accumulator before being fed to Sabatier reactor.
Gas Recovery/ Generation	None	None	None	None	None	None	None	Sabatier reactor for CO_2 reduction. Static Feed Water Electrolysis (SFWE) for oxygen generation. The SFWE uses a KOH electrolyte.
Trace Contaminant Control	Activated charcoal located in LiOH canisters upstream of the LiOH. Filters removed airborne particulates.	Similar to Mercury design	Similar to Mercury design	Similar to Mercury design	Activated charcoal canister located in the molecular sieve unit. Filters removed airborne particulates. Venting of atmosphere between missions avoided contaminant buildup.	Activated charcoal downstream of the LiOH. CO converted to CO_2 by ambient temperature catalytic oxidizer (ATCO). Filters removed airborne particulates.	Activated charcoal canister located in transfer tunnel between Spacelab and Orbiter. CO converted to CO_2 by ATCO. Filters removed airborne particulates.	Activated charcoal with a high-temperature catalytic oxidizer. Filters remove airborne particulates.
Trace Contaminant Monitoring	CO sensor[2]	No on-orbit monitoring	No on-orbit monitoring	No on-orbit monitoring	Drager tubes monitored buildup of CO and other trace contaminants.[28]	No on-orbit monitoring	No on-orbit monitoring	A CO monitor and a gas chromatograph/ mass spectrometer (GCMS) for detecting contaminants.

Table 1b - ECLSS on U.S. Spacecraft

Subsystem	Mercury	Gemini	Apollo CM	Apollo LM	Skylab	Orbiter	Spacelab	Space Station
Water Recovery & Management								
Water Supply Quality	Potable only	Potable only	Potable only	Potable only	Potable only	Potable only	Not applicable	Potable only
Water Processing	None. Vent waste water.	None. Vent waste water	None. Stored waste water and vented excess, or sent excess to evaporators for additional cooling.	None. Stored waste water. No overboard dumpling of wastes on lunar surface.	None. Stored waste water in tanks and vented when tanks full.	None. Store waste water in a tank and vent waste when tank is full.	Not applicable	Urine-vapor compression distillation (VCD). Potable and wash water multifiltration using sorbent beds.
Water Monitoring	No on-orbit monitoring	No on-orbit monitoring		No on-orbit monitoring	Iodine sampler. Water samples fixed with a linear starch reagent and compared to photographic standards.	No on-orbit monitoring	Not applicable	On-line TOC, pH, iodine concentration, and conductivity monitor for each water processor. Off-line batch microbial and chemical monitoring using mass spectrometry; filter cultures; and gas, liquid, and ion chromatography.
Water Storage and Distribution	One tank with flexible bladder. Squeezing an air bulb pressurized the bladder to deliver water (sphygmomanometer).[3]	One 7.3 liter tank containing a bladder pressurized with oxygen to deliver water. Empty tank was refilled from reserves in the service module.	Fuel cell by-product was principal source of potable water. Palladium and silver removed dissolved H_2. Potable tank used a bladder pressurized by oxygen to deliver water	Three (four on Apollo 15, 16 17) potable tanks, each with a bladder pressurized by nitrogen to deliver water. Potable water also used to cool spacecraft and extravehicular mobility units.	Ten cylindrical 600 lb. capacity stainless steel tanks fitted with pressurized steel bellows to deliver the water. One 26 lb capacity potable tank.[28]	Four 168 lb capacity stainless steel tanks fitted with metal bellows pressurized by N_2. Drinking water is from the fuel cell by-product.	Not applicable	Tank design similiar to the Orbiter, except air is used instead of N_2 to pressurize the metal bellows.

Table 1c - ECLSS on U.S. Spacecraft

Subsystem	Mercury	Gemini	Apollo CM	Apollo LM	Skylab	Orbiter	Spacelab	Space Station
Water System Microbial Control	Water quality depended on the quality of the public water system in Cocoa Beach, FL. Bacterial control depended on the residual disinfectant (chlorine) in the public supply.[29]	Chlorine added to the water before launch	Chlorine at a concentration of 0.5 mg/l maintained by adding 22 ml sodium hypoclorite solution every 24 h.	Iodine added before launch. No on-orbit biocide addition. Pre-flight analysis performed to predict when the iodine concentration would fall below 0.5 mg/l during mission. When this predicted time was reached a bacteria filter was added.	Iodine maintained between 0.5 and 6.0 mg/l by periodic injection of a 30 g/l potassium iodide solution.	Iodine from microbial check values (MCV). MCV passively adjusts iodine concentration between 1 and 2 mg/l.	Not applicable	Iodine from microbial check values (MCVs). Heat sterilization at 120° C for 20 min planned as part of water processing cycle.
Temperature and Humidity Control								
Atmosphere Temperature and Humidity Control	Separate suit and cabin condensing heat exchangers (CHX). Mechanically activated sponge water separator removed water from the CHX. Condensate rejected to water boiler for heat rejection. Pilot regulated suit and cabin temperature by adjusting water flow rate through the suit and cabin HX's with a needle valve.[30]	Suit CHX primary method for cabin temperature and humidity control. Wicks removed water from CHX by capillary action. Water-ethylene glycol coolant.	Separate suit and cabin CHX's. Wicks removed water from CHX by capillary action. Manual throttling of O₂ / coolant flow rate in suit loop to control temperature. Heat transport loop with MCS-198 coolant primary method for heat rejection.[31]	Water circulated through pressure garment assembly to cool astronaut. Water-ethylene glycol coolant.	Four CHXs, two operating at all times. Coolanol 15 coolant.	Centralized cabin liquid-air CHX using water coolant. Air bypass ratio around CHX adjusted to control temperature. Condensate removed by slurper bar and centrifugal separator.	Similar to Orbiter design	Similar to Orbiter design
Cabin Ventilation	Cabin fan	Cabin fan	Cabin fans. The fans were noisy, so the crew only operated them during short specified periods.[32]	Cabin fan	Three ventilation ducts with four fans each. Air distributed from circular diffusers with dampers mounted flush with the floor, and from rectangular outlets with dampers and adjustable flow vanes. Three portable fans with adjustable diffusers.	Cabin fan with ventilation ducts	Cabin fan	Cabin fans and separate local area ventilation fans

Table 1d - ECLSS on U.S. Spacecraft

Subsystem	Mercury	Gemini	Apollo CM	Apollo LM	Skylab	Orbiter	Spacelab	Space Station
Equipment Cooling	Cold plates and air cooling. Cabin gas absorbed heat generated by equipment and was cooled when it passed through the cabin CHX.	Similar to Mercury	Similar to Mercury	Similar to Mercury	Similar to Mercury	Air cooling, cold plates, and air/liquid equipment dedicated HXs. Avionics air loop separate from cabin loop, except in aft flight deck.	Air cooling, cold plates, liquid/liquid equipment dedicated HXs. Avionics air loop separate from cabin loop. Flow control valves set manually before flight.	Air cooling, cold plates, and equipment dedicated HXs. Avionics air loop separate from cabin loop in the habitation and laboratory modules, but combined with cabin loop in nodes and logistics module. Air flow controlled automatically.
Atmosphere Control and Supply								
Atmosphere Composition	100% O_2 at 5 psia (34.5 kPa).	100% O_2 at 5 psia (34.5 kPa)	100% O_2 at 5 psia (34.5 kPa). 60% O_2, 40% N_2 atm. during launch.	100% O_2 at 5 psia (34.5 kPa)	Mixed O_2/N_2 at 5 psia (34.5 kPa) total pressure. 72% O_2, 28% N_2 by volume.	Mixed O_2/N_2 at 14.7 psia (101 kPa) total pressure. 21.7% O_2, 78.3% N_2.	Mixed O_2/N_2 at 14.7 psia (101 kPa) total pressure. 21.7% O_2, 78.3% N_2.	Mixed O_2/N_2 at 14.7 psia (101 kPa) total pressure. 21.7% O_2, 78.3% N_2 volume.
Gas Storage	O_2 stored as a gas at 7500 psi (51.7 MPa) in two 1.8 kg. capacity tanks made of 4340 carbon steel with electrodeless nickel plating. One tank was primary supply, the other was backup.[30]	O_2 stored as a supercritical cryogenic fluid at 850 psi (5.86 MPa) in one spherical tank. Separate tank supplied the fuel cells. Two secondary cylindrical 5000 psi O_2 bottles. One small O_2 bottle attached under each ejectable seat for emergencies.[31]	O_2 stored as a supercritical cryogenic fluid at 900 psi (6.20 MPa) and 180 C_2 in two 145 kg capacity spherical Inconel dewar tanks. Tanks were common for ECLS and power systems. Tanks discarded during reentry, then O_2 was supplied from 1.7 kg capacity surge tank.[32]	21.8 kg of O_2 stored as a gas at 2700 psi (18.6 MPa) in descent stage. In ascent stage O_2 stored as a supercritical cryogenic fluid at 850 psi (5.86 MPa) in two Inconel bottles.[32]	O_2 and N_2 stored as gases at 3000 psi (20.7 MPa) in six bottles each, for a total of 2779 kg of O_2 and 741 kg of N_2	N_2 and O_2 stored as gases at 3300 psi (22.8 MPa). Four spherical N_2 tanks and one emergency O_2 tank. Metabolic O_2 supplied by the power reactant storage and distribution system, which uses supercritical cryogenic storage tanks.	N_2 stored as a gas at 3300 psi (22.8 MPa) in a spherical tank. O_2 source is a 100 psi (689 kPA) line from Orbiter.	Cryogenic stores of O_2 and N_2

Table 1e - ECLSS on U.S. Spacecraft

Subsystem	Mercury	Gemini	Apollo CM	Apollo LM	Skylab	Orbiter	Spacelab	Space Station
Waste Management / Fecal/Urine Handling	In-situ urine collection bag stored onboard. No provisions for fecal handling. No provisions for urine handling on first Mercury mission.	Feces collected in bags and stored. Bags taped to buttocks. Urine collected using urine transfer system, consisting of a rubber cuff connected to a flexible bag. Urine could be directed to boiler tank to assist with spacecraft heat rejection.	Feces collected in bags and stored. Bags taped to buttocks. Bags were needed to mix liquid bactericide with feces. Before Apollo 12, Gemini urine collection system was used. After Apollo 12, urine receptacle assembly, which did not contact the crewman, used. Urine vented.[32]	Fecal containment system identical to Apollo CM system. Primary difference was no overboard dumping of urine on lunar surface.	Feces collected in gas permeable bags attached under a form-fitting seat, then vacuum dried and stored. Urine collected using individual receivers, tubing, and disposable collection bags.[28]	Commode-Urinal - Feces collected in the commode storage container, vacuum dried, and held. Urine sent to a waste water tank which is vented when full.	Utilizes Orbiter facilities	Commode/Urinal- Feces collected in a bag and compacted in a cylindrical canister for biodegradation. Urine sent to the vapor-compression distillation unit to be recovered as potable water.
Fire Detection and Suppression / Suppressant	Water from the food rehydration gun.[14] Capability to depressurize cabin by manually opening cabin outflow valve.	Similar to Mercury design. Maximum of three cabin depressurizations could be accommodated by on-board oxygen supply.	Water from food rehydration gun and a portable aqueous gel (hydroxymethyl cellulose) extinguisher, which could expel 0.06 m of foam in 30 s. Capability to depressurize cabin	Similiar to Apollo CM design	Portable aqueous gel similar to Apollo. Capability to depressurize cabin.	Halon 1301. Two Halon tanks with distribution lines in each avionics bay. three portable Halon extinguishers. Capability to depressurize cabin.	Halon 1301. Halon bottle with distribution lines located in each equipment rack. Two portable Halon extinguishers. Capability to depressurize cabin.	CO_2. Centralized CO_2 bottles with distribution lines to powered equipment racks. Portable CO_2 extinguishers. Capability to depressurize cabin.
Detection	Crew senses[33]	Crew senses	Crew senses	Crew senses	Ultraviolet detectors	Ionization smoke sensors	Ionization smoke sensors	Photoelectric smoke detectors and UV/IR/visual flame detectors.

Table 2a - ECLSS on Soviet Spacecraft (Modified from Ref. 41, used with permission Society of Automotive Engineers, © 1990)

Subsystem	Vostok	Voskhod	Soyuz	Salyut	Mir 1
Atmosphere Revitalization					
CO$_2$ Removal	CO$_2$ removed through reaction with potassium superoxide (KO$_2$) in the oxygen regenerator (forming potassium carbonate and oxygen).[3]	Similar to Vostok design.	Similar to Vostok design. LiOH beds used to absorb about 20% of CO$_2$.[35]	Similar to Soyuz design.	Four-bed molecular sieve. Two regenerative silica gel desiccant beds and two regenerative molecular sieve beds containing adsorbent similar to Zeolite 5A. LiCl canisters used as backup.[36]
Gas Recovery/ Generation	Nonregenerative chemical cartridges of KO$_2$. KO$_2$ reacted with water to produce O$_2$ and KOH.[3]	Similar to Vostok design	Similar to Vostok design	Similar to Vostok design	CO$_2$ not utilized. CO$_2$ vacuum desorbed overboard. Water electrolysis using a KOH electrolyte for oxygen generation. Electrolyzed water from recovered urine supplemented by onboard stores.[36]
Trace Contaminant Removal	Activated charcoal and filters. Contaminants also removed through reaction with constituents in oxygen regenerator.[3]	Similar to Vostok design	Similar to Vostok design	Activated charcoal, high efficiency fiberglass filter, and catalytic chemical absorbents. Oxygen regenerator also removes contaminants[37]	Regenerated charcoal beds and catalytic oxidizers. Charcoal beds regenerated by vacuum for 6 hours once every 10 days. Impurities vented.[37]
Trace Contaminant Monitoring	Gas analyzer determined percent composition of O$_2$ and CO$_2$ in cabin atmosphere. No other on-orbit atmosphere monitoring.[3]	Similar to Vostok design	Similar to Vostok design	Similar to Vostok design. Several gas analyzers distributed around the station.[37]	Similar to Salyut design
Water Recovery and Management					
Water Supply Quality	Potable only	Potable only	Potable only	Potable only	Potable, hygiene, and electrolysis grade
Water Processing	None	None	None	Salyut 6, 7 - Potable water recovered from condensate. Waste water pumped into storage columns containing ion exchange resins and activated charcoal, then sent through filters containing fragmented dolomite, artificial silicates, and salt. Minerals added, including calcium, magnesium,[37] bicarbonate, chloride, and sulfate.	Three water purification systems: 1. Condensate recovered by same process used on Salyut 6, 7. 2. Wash/kitchen water recovered by system of filters and ion exchange resins. 3. Electrolysis water recovered from urine by vapor diffusion distillation.[36]
Water Quality Monitoring	None	None	None	None	Water analyzers[36]

Table 2b - ECLSS on Soviet Spacecraft

Subsystem	Vostok	Voskhod	Soyuz	Salyut	Mir 1
Water Storage and Distribution	Water held in a container made of two layers of elastic polyethylene film, hermetically sealed inside a metal cylinder. Low pressure created by the crewman's mouth induced water flow from the container. Each crewman allotted 2.2 l/day of water.[3]	Similar to Vostok design	Similar to Vostok design	Rodnik ("spring") system supplies water from tanks with a total volume of over 400 liters[37]	Similar to Salyut design. Tanks use pressurized bladders to deliver water.[36]
Water Supply Microbial Control	Silver preparation added to water, which was boiled before launch[3]	Similar to Vostok design	Similar to Vostok design	Water is heated and ionic silver is introduced electrolytically to a concentration of 0.2 mg/l[37]	Similar to Salyut design
Temperature and Humidity Control					
Atmosphere Temperature and Humidity Control	Liquid-air condensing heat exchanger. Condensate trapped by porous wicks between heat exchanger tubes. Temperature adjusted by automatic regulation of air flow rate through heat exchanger. Cosmonaut set temperature and humidity. Temperature range between 12–25 °C, relative humidity between 30%–70%. Humidity was controlled by the temperature of a coolant and an additional dehumidifier containing anhydrous silica gel and activated charcoal impregnated with LiOH. Dehumidifier operated cyclically. Air inlet to dehumidifier opened after humidity rose above 70%. Air inlet automatically closed when humidity reached 35 ± 5%.[38]	Similar to Vostok design.	Liquid-air condensing heat exchanger. Temperature adjusted by automatic regulation of air flow rate through heat exchanger. Liquid coolant was a water/ethylene glycol mixture. Cosmonaut set temperature and humidity of craft. Temperature range between 12–25 °C, relative humidity between 30–70%. Humidity controlled primarily by condensing heat exchanger. Condensate trapped by porous wicks between the heat exchanger tubes. Primary role of the chemical water adsorbants was control of the oxygen production rate of O_2 regenerator.[3]	Liquid-air condensing heat exchanger. Temperature set by cosmonaut between 15–25 °C. Coolant was antifreeze-type fireproof liquid. Porous wicks trapped moisture between heat exchanger tubes. Condensate collected in a moisture trap and pumped out manually by the cosmonauts.[39]	Liquid-air condensing heat exchanger. Two internal thermal control loops - a cooling loop and a heating loop - charged with "Temp" coolant. Redundant piping system included with each loop. Loop temperature controlled automatically.[36]
Cabin Ventilation	Cabin fan	Cabin fan	Cabin fan	Cabin fan. Cosmonauts controlled air flow rate between 0.1–0.8 m/s.[37]	Fans pull air through ducts to exchange gas between modules.[40]

Table 2c - ECLSS on Soviet Spacecraft

Subsystem	Vostok	Voskhod	Soyuz	Salyut	Mir 1
Equipment Cooling	Avionics is cooled by air that was passed through the heat exchanger	Similar to Vostok design	Similar to Vostok design	Similar to Vostok design	Avionics cooled by heat exchangers and air pulled from cabin. Condenser with freon removes moisture that condenses on the equipment.[36]
Atmosphere Control and Supply					
Atmosphere Composition	Sea-level atmosphere - O_2/N_2 mixture at 14.7 psi (101 kPa)	Sea-level atmosphere- O_2/N_2 mixture at 14.7 psi (101 kPa)	Sea-level atmosphere. O_2/N_2 mixture at a total pressure between 13.7–16.4 psi (94.4–113 kPa), with ppO_2 between 2.7 and 3.9 psi (10.5–15.2 kPa).	Sea-level atmosphere. O_2/N_2 mixture at a total pressure between 13.5–18.5 psi (93.1–128 kPa), with ppO_2 between 3.1–4.6 psi (21.4–31.7 kPa).	Sea-level atmosphere. Up to 78% N_2, 21–40% O_2. Maximum ppO_2 is 6.8 psi (46.9 kPa).
Gas Storage	Oxygen supply stored chemically. Emergency tanks of high pressure oxygen and air for suit ventilation and cosmonaut breathing. Cosmonaut's suit could be pressurized if the cabin depressurized. No N_2 storage. Cabin hermetic seal was designed for zero leakage.[40]	Similar to Vostok design	Similar to Vostok design	Oxygen supply stored chemically. Cylinders of compressed air for leakage makeup. No separate N_2 or O_2 storage.[38]	Backup oxygen stored chemically as $NaCeO_7$. N_2 is stored as a high pressure gas. Oxygen is produced from water electrolysis.[37]
Waste Management					
Fecal/Urine Handling	Urine and feces entrained in air stream and collected. Design of the urine/feces receiving unit permitted simultaneous collection of urine and feces when clothed in a space suit.	Similar to Vostok design	Similar to Vostok design	Each defecation is collected in a bag which is then stored in sealed metal containers which are ejected to space, about once a week. The urine collector, separate from the main commode, is a cup-and-tube device with a disposable plastic insert and filter.	Commode for urine and feces collection. Urine sent to water recovery processor after passing through an air/liquid separator.

Table 2d - ECLSS on Soviet Spacecraft

Subsystem	Vostok	Voskhod	Soyuz	Salyut	Mir 1
Fire Detection and Suppression					
Suppressant	Cabin depressurization capability	None	Same as Vostok design	Same as Vostok design	Portable extinguishers. Crew can open valves to extinguish fires in inaccessible areas. Cabin depressurization capability. [36]
Detection	Crew senses	Crew senses	Crew senses	CO_2 detectors doubled as smoke detectors [37]	Optical sensors [36]

has come a long way since that first Mercury flight, having since supported human life on Gemini, Apollo, Skylab, Spacelab, Space Shuttle, and soon on Space Station. Table 1 details the primary facets of ECLSS design for each of these U.S. spacecraft. The dates listed with each spacecraft give the period when it was being used for space missions.

1) Mercury (1960–1963)—The objectives of the Mercury project were to place manned spacecraft in Earth orbit, explore human reactions in orbit, test the possibilities of manual spacecraft control by the pilot, and safely recover astronauts and capsules from space. Mercury was a pressurized one-man capsule in the shape of a bell, with 1.56 m^3 of habitable space for the astronaut.[2] The Mercury ECLSS is composed of pressure suit and cabin subsystems. The pressure suit subsystem was primarily responsible for revitalizing the astronaut's atmosphere supply and for controlling his/her temperature and humidity level. The cabin subsystem controlled cabin ventilation, cabin temperature (the cabin heat exchanger did not remove water vapor), and atmospheric pressure. The space suit was normally unpressurized during flight.

2) Gemini (1964–1966)—The Gemini project, an extension of the Mercury project, was the second phase of the U.S. plan to land humans on the Moon. Its objectives were to test crew and capsule behavior for a nonstop 14-day orbit, develop the capability to rendezvous and dock with other spacecraft, perform extravehicular activities, develop methods for controlling spacecraft reentry flight paths, and provide a basis for scientific experimentation. Gemini was a pressurized two-man capsule with 2.26 m^3 of habitable space for the astronauts.[2] As with Mercury, the Gemini ECLSS was divided into the pressure suit and cabin subsystems. Gemini improvements over the Mercury ECLSS included supercritical oxygen storage instead of high-pressure storage, an integrated heat exchanger/water separator, and a mechanically activated sponge-type water separator.

3) Apollo (1968–1972)—The objectives of the Apollo project were to land a human on the Moon and return him/her safely to Earth, explore the Moon from the lunar surface and from lunar orbit, and demonstrate that humans can move about and work in an alien environment. The total Apollo space vehicle included two separate life support systems, one on the command module (CM) and one on the lunar module (LM). The CM ECLSS occupied 0.25 m^3 of the cabin and was capable of operating for 14 days. Oxygen and potable water from fuel cells were supplied from the Apollo service module, which was attached to the base of the CM. Launch safety was increased by using a 60 percent oxygen (O_2) and 40 percent nitrogen (N_2) cabin gas mixture during prelaunch and launch periods, although the suit circuit remained at 100 percent O_2. The ascent stage of the Apollo LM was a pressurized two-man craft with 4.5 m^3 of habitable space.[2] The third astronaut from the CM remained in the CM in circumlunar parking orbit until the ascent module returned from the Moon. In contrast to the Apollo CM ECLSS, the LM ECLSS had potable water from storage tanks instead of fuel cells, no overboard venting of urine on the lunar surface, and iodine bacte-

ricide instead of chlorine to avoid corrosion problems anticipated between chlorine and the LM sintered nickel sublimator plates. Unlike the situation in all previous spacecraft, there were no seats in the LM, so the astronaut had to be accommodated from a standing position.

4) Skylab (1973–1974)—The objectives of Skylab, the first U.S. space station, were to study the effects of long-duration space flight on humans; study the Earth, Sun, and stars; and perform experiments in a microgravity environment. Skylab was a three-person laboratory with a total habitable volume of 361 m^3 (Ref. 2). The crew lived and worked in the two-level orbital workshop, although most of the ECLSS equipment was located in the airlock module. New ECLSS techniques on Skylab included a mixed O_2 and N_2 atmosphere and two-canister molecular sieves instead of lithium hydroxide (LiOH) canisters to remove carbon dioxide (CO_2), a method of monitoring iodine concentration in the water supply, the storage of urine samples in a freezer for analysis on Earth, and ultraviolet fire detectors. Between missions, when Skylab was unoccupied, the atmosphere was depressurized to 13.8 kPa and allowed to decay down to 3.45 kPa until the next group of astronauts arrived. Depressurization removed trace contaminants from the cabin to reduce the chance of fire.

5) Space Shuttle Orbiter (1981–present)—The objective of the Space Shuttle Program is to replace expendable launch vehicles with a reusable transport to increase accessibility to space at a relatively low cost. Shuttle missions support private and commercial ventures in space, including the eventual construction of a permanent space station. The Orbiter is designed to carry an average crew of seven for a nominal mission of 7 days in a total habitable volume of 74 m^3 (Ref. 2). The Orbiter became the first U.S. spacecraft to use a standard sea-level atmosphere—a gas mixture of 22 percent O_2 and 78 percent N_2 at a total pressure of 101 kPa. Other Orbiter ECLSS innovations included Halon 1301 fire suppressant; microbial check valves to passively adjust iodine concentration in the potable water supply; and a commode for fecal collection and storage, to be used instead of simple bag collection.

6) Spacelab (1983–present)—The cylindrical Spacelab laboratory module, situated in the Space Shuttle cargo bay during a Spacelab module mission, provides a pressurized, shirt-sleeve environment for performing experiments in microgravity. Most of the Spacelab ECLSS is very similar to the Orbiter system and depends on the Orbiter for its metabolic O_2 supply. Cabin air is exchanged with the Orbiter through the Spacelab transfer tunnel. An avionics air loop, separate from the cabin air loop, is used for air-cooling rack-mounted instrumentation. Spacelab can remain operational throughout a Space Shuttle mission.

7) Space Station—The Space Station will serve as a research laboratory in space and potentially as a staging base for missions to the Moon, Mars, and beyond. The description of Space Station ECLSS below and in Table 1 is for a crew of eight for the fully configured Space Station. Space Station

will be composed of a number of pressurized elements, including laboratory modules, habitation modules, nodes, an airlock, and a logistics module. The planned ECLSS design will provide a closed system for air and water and will be more complicated than any ECLSS of the past, all of which were basically open systems. CO2 will be reduced to recover the useful O_2 atoms in the form of water. O_2 will be produced by water electrolysis, eliminating the need for O_2 resupply. Hygienic wastewater, urine, condensate, and CO_2 reduction water will be recycled to keep water resupply to a minimum. Long-term operation must accommodate simple on-orbit maintenance requiring little crew time. The above description pertains to a single design variant of Space Station. Some of the information presented in Table 1 may change before launch of the first station element. As the present work goes to press, the design of the entire station is undergoing review and revision and may change drastically.

C. ECLSS Design History on U.S.S.R. Spacecraft

The first human being in space was Yuriy Alexeyevich Gagarin, a Soviet Air Force pilot. Launched into Earth orbit aboard a Vostok capsule by an A-l rocket on April 12, 1961, Gagarin made one orbit of the Earth, completing the 108-min mission with little difficulty. The U.S.S.R. has far more experience with manned space flight than all other nations combined, particularly in the realm of long-duration missions. A number of cosmonauts have completed stays in space of well over 300 days. Since 1971, the Soviets have launched eight space stations, including the currently orbiting Mir station. Table 2 describes the ECLSS designs on the Soviet Vostok, Voskhod, Soyuz, Salyut, and Mir spacecraft. In Russian, the ECLSS is referred to as the Sistema Obespecheniya Zhiznedeyatelnosti (SOZh), meaning "Life Support System."

1) Vostok (1960–1963)—The spherical Vostok, with a habitable volume of approximately 3 m^3, was the first spacecraft to carry a human into space. The objectives of the Vostok program were to test human behavior under microgravity, test high acceleration and deceleration levels (8–10 g), test and further develop ground-controlled automatic spacecraft guidance, and make astronomical and geophysical observations.[2] The Vostok ECLSS was a simple semiclosed system with a 101-kPa air atmosphere. Cabin ECLSS equipment was responsible for CO_2 removal and the control of cabin odor, humidity, ventilation, temperature, and air supply.[3] The cosmonaut wore a space suit that was ventilated by cabin air and did not have the capability for air purification or humidity control. In an emergency, the suit could be supplied with air and O_2 from tanks mounted on the Vostok exterior.

2) Voskhod (1964–1965)—The spherical Voskhod capsule was basically an improved version of the Vostok with a rearranged interior to accommodate three crewmembers. To help make room for the cosmonauts, Voskhod became the first spacecraft in which the crew did not wear space suits. Objectives of the Voskhod program were to gather data on group crews and study human behavior outside the capsule.[2]

Voskhod 2 was equipped with two space suits and an inflatable decompression chamber, from which the first space walk was performed.

3) Soyuz/Soyuz T (1967–present)—Soyuz was designed primarily for docking with other space vehicles. Objectives of the Soyuz program were to perfect docking and crew transfer between capsules and Salyut stations, practice craft orbital transfer, and perform scientific observations and experiments.[2] Designed for 7-day missions, the Soyuz was a three-man vehicle with two pressurized compartments, one for living and working and the other for descent. Soyuz cosmonauts did not wear pressurized suits. After Soyuz 11, the crew was reduced to two to make room for pressurized suits. The hermetically sealed Soyuz cabin was designed for zero leakage. Soyuz T, a modified version of Soyuz, which retains the basic size and shape of the Soyuz craft, has a redesigned interior to accommodate three space-suited cosmonauts. Soyuz spacecraft are still used to ferry cosmonauts to and from the orbiting Mir space station.

4) Salyut Space Stations (1971–1986)—Salyut was the first spacecraft designed for extended missions in space and, thus, became the world's first space station. Since the beginning of the Salyut program, seven Salyut stations were placed in orbit. With the overriding goal of establishing a permanent presence in space, Salyut was considered the cornerstone of Soviet policy aimed at establishing human colonies on the Moon and Mars.

Designed for a crew of five, Salyut consists of three inseparable modules with a total usable volume of about 100 m^3 (Ref. 2). Each successive Salyut improved on the previous station, although the basic configuration remained the same. The ECLSS remained predominantly the same on the Salyut stations until Salyut 6, when a water regeneration system was added to recover condensate and wash water.

5) Mir Space Station (1986–present)—Currently in Earth orbit, the Mir space station is the third generation of Soviet orbital stations, although the design of its core is basically similar to that of Salyut 7. The Mir core, designed for a crew of six in a habitable volume of about 150 m^3 (Ref. 4), is the first space station designed to accommodate growth by the addition of modules. Mir uses several regenerative ECLSS technologies. O_2 is produced by water electrolysis, and CO_2 is removed by a four-bed molecular sieve system and vented to space. Wastewater is also recovered. Research is currently in progress to further advance the Mir ECLSS to increase the closure.

D. Summary

A summary of the ECLSSs on past, present, and planned spacecraft has been presented. The tabular summary allows for ready comparison of spacecraft ECLSS design and depicts how the ECLSS has evolved (and continues to evolve) from the early open systems to the nearly closed ECLSS space station systems planned for the l990s. As endeavors in manned space flight continue, the knowledge of how to sustain human life in space will continue to advance. The development of techniques for regenerating atmosphere and water will reduce dependence on resupply from Earth, increasing the chances for long-duration space voyages far from home. Future ECLSSs may be completely closed, with as little dependence as possible on outside sources for life-sustaining supplies. Closed-loop ECLSSs will pave the way for human settlements on the Moon and beyond, where regular resupply from Earth may not be feasible. ECLSS evolution will make the permanent human occupation of space more than simply a dream.

II. Common and Specific Mission Requirements

A. Overview

The basic architecture of the ECLSS can be divided into requirements that are common and those that are mission specific. An example of a common requirement is the cabin air ventilation flow range. An example of a mission specific requirement is provision of food supply refrigeration.

In this discussion, we will use the planned Space Station ECLSS as an example. The ECLSS is composed of six major subsystem groups,[5] which are interlinked with each other as well as with external interfaces. The definition of the ECLSS can be given by defining the six subsystem groups: temperature and humidity control (THC), atmosphere control and supply (ACS), atmosphere revitalization (AR), water recovery and management (WRM), waste management (WM), and fire detection and suppression (FDS).

The subsystem groups can further be described by listing the functions performed in them. THC consists of air temperature control, humidity control, ventilation, equipment air cooling, thermal conditioning, and airborne particulate and microbial control. ACS encompasses O_2N_2 storage, distribution and resupply, venting, relief, and dumping, as well as O_2N_2 partial and total pressure control. AR consists of CO_2 removal, CO_2 reduction, O_2 generation, and trace chemical contamination control and monitoring. WRM comprises urine water recovery, wash water processing, potable water processing, water storage and distribution, and water quality monitoring. WM encompasses fecal waste collection, processing or storage, and fecal return waste storage and handling. FDS comprises fire detection and fire suppression.

B. General Requirements

Requirements which the ECLSS must meet fall into four basic categories. The first and probably the most critical category is related to crew health and is defined by medical personnel. The next category is related to environmental control for equipment. The third involves general service provisions, which are typically dictated by either programmatic or system design considerations or overall system efficiency studies. The final category involves requirements derived from the extrapolations of other requirements in the first three cat-

egories or derived to protect ECLSS equipment.

The ECLSS requirements must be based upon the nominal human mass balance, as defined in Table 3. This table shows both input and output masses for food, liquids, and gases. Variations will depend primarily on activity levels and food water content. Table 4 shows a typical set of overall atmospheric requirements with footnotes to elaborate. Those requirements not specified here include electrical and electronic aspects (e.g., grounding and power stability specifications), material requirements (e.g., flammability and corrosion), structural and stress requirements (e.g., proof and burst design levels), special safety issues (e.g., sharp edge elimination and locknut safety wiring), noise or vibroacoustic requirements, and electromagnetic interference requirements.

C. Subsystem Group Requirements

The THC subsystem group must provide THC functions over the entire pressurized volume under normal operations. Adequate ventilation must be provided in all habitable areas, including intraelement and interelement airflow. As an integral part of the air circulation, both particulate and microbial control must be ensured. The ECLSS must be capable of providing air cooling to permanently mounted equipment (especially in enclosures such as racks). Refrigeration and freezer capability must be provided for food and other items requiring low-temperature storage. Table 4 gives specific temperature, humidity, and ventilation flow requirements. It should be noted that the system will be capable of temperature selection and control by the crew to a set-point value anywhere in the range of achievable temperatures plus or minus 1 °C.

Ventilation flow is provided to all human-occupied zones in a range of 5–13 m/min, with expectations of near-perfect mixing and with no short circuiting of flow, or dead spots, in the human-occupied volume. In addition, surface temperatures must be maintained above the local dew point to avoid condensation. Refrigeration is typically provided when non-thermally-stabilized food is utilized. The temperature of refrigeration is 5 °C. Typically, food freezers operate at −32 °C; however, lower temperature operating regimes may be desirable when the freezer is used for other purposes, such as quick freezing of biological specimens or storage for specialized science purposes. Table 4 also details microbial and particulate requirements. Although one typical set of particulate limits is given, the limits are generally a variable that may differ considerably from mission to mission.

ACS subsystem group functions provide methods of regulating and monitoring the air total pressure and selected partial pressures. Storage, distribution, and supply of O_2 and N_2 are provided. Vent, relief, and overboard bleed or dump capabilities are also provided as an ECLSS service. Sufficient N_2 for makeup of leakage and required repressurization must be provided, along with other support requirements, as necessary. O_2 for leakage, as well as metabolic makeup, with added resources as necessary to support contingencies, is a normal ECLSS-supplied service. Table 4 also provides total

Table 3 Nominal crewmember metabolic balance, nonextravehicular activity (kg/man-day)[a]

Input		Output[b]	
Food solids	0.62	Waste solids	0.11
		Urine	0.06
		Feces	0.03
		Sweat	0.02
Liquids (water)	3.52	Waste liquids	3.86
Drink	1.61	Urine	1.50
Food preparation	0.76	Sweat and respiration	2.27
Food H_2O content	1.15	Fecal H_2O	0.09
Gases	0.83	Gases	1.00
O_2	0.83	CO_2	1.00
Total	4.97	Total	4.97

[a]Assuming metabolic rate = 2700 kcal/man-day and respiration quotient = 0.87.
[b]The food and O_2 inputs are metabolized by the crewmember to produce 0.34 kg/man-day of metabolic water (reflected in the waste liquids total) and 0.45 kg/man-day of CO_2.

Table 4 Atmosphere requirements for Space Station (90-day)

Atmospheric requirement	Units	Operational	Emergency
CO_2 partial pressure	mmHg	3 max.	12 max.
Temperature	deg C	19–27	15–33
Dew point[a]	deg C	4.4–10	4.4–10
Ventilation	m/min	5-13	1.5–60.0
O_2 partial pressure[b]	kPa	19.5–22.4	15.6–23.5
Total pressure	kPa	98.6–101.3	98.6–101.3
Dilute gas	–	N_2	N_2
Micro-organisms	CFU/m[3c]	1000[d]	1000[d]

[a]Relative humidity shall be within the range of 25–75 percent.
[b]In no case shall the O_2 partial pressure be below 15.0 N/m[2] (2.3 psia) or the O_2 concentration exceed 23.8 percent of the total pressure.
[c]Colony Forming Units (CFUs).
[d]These values reflect a limited base. No widely sanctioned standards are available.

pressure as well as O_2 partial pressure requirements. In spacecraft atmospheres, monitoring of O_2 partial pressure and total pressure is a requirement.

The AR subsystem group conditions the air as necessary to provide a safe and habitable environment for the crew. Monitoring and control of atmospheric trace contaminants and odor are provided, as well as the removal of CO_2. The reduction of CO_2 and generation of O_2 are optional, depending on the level of closure desirable. Atmospheric trace contaminants and odors must be controlled, as necessary, to prevent crew exposure to levels exceeding maximum allowable concentrations. Crew generation of CO_2 during nominal periods is 1 kg/man-day. Breathable quality O_2 is supplied for metabolic makeup at a rate to meet use demands. The nominal use rate of O_2 is 0.83 kg/man-day. The trace contaminant level is controlled at or below the Spacecraft Maximum Allowable Concentration (SMAC).[6] Where near-real-time trace contaminant readings are necessary, sensors must be capable of detecting the SMAC for each constituent at accuracies within ±50 percent.

The WRM subsystem provides the collection, storage, and dispensing of water to meet crew and selected other needs.

Table 5 Nominal crewmember and cabin water balance, nonextravehicular activity (kg/man-day) (general requirements for U.S. crewmembers)

Input		Output	
Crewmember metabolic and food preparation:			
Drink	1.61	Urine	1.50
Food H$_2$O content	1.15	Sweat and respiration	2.27
Metabolized H$_2$O	0.35	Fecal H$_2$O	0.09
Food preparation, liquid	0.79	Food preparation, latent	0.04
Total	3.90	Total	3.90
Cabin:			
Clothes wash	12.46	Clothes wash	
		Liquid	11.86
		Latent	0.60
		Hygiene	
Shower	5.44	Liquid	6.81
Hand wash	1.81	Latent	0.44
Urine flush H$_2$O	0.49	Urine flush H$_2$O	0.49
Total	20.20	Total	20.20

Table 6 Water requirements (general standards developed for U.S. crewmembers)

Parameter	Units	Operational	Degraded	Emergency
Potable water	kg/man-day	3.1	3.1	3.1
Wash water	kg/man-day	23.3	9.1	1.4

Water chemical, microbial, and physical control must be accomplished in accordance with accepted standards. Processing of wastewater is optional. Urine, as well as fecal water, may be recovered. Microbial control of water may be accomplished by a number of means. In the United States, iodination is typically required, with an average level of 2 parts per million (ppm) normally used. Distribution services must include both purified water and wastewater. Dispensing must include provisions for the storage and/or disposal of unused waste, such as spent filters, resin beds, and brine recovery residue. Provisions for wet trash and fecal water recovery are optional.

Water thermal conditioning at the use or distribution point may be provided in lieu of central conditioning. Nominal metabolic input and output levels, including water balance, used in the design of Space Station ECLSS are given in Table 5. It should be noted here that food water content dramatically affects the overall water balance and may vary greatly depending on the onboard refrigeration and freezer provisions, crew preference, and medical considerations. Minimum water quantity requirements are given in Table 6, using the current Space Station design as an example. In all water reclamation systems, the capability should exist to recover from upset conditions, especially microbial contamination. On-line water monitoring and control are generally provided for the following parameters: total organic concentration, resistivity, pH, biocide level, turbidity, and temperature.

The WM subsystem provides for the collection, storage and/or processing, and disposal, if necessary, of human waste. This will include considerations of urine, its residue where applicable, and fecal matter. Fecal matter may be compacted and treated (or stabilized), where feasible. Urine will be stabilized and treated with biocide at the collection point where feasible. Urine excreted by a crewmember will nominally be 1.5 kg/day. Typical crew dry fecal matter output is 0.03 kg/man-day. Nominal water expected in fecal matter is 0.09 kg/man-day.

FDS functions include the means for detecting and suppressing fires internal to the pressurized volume. Fire suppressant capability must be restorable after discharge. For multielement or zoned applications, annunciation of fires in any element or zone must be made in all habitable elements or zones. Fire control strategy must include identification of fire location, and both fixed and portable fire suppressant capability must be provided. Sufficient suppressant must be stored onboard to ensure that the worst case and maximum number of fire events can be properly dealt with in a safe and timely fashion. Fires must also be detected early enough to ensure sufficient time either to fight the fire locally or exit the affected element safely while fighting the fire remotely. Where multielement configurations are employed, fire annunciation of a detected event and remote suppression discharge capability to any other element should be employed.

D. Test Verification

The requirements for verification generally are related to the maturity of the program, type of program, previous history of the equipment, and importance or criticality of the equipment. As a result, test requirements may vary greatly. In general, however, most equipment must undergo some form of development, qualification, and acceptance testing. The need for other testing, such as system-level tests, life testing, and prior flight testing, depends on a number of variables. One standard rule is that all items capable of functioning in an Earth environment will be exercised prior to flight.

E. Support to Other Systems

Typically, the ECLSS may provide utility services to other systems. These functions may include services from all ECLSS subsystem groups. For example, the THC subsystem group may provide equipment air cooling to all other systems as well as payloads. The ACS subsystem group may provide gases to the man-system functions (e.g., health monitors) or to payloads. In addition, other attached elements not part of the basic element may be provided by the ECLSS. For example, water or other ECLSS functions could be provided temporarily (e.g., to a transient transfer vehicle) or continuously (e.g., to a continuously docked module).

F. Special Subjects

Safety of the crew is of the utmost importance; consequently, the issue of crew safety in an emergency is of special interest. This condition has been referred to as "safe haven." The allowed environment during safe haven typically may be more relaxed than that required in the normal operating mode (Table 4), especially the life support parameters. Another source of special design requirements is the presence of animals in the pressurized volume in which the crew is also located. Separation of animal ECLSS function responsibilities must be carefully executed between the animal enclosure design and the ECLSS. Another example of special requirements might be the isolation of payload contaminants from the pressurized atmosphere. This is especially important when the payload complement utilizes toxic substances in its equipment. In this event, it is advisable to require a payload containment vessel design with dual-failure tolerance.

The determination of the correct closure approach is again mission-scenario dependent. In the case of a design, such as a small surface lander from a planet orbiting vehicle, a short-duration rover, or an Earth-to-Moon transfer vehicle, where mission times are short, an open-loop design will be indicated. However, in a longer duration flight, such as a planetary mission or a permanent planetary base, a closed-loop design may be more attractive. Other topics of interest are reliability and maintenance. Although optimization of these features is always desirable, it will be appropriate to specify them more rigorously on long-duration flights.

III. The Potential Role of In-Situ Resources for Life Support

The duration of mission, crew size, and distance from the Earth are the key parameters in determining the cost of human exploration of outer space. One way to reduce the cost of a mission is to provide a self-sufficient life support system with no resupply from Earth. In order to achieve this goal,

1) Mission closure of the life support system functions with the help of various regenerative support technologies is required.

2) Utilization of in-situ resources may be needed to produce products and by-products that can be used for life support, power, and propulsion.[7,8]

A. Extraterrestrial In-Situ Resources

The continuous supply of four important elements—carbon, O_2, hydrogen, and N_2—is needed for a self-sustaining life support system. The recovery and availability of these elements from various extraterrestrial in-situ resources are required to provide 0.9 kg/man-day of O_2, 25 kg/man-day of water, 0.6 kg/man-day of dry food, energy, and other expendable materials.[9]

Figure 1 illustrates the fact that regolith, subsurface, polar caps, atmospheric gases of extraterrestrial bodies, and solar energy are five major in-situ resources available in outer space. The resources in the regolith are concentrated in two different particle size ranges. The solar-wind-implanted particles of size below 20 μm are rich in hydrogen and N_2.[10] The particles larger than 20 μm are oxides of aluminum, calcium, chromium, iron, sodium, silicon, titanium, etc.[11,12] A useful by-product of regolith processing may be the possible generation of propellants, such as silane,[13] and recovery of uranium and thorium for thermoelectrical nuclear power plants.[14]

The availability of water is an important issue in planning the human exploration of outer space. Although O_2 is plentiful in the lunar and martian regolith, water and hydrogen are very scarce. The abundance of water in outer space is not well understood; however, it is anticipated that frozen water

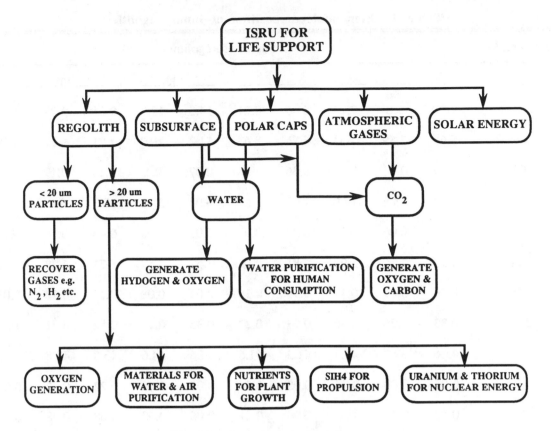

Fig. 1 In-situ resources in outer space.

and CO_2 are available at the subsurface and polar caps of Mars and on both moons of Mars, Phobos, and Deimos.[15,16] CO_2, along with small amounts of water vapor, N_2, and argon, is also available in the atmospheric gases to produce O_2 for life support.

B. In-Situ Resources on the Moon and Mars

There are a number of important in-situ resources available on the lunar surface:

1) The lunar regolith of particle sizes greater than 20 μm: The element composition data for the lunar regolith obtained from several locations are shown in Table 7.[11]

2) The lunar regolith of particle sizes larger than 20 μm: The concentration of hydrogen implanted from the solar wind varies from 124–184 ppm at a depth above 150 cm to 84–104 ppm below that depth.[17] A range of 17–106 ppm hydrogen in 17 bulk soil samples from all Apollo missions was reported.[18] The other solar-wind-implanted gases in the lunar fine are helium (0.5 g/g H_2), helium-3 (0.0002 g/g H_2), neon (0.05 g/g H_2), and argon (0.01 g/g H_2). For every gram of hydrogen recovered from lunar fines, 1.7 grams of N_2 are produced.

3) Extraction of nutrients from lunar soil to support agricultural activities is an area that requires more research. Table 8 presents a comparison of the concentration of essential nutrients needed for plant growth and the concentration of nutrients available in the lunar soil.[19]

4) For more advanced lunar settlements, the thorium and

uranium available in the lunar soil may be recovered to produce nuclear fuel to provide energy.

5) Since lunar soil is rich in O_2 and minerals (Table 7), propellants, such as liquid O_2, liquid hydrogen, and silane, also have potential for being manufactured on the Moon.

The important in-situ resources available on the Mars surface are as follows:

1) Martian soil, like lunar soil, is rich in O_2 and minerals.[20]

2) The atmospheric gases of Mars are rich in CO_2.[8]

3) It is believed that large quantities of frozen water and CO_2 are available at the martian polar caps.[15] Similarly, the presence of large quantities of frozen water and CO_2 is also projected on two martian moons, Phobos and Deimos.

4) Sunlight is available 24 h/day.[8] This is an important in-situ resource for the operation of energy-intensive regenerative life support technology.

5) Martian soil, like lunar soil, provides a raw material to produce micronutrients for plant growth.

6) Propellants, such as liquid hydrogen, liquid O_2, and silane, may also be produced from martian resources.

C. In-Situ Resource Utilization (ISRU) Technologies

Recovery of O_2 and other materials from regolith, recovery of hydrogen and N_2 from fine regolith, recovery of potable water from polar caps and the subsurface, generation of O_2 from water and CO_2, production of propellants, genera-

Table 7   Elemental composition of lunar regolith[11]

Element, %	Source of Regolith								
	Mare					High		Basin	
Al	7.29	5.8	7.25	5.46	8.21	14.3	12.2	9.21	9.28	10.9
Ca	8.66	7.59	7.54	6.96	8.63	11.2	10.0	7.71	6.27	9.19
Cr	0.21	0.31	0.24	0.36	0.2	0.07	0.1	0.15	0.19	0.18
Fe	12.2	13.6	12.0	15.3	12.7	4.03	5.71	10.3	9.0	6.68
K	0.12	0.06	0.22	0.08	0.08	0.09	0.06	0.46	0.14	0.13
Mg	4.93	5.8	5.98	6.81	5.3	3.52	5.59	5.71	6.28	6.21
Mn	0.16	0.19	0.17	0.19	0.16	0.05	0.08	0.11	0.12	0.08
Ma	0.33	0.26	0.36	0.23	0.27	0.35	0.26	0.52	0.31	0.3
O	41.6	39.7	42.3	41.3	41.6	44.6	44.6	43.8	43.8	42.2
P	0.05	0.03	0.14	0.05	0.06	0.05	0.05	0.22	0.07	0.06
S	0.12	0.13	0.1	0.06	0.21	0.06	0.08	0.08	0.08	0.06
Si	19.8	18.6	21.6	21.5	20.5	21.0	21.0	22.4	21.7	21.0
Ti	4.6	5.65	1.84	1.29	2.11	0.34	0.29	1.02	0.79	0.97

tion of electrical energy, and production of food are seven major functions that could be utilized to produce materials for life support.

For producing O_2 and other materials from regolith, the regolith may be magnetically processed to separate pyroxene and olivine, followed by electrostatic processing to separate anorthite from ilmenite. In hydrogen reduction processing, ilmenite is reduced in the presence of hydrogen at 923–1273 K. Water is further electrolytically processed to produce hydrogen and O_2. The by-products are iron and titanium dioxide.

In the magma electrolysis process, ilmenite is melted at 1640 K and then electrolyzed to produce O_2. The by-products are iron and titanium dioxide. In the carbochlorination process, anorthite, along with carbon and chlorine, is reacted at temperatures in the range of 848–1043 K. The gaseous metal chlorides, along with carbon monoxide (CO), are passed through a series of condensers. The first condenser removes aluminum trichloride at 363 K, and the second condenser removes CO from silicon tetrachloride and calcium chloride salts at 243 K. The CO is further processed in a Bosch reactor and water electrolysis units to produce O_2.

In a carbothermal process, the magnesium silicate part of the beneficiated regolith is reacted with methane at 1878 K. Water is electrolyzed to produce O_2 and hydrogen. The magnesium oxide and silicon are by-products of this process. In an acid leach process, the mare regolith (unbeneficiated) is processed with hydrofluoric acid at 283 K. The electrolysis of water and iron hexafluorosilicate produces O_2. Silicon tetrafluoride is processed to recover hydrogen fluoride. The by-products are iron, aluminum, magnesium, calcium oxide, and titanium dioxide. In a vapor-ion distillation process, regolith is vaporized and ionized, followed by selective condensation to obtain products as shown: O_2: 54 K; aluminum: 923 K; titanium: 1943 K; iron: 1890 K; and magnesium: 922 K.

Hydrogen may be produced from regolith fines through the use of microwave energy to heat the regolith to 873–1273 K to release adsorbed hydrogen from the materials.[21] Water could be produced from frozen polar caps and subsurface reservoirs, with additional processing to produce potable quality water. The membrane-based reverse osmosis and the adsorbent-based multifiltration are the technologies most commonly used for water purification.[22] To generate O_2 from water and CO_2, the static feed water electrolysis and solid

Table 8   Comparison of essential plant growth nutrients and lunar regolith availability

Nutrients	Plant concentration, percentage weight	Lunar concentration, percentage weight
Carbon	18	0.011
Hydrogen	8	0.0055
Oxygen	70	40
Nitrogen	0.3	0.01
Phosphorous	0.07	0.4
Potassium	0.3	0.4
Calcium	0.5	9.0
Magnesium	0.04	6.0
Sulfur	0.07	0.5
Iron	0.01	9.0
Manganese	0.001	0.2
Boron	0.001	0.002
Molybdenum	0.00001	0.0001
Copper	0.0002	0.0013
Zinc	0.0005	0.0028
Chlorine	0.02	0.0026

polymer electrolysis are the most commonly used methods for water electrolysis.[22] High-temperature metal oxide membranes may be used to electrolytically reduce CO_2 to O_2 and CO.[22] The membrane provides selective transport of ions, thus facilitating the separation of O_2 from CO. Propellants such as O_2 and hydrogen could be cryogenically liquefied to produce liquid hydrogen and O_2.

Photovoltaic methods are a prime candidate to produce electricity on Mars, since adequate sunlight is available. On both the lunar and martian surfaces, the combination of photovoltaics and regenerative fuel cells is a candidate for electrical energy generation. Membrane-based and alkaline fuel cell systems may be used for the generation of electricity. The possibility of using in-situ thorium and uranium as nuclear fuel also exists. However, electrical power generation using space-derived nuclear fuels has yet to be demonstrated to be feasible.

D. In-Situ Resource Usage (ISRU) for Extra-Terrestrial Habitats

The significant in-situ resources available on the lunar surface for physical-chemical life support systems are lunar regolith for O_2 generation and solar energy for power genera-

tion. The systems for mining lunar regolith and processing it to generate O_2 have yet to be developed. Therefore, it is unrealistic to predict weight savings in physical-chemical life support systems that could be achieved by lunar regolith utilization. Such predictions would have to trade the weight of mining and processing equipment against that of the life support system.

Mars is an excellent site for ISRU. It is a source of O_2, N_2, hydrogen, CO_2, and water, in addition to available solar energy. For a Mars expedition mission, it is conceivable that a physical-chemical life support system could function almost totally from ISRU. A major contributor to the total life support system weight, the weight of the storage subsystem (consumables and makeup supplies), could be drastically reduced with the help of ISRU technologies.

IV. Reliability of Physical-Chemical Life Support Systems for Long-Term Nonresupply Missions

A. Overview

Future human space missions will require the development of physical-chemical life support systems capable of sustaining future astronauts in space for much longer durations than

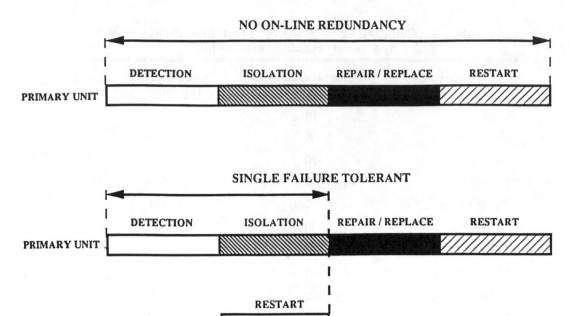

Fig. 2 Time to recover from a fault: No redundancy vs. single failure tolerance.

previous missions. Since the emphasis in these missions will likely be directed away from orbit above the Earth to permanent lunar or planetary bases or interplanetary flights, the next generation of life support systems must provide highly reliable service while meeting weight, power, volume, resupply, and cost constraints. Although life support systems for lunar or planetary bases will evolve to make the best use of available resources, transfer vehicles designed to ferry astronauts to and from these remote outposts may use ECLSS technology first developed for Space Station and Mir. Based upon flight experience with the Space Station and Mir programs, repair and redundancy strategies should be well established for long-term space endeavors. A conceptual life support system with estimates of space weight and repair and redundancy strategies is presented.

B. Statement of the Problem

The mission parameters for a human mission to Mars are used to derive a set of generic requirements applicable to the development of a long-term ECLSS. Although the duration of a human mission to the outer planets in the solar system would be much longer than for a visit to Mars, requirements governing the development of an ECLSS for an Earth-to-Mars transfer vehicle should be similarly relevant to any interplanetary mission. NASA's 90-Day Study on Human Exploration of the Moon and Mars outlined a plan to establish a lunar outpost and perform a human visit to Mars early in the next century.[23] The lunar outpost, along with Space Station, may be used as a development and staging area for the exploration of Mars. The total round-trip duration for manned visits to Mars early in the next century is expected to range between 500 and 800 days, depending on the trajectory of the

vehicle and the stay time in the martian system. Crew sizes for these early missions are expected to be small (four to five astronauts). The only mission resupply identified is a preplanned rendezvous with a cargo vehicle in orbit around Mars. The mission parameters are summarized as follows: 1) mission duration of 1–3 years, 2) no unscheduled or contingency resupply, 3) limited mission abort/rescue options, 4) crew size of four, and 5) design to cost.

The mission duration, as well as the resupply and emergency constraints, will require that the ECLSS be designed within an established reliability requirement. Through analysis and testing, it will have to be demonstrated with a high degree of confidence that the ECLSS can operate satisfactorily over the mission duration. Some hardware will be designed to survive the mission with minimal repair, whereas other components may be replaced several times. Designing to cost may result in the use of life support equipment derived from Space Station and Mir to a large extent. This could minimize development costs and possibly minimize life testing because of the available flight experience. The reliability and maintainability design is key to meeting this requirement, as the number of spares will represent a significant portion of the launch weight.

C. Reliability and Maintainability Design Approach

Central to the design of a life support system for long-term space missions are reliability and maintainability considerations. Repair and redundancy strategies, system data base development, reliability allocations, spare requirements, and life testing must all be addressed to ensure an adequate design. Two basic strategies exist in the design of reliable systems.[24,25] First, a system can be designed to survive a given

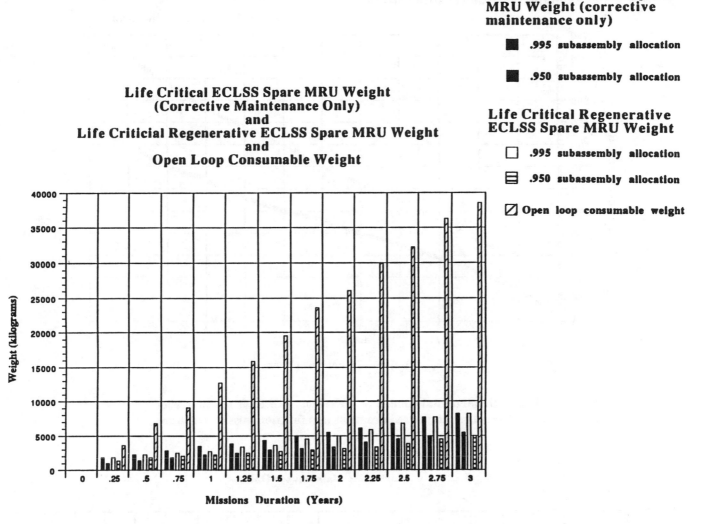

Life Critical ECLSS Spare MRU Weight (corrective maintenance only)

■ .995 subassembly allocation

■ .950 subassembly allocation

Life Critical Regenerative ECLSS Spare MRU Weight

□ .995 subassembly allocation

▤ .950 subassembly allocation

▨ Open loop consumable weight

Life Critical ECLSS Spare MRU Weight (Corrective Maintenance Only) and Life Criticial Regenerative ECLSS Spare MRU Weight and Open Loop Consumable Weight

Fig. 3 Estimated weight of life critical ECLSS MRU spares for two reliability requirements as a function of mission duration. Comparison of critical regenerative ECLSS space MRU weight and open loop consumable weight as a function of mission duration.

mission duration with little or no repair. Backup assemblies are available in the event of failure; and, in the case of manned missions, only the most critical spares are provided. A second approach is to design a maintainable system or, in other words, a system that can be restored after failures. The maintainable system approach is more practical for human missions of longer duration where crew intervention is possible. The maintainable system design must account for all of the necessary spares. In this design approach, redundancy is implemented primarily to circumvent the temporary loss-of-time critical functions.

D. Repair and Redundancy Strategy

Future space vehicles will comprise a number of different systems, such as life support, power, propulsion, and data management. Each system can be divided into a number of subsystem groups, with each subsystem group providing sev-

eral related functions. In the ECLSS architecture, for example, all water reclamation and management functions for the recovery, monitoring, and distribution of potable and wash waters are grouped under one subsystem group. Furthermore, each group is subdivided into a number of subassemblies. In the case of the ECLSS, a subassembly generally provides all or part of a single function, such as CO_2 removal, avionics cooling, or wash water recovery. To facilitate maintenance and repair, each subassembly is further divided into a number of replaceable units and components. Subassemblies are maintained through the replacement of specially defined subcomponents called mission replaceable units (MRUs). Each subassembly is divided into a number of MRUs; MRU selection is optimized against individual mass and predicted failure rate. Other factors influencing MRU selection include the number and type of connections (i.e., electrical, mechanical) and accessibility within the subassembly.[26] Repair below the MRU level is permitted through the use of another replace-

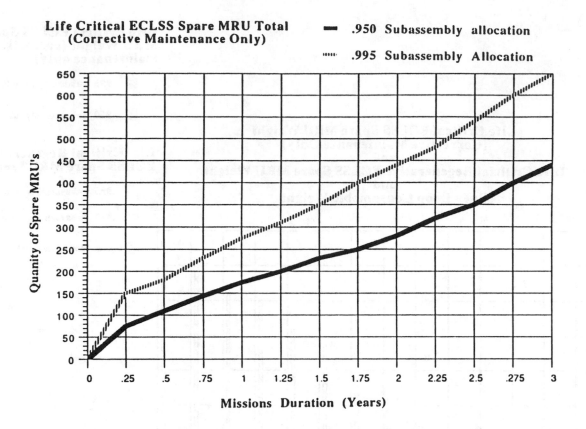

Fig. 4 Estimated total number of life critical ECLSS MRU spares for
two different reliability requirements as a function mission duration.

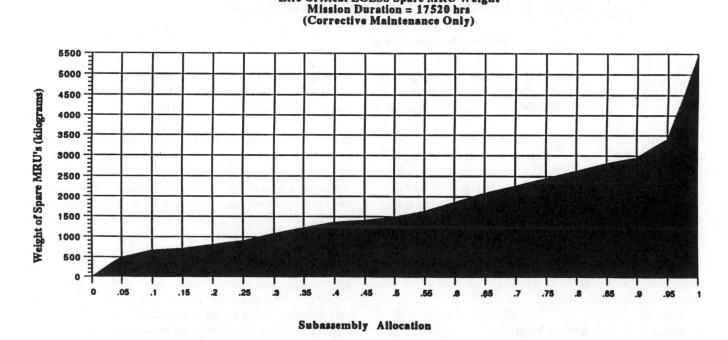

Fig. 5 Weight of life critical ECLSS MRU spares as a function
of subassembly reliability allocation for a two year mission.

able subcomponent, called a mission replaceable component (MRC). MRCs allow for the use of common parts, primarily sensors (although others are possible), between MRUs. A failed MRU that would otherwise be rendered useless can be returned to active service through the replacement of a much less complex part, the MRC.

On-line redundancy of life support subsystems will be implemented to minimize the effects of a disruption of service due to failure. The level of failure tolerance will be dependent upon the criticality of the function. Recovery from a failure occurs in four steps: 1) detection, 2) isolation, 3) repair, and 4) restoration. As shown in Fig. 2, the presence of an on-line backup unit can reduce the total recovery time, since the redundant system can be started while the primary one is repaired. The life-critical nature of most ECLSS functions demands at least single-failure tolerance, with dual- or triple-failure tolerance preferred to cover protracted repair times or multiple failures.

E. Reliability Allocations and Spare Requirements

Program reliability requirements for long-term space missions will likely be defined at the system or subsystem level. Through maintenance, the ECLSS will be required to provide service with limited interruption for the duration of long-term space missions. Since the ECLSS is a complex system comprising different subsystems and subassemblies, the reliability and maintainability design approach becomes a question of how to allocate the high-level reliability requirements down to the lowest components in the system. One method would be to envision each high-level component, such as a subsystem or subassembly, as a number of low-level components, such as an MRU, connected in series. The low-level reliability requirements are derived such that the higher level requirement is met. Using the basic laws of probability,[24,25] reliability requirements are applied in succession at the subsystem, subassembly, and MRU levels. Significant resource reductions are possible if low-level reliability requirements are optimized with regard to weight (i.e., a higher reliability requirement should be allocated to a lighter component, such as a sensor, rather than to a heavier component, such as a compressor).

Using this approach and a data base constructed from Space Station reliability and mass property data,[27] estimates of spare weight were computed parametrically for life-critical ECLSS hardware against mission duration and subassembly reliability requirements. For demonstration purposes, each life-critical ECLSS subassembly was assumed to have a reliability allocation of either 0.995 or 0.950, meaning a 99.5 percent or 95.0 percent probability of success over the given mission duration. As expected, the weight of spares required to meet a given requirement increases with increasing mission duration (Fig. 3). Also, the total number of spare MRUs required to meet a given requirement was computed and is shown plotted against mission duration in Fig. 4. The dependence on the subassembly allocation is shown in Fig. 5 as the weight of

spare MRUs required to support a mission of 2 years in duration, plotted parametrically against subassembly allocation. Again, the allocation of reliability requirements down to the MRU level was not optimized with regard to individual MRU weight. Weight savings are possible if heavier MRUs are allocated a lower requirement whereas lighter MRUs are designed to a more stringent requirement.

In light of the apparent excessive weight of spares needed to support a regenerative ECLSS, a comparison against consumables required for an open-loop ECLSS is shown in Fig. 3. The weight of the consumables is based upon a crew size of four and assumed requirements of 2.6 kg/man-day of drinking water, 5.4 kg/man-day of wash water, and 0.8 kg/man-day of O_2. Although the weight of tankage is not included in the comparison, the regenerative system shows a clear advantage in launch weight. The installed weights of both systems, as well as other penalties, such as power, would have to be addressed for a complete trade.

F. System Data Base

A reliability and maintainability data base is essential to the design of long-term ECLSSs. Reliability and maintainability data, such as component failure rates and mean time to repair (MTTR), will be used in system design trade-off and analyses, along with weight, power, and volume estimates. Future ECLSS data bases will make extensive use of Space Station and Mir flight experience, as well as aircraft and submarine data. As system development progresses, the data base will be continually updated and validated against ground test data.

The data base will likely be organized at the MRU level. Each MRU field will contain entries for a predicted failure rate mean time between failures (MTBF) and MTTR. The MTTR projections will reflect the actual time required to remove and replace an MRU with an identical MRU, as this will be the normal method of repair. The MTTR will account for such factors as number of connections, connector type (i.e., electrical and/or mechanical), and MRU accessibility within the subassembly.[26] The data base will also contain entries for the MRU duty cycle and estimates for the MRU weight and volume. The weight and volume entries will be used to support logistics analyses to determine the total launch weight and volume of spares required for a mission of given duration. The data base may also include entries to indicate the changeout frequency of consumable MRUs, such as particular filters or sorbent beds.

A number of data base entries will be quantities derived from information contained elsewhere in the data base. Key among these will be estimates for the number of spare MRUs. As illustrated earlier, system reliability requirements will be allocated to the MRU level. The estimates for crew maintenance hours are computed from the individual MRU failure rates and MTTR predictions.[26,27] As crew time is a critical resource like weight or power, the ECLSS design must ensure that an inordinate amount of time is not consumed for

Table 9 Example ECLSS Data Base

Mission duration   17,520 h
Subassembly reliability goal   0.995

MRU description	Subsystem	Subassembly	Qty.	Unit mass, kg	Total mass, kg	MTBF, h	Failures 10^6, h	Allocation	Total units	Spare units	Spare mass, kg
Water separator	THC	Cabin	1	7.26	7.26	38,183	26.190	0.9992	7	6	44.20
Cond. heat exchange	THC	Cabin	1	17.83	17.83	100,000	10.000	0.9992	4	3	51.29
Temperature sensors	THC	Cabin	1	1.81	1.81	150,000	6.667	0.9992	3	2	4.02
HEPA filter	THC	Cabin	1	6.80	6.80	832,639	1.201	0.9992	2	1	5.65
Check valves	THC	Cabin	1	6.80	6.80	620,732	1.611	0.9992	2	1	6.66
Cabin fan	THC	Cabin	1	19.32	19.32	41,752	23.951	0.9992	7	6	108.57
Totals			6	59.83	59.83	14,364[a]	69.62				220.39

[a]Mean time before failure for total system derived from test data and is not a total of numbers appearing above it in the column.

maintenance when compared to other activities. An example data base is provided in Table 9.

G. Life Testing

A test program must be implemented to qualify the long-duration ECLSS before flight and to validate and/or partially generate the reliability and maintainability data base used in the design of the system. Life testing of subassemblies and lower components will be used to validate predicted component failure rates contained in the ECLSS data base or to obtain new failure rates where existing data are nonexistent or suspect. Additional tests using form and fit mockups or flight quality hardware may be conducted to validate MTTR predictions.

The keys to implementing a successful life test program are determining the number of trials necessary to establish the average failure rate of a given subassembly or MRU and deciding which subassemblies or MRUs to test. Obviously, resources to conduct extensive life tests on every component in the system will not be available. It will be necessary, through similarity or existing flight data, to waive life testing on some components in the system. Extensive flight data will likely exist for a number of ECLSS components, including air and liquid heat exchangers, fans, and sorbent beds. Of course, new technologies with no previous flight experience will receive high priority for ground testing to substantiate failure rate predictions contained in the engineering data base.

References

[1]Sharp, M.R. *Living in Space*. Garden City, N.Y., Doubleday & Company, Inc., 1969.

[2]Silverstri, G. *Quest for Space*. N. Y., Crescent Books, 1986.

[3]Popov, I.G. Food and Water Supply. In: Calvin, M. and Gazenko, O.G., Eds. *Foundations of Space Biology and Medicine*. Washington, D.C., NASA, 1975, Vol. III, pp. 23, 34, 36, and 37.

[4]Bluth, B.J. Soviet Mir Space Station Complex–A presentation. Space Station Freedom Program Office. Reston, Virginia, Apr. 1989.

[5]Humphries, W.R.; Schunk, R.G.; and Reuter, J.L. Space Station Freedom Environmental Control and Life Support Systems design–A status report. Paper presented at International Conference on Environmental Systems, Williamsburg, VA, 1990.

[6]National Aeronautics and Space Administration. Flammability, odor and offgassing requirements and test procedures for materials in environments that support combustion. NASA Handbook 8060.1b, Washington, D.C., NASA Hq., 1971.

[7]Mendell, W.W., Ed. *Lunar Bases and Space Activities of the 21st Century*. Houston, Lunar and Planetary Institute, 1984.

[8]Powell, F.T. Local resources utilization and integration into advanced mission's LSS. In: *Materials of 18th Intersociety Conference in Environmental Systems*, San Francisco, July 11–13, 1988.

[9]Ferrall, J.F.; Rohatgi, N.K.; and Seshan, P.K. Physical-chemical closed-loop life support systems analysis and assessment. In: FY '89 Annual Report, Pasadena, Calif., NASA Jet Propulsion Laboratory, 1989.

[10]Carter, J.L. Lunar regolith fines: A source of hydrogen. In: Mendell, W.W., Ed. *Lunar Bases and Space Activities of the 21st Century*. Houston, Lunar and Planetary Institute, 1984, p. 571.

[11]Phinney, W.C.; Criswell, D.; Drexler, E.; and Garmirian, J. Lunar resources and their utilization. In: O'Neill, G.K., and O'Leary, B., Eds: *Space-Based Manufacturing from Nonterrestrial Materials*, Progress in Astronautics and Aeronautics, vol. 57, AIAA, New York, 1977.

[12]Lockheed Missiles & Space Company. Lunar base controlled ecological life support system. Interim report, Lockheed Missiles & Space Company, Inc., Sunnyvale, Calif., October 13, 1990.

[13]Rosenberg, S.D. A lunar-based propulsion system. In: Mendell, W.W., Ed. *Lunar Bases and Space Activities of the 21st Century*, Houston, Lunar and Planetary Institute, 1984, p. 169.

[14]Buden, D. and Ahgelo, J.A. Nuclear energy–Key to lunar development. In: Mendell, W.W., Ed. *Lunar Bases and Space Activities of the 21st Century*. Houston, Lunar and Planetary Institute, 1984, p. 85.

[15]Cordell, B.M. The moons of Mars: A source of water for lunar bases and LEO. In: Mendell, W.W., Ed. *Lunar Bases and Space Activities of the 21st Century*. Houston, Lunar and Planetary Institute, 1984 p. 809.

[16]Clifford, S.M. Polar basal melting on Mars. *Journal of Geophysical Research,* vol. 92, no. B9, p. 9135.

[17]DesMarais, D.J.; Hayes, J.K.; and Meinschein, W.G. The distribution in lunar soil of hydrogen released by pyrolysis. In: *Proceedings, 5th Lunar Science Conference*, Houston, Lunar and Planetary Institute, 1974, p. 1811.

[18]Bustin, R.; Kotra, R.K.; Gibson, E.K.; and Nace, G.A. Hydrogen abundances in lunar soils (abstract), *Lunar and Planetary Science*, 1984, vol. XV, p. 112.

[19]Henninger, D.L.; Langle, C.W.; and Ming, D.W. Lunar agricultural soil. In: *Lunar Bases and Space Activities of the 21st Century*, Houston, Lunar and Planetary Institute, 1988.

[20]National Aeronautics and Space Administration. Space and planetary environment criteria guidelines for use in space vehicle development. NASA TM 82479, Huntsville, AL, NASA Marshall Space Flight Center, 1982.

[21]Tucker, D.S.; Vaniman, D.T.; Anderson, J.L.; Clinar, F.W., Jr.; Ferber, R.C., Jr.; Frost, H.M; Meek, T.T.; and Wallace, T.C. Hydrogen recovery from extraterrestrial materials using microwave energy. In: Mendell, W.W., Ed. *Lunar Bases and Space Activities of the 21st Century*, Houston, Lunar and Planetary Institute, 1984, p. 583.

[22]McDonnell Douglas Space Systems Company. Space

Station ECLSS evolution study, Report to MSFC. NASA-36407 Huntsville, AL, NASA Marshall Space Flight Center, June 20, 1989.

[23]National Aeronautics and Space Administration. Report of the 90-Day Study on Human Exploration of the Moon and Mars. Washington, D.C., internal NASA document, Nov. 1989.

[24]Doty, L.A. *Reliability for the Technologies.* New York, Industrial Press, 1985.

[25]United States Army. Engineering Design Handbook: Reliability Production. AMCP 706-197, Washington, D.C., Department of the Army, Jan. 1976.

[26]Boeing Aerospace. Space Station Freedom program maintainability plan. DR LS02, Huntsville, AL, Jan. 1990.

[27]Boeing Aerospace. Space Station Freedom program maintainability allocation report. DR LS01, Huntsville, AL, Apr. 1990.

[28]Hopson, G.D.; Littles, L.W.; and Patterson, W.C. Skylab environmental control and life support systems. ASME Paper 71-AV-14, Life Support and Environmental Control Conference, San Francisco, Jul. 12-14, 1971.

[29]Willis, C.E., and Schultz, J.R. Spacecraft water system disinfection technology: Past, present and future needs. Society of Automotive Engineers (SAE) Paper 871487, 17th Intersociety Conference on Environmental Systems, Seattle, Jul. 13-15, 1987.

[30]Samonski, F.H. Jr. Technical history of the environmental control system for Project Mercury. NASA TN D-4126I, Washington, D.C., NASA Hq., 1967.

[31]Watkins, H.D. Basic Gemini ECS keyed to 14-day flight. *Aviation Week & Space Technology.* Aug. 19, 1963, pp. 52–69.

[32]Johnston, R.S.; Dietlein, L.F.; and Berry, C.A., Eds. *Biomedical Results of Apollo.* NASA SP-368, Washington, D.C., NASA Hq., 1975, pp. 91, 93, 94.

[33]Mackowski, M.J. Safety on the space station. *Space World*, Mar. 1987, pp. 22–24.

[34]National Aeronautics and Space Administration. *Skylab Operational Data Book.* MSFC-01549, Huntsville, AL, NASA Marshall Space Flight Center, Dec. 1970.

[35]Hamilton Standard. Final Report–Soviet space life support systems. U.S. Government Contract 85-N987400-000, Windsor Locks, CT, Nov. 1985.

[36]Bluth, B.J., and Helppie, M. Soviet Space Stations as Analogs, 2nd Ed. Report under NASA Grant NAGW-659, Washington, D.C., NASA Hq., 1986.

[37]Sisyakan, N.M., and Yazdovskiy, V.I., Eds. *The first manned space flights. Scientific results of biomedical research conducted during flights of Vostok and Vostok-2.* Moscow, Nauka, 1963 (in Russian, Translation: N63-15658, Air Force Systems Command Foreign Technology Division, Wright-Patterson AFB, Ohio, 1962).

[38]Pochkayev, I.; Serebrov, A.; and Ulyanov, V. The Mir Space Station. *Aviatsiya i Kosmonavtika*, Nov. 1986, pp. 22–23 (in Russian, Translation: *U.S.S.R. Space Life Sciences Digest* , CR-3922(12), Issue 10, Washington, D.C., NASA Hq., 1987).

[39]Gilberg, L.A. *Living and Working in Space.* NASA Technical Translation, NASA TT F-17075, Washington, D.C., Jul. 1976.

[40]Voronin, G.I.; Genin, A.M.; and Fomin, A.G. Physiological and hygienical evaluation of life support systems of the Vostok and Voskhod spacecraft. In: Bjurstedt, Hilding, Ed. *Proceedings of the Second International Symposium of Basic Environmetal Problems of Man in Space.* New York, Springer-Verlag, 1967.

[41]Diamant, B.L., and Humphries, W.R. Past and present environmental control and life support systems on manual spacecraft. Society of Automotive Engineers (SAE) Paper 901210, 1990.

Chapter 16

Biological Life Support Systems

G. I. Meleshko, Ye. Ya. Shepelev, M. M. Averner, and T. Volk

Since the publication of the first joint work on space biology and medicine in 1975, the status of the problem of the man-rated biological life support systems (BLSS) has altered substantially. What is most important is that the inevitable need for the BLSS for future space programs demanding long-term autonomous human survival far from Earth has become increasingly obvious and has been generally acknowledged. This has led to increased international collaboration and to a substantial expansion of the geography of BLSS research, which is now being conducted in Canada, Japan, and many European countries.

The United States is implementing a program to develop the Controlled Ecological Life Support System (CELSS) for use on Space Station. The CELSS will include a number of BLSS subsystems, especially higher plant subsystems, combined with a physical-chemical regeneration system.

The first ground-based models of the BLSS for humans were developed in the Soviet Union. In the Russian Federation, a new phase in the study of this problem has begun— the study of individual BLSS components and technologies as they function in space with the participation of Mir crews. As a result, this area has now graduated from the status of an intriguing problem to be solved in the distant future to that of an extensive program involving genuine experimental developments.

The use of the principle of the biological substance cycle to support the vital processes of cosmonauts was first proposed by K.E. Tsiolkovskiy as early as 1911.[1] Less than 50 years later, at the start of the space era, the creation of a man-rated BLSS had become a practical goal.

Early discussions of the feasibility of such systems were published in the United States[2-4] and then in the U.S.S.R.[5-8] These discussions gradually generated the conviction that BLSSs were essential to the future of cosmonautics. BLSS concepts that resembled the modern ecological understanding of the term were proposed in the U.S.S.R. in 1963,[8] and were more fully developed in 1966 on the basis of empirical data.[9]

Initial theoretical designs of different variants of bioregenerative systems were based on the data available at the time regarding laboratory and industrial cultivation of one-celled algae, including *Chlorella*. It was believed that these algae could use human waste products as a food source and that their biomass could satisfy human needs for the major nutrients. These ideas led to empirical attempts to create BLSSs for regenerating the atmosphere through *Chlorella* photosynthesis.

American scientists conducted the first experiments using animals (mice) soon after the appearance of the first man-made Earth satellites.[10-12] These experiments were terminated because of the low productivity of algae cultures, which resulted in the accumulation of excess carbon dioxide and failure to produce sufficient oxygen. In 1961, at the USAF School of Aviation Medicine, a 50-h experiment using monkeys was conducted and had a similar result. Experiments conducted by Soviet researchers in 1960 with rats and dogs, lasting 6–8 days, and then with humans (two experiments, each lasting 1-1/2 days) were equally unsuccessful.[13] Despite their failure, these experiments were historically significant, since they were the first to establish the possibility of directly yoking human gas exchange to photosynthesis by a single species of plant—*Chlorella*. Somewhat later in the United States, the Boeing Corporation attempted to support human gas exchange for a period of 6–56 h.[14]

After the first unsuccessful experiments, scientists were pessimistic about the efficacy and feasibility of using bioregenerative systems on spacecraft. This skepticism was not surprising, since they had hoped to be immediately able to incorporate the results of their initial experiments in the design of spacecraft life support systems, and this was not possible. These negative conclusions were based on the results of the first essentially empirical period in the development of the BLSS and clearly resulted from direct attempts to create working models of systems without sufficient theoretical and experimental grounding. A contributing factor was the fact that the creation of the BLSS was understood from the very beginning as an applied or even an engineering problem, rather than as a component of the fundamental scientific problem of creating closed ecological systems, the underlying laws of which remain less well understood than those of natural ecosystems. To a significant extent, this discredited the area itself, and BLSS research was curtailed significantly and, subsequently continued only in the U.S.S.R.

The Russian portions of this chapter were translated into English by Lydia Razran Stone.

Many years of work were required to develop the theoretical and empirical rationale for the basic principles underlying the structural and functional organization of the BLSS; to identify ways to substantially increase the efficiency of algae in the system; and, especially, to create a completely new technology for their continuous cultivation. In addition, this technology had to be suitable for use, along with other components of the BLSS, including man, in a closed ecological system. Only after these problems were solved in the 1970s was it possible to return to experimental modeling of a man-rated BLSS. Experience with research on such models is described in Section IV.

The BLSS, as the term is currently understood, is designed to create and maintain a living environment for humans that is maximally appropriate to their needs, which are the products of evolution. Of course, this objective encompasses the traditional requirement for all life support systems (i.e., providing the major requirements for life—oxygen, water, and food), but it is not limited to them. The current concept of the future capabilities of the BLSS adds a completely new criterion—the goal of complete biological adequacy of the human living environment; and this goal cannot be achieved using nonbiological methods of life support.

The BLSS functions primarily through the utilization of a biological substance cycle created by the combined metabolic activity of plants; animals; micro-organisms; and humans themselves, who become an essential component of the system. These functions can be realized most fully through the use of biological structures characteristic of natural ecological systems—structures that have the properties of self-regulation; self-repair; adaptation; and, ultimately, the capacity for long-term autonomous survival in a state of stable equilibrium. These properties should serve as criteria for evaluating artificial ecosystems created as man-rated BLSSs.

Thus, we consider the BLSS as a kind of functional analog of natural ecosystems with respect to their organization, which is based on matter and energy linkages among individual functional components (subsystems) joined in a functionally integrated system. Individual BLSS subsystems are considered in Section II.

In the first edition of this work in 1975,[18] it was noted that, if a BLSS is conceived as an integrated biological system with a relatively closed biological substance cycle, it is easier to assess the potential for utilizing individual biological subsystems for regenerating certain substances in mixed biological-physical or biological-chemical systems. Today, we can point to the NASA CELSS Program, which is already conducting large-scale exploratory development and research and development on a component containing higher plants and other biological subjects in the non-biological LSS of Space Station. The CELSS Program is discussed in Section III.

In this chapter, in addition to presenting material directly relating to the BLSS, we also discuss new experimental data and ideas reflected in the recent scientific literature. One such idea is the general theory of habitability of extrabiospheric

environments and, in particular, the significance of this concept for the development of man-rated life support systems that will support high levels of autonomy for space missions. This concept is discussed in section I. We also deem it essential to reconsider the biological effects of weightlessness from a broad ecological perspective, since BLSSs on spacecraft must function in microgravity. Weightlessness as a condition under which the BLSS is implemented is addressed in Section V.

Section VI describes mathematical modeling of biological systems.

The bulk of the material in this chapter was written by G.I. Meleshko and Ye.Ya. Shepelev (Institute of Biomedical Problems, Russian Federation Ministry of Health, Moscow). The material on the CELSS program was written by M.M. Averner (NASA, U.S.A.) and the section on mathematical modeling of BLSS was contributed by T. Volk of New York University (U.S.A.).

Fundamental Concepts and Terms

1) *Abiotic environment*: that part of an organism's living environment consisting of nonbiological factors.

2) *Autotrophs*: organisms capable of synthesizing organic substances from carbon dioxide, water, and mineral salts. On the basis of the energy source used in this process, autotrophs are subdivided into photoautotrophic organisms, which utilize the electromagnetic radiation of visible light; and chemoautotrophs, which obtain energy by oxidation of minerals, iron, sulphur, hydrogen, and nitrates.

3) *Biotic environment*: all the living elements of an organism's environment.

4) *Biomass*: the sum of all the substances comprising the body of an organism or set of organisms.

5) *Biosphere*: all portions of the lithosphere (solid envelope of the Earth), hydrosphere, and atmosphere linked (now or historically) with the activity of terrestrial organisms.

6) *Biocenosis*: functionally linked set (community) of organisms inhabiting a common territory or aquatic area.

7) *Biogeocenosis*: the biocenosis combined with the abiotic factors of the environment. This is the fundamental structural and functional subdivision (unit) of the biosphere that is responsible for a particular type of biogeochemical activity—the substance cycle.

8) *Heterotrophs*: organisms not capable of primary synthesis of organic substances and thus requiring the supply of such substances from without.

9) *Biological life support system*, or BLSS: "artificial" set of organisms and abiotic factors assembled in a limited territory. This system is a single functional community of autotrophs and heterotrophs, including humans, existing in a state of dynamic equilibrium within a relatively closed substance cycle regulated mainly by intrinsic control mechanisms.

10) *Population*: set of individuals of a single species inhabiting a relatively isolated homogeneous territory or aquatic area.

11) *Ecological system*: Unlike biogeocenosis (q.v.), which is defined as a unit of the biosphere, this term is applied to biological systems of any size—from the ocean to a particular puddle or from the forest to a stump. The absence of a size marker makes it possible to use the term more broadly than biogeocenosis, and it has been applied to the BLSS. However, this term refers only to biological systems and, in the ecological literature, is not used to refer to nonbiological systems.

12) *Closed ecological system*: hypothetical system based on a closed biological substance cycle without exchange of material beyond the enclosure of the system.

I. Biological Life Support Systems and Habitability

We have included this section in what might seem to be a narrowly specialized chapter on BLSS because creation of a life support system is often reduced to a set of purely technological (for physical-chemical systems) or biotechnological (for BLSS) problems, without considering the ecological problems associated with the major element of these systems—the human. Such ecological problems ultimately involve the theory of spacecraft habitability; i.e., the living conditions of the space crewmembers, who are the most important component of the life support systems being designed.

Any BLSS concept is derived from current ideas about the living environment humans need and the concept of habitability that underlies these ideas. As we are on the threshold of a new phase of manned space flight, it would be useful to consider an issue that, at first, might seem to be obvious; i.e., the purpose and specifications of man-rated life support systems. Each time such a system is designed, specifications are derived from current ideas about the necessary and sufficient conditions and components of a living environment as applied to specific space programs. However, these ideas inevitably change over time, as the duration and autonomy of space missions increase and as our understanding of the human living environment deepens.

If we base our concept of habitability solely on the standard list of physical and hygienic requirements for life, then it is sufficient to consider the following as goals of a life support system: to support certain physical-chemical parameters of the environment; to provide certain amounts of consumable substances (oxygen, water, and food); and to dispose of waste products for a certain period of time. However, if we base our concept of habitability on the requirement for a biologically complete environment, one that will not, in principle, curtail the life span of a human living in it, then the life support system must meet ecological requirements derived from this requirement. Such an environment must meet the needs developed by humans over the course of evolution (which are still not thoroughly understood) and share the major properties of the natural environment. The only life support system that can meet these needs is one based on a biological substance cycle, which is the only validated mechanism on our planet for sustaining life over a prolonged period of time.

We have failed to find in the literature a comprehensive discussion of the current tacit understanding of the concept of habitability. It is possible that there is no such understanding and that, in its stead, we have empirical practice. There is also no unambiguous generally accepted definition of the term "habitability" itself. It seems possible to define "habitability" as the totality of environmental conditions (physical, chemical, biological, and social) that make the environment suitable for human survival and activity, either indefinitely or for a specific, limited period of time (limited habitability). Obviously, at the current stage of manned space flight, we are dealing with limited habitability. Our definition of habitability is future oriented: the future goal of space medicine is implicit in it—to decrease constraints on the period of time that humans can remain in space (of course, without ill effects), and to transform the limited habitability of current spacecraft into unlimited, true habitability. From this point of view, our strategy in the medical support of future space programs must involve determining what level of inadequacy is acceptable for an artificial spacecraft environment (as compared to the natural environment on Earth).

In the U.S.S.R., we have been working on certain aspects of the ecological concept of habitability and its initial assumptions for a long time. This work is described in a number of sources.[15–19] In its most general form, it is presented in a paper by O.G. Gazenko, A.I. Grigoryev, et al.[20]

The major aspect of the ecological concept of habitability is the biological completeness of the living environment. The concept of biological completeness (i.e., the full adequacy of the living environment to meet the evolved needs of humans) developed gradually. It was derived from a number of sources as we became increasingly aware of the advantages of conceiving of nature as an integral whole and began to recognize the power implicit in the principle of the organism's unity with its environment. It is interesting that the most profound treatment of this principle is encountered outside of biology, in the ideas of the geologist and chemist, V.I. Vernadskiy,[21] who considered the unity of the organism-environment system not merely in the context of individual organisms but on a global scale.

The concept of the biological completeness of the environment was first advanced with regard to the environment of the roots of plants in a discussion of the possibility of directly utilizing the products of physical-chemical mineralization of organic wastes in artificial ecological systems.[9] This idea was derived from the notion of the soil as a complex natural body in which the destruction of organic substances occurs simultaneously with soil-transforming processes involving many soil organisms and root systems. As a result of this process, plants obtain not only the mineral substances known in agrochemistry but also a whole set of physical, mineral, organic, and biological environmental components maximally suited to the linkages and needs developed through evolution. The biological completeness of the environment is a direct consequence of its natural, biogenic origin. Thus, the introduction of the physical-chemical mineralization of organic wastes into a biological substance cycle, or the use of hydroponics to cultivate plants in a BLSS, cannot qualify as adequate, since they fail to supply a biologically complete environment to the roots of the plant.

Later, the concept of biological completeness was derived independently in hydrobiology with regard to drinking water. Here, biological completeness can be defined as the capacity to serve as the living environment of aquatic organisms and is a consequence of the fact that natural bodies of water contain the biologically active primary and secondary by-products of the vital functions of hydrobionts.[22] Here, too, the biological completeness of the environment is associated with its biogenic origin. It is obvious that, *a priori,* water regenerated by physical-chemical methods cannot possess this fundamental property of naturally occurring water. As we will argue below, such artificially reclaimed water does not possess the properties of a biologically complete living environment for aquatic organisms.

Everything that was said with regard to soil and water can be logically extended to the general concept of biological completeness of any natural environment to the organisms that inhabit it. In essence, this is an *a priori* property of the natural environment and does not require further empirical proof. The completeness of the natural environment follows from the long period of joint evolution of terrestrial organisms and the biosphere in the presence of the Earth's geophysical fields. At each moment during the evolution of the biosphere, terrestrial organisms manifested the maximum attainable level of adaptation to their environment and to assimilation of available material and energy resources, and there existed the maximum possible number of energy, trophic, and signal (informational) linkages between the organism and its environment. Taken as a whole, this situation also defines the concept of the biological completeness of the living environment. Of course, all this applies to humans as well, regardless of their ability to optimize their individual physical environments with the help of shelter, clothing, etc.

Thus, biological completeness of the environment may be defined as the extent to which the environment meets the evolved needs of an organism, enabling the organism to survive for an unlimited time in this environment. We apply this concept both to the environment as a whole and to its major components—the natural atmosphere, natural water, and soil and also to the size and configuration of the living environment (a "social" factor of varying importance for different organisms). The key feature of this definition (as is the case for the definition of the concept of habitability described above) is that there is no time limit on habitation. This is a critical point for the development of future BLSSs, in which habitation may continue over a number of natural generations. An axiom can be derived here: The standard for biological completeness against which every artificially generated living environment must be evaluated is the natural environment and its most important components—the atmosphere, water, and soil (as the environment of plants and the locus of interactions between biotic and abiotic elements).

Table 1 Critical period for onset of deprivation effects for a number of environmental factors

Factor	Critical time
Oxygen	$n \cdot 10^{-2}$ (min)
Water	$n \cdot 10^{1}$ (days)
Food	$n \cdot 10^{2}$ (weeks)
Vitamins, minerals	$n \cdot 10^{3}$ (months, year)
????	$n \cdot 10^{m}$ $(m \geq 4)$ (years, generations)

The importance of applying the appropriate concept of habitability to the development of life support systems should become particularly obvious in the near future, when we will be preparing for such inevitable space programs as interplanetary flights and planetary bases. Such programs will compel humans to spend many years cut off from contact with the Earth's biosphere. Under these conditions, an appropriate understanding of the concept of habitability may turn out to be decisive with respect to the biomedical reliability of the space programs themselves. We are approaching an era when concepts from theoretical biology and even natural philosophy must become organizing factors in the development of far-reaching programs of human extraterrestrial activity. To put it simply, when scientists and managers plan programs that require humans to live and work away from the Earth, they must clearly understand the factors of which these humans will be deprived and what the consequences will be.

Although habitability has not been formally defined, the operational definition in use today may be inferred from the fact that the standards for ambient conditions on manned spacecraft are based on traditional physiological and hygienic requirements for such an environment. The current implicit definition of the concept of habitability encompasses a limited number of natural factors that are of critical importance for life support. The most important of these factors are presented in Table 1, in which we have attempted to compare incommensurate environmental factors by citing the time that must elapse before adverse consequences of disrupted human-environment linkages manifest themselves.

The broken line in this table marks the bounds of our knowledge of the major environmental factors critical to human survival. This knowledge underlies the way in which standards are set for living conditions in inhabited spacecraft.

The upper portion of Table 1 contains only factors the deprivation of which leads to critical problems for humans that become manifest in 1 year or less; i.e., approximately 2 percent of the length of a generation or less than 5 percent of the working life of a cosmonaut. However, this does not mean that no other environmental factors are critical to human life with deprivation effects that become manifest only after more than a year, within a single generation, or even in subsequent generations.

Potential factors of this sort that today are not considered in habitability include geophysical fields—magnetic, gravitational, and electrical; the constant generation and motion of atmospheric charged particles of various origins (aero-ions) associated with the Earth's electrical field; aerosol particles, including bacteria, spores, and plant pollen; and ultraviolet radiation and its associated photochemical activity.

Furthermore, the current understanding of the environment still does not encompass its most important characteristic from the standpoint of the theory of habitability—the biogenic essence of the natural environment. After all, the natural atmosphere is qualitatively very different from our models of the "space atmosphere" (nitrogen + oxygen + carbon dioxide), whereas natural water is far from being merely a substance with the chemical formula H_2O (which, incidentally, in its pure form is harmful to all living things).

Science, of course, does have some understanding of many factors not covered in the table, but this knowledge falls within the purview of a number of separate disciplines (i.e., atmospheric physics and chemistry, hydrology, hydrobiology, ecological physiology, medical geography, and health resort science) and has not been integrated into a unified body of knowledge concerning the natural factors of the human environment, a science of terrestrial human ecology. This is a significant problem for the development of our future concepts of habitability and human ecology.

It is well known that the normal components of the Earth's atmosphere include hundreds of organic substances, mainly released by plants and soil micro-organisms. In traditional toxicology, these are usually called "harmful contaminants." Typically, no one even considers whether any of these permanent components of the atmosphere may be beneficial or even essential to humans. This is true of every discipline except health resort science, the science of natural therapeutic factors. As early as the 1920s, N.G. Kholodnyy[23] began to work actively on this problem. He hypothesized that the volatile substances released by plants are physiologically active and serve vitamin-like functions essential for normal vital activity when inhaled by humans or animals. He proposed that they be called "atmovitamins," or respiratory vitamins. Here, we have an example of an idea that was ahead of its time and is acquiring new prestige only today, not merely within the study of human terrestrial ecology but also in human space ecology as it pertains to the BLSS. Any program that develops our future concept of habitability for extrabiospheric manned spacecraft intended for multiyear autonomous habitation should encompass the further development of this idea.

Aside from gaseous components, the Earth's atmosphere contains a large number of aerosols and multimolecular compounds, which are organic as well as inorganic in nature. Aerosol particles have diameters ranging from submicrons to microns. In the submicron range, these particles have been shown to be associated with changes in the physical properties of the major components of the atmosphere and increases in their chemical and catalytic activity.[24] If such particles are ionized in the Earth's electrical field, then they become aero-

Table 2 Amount (in tons/year) of products of certain mass-exchange processes emitted into the biosphere[25]

Substance	Amount emitted into atmosphere, tons/year
Vapors from natural or man-made aerosol-forming substances	1×10^9
Ions emitted with transpirational water of plants	1.2 to 1.4×10^9
Spores and plant pollen	1.6×10^9
Volcanic emissions into the atmosphere	2.3 to 3×10^9

ions—an independent and active ecological factor in the living environment of terrestrial organisms. The absolute quantities of biogenic and abiogenic emissions of a number of substances in the atmosphere are given in Table 2.[25]

It will be noted that the amounts of substances emitted as a result of a number heterogeneous processes are surprisingly similar. Only global processes (i.e., the production of plant biomass and oxygen) release orders of magnitude more substances into the atmosphere, with emissions reaching 2.32×10^{11} metric tons/year.[26]

Air is the single component of the Earth's natural environment with which living things are in contact every second of their lives. This is not true of either water or food. The fact that, in a year, approximately 5000 m^3 of air pass through the lungs provides some idea of the magnitude of the flow of various organic and mineral components of the atmosphere through the human body. Currently, science does not have even an approximate estimate of the true ecological significance to humans of these permanent components of the natural atmosphere. Space medicine has devoted even less attention to this issue.

Thus, even a superficial review of findings concerning the physical, chemical, and biological components of the natural atmosphere does more than merely demonstrate the complexity of its composition. It is completely obvious that the pathways of many of the biosphere's biological and geochemical cycles (and, thus, the interactions among various terrestrial forms of life, including humans) cross and recross in the biosphere. This, alone, is enough to demonstrate that the traditional substitution of a mere mixture of nitrogen, oxygen, and carbon dioxide for the Earth's natural atmosphere on manned spacecraft is only an interim solution. Such a substitution cannot be relied upon in future space programs involving interplanetary flights, in which human contact with the biosphere will be severed for a number of years. In science, which has become so compartmentalized, there is currently a trend to return to earlier, more holistic ideas of nature as a unified entity. In this context it is extremely appropriate to resurrect the old-fashioned but profound idea that what humans breathe is air and not the oxygen that science puts such faith in today.

Natural water is also a complex substance with many components. All the forms that it takes on the Earth are, or have been, the living environment of a variety of organisms, and many of its properties are associated with living matter. Water regenerated from various substances by means of various physical-chemical methods, even when it fully meets standards for potable water, cannot support aquatic organisms.[27] For this reason, scientists concerned with hydrobiology were long ago forced to formulate the concept of biologically complete water, which they identified with the presence of metabolic products of aquatic organisms (lipids, free fatty acids, products of lipid peroxidation, fat-soluble vitamins, free radicals, etc.). Most of the results in this area were obtained by hydrobiologists at Moscow State University.

All of this demonstrates that the environments we have been creating on spacecraft are, unfortunately, only surrogates for the natural environment. It shows the extreme complexity of the composition and origin (biogenic and abiogenic) of the natural atmosphere and natural water and how inextricably related they are to the vital activity of the organisms that inhabit them.

It is obvious that on Earth there are no alternative, nonbiological mechanisms that could reproduce the natural environment in all its biological richness. It is also obvious that, like all other living things, humans are, in principle, unable to live in an artificial, abiogenic environment for longer than the limited period made possible by the inertia of biological systems. This assertion does not require empirical verification, since it follows logically from the fact that living things evolved by adapting to their environment. The requisite proof was long ago furnished by the history of the biosphere and the entire history of the development of humans as components and products of the biosphere. The entire history of the development and evolutionary consolidation of the unity of life and its environment has served as a continuous "experiment" in the actual, scientific, and not merely philosophical sense of the term. Recognition of the practical constructive power of this principle of unity and acknowledgement of the place of human beings as components and products of nature on the Earth must form the basis for deriving the fundamental principle underlying modern human ecology and the concept of habitability associated with it.

These ideas about the natural environment and the place of human beings within it have enabled us to derive the following empirical propositions that may be used as the axiomatic basis for deriving future concepts of habitability, given the new conditions under which this concept must be applied—the severance of human contact with the biosphere for a number of years.[20]

1) Our knowledge of the natural environment of humans is inadequate. It does not include the full set of the environment's properties as a complex, multicomponent, biogenic, self-regulating, and self-repairing system.

2) The natural environment has been the arena of the adaptive evolution of life on Earth. This fact establishes its *a priori* adequacy to meet the needs of living things (which developed through evolution) and distinguishes it in principle from any artificial, abiogenic environment.

3) The natural environment of the Earth is the only one that has been evolutionarily tested and demonstrated to be suitable *a priori* for the unlimited long-term survival of humans. No possible abiogenic version has this sort of *a priori* validity. For this reason, the natural environment must serve as the absolute standard for a living environment for humans, as well as other living things.

4) The duration of human habitation of any artificial, abiogenic environment is theoretically limited; the greater the lack of correspondence between this environment and its natural prototype, the greater are these limits.

5) The manned spacecraft environment can be made biologically complete only if it has been formed through biological mechanisms analogous to those through which natural ecosystems are formed.

For a long time to come, the quality of life and the complete satisfaction of human needs on space stations will continue to depend on the limited capacities of space technology; space medicine, therefore, will have to accept the reality that technological considerations have first priority. But this reality is, in principle, temporary. The inevitable increase in the technological capacities (including power supplies) of spacecraft will diminish the attention that must be paid to technological limitations, and the emphasis that can be placed on human needs and requirements will gradually increase. At the same time, the issue of habitability will be extended to encompass an increasing number of properties of humans themselves, as well as their living environment.

For the present, one thing is clear: It is theoretically possible for humans to live and work in space for an arbitrarily long period of time. In principle, the duration of severance of human contact with the Earth may be increased in direct proportion to how representative a subset of human biospheric linkages have been incorporated into the actual BLSS. In this chapter, however, we do not touch on the biosocial and psychosocial aspects of the problem, which will become increasingly significant with increasing duration of isolation from the Earth. These aspects require a separate analysis.

II. Structural and Functional Organization of the Biological Life Support System

An ecological approach to development of the BLSS dictates that the functional structure of the system developed should be based on the structure of natural ecosystems. Figure 1 presents a model of the trophic linkages among the major components of an ecological system, showing its various trophic levels. The first level comprises the "energy gates" of the system, through which energy enters from without. This provides the basis for the existence of the entire system. This level is formed of photoautotrophic organisms, which reproduce their mass from inorganic substances (e.g., water, carbon dioxide, and minerals), utilizing the electromagnetic energy of light. The second level comprises herbivorous animals, which, in turn, serve as food for the carnivorous animals (primary, secondary, etc.) that form the third and subse-

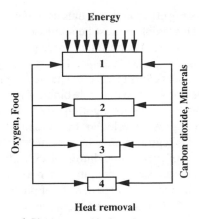

Energy

1. Photoautotrophic Organisms
2. Herbivorous Animals
3. Carnivorous Animals
4. Mineralizing Microorganisms.

Fig. 1 Trophic linkages in an ecological system.

quent trophic levels, the number of which depends on the length of a specific food chain.

Typically, many competing or complementary species occupy each trophic level. Ultimately, the last stage of the trophic chain comprises various soil organisms (invertebrates, fungi, protozoa, and bacteria), which complete the decomposition of organic substances and transform them into the mineral compounds that are used by plants in the next cycle of synthesis of organic substances and accumulation of energy. The passage of substances from one trophic level to the next entails loss of a significant amount of energy; Fig. 1 depicts this passage by a progressive decrease in the area of the rectangles representing the various trophic levels.

In an actual BLSS, photoautotrophic organisms may be represented by higher plants and one-celled algae. The next trophic level, that of heterotrophic organisms, comprises humans and those herbivorous animals that can be a source of human food. The final stage of mineralization and return of unused organic substances and wastes to the system is realized by heterotrophic micro-organisms, which perform this function in a community with algae and higher plants or in special microbiological reactors. All these structural subsystems of the BLSS are called the functional components of the BLSS. Such components can be defined as relatively isolated populations or communities of organisms realizing a particular stage in the substance cycle of the system.

A. Photoautotrophic Component

The key process of synthesizing organic substances by using light energy occurs at this level. In its general form, this occurs in accordance with the formula

$$nCO_2 + nH_2O \longrightarrow n(CH_2O) + nO_2$$

Absorbing light energy, in the form of the chemical bond energy of organic substances, is expended in the subsequent

trophic chains of the system. This formula depicts the biological regeneration of the atmosphere—replenishment of oxygen and elimination of excess carbon dioxide—through photosynthesis. Only a small portion of the spectrum of light radiation (the 380–710-nm waveband) can be used by plants for photosynthesis. This waveband is called photosynthetically active radiation (PAR).

The light energy that is bound in organic substances may, in theory, reach 20 percent of that absorbed by the plants, and this value is used as an indicator of the energy efficiency of photosynthesis. Under actual conditions, this value is significantly lower. For one-celled algae in the laboratory, it fluctuates within the range of 7–12 percent. In higher plants, efficiency is 0.2–1.5 percent under natural conditions and reaches 4–14 per cent under laboratory conditions.

The photosynthetic component not only provides the basis for the existence of the BLSS but also determines its overall structure and functional capacities. If it is based on one-celled algae alone, the BLSS fully solves the problems of regenerating the atmosphere and water and stabilizing organic components and atmospheric microflora; however, it produces only a small fraction of the food required. Under these conditions, the photosynthetic component has minimal mass and volume. If this component consists exclusively of higher plants, then it is capable of producing the requisite amount of food but has less influence on the atmosphere. In addition, a photosynthetic component consisting of higher plants would have to have high mass and would occupy considerable space. Of course, in developing the actual BLSS, we may consider the advantages and shortcomings of each of these particular photosynthetic components and choose to combine them in order to optimize the human living environment, given the limitations of space technology.

1. Higher Plants

Higher plants will probably compose the major portion of the photoautotrophic component in a man-rated BLSS. Aside from regenerating the atmosphere, higher plants provide the vegetable component of the diet. The diverse nutritional requirements of the human diet ordinarily satisfied by vegetables are not readily satisfied by any other source on spacecraft. Since BLSS began to be considered, the issue of proper criteria for selecting plant and animal species for a BLSS has been discussed repeatedly in the literature. This question is typically formulated in terms of absolute criteria, which are not ranked for importance and are meant to apply to any BLSS, regardless of purpose. The main criteria cited are high productivity per unit weight, high efficiency of energy use, maximum proportion of edible biomass, compatibility with other BLSS components and humans, adaptability to cultivation under conditions imposed by space flight, and stability under exposure to extreme environmental factors.

The most general criteria for selecting plants for space greenhouses are cited in Hoff et al.,[28] with each plant species assigned an overall numerical rating, which is important for

Table 3 Two variants of crops proposed for space greenhouses
[From Ashida et al.[30] and Midorikawa et al.[31]]

Culture	Specific area of the crop, m^2/man	
	Ashida et al.	Midorikawa et al.
Rice	16.5	18.8
Wheat	19.25	–
Potatoes	5.5	–
Sweet potatoes	5.5	–
Sugar beets	2.75	–
Lettuce	2.75	1.8
Tomatoes	2.75	–
Peanuts	2.75	–
Soybeans	2.75	16.6
Strawberries	–	1.3

estimating the intrasystemic efficiency of the higher plant component. Similar data are also provided in a paper by F. Salisbury.[29] Current ideas about what plant species should be selected for space greenhouses vary with regard to the variety of nutrients they provide for the human diet, as is illustrated in Table 3.[30,31]

Column 2 of this table is of particular interest here. The assumption is made in this work that a necessary and sufficient human diet (2940 kcal per day, according to the authors' data[31]) can be provided primarily by rice and soybeans. Although the adequacy of this particular diet is doubtful, this work does implicitly raise the possibility of a vegetarian diet (as does the other work incorporated in this table) and, thus, provides the impetus for an open scientific discussion of this issue.

The issue can be reduced to the following question: Is there some essential minimum of "animal products" that must be included in the daily human diet, and, if so, what is this minimum? Space medicine has not yet considered this issue and, thus, can provide no answers, even with respect to traditional animal foods. How does science evaluate nontraditional animal products, starting with the biomass of plankton, including infusoria? Does the concept "products of animal origin" (apart from the vagueness of the term "origin") have any real biological (including biochemical) significance? After all, vegetarianism has been flourishing for centuries.

Today, these questions have moved from the purely theoretical realm and become practical interests of space medicine, since they relate directly to the structure and functions of the BLSS. The question of the necessary percentage of animal products (even traditional animal products) in the human diet has no definite, scientifically based answer. At the same time, it is well known that decreasing the proportion of the heterotrophic component of the ecosystem (BLSS) in-

creases its energy efficiency and, thus, is preferable from this standpoint. This problem must be addressed by space biology and medicine to support future space programs.

Since mission volume, mass, and energy are always limited, the foremost factors in selecting particular plants for the BLSS are their production of edible biomass per unit volume and mass, requirements for light energy, nutritional value, and duration of growth cycle. For this reason, most early investigations concentrated on achieving maximum increases in productivity of particular cultures. NASA CELSS studies addressed conditions for obtaining the maximum yield of wheat through increases in the density of planting, intensity and duration of illumination, temperature, levels of carbon dioxide and humidity, and feeding with a nutrient solution. Calculations have shown that the mass and dimensions of the system were more limiting than energy. Thus, it was decided to attempt to obtain maximum yields per unit space per unit time, even if this meant lowering the efficiency of light use, which is unavoidable for high intensities.[32]

Using this approach, with illumination at the level of atmospheric sunlight (2 cal/m^2/min total radiation), the maximum acceptable density of planting, the maximum level of carbon dioxide compatible with human needs, and optimal ambient conditions (temperature and humidity), Bugbee and Salisbury[32] obtained a yield of short-stem wheat of up to 60 grams/m^2/day, which exceeds record agricultural yields by a factor of 4. The harvest index (percentage of edible biomass in the total yield) was approximately 45 percent.

These experimenters believe that the productivity of wheat may approach that of one-celled algae; however, attainment of an analogous yield of rice and soybeans would undoubtedly be more difficult. Rice and soybeans are short-day plants and require a long period of darkness, which decreases the daily amount of radiation absorbed and the rate of growth.

The issue of the area (and, indirectly, the volume) required for the plants in a space greenhouse is extremely important for a BLSS and is a function of the plants' productivity. For example, given the productivity of wheat of 60 grams/m^2/day obtained under laboratory conditions by Bugbee and Salisbury,[32] 13 m^2 of sown area are sufficient for one person. For a lunar base, considering the duration of solar illumination on the surface of the Moon, the area required is estimated at 40–50 m^2 per person.

It should be noted that none of these theoretical calculations consider experience in growing plants, including wheat, as a component of truly closed systems. Experience has shown that, under such conditions, it is not always possible to obtain yields analogous to those obtained under open cultivation conditions.[33,34] The reasons for this are still unclear and require careful study, since they may make it difficult or impossible to implement certain designs. It is important that these considerations apply not so much to total biomass as to the specialized plant organs producing edible biomass, such as edible roots and especially reproductive organs (grains and oil-bearing crops). The course of plant morphogenesis and embryogenesis under different ambient physical conditions, in closed ecosystems with close interaction of all BLSS components in an extremely limited space, tends to reveal the incompleteness of our understanding of these complex processes and functions. In any event, in the BLSS models we have studied,[34] we observed occasional periods during which grain failed to form in wheat plants. This failure had no obvious relationship to other components of the system or cultivation conditions.

Plant cultivation methods remain an important problem for a BLSS. It has been established indirectly that the best methods are hydroponics, which permit strict control of the delivery of minerals to plants, and even aeroponics, which minimize the amount of nutrient solution. In this connection, F. Salisbury's statement to the effect that, given efficient hydroponics, the root system of the plant comprises a total of 3–4 percent of the total dry biomass, compared to 30–40 percent in a plant growing in soil,[29] is of interest. However, the difficulty of using free liquids in weightlessness compels consideration of substrate methods of cultivation, using salt-saturated substrates of artificial (ion exchange resins) or natural origins. A natural salt-saturated substrate (natural zeolite) was used in the Soviet space greenhouse flown on Mir starting in June 1990.

The unique conditions associated with the construction of lunar and planetary bases also suggest that substrate methods may be the most promising. If it is possible to reproduce the natural process of soil formation to create fertile soil on the Moon and other planets by analogy to the soil formation process on the ancient Earth, the planet's own soil could be used for plant cultivation. At the Institute of Biomedical Problems in Moscow, this possibility was subjected to experimental testing in a 3-year (1981–1983) experiment involving systematic introduction of wheat straw into an inert substrate containing 10 percent natural straw by weight, using humus in a hotbed as a control. It was found that a stable soil biocomplex formed in the inert substrate during the first year. After this period, the total dry mass of the substrate did not increase; and the rate of decay of straw corresponded to the rate of its introduction into the substrate, as well as to the rate of formation in a greenhouse of comparable area. The level of organic substance in the newly formed soil stabilized at a level of approximately 6 percent of the total dry mass of the substrate.[35]

This process would appear to be the most natural route for processing and utilizing any other organic wastes in the BLSS, involving not only soil microflora but also substances emitted by the roots. Processes of mineralization of organic substances are accompanied by processes of secondary biosynthesis of complex humic compounds, the importance of which (for soil fertility) have long been recognized. This natural combination of biological mineralization and utilization of natural wastes in the area of the root, with formation of biologically complete substrates, approximates a functional analog of natural soil. This is fully consistent with the concept of the biological completeness of the living environment in the BLSS—in this case, the living environment of plants.

With all its advantages, a photoautotrophic component based solely on higher plants has an important shortcoming—the high inertia associated with the long cycle of plant development, which, as a rule, exceeds 30 days. This means that a long period is required to restore the normal functioning of the higher plant component if it is damaged in an emergency or accident. Moreover, the total gas exchange ratio of higher plants (CO_2:O_2), is close to 1 and, therefore, is nowhere near the respiratory quotient of humans, giving rise to the problems of excess oxygen and carbon dioxide deficit.

2. One-Celled Algae

In a closed-substance-cycle system, algae fulfill the same air revitalization function as higher plants, enabling energy to enter the system from without. Of greatest interest for closed ecological systems are green and blue-green, one-celled algae (cyanobacteria). The small size of the individual cells, their relatively simple morphology, high rate of reproduction, short developmental cycle, high level of photosynthesis per unit of biomass, and high stability under exposure to adverse environmental factors work together to enable intense cultivation with automatic stabilization of ambient conditions. The algae that have been studied most often are those of the *Chlorella* family. This species was the first candidate for a photosynthetic (photoautotrophic) component of a BLSS, and its use for this purpose was widely discussed in the literature as early as the 1950s. The Institute of Biomedical Problems constructed the first models of biological atmosphere regeneration systems using *Chlorella*.[13] Subsequently, a functional component of a closed-substance-cycle system using *Chlorella* was developed. Scientists derived principles for obtaining high productivity and developed a technology involving continuous cultivation with a closed cycle of nutrient medium balanced for utilization of mineral elements by cells. This is the only possible method for closed-substance-cycle systems. This technology provided optimal conditions for the formation of a stable bacterial community concomitant with the algae and maintained the stability of the nonsterile algae culture as an algo-bacterial cenosis. The first experimental models of a man-rated BLSS had this system as a component and demonstrated the capacity of algae in a community with bacteria to play a number of unanticipated roles in generating a living environment suitable for humans.

An in-depth study of BLSS models based on photosynthesis by one-celled algae (*Chlorella*) has shown that the traditional comparison of one-celled algae and higher plants using physiological and technological criteria is insufficient for determining their roles and functions in a man-rated BLSS as a closed ecosystem. Additional ecological criteria are required. Using these criteria, it was found that, within the BLSS models studied, an "algae culture" is not actually a "culture" (as, for example, wheat) but is a relatively independent autotrophic-heterotrophic aqueous ecosystem with concomitant heterotrophic microflora composing an integral part. This is why system models based on *Chlorella* remained stable

Table 4 Composition of the biomass (percent of dry weight) of various species of one-celled algae

Type of algae	Protein	Fat	Carbohydrate	Ash
Chlorella	53.2	20.7	19.1	5.7
Chlamydomonas	34.1	8.8	54.5	4.5
Closteriopsis	34.3	16.9	46.2	4.6
Euglena	56.0	22.0	18.2	4.5
Spirulina	57.5	12.0	22.5	7.8

over time and, in addition to playing their assigned roles of regenerating air and water, also significantly increased levels of organic, bacterial, aero-ion, and aerosol components in the atmosphere. In other systems, functions such as these must be performed by special devices. The weight, volume, and power requirements of these devices are typically not counted in comparative evaluations, which is a mistake.

The major shortcoming of BLSS models based on *Chlorella* photosynthesis is the low closure of trophic linkages in the system. The biomass synthesized by *Chlorella*, despite its high caloric value, cannot serve as a major component of the human diet, as was proposed very early in work on this problem. In the system models that have been created, this biomass has been used in the diet in only small quantities, about 10 percent of the total weight of the diet. This is because the cell walls of *Chlorella* cells resist decomposition and the biomass contains high levels of protein and nucleic acids and low levels of carbohydrates. However, there are ways to optimize the composition of the biomass and increase its proportion in the human diet. This may be accomplished by including in this component other forms of one-celled algae with biomass composition different from that of *Chlorella*.

Various forms of algae with biomass composition differing from that of *Chlorella* have been studied at the Institute for Biomedical Problems (see Table 4). By selecting a community of algae having biomass with different compositions, it is possible to attain a more optimal overall biomass (with respect to the composition of the diet) and, thus, to increase the closure of the trophic linkages in models of this type (i.e., those without animals). However, the issue of the food value of algae and their possible use in the human diet cannot be considered entirely closed, despite a substantial amount of research in Japan, the United States, and the U.S.S.R.

Higher plants must comprise the major portion of the photoautotrophic component with respect to the amount of participation in the total substance cycle. However, the inclusion of one-celled algae significantly improves performance with respect to biomass composition, as well as enhances the dynamic properties of the system. One-celled algae, because of their high reproduction rate and the relative simplicity of the technology for growing them, are the least inert component in the system for regulating the photoautotrophic component and increasing its "repairability" after

emergencies have damaged it. Since inclusion of one-celled algae is the most feasible way to maintain the productivity of the photoautotrophic component (e.g., with respect to gas exchange) within the required range of values, the minimum proportion of algae used in this component should be that required to perform this function. The maximum proportion of one-celled algae in the photoautotrophic component will evidently be determined by the extent to which their biomass can be used in the diet of humans and animals.

B. Heterotrophic Component

In the first, necessarily simplified BLSS variants, the major function of the heterotrophic component, as the metabolic complement of plants, was performed by humans. However, the diet of these humans required the inclusion of other heterotrophs to produce animal protein. Animals selected for a BLSS have to meet the generally accepted criteria of high productivity per unit weight, energy efficiency, minimal proportion of nonusable biomass, etc. However, there are also special system requirements—minimal food competition with humans and maximal ability to consume plant wastes inedible by humans. In general, the preferable species are those whose own weight is low, both because of the high specific metabolic rate of smaller species and the fact that, because of the large number of individuals in the population, the function of the component as a whole is not severely disrupted by the accidental death of a few individuals.

The range of choice of species for the heterotrophic component is very great and, in principle, encompasses the entire animal kingdom, from protozoa to mammals. One of the first overviews of this subject, performed by Yazdovskiy and Ratner[36] covered almost this entire range. Serious consideration of fish in this role[37,38] has typically led to their rejection on the grounds of the great weight of the water required to maintain them. However, if we consider the need for some amount of shock-absorbing substances in the major flows of the cycle, then the use of such amounts of water can only be considered beneficial to the system.

With respect to invertebrates, the Institute of Biomedical Problems investigated the physiological and ecological characteristics of slugs for use in a BLSS. The proportion of edible biomass reached 75 percent, while the protein level approached 50 percent. These parameters are substantially higher than those for traditional agricultural animals and are of interest for future variants of the BLSS.[39]

At present, development of the heterotrophic component is at the stage of theoretical consideration and ground-based experimentation. The first attempts to study the issue of raising food animals under actual space-flight conditions revealed unique and unforeseen problems associated with weightlessness, problems which are more difficult to solve for animals than for humans.

Scientists at the Institute of Biomedical Problems (Moscow), in collaboration with specialists from Czechoslovakia, investigated the use of birds in a BLSS not only as a direct source of food but also to produce secondary food products—eggs. The results of experiments on Mir showed that for this highly organized free-living species, new problems associated with motor behavior arose in weightlessness.[40] In the absence of gravity, the whole set of innate sensorimotor reflexes and individual "skills" developed under terrestrial conditions becomes inappropriate. This poses new problems in the technology of animal maintenance in weightlessness—restraint in space, feeding, breeding, and others—complicating the issue considerably. This suggests a new, unexpected criterion for selecting animals for a BLSS: their constant association with a substrate in order to eliminate the problems of orientation and motor behavior in microgravity.

These first orbital experiments showed that developing a heterotrophic BLSS component using traditional agricultural animals and birds may be far more complex, even immeasurably more complex, than developing a component using nontraditional sources of animal products.

C. Organic Waste Processing Component

Major sources of waste in a BLSS are humans and the photoautotrophic component, which produces a significant proportion of the inedible biomass. The function of the organic waste processing subsystem of the BLSS is to decompose this waste and return the waste substances to the overall cycle through the photoautotrophic component. Inedible plant biomass, cooking wastes, fecal matter, and liquid wastes in the form of wash water and urine, comprise the bulk of such wastes. As the heterogeneity of species increases and the structure of the higher plant component approaches that of the human diet, the absolute and relative amounts of inedible biomass can only increase. This essentially makes the system an open one; and, if all the biomass is not returned to the cycle, then equivalent supplies of carbon dioxide and water have to be provided to compensate for losses of carbon dioxide, oxygen, and hydrogen.

The development of this component of the BLSS has not advanced significantly since the publication of the first edition of this work. As was the case then, we are concentrating on the processes of bacterial decomposition of organic wastes in aerobic conditions in special fermenters, with emission of carbon dioxide and water and subsequent utilization of some mixture of the products of decay by higher plants. However, this method has still not advanced beyond the stage of exploration in ground-based experiments; and, more important, the compatibility of higher plants with this component for processing wastes, as well as the products thus produced, has not been studied under closed conditions.

The only new approach to this problem noted here is the attempt to provide bacterial decomposition of plant wastes right in the substrate, with the plants themselves participating in the process in an analog of natural soil processes. This was described above in the section on higher plants.[35]

During the earliest period of work on BLSSs, in the 1960s, the idea arose that the final stages of the cycle (i.e., the transformation of organic substances by mineralizing organisms) could be replaced by physical-chemical processes for decomposing organic substances. At that time, conditions of high-temperature incineration, catalytic oxidation in a liquid environment, and "wet oxidation" at high temperatures and pressures began to be intensively studied. It became clear that decomposition and mineralization of organic substances into component elements and their oxides would make them difficult to utilize by the higher plant component; i.e., to return them to the cycle. This pertained especially to the major biogenic elements, phosphorus and sulphur, which are lost in the form of oxides during incineration in the gas phase and to nitrogen generated in its free state, a form which could not be assimilated by plants. A number of oxides of ash elements are relatively insoluble.

Nevertheless, in the United States and Japan, interest in these processes has recently revived in connection with the CELSS Program. Takahashi[41] describes a method of wet oxidation of wastes at a temperature as high as 700 °C and a pressure as great as 250 atm. However, this work gives no indication that the products obtained were used by higher plants.

While on the subject of the potential use of physical-chemical decomposition of organic wastes in BLSS, we should note that these processes are not functionally equivalent to the natural processes of biological decomposition of organic substances in nature, particularly in the soil. Biological decomposition in the soil results from the combined and interrelated activity of soil organisms and substances emitted by plant roots to produce products appropriate to the trophic needs of plants and to synthesize humus, which supports the natural fertility of plants. This is the way nature solves the problem of integrating the processes of mineralization and utilization of organic wastes in terrestrial and aquatic ecosystems. This is also precisely how we solved the problem of mineralization and utilization of the major components of urine, mainly nitrogen, in algae reactors in our model BLSS and, at the same time, facilitated the recovery of water excreted in urine.

In conclusion, it should be noted that, in the relatively well-developed BLSS, organic wastes may also be utilized by elements of the heterotrophic component—traditional or nontraditional producers of animal biomass or specially introduced saprophages. For example, we studied the physiological and ecological characteristics of the ordinary housefly, which, in the larval stage, consumes solid human wastes and can serve as food for domestic birds,[42] whereas the residual product is an effective, biologically active supplement to the substrate for growing higher plants.

In general terms, this is the structural and functional organization of the BLSS, in which each of the functional components (subsystems) is responsible for one portion of the overall cycle (Fig. 1) that unites these components into a single, functionally integrated, biological system. Using these components, which are necessary to any ecosystem, one can construct different BLSS variants that resemble natural ecosystems, with their characteristic stability based on the internal interactions of parts to a greater or lesser extent. We merely note that each functional component of the BLSS reveals its true functional parameters (the productivity, quantity, and quality of biomass produced; the relationship to its environment; and others) only when it operates within a specific BLSS model that includes humans and other components. Research with such models has shown that, in general, the characteristics of a potential BLSS component tested in open laboratory facilities do not correspond to those shown during joint functioning with other BLSS components in a closed environment.

There is another aspect of the use of these components of a BLSS. They may act as independent components within a nonbiological system and be used to supplement life support systems based on stored supplies or physical-chemical regeneration. Recently, there has been a trend to use components this way; and this has given rise to the idea of a new class of life support system—mixed (hybrid) systems incorporating processes particular to both physical-chemical and biological regeneration, which had previously been considered alternatives. The category of hybrid systems also covers a variety of systems transitional between the two pure types as the functions of the biological components increase. Of course, inclusion of isolated biological components (e.g., a facility for growing edible plants or maintaining animals) in a physical-chemical system does not make this system biological, although it suggests the potential for development into a biological system in the future.

III. Hybrid Biological-Physical-Chemical Life Support Systems (Controlled Ecological Life Support Systems)

NASA, with the participation of scientists from Japan, Canada, and a number of European nations, is developing the best known of these projects, the CELSS program, for Space Station, lunar bases, etc. [Note: As used in this section, the term "ecological" in CELSS refers to the human living environment and does not correspond to the concept of a biological (ecological) life support system, as the term is used elsewhere in the current chapter.]

The CELSS concept is based upon the integration of biological, physical, and chemical processes to develop safe and reliable life support systems that will produce palatable food, potable water, and a breathable atmosphere by recycling metabolic and other wastes. The central feature of a CELSS is the use of green plant photosynthesis to produce food, with the resulting production of oxygen and potable water and removal of carbon dioxide. For additional information, see Refs. 43-45.

A CELSS is an integrated set of biological and nonbiological subsystems that function through processes of regeneration and recycling to sustain human life. The essence of the system is the production of biomass that can be converted into food, while generating minimal inedible residue, which must be further processed as waste matter before it can be

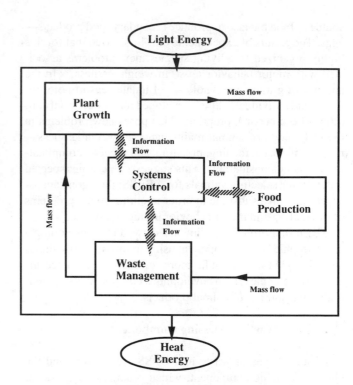

Fig. 2 Prototype ecosynthetic life support system showing inputs, outputs, and internal linkages between functional components.

recycled. The major functions of the CELSS subsystems are biomass production, food processing, waste processing, and system monitoring and control. Because these subsystems are interactive and interdependent, a total systems approach is critical. Figure 2 shows the proposed structure of linkages between the plant growth subsystem and others. Because volume, weight, and energy are all at a premium in space, a particular crop's desirability is judged partly on the basis of how much edible food it can continually produce in a given volume and the amount of light, nutrients, and growing time it requires. Thus, much of the early research in this area focused on maximizing the productivity of specific crop plants. The results of NASA's studies of wheat are summarized in Section II.A.1.

A. Food Production Subsystem

A necessary function of any life support system is to supply appetizing and nutritionally adequate diets for the crew. In theory, these diets could consist solely of vegetables or of vegetables combined with animal proteins or nontraditional foods (i.e., carbohydrates derived from cellulose degradation). Plant combinations that provide suitable diets are selected on the basis of harvestability, palatability, processing requirements, nutritional content, growth habitat, and power requirements. Mathematical models incorporating these characteristics are being developed to determine optimal plant combinations. Preliminary calculations indicate that 99 percent of the crew's nutritional requirements could be met with only three or four plant types (for example, legumes, grains, and vegetables).

Although most crops to date have been chosen for their high ratio of edible food to total biomass, researchers continue to explore methods of converting inedible biomass to food. Candidate techniques include microbial, chemical, and enzymatic processes. Microbial food sources, particularly yeast and algae, are candidates for nutritional supplements.

Biomass generated by crop plants will require processing to make it suitable for human consumption. Studies are now underway to define systems that will harvest, preprocess, store, and convert plant biomass into edible forms. Related research focuses on general food processing methods and examines microbial, chemical, and enzymatic systems as candidate techniques for food conversion. Techniques have been developed to recover a pure protein concentrate from algae grown under controlled conditions.

B. Waste Management Subsystem

In a completely closed environment where all foods are grown onboard and all wastes are recycled into foods, the material balance for the necessary chemical elements can be closed in a manner analogous to that which occurs on Earth. For additional information in this area, see Refs. 41 and 46-48.

Carbon, oxygen, and hydrogen, the three major elements involved in human and animal metabolism appear in the form of carbon dioxide, water, and partially oxidized organics in feces, urine, and exhaled breath. If only carbohydrates, the molecules of which comprise carbon and water, are subject to oxidation in the human body, then the net effect of human and animal metabolism and subsequent oxidation is the exact inverse of photosynthesis.

Water that is not utilized in metabolic processes is essentially used as a carrier fluid within the living components and is used externally in waste processing subsystems. Thus, physical separation processes should be sufficient to recycle water in wastes for use as drinking water, sanitary water, and wash water.

The nutrient solutions used for growing plants in controlled growth chambers invariably contain 12 to 16 elements that are present as inorganic salts and the organic chelating agents needed to maintain some of the ions in solution. These elements (which act as plant nutrients) appear in the waste streams in the forms of spent nutrient solutions, inedible vegetation, uneaten foods, food processing wastes, human and animal metabolic wastes, and animal processing wastes. One major function of the waste processing system is to recover the plant nutrient elements from the various waste streams and convert them back into forms that plants can reassimilate into the food chain.

The functions of the CELSS waste processing subsystems are to convert all wastes into the inputs required to sustain life and to remove contaminants that may be harmful or impair functioning of the living components of the habitat. The major inputs required to sustain human life are food, oxygen, drinking water, sanitary water, and wash water. The major waste outputs include a) solids (human and animal feces, inedible vegetation, uneaten foods, food processing wastes, and animal processing wastes); b) liquids (human and animal urine, spent nutrient solutions, and spent wash water); and c) gases (oxygen from plants, carbon dioxide from humans and animals, water vapor, and off-gases).

The following subsystem technologies have been researched and developed to varying degrees:

- Oxidation of organics by incineration
- Wet oxidation of organics
- Biological oxidation of organics
- Integrated algal bacterial systems
- Higher plants grown on urine
- Wash water recycle
- Atmosphere decontamination
- Carbon dioxide and oxygen extraction
- Recovery of plant nutrients and trace metals from solid and liquid waste streams

None of these technologies has been studied previously in terms of adaptability to the specific requirements of the CELSS concept. For example, the three alternative oxidation processes (incineration, wet oxidation, and biological oxidation) are well-developed technologies for terrestrial applications; the first two have also been researched by NASA for limited space applications. However, even for what are normally considered "well-developed technologies" on Earth, significant research and development are required to determine how readily they can be adapted to a CELSS waste treatment process.

Precise measurement and characterization of system inputs, outputs, and operating parameters are required to obtain detailed mass and energy balances. These data are needed to establish the engineering interfaces and the design of accompanying subsystems. For example, the concentrations and types of organics in the off-gas, which are functions of operating temperature and mode of operation, will define the need for subsequent catalytic oxidation of the off-gas. The degree to which nitrogen is formed during the oxidation of organic nitrogen will determine the need for a separate nitrogen-fixing subsystem in the overall processing scheme. The forms and concentrations of metals in the ash, which may be a function of oxidation temperature, will have ramifications for the methods used to solubilize and separate the ash components in the preparation of plant nutrients.

C. Systems Control

The success of a life support system depends upon the integration of the biological and nonbiological processes and subsystems into a reliable and predictable system. To accomplish this goal, system monitoring and control strategies and technologies need to be developed and tested. Initial research has focused on conducting a number of theoretical studies based upon the application of engineering control theory.

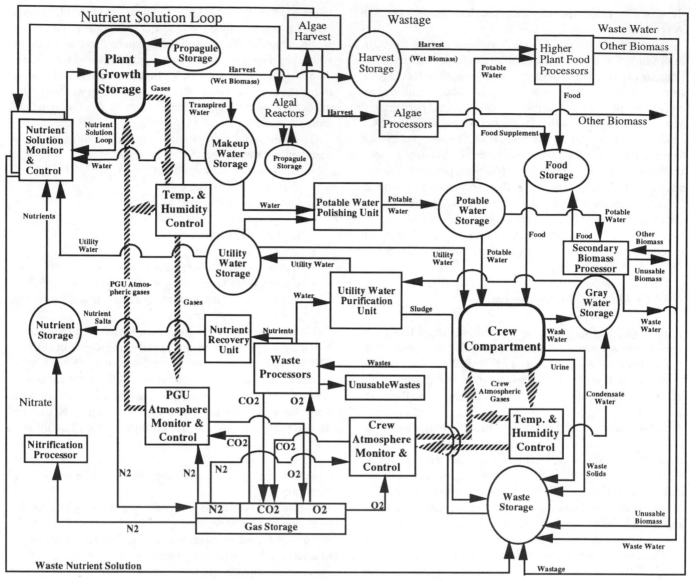

Fig. 3 CELSS initial reference configuration.

The results of the initial research in this area have focused on the production of mathematical models that could be subjected to various system control approaches. A critical conclusion from these studies is the demonstration that certain ecosynthetic life support systems may well be susceptible to long-term failure modes and that the design of control systems to deal with such failures will be crucial to mission success.

D. Initial Reference Configuration for the Controlled Ecological Life Support System

Figure 3 shows a prototype CELSS reference configuration. This configuration will be used for future CELSS investigative efforts and will highlight those subsystems that require intensive planning and research, particularly for a ground-based human-rated CELSS test bed. The evaluation criteria to be applied to a successful ground-based test will address not only the maintenance of air, water, and food production within acceptable limits but also the practicality of achieving the specified results and the resilience of the system across a wide variety of failure modes. Therefore, the test system will incorporate, to the maximum possible extent, the modularity and flexibility desired for an operational system. The crew interfaces will be developed to the extent that only minor enhancements will be needed to adapt the CELSS for operational use. Amendments will be made to the reference configuration as necessary, but its general structure will remain similar to that described herein.

The functions of the CELSS include atmospheric pressure and composition control, temperature and humidity control, atmosphere revitalization, water management, food production, and waste management. Requirements for the proof-of-concept test involve maintaining those functions for a specified time at predetermined performance levels.

The overall system design emphasizes modularity in the

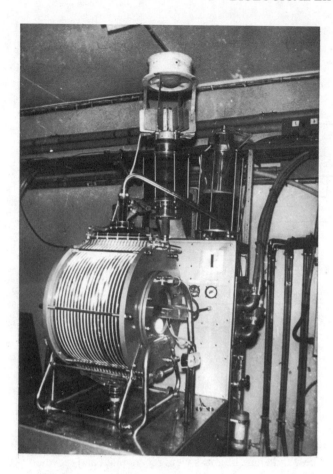

Fig. 4 Photosynthetic reactor (gas exchanger).

processors (plants, waste, and crew) that interact through connections to material reservoirs (storage tanks and cabin atmospheres). The system will also allow operation in a number of alternate modes to allow maximum flexibility in coping with single-point failures. System-level control of the CELSS will be enabled by reference to a computer-based emulation model, which will have a simplified crew interface and mode selection.

In conclusion, it should be said that hybrid biological-physical-chemical systems are sure to be the first actual instances of the partial use of the biological method of regeneration in a life support system.

IV. Experimental Biological Life Support System Models

After the first attempts in the 1960s in the U.S.S.R. to create a BLSS based on photosynthesis of one-celled algae (see Sections II.A.1 and II.A.2), a long period of research was required before these endeavors could resume at a new level of algae productivity, using a continuous noncirculating flow method of cultivation. Even more important, the new systems were based on a new level of understanding of the problem of the BLSS itself, not as an applied technological task but as an independent ecological problem—the creation of

artificial closed ecological systems, of which the BLSS is an example.

At present in Russia, various BLSS models have been developed and studied, from the simplest, based on one-celled algae, up to models including (or exclusively based on) higher plants and components of a system for mineralization and utilization of organic wastes. The best known and most highly publicized data are those generated by "man-higher plants" models studied in the Institute of Biophysics of the Siberian Division of the Russian Academy of Sciences (Krasnoyarsk) using the Bios-3 facility.[49,89–91]

In this chapter, however, we will concentrate on less widely known data concerning the environment generated in the BLSS models, human physiological reactions to this environment, the closure of these models with respect to mass exchange, their stability, and other aspects of their correspondence (or lack thereof) to the major properties of natural ecosystems. These data were obtained in the Institute of Biomedical Problems of the U.S.S.R. (currently Russian) Ministry of Health (Moscow).[50,51]

A. Models of the Biological Life Support System Based on One-Celled Algae

The major functional component of this model is a nonsterile, noncirculating culture of the one-celled algae, *Chlorella vulgaris*, in a photosynthetic reactor (Fig. 4). The reactor is cylindrical in shape with xenon luminescent lamps of 6 kW along its long axis. The light falls directly on the base of wedge-shaped light guides made of acrylic plastic and is directed into the center of the algae suspension, which is located between the light guides and the outer wall of the cylinder. The volume of the suspension in the gas exchanger is approximately 15 liters, with a working density of 10–12 grams of dry substance per liter. The working density is supported at the appropriate level through automatic removal of a portion of the suspension at a signal from a photoelectric density sensor, with simultaneous addition of a nutrient medium balanced for mineral elements, along with condensate of water vapor from the inhabited module. Air is blown through the reactor at a rate of approximately 200 L/min. Human gas exchange is supported by three, or (less frequently) two, such reactors. After passing through the reactors, the air enters a pressurized cabin inhabited by humans, which has a free volume of 5 m³. A flow chart of the structure of this model is presented in Fig. 5.

Aside from humans and *Chlorella,* the model contains units for biological mineralization and dehydration of urine and for drying solid human wastes and unusable *Chlorella* biomass for return of free water to the overall cycle. These units are used, also, when a higher plant component is added to this model.

The component for biological mineralization of urine is designed for regeneration and repeated use of the water and nitrogen excreted by humans in urine, and also of the carbon dioxide that forms when urea decomposes. The process in-

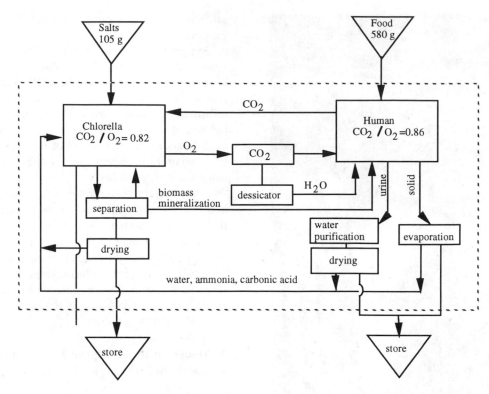

Fig. 5 Functional structure of a "human-*Chlorella*-mineralization" model.

volves preliminary processing of urine in a special fermenter by urobacteria, followed by distillation of water and ammonia in an evaporator. Water vapor containing ammonia and other components is either fed into the algae reactor directly or is passed through a cell containing nitric acid, where the ammonia is bound into ammonium nitrate and is fed into the algae suspension as a component of the corrective solution to compensate for loss of nitrogen from the medium. Dehydration of unusable biomass (after centrifugation) and feces occurs at a temperature of 70–80° in an air stream and then enters the algae reactor without undergoing any cleaning.

1. Material Balance in the Biological Life Support System Model

The human and algae food chain in the models under discussion have remained almost completely open. System inputs from without included mineral salts for the algae and food for the humans with a total energy value of 2450–2700 kcal/day, to which were added 50 grams of dry biomass from harvested *Chlorella*. The nitrogen fed to the algae was partially provided by nitrogen in urine, approximately 10 percent of which was returned to the human diet in the biomass of *Chlorella*. The unusable algae biomass and solid human waste exited the system (see the flow chart in Fig. 5) after dehydration.

The model provided a complete water regeneration cycle. The water generated by the cycle was used as drinking water, in food preparation, and for hygienic purposes by the humans and was consumed by the algae in the process of photosyn-

thesis. Human transpirational water and free water from urine, feces, and algae biomass were regenerated and recycled. All the water entered the photosynthetic reactor in the form of gas and was output as condensate in an amount corresponding to the amount consumed. The condensate obtained was subjected to further cleaning through sorption, disinfection, and saturation with mineral salts, using a method developed at the Institute of Biomedical Problems and employed on space station Mir.[52] The water obtained met hygienic standards for potable water.

However, a fully closed water cycle was not possible in this system because water entered from without in the food ration and, in combination with organic substances, left the system in the form of dried fecal residue and algae biomass. These external "inputs" and "outputs" essentially were balanced, allowing the system to function without addition of water to the initial supply. The loss from the system because of bound water in food and discarded wastes amounted to approximately 9 percent of its daily turnover. The 91 percent closure of the water cycle thus attained is probably the maximum possible level for a system with external supplies of food and disposal of dry residue of organic wastes.[51]

The model achieved complete regeneration of oxygen. The productivity of the photosynthetic reactors was initially made to correspond to the oxygen consumption rate in the system by selecting the level of illumination for the algae culture. This correspondence was stable throughout the experiments (up to 30 days) and did not require corrective adjustment (Fig. 6, curve 1). However, concentrations of carbon dioxide in the system increased continuously (Fig. 6, curve 2) and the ex-

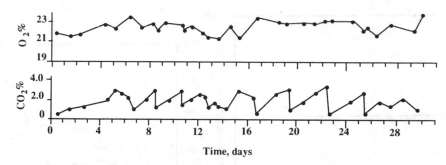

Fig. 6 Dynamics of oxygen and carbon dioxide levels in the atmosphere.

Table 5 Percent of substances regenerated in two BLSS models

Substance	Consumed, grams/day	Man-algae-mineralization model Regenerated		Man-algae-mineralization-higher plants model Regenerated	
		Grams/day	Percent	Grams/day	Percent
Oxygen	755	755	100	755	100
Food	530	50	9	138	26
Water	3400	3400	100	3400	100
Total	4685	4205	90	4293	92

cess had to be absorbed by chemical absorbers approximately once every 2-1/2 days.

This gas exchange imbalance occurs because the assimilation coefficient of algae (amount of absorbed carbon dioxide per unit of emitted oxygen) is determined by the composition of the biomass synthesized by the algae, whereas the inverse ratio of these gases in human respiration (respiratory quotient) is determined by the composition of food assimilated, which differs significantly from the composition of the algae. Evidently, complete gas balance can be attained only in rather complex multispecies systems, in which the entire output of the photoautotrophic component is fully utilized in the trophic chains of the heterotrophic organisms. In the models studied, excess carbon dioxide equaled 5–7 percent of its daily turnover.

Despite the simplicity of the biocenotic structure of the "humans-algae-mineralization" models studied, they are able to regenerate the oxygen and water in amounts that fully meet human needs. However, they can meet the need for food only partially (up to 10 percent of total mass). The total amounts of regenerated substances produced in such a system are presented in Table 5. This system, which produces approximately 90 percent of the quantity of substances consumed, is evidently close to the maximum possible efficiency for systems with analogous structures; i.e., those in which the photosynthetic component is represented by only one species of plant, which makes up only a small proportion of the diet. In models such as this, having incomplete closure with respect to trophic linkages, it is important to keep the substances input to and output from the system in balance. This maintains the

material and, thus, the functional equilibrium of the system over time.

Significant characteristics of the models being studied are the small air volume of the system (5 m^3 per person), the low initial supply of oxygen (1 m^3 per person), and the low initial supply of water (52 liters per person), including that used in the algae suspension. These system parameters are of great importance, since they determine the duration of recovery cycles for water and oxygen, the major system components. Because of the system's low volume and the small initial amounts of regenerable substances needed, speed of regeneration is high so that, during a typical experiment (30 days), up to 15 cycles of oxygen and almost 2 cycles of available water are regenerated. Some data suggest that renewal of the supply of oxygen in the Earth's atmosphere requires 2000 years. This comparison demonstrates one property that makes small-scale models with relatively small initial supplies of regenerable substances useful for experimental ecology.

2. Volatile Components of the Atmosphere

Volatile contaminants in the atmosphere are an important factor in the habitability of a BLSS. The atmospheres of autonomously functioning BLSS subsystems (for algae suspension, urine mineralization, and dehydration of solid wastes and algae biomass) have been found to contain dozens of organic compounds, the predominant ones being hydrocarbons (C_1–C_5), aldehydes, ketones (C_3–C_5), carbonic acids, alcohols, and complex esters. Many compounds remain unidentified.

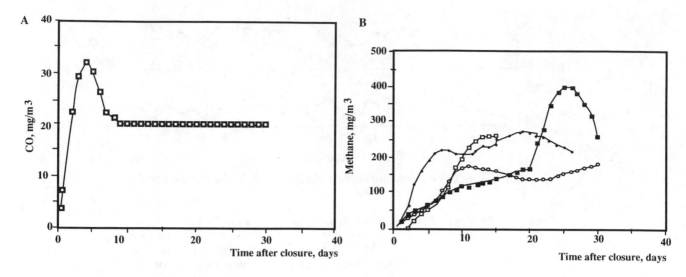

Fig. 7 Dynamics of concentration of carbon monoxide (A) and methane (B) in the atmosphere of the model studied (for methane, each trial is plotted separately).

When individual components are linked to form a single system, the water-soluble contaminants in the atmosphere have been found to consist primarily of aldehydes and ethyl alcohol in concentrations up to 0.5 mg/L. The less soluble components (carbon monoxide and methane) accumulate in the atmosphere, and stabilize at a certain level. The equilibrium concentration for carbon monoxide was approximately 20 mg/m^3 (Fig. 7A), and for methane 150–250 mg/m^3 (Fig. 7B). There are two phases in the pattern of change of these components over time: an accumulation phase and a stationary phase. Time required for carbon monoxide to reach the stationary phase was found to be 4–6 days after closure of the system, with inclusion of humans (Fig. 7A); for methane, time required was 7–10 days (Fig. 7B). Occasional jumps in the levels of certain volatile components were transient and associated with disruption of the thermal regime for drying organic wastes.

The dynamics of concentrations of volatile components in the atmosphere of the BLSS demonstrates that the system must have certain mechanisms for binding these components. Evidently, the photosynthetic reactor, with its algobacterial community, acted as a hydrobiological filter for removing volatile components from the atmosphere. These substances not only dissolved in the liquid medium but also were utilized in the suspension of algae and concomitant microflora and were thereby drawn into the overall cycle.

It must be noted that the general results of the combined gas-forming and gas-absorbing activity of the functional components of the system were studied in the absence of any filtering or absorbing devices. In a number of cases, this caused standards for acceptable concentrations of certain contaminants (e.g., carbon monoxide) to be exceeded temporarily. However, had filters been used, it would not have been possible to identify the system's tendencies and capacities to stabilize volatile components in the regenerated atmosphere.

The capacity of the algae suspension to assimilate volatile atmospheric components was not studied specifically but potentially could be very large. For example, the suspension assimilated the nitrogen in urine after urea decomposed producing ammonia. Thus, the use of one-celled algae in a BLSS revealed the system's unanticipated capacity to stabilize volatile components when the atmosphere was regenerated without special filters.

Investigations of these models revealed an additional unanticipated function, optimization of the composition of charged components of the atmosphere—aero-ions. Throughout all the experiments, light, negatively charged ions with a coefficient of unipolarity of approximately 0.6 and a total concentration of 1.3–1.5 x 10^3 ion/mL were predominant in the system's atmosphere. This type of ionization is characteristic of the atmosphere of coastal regions and open areas covered with vegetation and is not observed in the atmosphere of inhabited enclosures with non-biological LSSs. This is of great significance from the standpoint of the quality and adequacy of the human living environment formed in the BLSS. A detailed analysis of this issue was presented in a work by A.V. Anisimov, a scientist of the Institute of Biomedical Problems.[53]

3. Micro-Organisms in the Biological Life Support System

Still another unanticipated function of a system based on one-celled algae was discovered when microbial composition and dynamics were studied in the atmosphere of these BLSS models.

Microbiological issues are among the most important in space medicine with respect to flights of spacecraft and space stations (see Chapter 4 of this volume). In a BLSS, as a closed ecosystem, a new aspect of space microbiology becomes salient. This is the case because the human indigenous microflora that predominate in spacecraft environments are only a fraction of the total microecosystem of a BLSS. Each BLSS

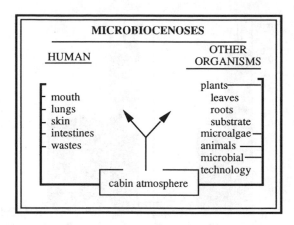

Fig. 8 Structure of a microbial community in a BLSS.

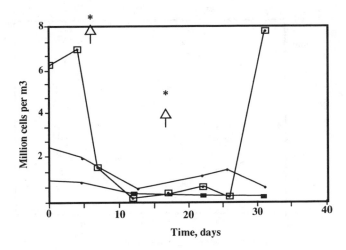

* indicate points at which bacterial count increased due to short periods of depressurization of the system

Fig. 9 Dynamics of total bacterial count in the atmosphere of a BLSS in two experiments (curves 1 and 2) and *Staphylococci* count (curve 3).

component may have concomitant microflora that coexist with one another in complex and unanticipated interrelationships and form a kind of system within the larger BLSS macroecosystem, which itself may be studied from an ecological standpoint.

The literature on BLSSs includes valuable information on the microflora of the individual components of the ecosystem, one-celled algae[54] and higher plants.[55,56] However, with the exception of work by J.I. Gitelzon et al.,[57] these studies remain isolated and have not influenced the study of the microecosystem as an integrated component of the BLSS and an independent ecological factor.

Our own investigations have also concentrated on the microflora of individual biotopes of the BLSS. However, they can provide the foundation for an initial attempt to conceptualize the problem of the overall microbiology of the BLSS. The structure of the microbiocenosis of the BLSS is depicted schematically in Fig. 8. The BLSS microflora represent a system of relatively isolated but ultimately interrelated communities of micro-organisms occupying various ecological niches in human biotopes, other functional components of the ecosystem, and the equipment and interior of the spacecraft. Isolation of individual biotopes is relative and does not prevent cross-exchange among their microcenoses. For example, representatives of intestinal microflora are periodically found among the microflora of the spacecraft interior, the nasopharynges of crewmembers,[58] and the root areas and nutrient media of the higher plants.[59]

The associations among various microbial communities may take the form of a systematic incursion of alien flora, followed by their inevitable elimination in a developing community. But the association may also be more complicated, taking the form of competition or symbiosis and complementary functions in the assimilation of ambient trophic resources, when complex substances must be decomposed through the action of various micro-organisms with different types of metabolism. The latter situation is most likely in organic waste collectors but is possible, also, in biotopes of the interior, which is full of decay-resistant polymer materials with various chemical structures.

The atmosphere plays an important role in the microecosystem of the BLSS. It is a kind of central "communications center," the arena of communications among microbial communities of various biotopes. Thus, atmospheric microflora may carry information about the state of these communities. Moreover, the atmosphere is the source of organic hydrogen for micro-organisms growing on inert substrates having only limited trophic resources or none at all. Here, we are referring to various structural and decorative materials, on which, according to A.N. Viktorov's data,[60] stable fungal communities of micro-organisms are established (see, also, Chapter 4 of this volume). One must assume that atmospheric moisture and the organic components of the atmosphere provide sufficient resources to sustain such communities. The role of these factors as sources of nutrition for atmospheric microflora was first noted by N.G. Kholodnyy.[61]

In the BLSS models we studied, the qualitative and quantitative composition of the system's microbiocenosis was determined by at least three interacting sources of microflora: human indigenous microflora, the microcenosis of the nonsterile cultures of algae, and microflora of the urine collector and mineralization fermenter. Typical overall population dynamics for bacteria in the atmosphere of the inhabited system are presented in Fig. 9, which depicts data from two experiments. This figure shows that the initial number of microflora decreased after closure of the system and stabilized at a rather low level—approximately 10^3 cells in 1 m^3 of air. This level is one to two orders of magnitude below that typically observed in ground experiments with non-biological LSSs or on manned flights on Salyut space stations.[58] The two points in the figure where one can see sharp increases in the number of microflora were associated with periods of short-term depressurization of the inhabited cabin (indicated by arrows) in one of the experiments. In the other experiment, a similar increase occurred at the end of the experi-

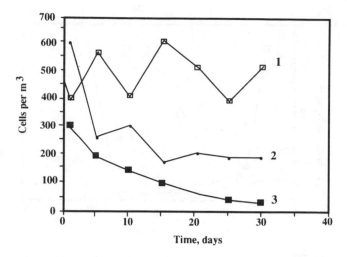

Fig. 10 Dynamics of the number of hemolytic *Staphylococci* in the atmosphere of an office (1), inhabited cabin (2), and greenhouse (3) modules of a BLSS.

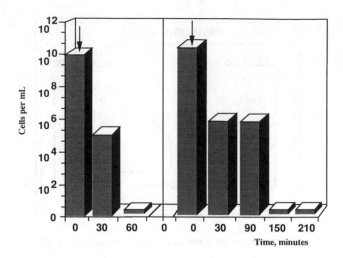

Fig. 11 Elimination of pathogenic *Staphylococci* in an algae suspension (arrows indicate the point at which *Staphylococci* were introduced into the suspension).

ment, when an air sample was taken several minutes after the inhabited cabin was opened. This short period was sufficient to allow incursion of microflora from the surrounding environment. It is important that in the BLSS, after temporary depressurization of the system, the bacteria immediately return to their initial level, demonstrating the existence of internal mechanisms for stabilizing the bacterial community in the face of external disturbances. The progressive divergence in the levels of bacterial contamination of pressurized BLSS modules (e.g., inhabited greenhouse) and the atmosphere of an office environment are shown in Fig. 10.

In models of the BLSS based on one-celled algae, the microbiocenosis that forms spontaneously in the algae culture plays a significant role in generating the atmosphere. The limited levels of volatile organic components in the atmosphere, as discussed above, are largely due to the microflora associated with the algae. The dynamics of changes in the levels of methane in the atmosphere presented in Fig. 7B are of special interest here. The absorption of methane and its stabilization in the atmosphere, which occur later than the analogous processes for carbon monoxide, indicate that the responsible process develops after the closed system starts to function, attesting to the capacity of the established bacteriocenosis to undergo adaptive changes in structure when new trophic resources appear. It is evident that a new ecological niche begins to form, consisting of methane-oxidizing bacteria and members of the extensive *Pseudomonas* group, typically the predominant representative of microflora in an algae reactor. This could be the result either of selection and increase in forms already capable of methane oxidation or of the appearance of active enzymatic systems in previously inactive forms of bacteria. This empirical demonstration of self-adjustment (self-modification) exemplies one of the fundamental properties of ecological systems, which is realizable even in a biocenotic structure as simple as the BLSS models studied.

With respect to species composition, the predominant microflora in the BLSS are forms that are functionally (trophically) associated with the skin and mucous membranes of the human upper respiratory tract (as a natural ecological niche). The dynamics of levels of the major groups of microorganisms are analogous to the dynamics of total levels but are less pronounced. An important feature of the behavior of atmospheric microflora in the BLSS is the decrease in the proportion of pathogenic forms of bacteria, particularly hemolytically active forms of *Staphylococci*. The practical importance of this phenomenon for general habitability considerations required that it be experimentally verified.

To accomplish this, at the end of one of the 1-month experiments on BLSS models, a culture of algae in the photosynthetic reactor was inoculated with measured amounts of labeled (phagotyped) strains of hemolytic *Staphylococci*, after which their levels in the suspension and atmosphere were measured (work performed by G. O. Pozharskiy). It was established that, as early as 2–4 h after inoculation (depending on the amount of bacteria added), no bacteria were evident in either the algae suspension or the atmosphere (Fig. 11). This effect is consistent with the general fate of the majority of species artificially introduced into ecosystems, which fail to find suitable ecological niches or else encounter unforeseen competition, ultimately leading to their displacement by local forms. In this case, the phenomenon occurred relatively rapidly—within a single microbial generation. This provided a very clear example of the ecological stability of the leading microbiocenosis of algae in the BLSS and its important role in the formation of a microbiologically wholesome atmosphere for human habitation.

It is obvious that the mechanism underlying the stabilization of the number and species composition of microflora (through ecological self-regulation of the microbiocenosis) that is characteristic of this model would not be possible in a system where human microflora failed to encounter ecological resistance from other microcenoses and, thus, were able to grow progressively without experiencing pressure from the biological environment. This is precisely what occurs when humans are isolated in systems with non-biological LSSs. Under these conditions, the prospects for the success of a long-term, possibly multiyear, exposure of humans to their own microflora seem ecologically dubious, given the high adaptability of micro-organisms and the lesser flexibility of the human immune system. For this reason, special sanitary and microbiological measures would inevitably be required (see Chapter 4 of this volume).

4. Biological Life Support System Reliability Issues

Like natural ecosystems, the BLSS can survive independently in a state of long-term dynamic equilibrium. This feature resembles the concept of system reliability. In the literature, we often encounter the statement that biological systems are relatively unreliable, especially when compared to physical-chemical systems. One must bear in mind that BLSS reliability has two aspects: the technological and the biological. The technological aspect relates to the reliability of the numerous units and assemblies of the BLSS and is subject to analyses based on existing theory and methods for evaluating the reliability of technological systems.

At present, the theory and methods needed for evaluating the reliability of biological systems do not exist. However, a good candidate for a reliability criterion is long-term, stable survival of living systems at all levels of biological organization—from individual organisms with their characteristic lifespans, which are a species attribute, to populations, biocenoses, and ecosystems with long-term stability of survival on a historical scale—encompassing an enormous number of generations of the leading species in natural ecosystems. Yu.M. Svirezhev and D.O. Logofet performed a mathematical analysis of the stability of such systems.[62]

The stability of living systems is based on such properties as multiple levels of redundancy, self-propagation, self-repair after damage, self-regulation with respect to changes in external conditions, and adaptivity of structure and function. For this reason, the concept of system reliability developed in engineering is not really appropriate to living systems, especially since the engineers define reliability in multiple ways. For example, distinctions are drawn between Lyapunov reliability and Lagrange reliability.[62] Certain qualitative ideas concerning reliability in a BLSS are presented in a work by the present authors.[63]

With respect to the BLSS, it seems more appropriate to use the concept of stability, which we define as the capacity of a biological system at any level for long-term survival, under a certain range of conditions, while maintaining major functional characteristics within a normal range of fluctuations. From this point of view, we will consider the BLSS models studied.

One of the major results of the study of "man-algae-micro-organisms" models obtained in five experiments lasting

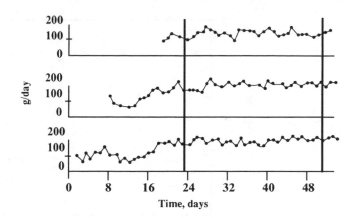

Fig. 12 Productivity of algae in three photosynthetic reactors operating in parallel (vertical lines delimit period in which the reactors were operating as a BLSS component).

29–31 days was their capacity for long-term stable functioning with the use of the technology and methods of algae cultivation described above, along with their low need for external regulation. Throughout the 1-month periods during which the models functioned, aside from the already noted imbalance of gas exchange (which is inevitable for such systems), no other signs of instability were observed that suggested time limits for their existence. The duration of the experiments was limited to a month only because of the unacceptability of confining humans in a space of 5 m^3 for an indefinite period.

All the major functional characteristics of the models stabilized immediately or after a transitional process varying in duration, after which no further major changes were noted. The duration and nature of the transitional processes during the initial period of BLSS functioning must be considered when life support systems are actually used.

The 15 complete oxygen regeneration cycles occurring over a period of a month provide reliable evidence for the stability of the processes in these models, since a system's stability is more appropriately measured in terms of number of cycles of substance regeneration occurring in it (the major result of the system's operation), rather than the duration of the test according to the calendar. After all, these 15 cycles of oxygen regeneration in a system 10 times the size (50 m^3), would take 10 times as long (300 days). This example demonstrates the fundamental principle of functional similarity of regenerative systems, which enables comparative evaluation of various BLSS models with different biocenotic structures and provides a method for accelerated testing of such systems. The issue of similarity of BLSSs is discussed in more detail in Ref. 18.

The stability of the functional characteristics of the models studied is primarily a result of the stability of the characteristics of the algae cultures performing the major functions in the systems. Among these characteristics are productivity (Fig. 12); composition of biomass (Fig. 13); and age structure of the population (Fig. 14), which remains stable for doz-

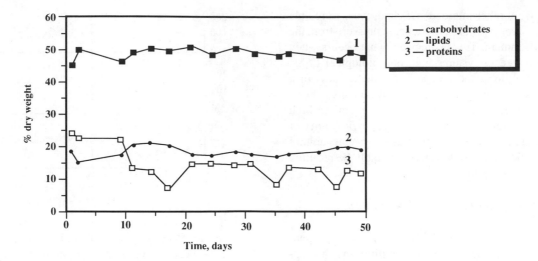

Fig. 13 Composition of *Chlorella* biomass in percent of dry weight during continuous independent cultivation and as a component of a BLSS model (delimited with vertical lines).

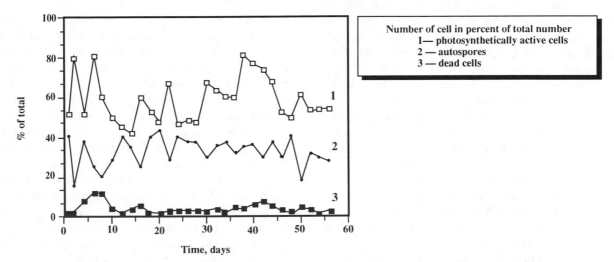

Fig. 14 Age structure of the population of *Chlorella* during continuous cultivation.

ens of cell generations. Except for normal fluctuations around the mean, these parameters undergo no changes. When accidental deviations from the optimal cultivation conditions occurred during the experiments (technical aspect of reliability), the cultures utilized self-repair mechanisms. Although the age group of cells most sensitive to disruption of ambient conditions (e.g., overheating) died, after conditions returned to normal, the culture recovered through the survival of the age group most tolerant of this factor. This is one of the intrapopulation mechanisms for maintaining stability.

The literature frequently discusses the potential genetic instability of systems based on organisms with short developmental cycles, in which a large number of generations must function. With respect to the BLSS, this issue is discussed in the work of J. Cook.[64] It is important to note that the use of the identical strain of *Chlorella* for a period of 25 years in our laboratory unimpeachably demonstrates the genetic stability of BLSSs based on one-celled algae.

The different manifestations of stability of the BLSS model

discussed immediately above are inherent in various structural levels of the system. For this reason, it is natural to base analyses of stability of biological systems on their hierarchical multilevel structure. One can then identify the role of various mechanisms for supporting stable system functioning. These mechanisms operate at various levels of biological organization: the ontogenetic ("organism"), population, biocenotic, and ecosystem levels. This approach to ecosystem stability is clearly the most natural and, thus, can facilitate future systematic study of the stability of BLSSs varying in biocenotic structure.[63]

The ontogenetic level of stability is determined by an organism's inherited traits and realized through the mechanisms of homeostatic, adaptive, and defensive reactions. These may be readily modified or may be relatively stable (adaptive modifications or adaptations). The adaptation of enzyme systems to changes in the trophic environment characteristic of micro-organisms is evidently of the latter kind.

At the population level, there are other mechanisms for

supporting stability. It is well known that resistance to changes in environmental conditions varies in individuals differing in age. Since the population consists of individuals at various stages of ontogenesis, the probability of this population maintaining a steady state under altered conditions is greater than it would be in a culture of individuals all of the same age. Figure 14 shows the age structure of populations of *Chlorella* under continuous cultivation.

At the level of biocenoses and ecosystems, there are still other mechanisms for supporting stability. An important factor here is species diversity. In ecology it is virtually universally accepted that species diversity is directly tied to community stability. This would truly be the case if differences among closely related species were not only morphological but also functional; i.e., if they played different roles in the overall substance cycle. Evidently, the situation here is more complex. Metabolic diversity of the functions of organisms and diversity of complementary ecological niches, and not the number of diverse units (species) in the system, are the important factors for stability of biological systems. In this case, functional diversity can be interpreted in terms of degree of closure of the cycle and, thus, degree of autonomy and stability of a given ecosystem.

Species diversity of communities (to the extent to which functional differences are involved) creates the conditions for development of different types of symbiotic relationships, increasing the stability of the system. This is, for example, the situation in a nonsterile algae culture, where concomitant microflora solve the problem of disposing of the metabolic products of algae and, most likely, release vitamins and other biological substances needed by the algae into the common medium. This, of course, makes such a culture more stable than a sterile culture.

Thus, in a complex system, each individual organism, which has its own mechanisms to support stability, is also protected by the defense mechanisms characteristic of the higher levels of biological organization—populations, biocenoses, and ecosystems—whereas the stability of higher levels is based on the mechanisms supporting the stability of each subordinate level.

B. Biological Life Support System Models Including Higher Plants

Models of BLSS including higher plants have been studied in the Institute of Biophysics of the Siberian Division of the U.S.S.R. (now Russian) Academy of Sciences (Krasnoyarsk) and the Institute of Biomedical Problems of the U.S.S.R. (now Russian) Ministry of Health (Moscow). Materials relating to the first group of such models have been published extensively[49] and are cited in the American literature.[89–91] We will not repeat this information but will present certain other data related to a less publicized model studied in the Institute for Biomedical Problems. This model included all components of the aforementioned "man-algae-micro-organisms" model, including units for dehydration of organic

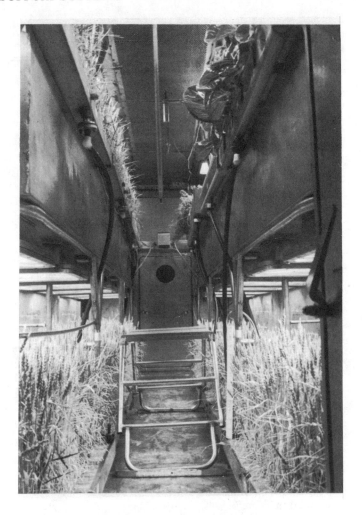

Fig. 15 Interior view of two-tier BLSS greenhouse. In the background is the pressurized hatch into the inhabited module.

wastes and mineralization and evaporation of urine. The higher plant subsystem was enclosed in a pressurized environment that included a greenhouse and hydroponic units with a two-tier 15-m^3 growing area (Fig. 15). The greenhouse shared an air supply with a 27-m^3 inhabited module and a 36.5-m^3 air conditioning (dehumidifying and warming) system. The total air volume of the pressurized area was 95 m^3. Wheat occupied 11.25 m^3 of the growing area of the greenhouse, with the balance devoted to vegetables. The plants were illuminated around the clock with 6-kW xenon lamps equipped with water filters. The vegetable crop received 60–80 W/m^3 PAR and the wheat crop received 125–185 W/m^3 PAR of illumination. The plants were cultivated without a substrate with periodic feeding of nutrient solution in the area of their roots. The solution was corrected twice a week, and any losses were countered using condensate collected in the air conditioning system. The majority of the condensate came from the transpirational water of the plants. More detailed information about this model is presented in a work by I.Ye. Ivanova et al.[34]

The design of the experiment included preliminary opera-

Table 6 Productivity of plants (M±m)
[From Ivanova et al.[34]]

Culture	Condition	Increase in dry biomass, g/m²/day	
		Total	Edible
Wheat	Control	25.8 ± 2.4	5.3 ± 0.7
	Experimental	32.8 ± 1.9	4.7 ± 1.3
Peas	Control	12.8 ± 1.9	3.5 ± 0.9
	Experimental	12.9 ± 3.8	2.3 ± 1.2
Beets	Control	8.4 ± 1.1	3.4 ± 0.8
	Experimental	5.0 ± 3.1	2.3 ± 1.5
Carrots	Control	11.0 ± 4.2	6.0 ± 3.9
	Experimental	9.7 ± 4.2	6.3 ± 3.1
Cabbage	Control	16.0 ± 4.3	14.4 ± 4.2
	Experimental	14.2 ± 4.4	12.9 ± 4.2

tion of the greenhouse in a stationary conveyor mode until the first crops were harvested (control period), after which a single human subject was introduced into the inhabited module. After 15 days, the air supply for this system was joined with that of a "man-*Chlorella*-micro-organisms" system that was already in operation so that they formed a single system including two humans, which then operated for 45 days.

The results obtained on the productivity of the plants are presented in Table 6.

The harvest index of all the plants, except carrots, was lower in the experimental period than in the control period. Here, it should be mentioned that the productivity of plants under greenhouse conditions, even in the absence of a pressurized environment, is significantly below that for open plant growth devices and phytotrons. This phenomenon, observed consistently throughout many years of work, has yet to be explained. An analogous phenomenon was noted by G.M. Lisovskiy.[33]

It is noteworthy that the vegetable culture yields did not decrease during the last period of the experiment, when they were subject to the greatest stress, because the atmosphere was shared with two human subjects; *Chlorella;* and all the other subsystems, including urine evaporation and waste dehydration.

Analysis of wheat yield revealed a pattern of results that was not completely clear. The total yield with respect to biomass during the experimental period increased compared to the period of autonomous growth; however, the grain yield fluctuated sharply, and periods of normal or greater yields compared to control were interrupted by periods of sharp decline or virtual absence of yield (the ears were barren of grain, Fig. 16). There were 4 such periods in the 10 wheat growth cycles occurring during the experimental period. According to Lisovskiy,[33] a similar phenomenon occurred in a

pressurized closed system including humans in the Bios-3 facility.

One thing, however, is clear: The reason for the barrenness of the ears in these experiments is not associated with the period of operation of the greenhouse as part of the complete BLSS. The lack of grain is the final result of embryonal damage to the development of the reproductive organs, which are established in the early stages of ontogenesis, 35–40 days before a grain harvest is obtained. Thus, the period responsible for the lack of grain occurred, for the first three of four cases, during the control period; and the cause of the harvest failure could not have been associated with one of the other components of the model, which were only introduced later. Overall, the higher plant component synthesized 432 grams of dry biomass daily, including 86 grams of edible substance (20 percent), of which 54 grams were wheat and 32 grams were vegetables.

In this experiment, in order to maximize use of plant biomass, nontraditional portions of the plant were included in the diet, including the tops of carrots, beets, peas, and cabbage. The vegetable mass was chopped mechanically and juice was extracted, the amount of which reached 60 percent of the initial moisture level of the wastes. Pulsed electrical blending of the initial mass increased the yield of juice to 80–85 percent of the free water contained. The dry substance of the juice comprised 40 percent carbohydrate and 18–30 percent protein.[65]

The actual daily diet of the subjects included a mean of 137 grams of dry biomass substance produced in the system, including 50 grams of *Chlorella*, with a total energy value of 454 kcal/day. This comprised 26 percent of the diet by weight and 19 percent of the calories. The protein produced in the system comprised 33 percent of all dietary protein (37 grams), of which 20 grams were *Chlorella* biomass. As a result, the level of regeneration of substances was somewhat higher than that of the previous model (Table 5).

Inclusion of higher plants in the photoautotrophic component, as anticipated, increased the total assimilation coefficient of the photoautotrophic component and brought it closer to the human respiratory quotient, so the rate of accumulation of carbon dioxide in the atmosphere decreased to 1 percent of the rate of emission by humans.

In this experiment, before the Chlorella and higher plant components were merged in a single system, each component had been demonstrated capable of supporting the gas exchange of one human. The greenhouse for the plants had a growth area of 15 m², and the illuminated surface of the *Chlorella* suspension ranged from 8 to 12 m². Illumination levels were comparable. A more important difference between requirements for the plants and algae was that the greenhouse required a total volume of more than 30 m³, whereas the *Chlorella* reactor occupied a volume almost an order of magnitude smaller. This may be significant when we determine the desirability of including algae in the first space BLSS versions, when all restrictions, including volume, will be stringent.

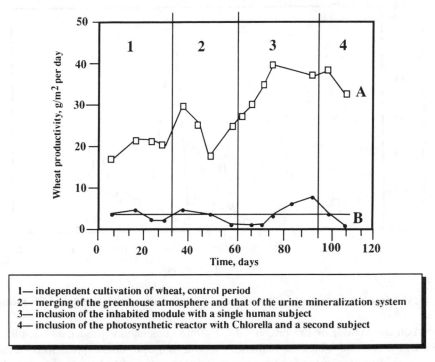

1— independent cultivation of wheat, control period
2— merging of the greenhouse atmosphere and that of the urine mineralization system
3— inclusion of the inhabited module with a single human subject
4— inclusion of the photosynthetic reactor with Chlorella and a second subject

Fig. 16 Dynamics of wheat productivity with respect to total biomass (A) and grain (B) during various stages of BLSS model formation.

Thus, introduction of higher plants into a BLSS based on algae increased the closure of the food and gas exchange cycle. Evidently, further potential for increasing the closure of the system is not very high, since it would require additional production of essential nutrients that represent a comparatively low proportion of the total dietary requirements of humans. At the same time, each additional increase in food production, including animal products, will be obtained at an increasing cost with respect to area, volume, and energy and will require production and processing of an increasingly greater amount of plant biomass and other wastes not utilized in the system. Thus, the degree of closure of the models studied in the U.S.S.R., evidently, is not far short of that which will be attainable and profitable for actual BLSS on spacecraft in the near future.

1. Microflora in Higher Plant Biological Life Support System Models

The inclusion of higher plants in system models led to a qualitative change involving fungi in the composition of microflora in the inhabited module, as has been noted by Tirranen.[55] Before humans were included in the system, fungi in the greenhouse were represented by *Penicillium*. After inclusion of humans, mold spores of the genus *Aspergillus* appeared; by day 10, after closure of the greenhouse, these comprised more than one-half of all fungi. After inclusion of the greenhouse in the "man-algae-micro-organisms" system and by the end of the experiment with the unified system, the *Aspergillus* genus comprised 70–90 percent of the fungi. The major areas where these fungi multiplied were the stalks and

ears of wheat. Fungi of the root area of the wheat plants consisted exclusively of members of the genus *Aspergillus*, which were not identified in the atmosphere of the inhabited area.

The predominant bacterial flora of the nutrient solution for the most important plant, wheat, were members of the genus *Pseudomonas*. After inclusion of humans in the system, these were joined by *Ps. Fluorescens, Ps. ureae,* and *Ps. aeruglinosa*.[66]

The dynamics of the total level of bacteria in the nutrient solution clearly were a function of the composition of the system model at various stages of the experiment (Fig. 17). After a prolonged period of stability, with a rather low level of bacterial flora during the period of autonomous plant growth, the introduction of a new component into the system (mineralization components, humans, and *Chlorella*) brought a sharp increase in bacteria, followed by a decrease until the next disturbance. Thus, throughout the almost 100-day period of microbiological monitoring, the bacterial flora of the nutrient medium reacted to disturbances as a single microbiocenosis and clearly displayed the capacity for self-regulation of bacterial level.

C. Status of Humans

In all BLSS model experiments the health status of the human subjects was studied not only to ensure their safety during the experiments but also as the major composite indicator for evaluating the appropriateness of the system's environment. A number of studies were directed at identifying possible physiological reactions of human subjects to anticipated abnormalities of the environment (increases in the level

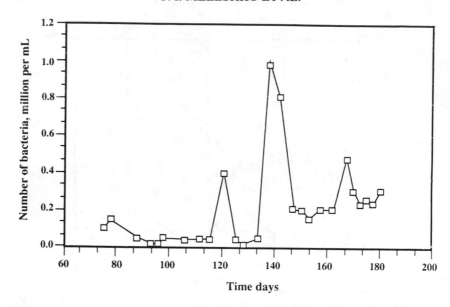

Fig. 17 Dynamics of bacteria content in the nutrient solution of wheat during BLSS model formation.

of carbon dioxide and carbon monoxide) or to unexpected properties of the environment that could affect the immune response. These data on human physiological status have independent significance as important indicators for evaluating the quality of the environment.

Here, we cite data in summary form from all experiments with BLSS models conducted in the Institute of Biomedical Problems.

A common phenomenon in all experiments was an increase in the level of carboxyhemoglobin in the blood of subjects, starting 4–5 days after the experiments began. In an experiment where the level of carbon monoxide in the air was increased during certain periods (reaching 30 mg/m^3), the level of carboxyhemoglobin increased from 5.5 percent during baseline to 14.5 percent on day 5 of the experiment. The quantity of hemoglobin did not show any systematic change and fluctuated throughout the experiments within 3–5 percent of the mean, although the number of erythrocytes sometimes increased toward the end of an experiment. The increase in carboxyhemoglobin was associated with a decrease in the level of the enzyme catalase in erythrocytes starting during the first few days of the experiment. By days 15 through 20 in one experiment, the catalase level had decreased by 30–50 percent of the mean baseline value. The number of erythrocytes by the end of this experiment had increased by 20–25 percent baseline, which can be understood as a compensatory reaction to a partial blockade of the respiratory function of hemoglobin by carbon monoxide.

The only change noted in the examined morphological parameters of peripheral blood was an increase in the number of eosinophils, which, in some cases, reached a level 3–5 times that of the baseline. Both depression of catalase activity of erythrocytes and marked eosinophilia suggest the presence of carbon monoxide intoxication induced by increased levels of carboxyhemoglobin in blood. However, the complete absence of any complaints, not to mention any objective symp-

toms associated with such intoxication, is difficult to explain. One of the possible explanations for this lack of symptoms of carbon monoxide intoxication may be associated with the gradual increase in levels of carbon monoxide in the atmosphere of the system throughout the first 2 days and the possible triggering of adaptive and/or compensatory processes.

Returning to the eosinophilia, we must also consider another interpretation, this one associated with a possible allergenic effect of the environment. Given the close association of humans and the biological components of the system, exacerbated by the limited area and common atmosphere for all components, one could reasonably expect allergenic or immunogenic phenomena. This aspect of human participation in a BLSS has not been studied. For this reason, in our experiments, under the supervision of I.V. Konstantinova and V.M. Shilov, we studied the status of natural, cellular, and humoral immunity in humans, including active and passive mechanisms. The study of the phagocyte activity of neutrophils, bactericidal activity of blood, and lysozyme activity of saliva in the subjects demonstrated that their participation in these biological systems was not accompanied by any shifts in natural immune status.

Reactivity of lymphoid cells (PHA-blast transformation of lymphocytes) was evaluated on the basis of rate of inclusion of labeled uridine in ribonucleic acid (RNA) synthesis. Here, the results were ambiguous: While, in some cases, there was a significant decrease in lymphocyte reactivity toward the end of the experiments, in other cases, the immune response of lymphoid tissue was unaltered. It is possible that individual differences in the immune systems of the subjects during the experiments were manifested here.

Close contact between the humans and the biological components of the systems and their concomitant microflora, volatile compounds in the atmosphere, and plant pollen naturally raise the possibility of allergenic effects of the environment. We have previously encountered marked food aller-

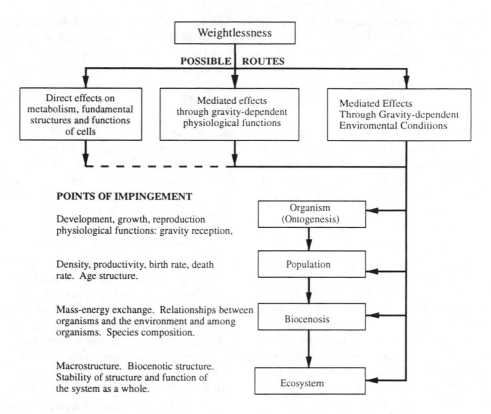

Fig. 18 Possible routes of the effects of weightlessness on living systems and points of impingement at various hierarchical biological levels.

gies after dietary intake of 50–150 grams of *Chlorella* biomass.[67] A similar result was also noted by American authors; however, this was during the period before the technology for cultivating algae was fully developed and still involved long periods of biomass accumulation in experiments. This allowed autolysis to occur, so the composition of the final product used as food was not controlled. In our experiments, *Chlorella* biomass (50 grams of dry weight) was included in the diet immediately after it was obtained from the photosynthetic reactors. The biomass then underwent thermal processing (30 min of boiling), which eliminated confounding factors to permit study of the issue of allergenic properties of *Chlorella* biomass, particularly its proteins, and the protein of concomitant bacteria. This could have been one explanation for the aforementioned eosinophilia. For this reason, under the direction of I.V. Konstantinova, we studied the allergic sensitivities of subjects to possible natural allergens in the systems. We performed allergy tests to bacterial allergens and a water extract from *Chlorella* homogenate but failed to detect sensitivities of the subjects to these allergens.

On the whole, the status of the subjects remained satisfactory throughout the course of the experiments. Toward the end of the period, a slight asthenization (debility) was noted; this could be attributed to the low motor activity and restricted living space, although a set of physical exercises had supported energy expenditure to match the calories in the diet.

Thus, the results of the study of health status of humans, including immunological status, failed to reveal anything not characteristic of healthy individuals in natural environments. The most important composite indicator of the adequacy of the human living environment failed to reveal any sign that the BLSS models studied were unwholesome. In the future, this conclusion will be most important for evaluating experimental models of the BLSS in which the human environment is formed through the activity of only one plant species ("human-algae-micro-organisms") or a small number of higher plants with concomitant microflora.

V. Weightlessness as a Condition of Biological Life Support System Implementation

When working on the problems of the human BLSS, we must assume that for a long time to come (although not forever) weightlessness will be an obligatory condition of space flight. For this reason, all aspects of this issue must be considered from the point of view of the possibility of functioning in microgravity.

Modern gravitational biology, which focuses on the study of the individual organism and its subordinate levels (cellular and subcellular), cannot answer the questions of whether ecological systems can exist in weightlessness, since the decisive factors are the levels above that of the organism—population, biocenosis, and ecosystem. This inspired us to reconsider, if only theoretically, the whole issue of the biological or other significance of weightlessness and possible points of impingement on various hierarchical levels of living systems.

At this stage, it was important to acknowledge that the concept of the biological significance of weightlessness is, in principle, ambiguous. The effects of weightlessness at various levels of biological organization, from the single organism to the ecosystem, may be realized through different routes and different mechanisms. The ideas generated by this analysis are schematically presented in Fig. 18.

The first route—the direct effects of weightlessness on components of biological processes of metabolism, development, growth, and reproduction—has not been persuasively demonstrated. The conclusion that there are no specific effects of weightlessness on these fundamental life processes is being increasingly substantiated. It has been argued that there does not even exist a theoretical rationale for such effects,[68] and we fully concur with this.

The second route is not direct but mediated through changes in the conditions under which the gravity-dependent functions of the organism are realized. Here, we are referring particularly to gravity reception and the associated reactions of circulation, antigravity, and motor functions and associated processes of fluid-electrolyte metabolism. The major relevant data here were obtained from research on long-term human space flights. This research has revealed not only the effects of weightlessness but also its mechanisms realized through gravity-dependent physiological functions.

The third route for the effects of weightlessness is also indirect. Effects are mediated through change in gravity-dependent factors of the environment; that is, through ecological factors. Here, we refer to the gravity-dependent stratigraphic distribution of gases, liquids, and solids, which determines the position of the organism within the medium it inhabits, its motor behavior, the distribution of trophic resources in the environment, and the processes of mass transfer. The absence of sedimentation and thermal convection take on significance here. This route becomes important at the level in which organisms exist in dense populations in the presence of intrapopulation gradients of environment and food resources and competition for these resources. In considerably larger ecosystems, this route becomes absolutely inevitable, since the initial conditions for the appearance and evolution of life on Earth were the gravitationally organized macrostructure of the biosphere and strict limitations on the main living environments—the atmosphere, hydrosphere, and upper layers of the Earth.

The schema in Fig.18 facilitates discussion of another aspect of the possible effects of weightlessness, the issue of the substrate itself, and the points at which it impinges on living systems at various hierarchical levels. Each of these levels is associated with inherent criteria of status. Each level transforms significant changes occurring in the lower levels into its own criteria of status, providing information about this level with its points of impingement and the mechanisms through which the effects of weightlessness are realized.

As is well known, life on Earth is discrete and quantum in nature; and its elementary units, its "quanta," are individual organisms, each with its own sublevels and subsystems, the numbers of which depend on the complexity of structure. The individual organism is also the direct recipient and detector of the effects of any external factors. This is the first and lowest hierarchical level of life and includes all stages of ontogenesis of the individual, from fertilization of the ovum to the adult organism containing the seeds of the next generation. All this composes the ontogenetic level, inexactly referred to as the "organismic"—the first level at which weightlessness impinges on living systems. Points of impingement of weightlessness can, in theory, include all the defining characteristics of life usually cited in definitions: food consumption and metabolism, growth, development, and reproduction. These are characteristic of any organism at any stage of evolutionary development. The ultimate, ecologically significant result of changes occurring at this level may be alterations (more likely decreases) in the viability of the individual, in individual life span, and in reproductive capacity.

However, individuals can only exist in isolation under artificial conditions. In nature, they do not simply exist but coexist with others like them in populations, biocenoses, etc. It follows that the effects of weightlessness at the ontogenetic level can lead to changes at other, higher hierarchical levels. However, this can also fail to occur, since changes at the level of the individual may be balanced through genetic, morphogenetic, and physiological regulation or through the mechanisms of population, interpopulation, and biocenotic regulation that protect every ecosystem.

At the population level, the effects of weightlessness are manifest in the major criteria of population status (density, productivity, age structure, birth rate, and death rate), which reflect not only the current status of the population but also its future prospects.

At the level of biocenoses and ecosystems, the potential effects of weightlessness are still more numerous and heterogeneous and their manifestations are more complex and difficult to predict, since, at these levels, there are complex interactions among many populations. Furthermore, the living environments, which themselves may be altered by weightlessness, typically include all forms of matter—solid, liquid, and gas. Criteria of system status at these levels become more and more general and ultimately amount to preservation or disruption of the stability of the structure and functioning of the ecosystem as a whole.

Thus, the superorganismic levels of living systems not only are subject to the effects of weightlessness but also can serve as tools for evaluating the ecological significance (or lack thereof) of changes occurring at the ontogenetic level. This level is the arena for accumulating adaptive changes and eliminating changes that do not affect the relative viability of individuals in populations and biocenoses.

This discussion has demonstrated the need for a new phase in the development of gravitational biology, in which we focus on the study of living systems at various hierarchical levels of biological organization. In other words, the study of individual changes at the ontogenetic level may be expanded to the study of the long-term fate of these changes in populations, biocenoses, and entire ecosystems.

The major practical conclusion of this analysis of the role of gravity is that the in-flight success of the models of closed ecosystems that have been tested on the ground for space flight cannot be predicted reliably without studying their major performance characteristics in weightlessness. For this reason, we could not content ourselves with a theoretical analysis of the problem but were compelled to move on to its experimental study, despite the drastic increase in the methodological and technical difficulties of conducting such experiments in space.

Even before this, however, we were compelled to confront the possibility of incorrect interpretation of the effects of weightlessness in our study of populations of one-celled algae. In our first experiment with heterotrophic cultures, we found a 50 percent increase in the number of cells in weightlessness compared to control; and, in the second, longer experiment, we found an almost 2-1/2-fold increase compared to control. Similar results were obtained by other authors in the study of the growth of bacteria.[69] Subsequent analyses revealed that, in weightlessness, the algae suspension was distributed along all the internal walls of the rectangular vessel (the "IFS-2" device), whereas, in the ground-based control, it was naturally confined to one wall, the bottom. As a result, the area of air contact in flight was several times greater than in the control. This significantly improved gas exchange conditions for the flight culture and was sufficient to explain the increase in the growth rate of this culture compared to the control (which, therefore, was not an appropriate control).

In subsequent experiments in this series, we used vessels for the ground-control conditions, in which the area of the bottom corresponded to the sum of the interior surfaces of the flight vessels; under these conditions, the rate of growth of the experimental culture did not differ from that of the ground control.[70] In these experiments, the objects of study were *Chlorella* cultures. By the end of the experiment, these cultures contained 10^8–10^9 cells per milliliter; i.e., billions of cells. Actively growing cultures of this size may be considered closed populations.

The population characteristics of the algae studied in flight were unchanged. The number of dead cells and cells with reduced viability remained within normal limits. Ratios among various age groups in the populations also were unchanged. The age structure in all experiments was characteristic of rapidly growing populations, with young individuals dominating. This was typical of the first two to three generations in shorter experiments, and of the fifth generation in the 15-day experiment.[71]

Subsequently, these results were confirmed with actively growing autotrophic cultures of *Chlorella* that served as components of a microecosystem in which the algae supported the gas exchange of the heterotrophic components of the system (fish and micro-organisms) and supported the trophic needs for the organic substance of the concomitant microbiocenoses.[72] Within the ecosystem, the algae also retained their physiological and population characteristics and supported the functioning of the community for the duration of the experiments.

Thus, analysis of the physical (mechanical) conditions of the environment in experiments and introduction of technologically appropriate controls made it possible to establish that the significant acceleration of algae growth in weightlessness found in our initial experiments was not the result of direct effects on mechanisms of growth, development, and reproduction of the cells. Rather, it was mediated by changes in the physical conditions of the environment, which influenced an important ecological factor—conditions of gas exchange between the suspension and the atmosphere. This result demonstrates the potential practical significance of such studies for BLSSs, since the cultivation technologies of various systems may themselves be affected by weightlessness.

The multifaceted role of weightlessness can be observed, also, in studies of the characteristics of embryonal development in quail. In 1979, a joint Soviet-Czechoslovakian experiment was performed involving incubation of quail eggs on biosatellite Cosmos 1129. For technical reasons associated with the biosatellite flight, the period of in-flight incubation was 11-1/2 days, instead of the 18 required for full embryogenesis. The experiment demonstrated that it was possible for an embryo (in some cases, at least) to undergo normal development while exposed to space during the initial critical stages of embryogenesis (which comprise 70 percent of the gestational period). However, the significant number of embryos that failed to develop (35 percent) was striking, as was the high frequency of morphological developmental anomalies, although there were other obvious potential causes [long-term (up to 20 days) storage of the eggs before the beginning of incubation, high temperature (23–28° C) during the last 10 days of storage; and decrease of humidity to 30 percent during the last half of incubation].[73]

A complete incubation cycle of quail eggs occurred on Mir in March 1990 in a Soviet-Czechoslovakian experiment using a second generation incubator manufactured in Czechoslovakia. For the first time, eight normally developed, viable chicks with active motor, vocalization, and appetitive behavior were hatched in weightlessness, a result which definitively supports the conclusion that normal embryogenesis is possible under such conditions.[74] However, even in this experiment, the hatching rate of the chicks was lower than normal, and the number of developmental anomalies in the embryos during various stages was elevated, although (unlike the case in the first experiment) conditions of egg storage before incubation were not adverse and incubation was not interrupted. During flight, there were cases in which the embryo occupied a longitudinal position in the egg and the chick developed in the egg with the head at the narrow end, which prevented them from emerging from the eggs without help. This did not occur in the control condition. Similar anomalies were reported in Ref. 75.

In interpreting the results of experiments on the incubation of eggs in weightlessness, we are evidently dealing with qualitatively different categories of functions. The mechanisms of morphogenetic processes in the course of development of the embryo appear to be rather rigidly determined genetically during all the critical stages and, in themselves, are not affected by weightlessness. This has also been demonstrated with mammals.[76] However, weightlessness may change external conditions for realization of embryogenesis in the egg itself. This seems highly likely when one considers the well-known gravity dependence of the macrostructure of eggs, the components of which (yolk, albumen, air chamber and the embryo itself) normally occupy positions determined by gravity, with an embryo's position fixed with respect to the other components of the egg macrostructure, especially the air chamber. In weightlessness, this internal structure may be retained or disrupted, which may, in turn, disrupt the conditions for embryo metabolism and respiration. In the latter instance, development may halt or be disrupted in some further way, thus becoming an example of the indirect effects of weightlessness.

The first 2–4 days in the lives of the viable chicks hatched in weightlessness revealed a new problem associated with weightlessness, which is important for the practical implementation of a BLSS. During this time, the birds were unable to develop the skills needed for active orientation and maintenance of body position in space. They constantly "floated" within their enclosure, and their chaotic tumbling was exacerbated by increasingly sharp movements of the wings and feet, despite the presence of a guiding air stream intended to propel them toward the grid floor so they could grasp it with their claws. Although they actively pecked food from the cosmonauts' hands, they could not be kept in the vicinity of their feeding dish and it proved impossible to maintain them onboard the station since they could not eat by themselves.

Analyses of videotapes showed that the development of motor skills appropriate to weightlessness was impeded by the innate reflex of pushing off from surfaces, which is natural and expedient for neonates in gravity. It is obvious that this introduces a completely new problem, that of developing appropriate motor behavior in the neonate in an agravitational environment, behavior that is incompatible with instinct. This problem, which can be solved for humans by instruction and training, may become one of the limiting problems for the realization of the BLSS in space and will apply, of course, not only to birds but also to all other free-living organisms.

Further observations were performed on adult birds. In July 1990, three females and one male quail, aged 60–65 days, were delivered to space station Mir. They spent 8 days in flight, including a day of flight in the transport spacecraft. On arrival at Mir, they were placed in the animal enclosure previously used for the chicks, in individual restraining slings that kept them near their feeding dish. Their specially developed feed of a pastelike consistency contained the amount of liquid they needed, so that it was not necessary to develop a special device to supply them with water. Active consumption of food began during the first minutes after the birds

were transferred to the chamber from the transport container, which should be of interest to physiologists studying vestibulo-autonomic responses.

Before flight, the birds had been in the stage of active oviparity. During flight, egg laying immediately ceased in all three females. (The last egg was laid by one of the females in the transport spacecraft, and a normal chick hatched from it on the ground.) This was consistent with a morphologically pronounced hypotrophy of the ovaries and oviducts observed immediately postflight. These disorders, noted also in birds of the synchronous control, were attributable to a pattern of nonspecific stress reactions and turned out to be reversible. By days 7 and 8 after landing (and at the same period in the synchronous control), egg laying resumed; and the first eggs laid after flight hatched completely normal, viable offspring. As of this writing, these hatchlings have produced several generations of offspring.

The birds' motor behavior is of some interest. During their time in orbit, one bird was twice freed from the restraining sling and released into the space of the station's work module. The videotape showed that after it had been released from the cosmonaut's hands, it hung motionless for a few seconds but, after the first movement, began to rotate randomly. However, unlike the chicks, the adult bird was soon able to perform short flights until it touched the wall of the module, which it had no way of grasping. On one of these flights, the bird returned to the enclosure and immediately began to peck at its food.

Of course, these observations are not sufficient to assess the potential and actual adaptation of motor behavior to weightlessness in birds. However, there does appears to be a difference, in principle, between the adaptive potential of adult birds and neonates. Adult birds already possess the initial basis for adaptation in the form of established, tested, individually acquired motor skills, although these were developed in a gravitational environment; and, here, we may speak about the adaptation of existing skills to new conditions.

A neonate chick still does not have any individually acquired skills. Thus, it has no initial base that could be adapted, and the innate base (unconditioned reflexes and instincts) is clearly inappropriate to the conditions in which it was born. It is possible that here it would be better not to speak about adaptation but, rather, about a completely new problem: the initial formation of motor skills in an inappropriate environment, from an existing base of clearly unsuitable, unconditioned innate mechanisms. It is clear that this problem is relevant to animals other than birds. One might argue that even human infants will have to confront this problem.

To evaluate the significance of weightlessness for the BLSS over the long term, a general prediction can be derived: As we progress from experimental prototypes and ground-based modeling of closed ecological systems to their practical use in spacecraft, we will increasingly have to consider the effects of weightlessness when selecting biological subjects, develop technologies for cultivating them, and design species and biocenotic structures and food chains for planned ecosystems. It is already quite clear that weightlessness effects will be realized not through primary changes in fundamental vital processes in organisms but through a variety of indirect effects at all levels of biological organization. Such indirect effects ultimately alter the unity of organisms and environment that have developed through evolution, a unity which is an invariant condition for life on Earth in all its manifestations.

All this implies that the problem of the man-rated BLSS cannot be solved merely by balancing the material and energy flows that form the basis of every ecosystem. In studying or designing these flows, we cannot completely abstract them from their carriers—specific organisms with active, individual, and species-specific relationships to the environment, including gravity. These relationships range from spatial orientation in plants to the sensorimotor bases of appetitive, sexual, and other forms of motor behavior in animals at various phylogenetic levels. In microgravity, all this may be disrupted to the extent that it could interfere with the stability of the BLSS as an ecosystem. This situation fully justifies the need for a new, *ecological* phase in the development of traditional gravitational biology, which has accomplished virtually all its original objectives, since it has already provided convincing evidence that fundamental vital processes are independent of gravity. However, it has stopped short of considering the ecological aspects of the individual effects of gravity it has found, including implications for the problem of closed ecological systems. This will require different approaches, subjects, and methods of research.

VI. Mathematical Modeling of Biological Life Support Systems

Before full BLSSs are constructed, mathematical models will be built to explore various aspects of the dynamics of the system and to test the influence of different configurations, the addition of alternative components, and operation during and after various failure modes. Perhaps the most crucial function of the mathematical models at this early stage of development is their ability to formalize and communicate the experimental findings from the disciplines dealing with BLSS components, such as nutrition, crop growth, engineering, and control theory.

These disciplines correspond to the major physical components of the BLSS: the human inhabitants, crops, recycling, and control systems. Each presents its own unique challenges involving modeling and will be examined in turn. These include diet models, crop growth models, engineering models, and models of system dynamics. Finally, we must also ask how these disciplines fit together into the larger picture.

A. Diet Models

Models of human nutrition serve as foundations for the design and analysis of closed life support systems. One of the most sophisticated nutritional modeling studies for closed

systems thus far in the United States is NASA's diet design study.[77] This study specified gross diet requirements for protein, lipid, and total energy. In addition, it included essential amino acids, fatty acids, vitamins, and many minerals.

Allowable values for all these substances were set with minima in all cases and with maxima in many cases; for example, total protein and fat-soluble vitamins. These values were matched with a range of foods, including legumes, roots, tubers, seeds, grains, and leafy vegetables. Protein diets comprised both raw and processed foods. The modeling goal, expressed mathematically, was to meet the dietary requirements and minimize total biomass. Wade[77] solved this linear programming problem by applying the simplex method to various food groupings. Various minimized diets were calculated. One diet consisted of spinach, sweet potatoes, rice, sunflower seeds, and wheat sprouts. An important finding of this study was that for any result, given input restrictions on groupings, there were always other diets in which the mix of food had substantially more variety with only slightly more total biomass.

Further efforts along these lines are progressing at Ames Research Center in California.[78] Expert systems can help in coupling potential diets to other requirements for optimizing the design of the entire system. In these studies, the crucial role played by diet models is evident: By specifying the diet, one specifies the crops that are grown and, ultimately, the areas, volumes, and mass flow rates of matter and energy for the particular crops. The design of a diet effects the design of all other parts of a BLSS.

B. Crop Growth Models

Modeling the life cycles of higher plants will be an important part of the closed system design. First of all, crop growth models aid the design of effective crop growth experiments by maximizing the information gained. Since many environmental variables influence crops, such as light quality and quantity, relative humidity, temperature, partial carbon dioxide and partial oxygen pressure, and nutrients, models can reduce the number of experiments required by helping experimenters define the most important questions. For example, Volk and Bugbee[79] found the leaf emergence rate in wheat to be relatively insensitive to cultivar differences and developed a generic response surface to light and temperature; this allows the researcher to focus on other aspects of growth and development during trials of candidate cultivars.

As another example, Bugbee and Salisbury[32] have developed a five-part analysis of crop growth in terms of efficiency in the conversion of photosynthetic photon flux (PPF) into edible biomass. The five steps are 1) conversion of energy to PPF; 2) percentage of absorption of PPF by crops; 3) photosynthetic efficiency (moles of carbon dioxide fixed per mole of PPF absorbed); 4) respiratory carbon use efficiency (losses); 5) harvest index (percentage of edible biomass). Bugbee and Salisbury can evaluate the maximum potentially achievable values and compare these values with their experimental results. This modeling procedure allows them to isolate and set priorities on potential areas for improvement.

A second important function of crop growth models in BLSS design is to provide the input and output flows of matter and energy required for coupling to models of other components of the system, such as waste processors, food processors, and gas exchangers. Carbon dioxide, oxygen, and water flow rates are the major mass flows to be specified by crop growth models. Although there is an extensive literature on crop models for field agriculture (for example, see the work from Groningen, Netherlands), models for crops in closed systems need to be different. For example, closed system models need to be able to evaluate the transpiration rate of water at high carbon dioxide levels, as well as provide rates of oxygen production by the crops. One approach to oxygen production was developed by Volk and Rummel[80] by accounting for oxygen production and consumption associated with the biosynthesis of various tissue components of edible and inedible biomass (protein, carbohydrate, lipid, fiber, and lignin). Volk and Cullingford[81] used this approach in a generic model for the growth of wheat, soybeans, and potatoes and showed the corresponding flows of carbon dioxide and oxygen during the crop life cycle. Because they define explicit material flows, crop models are key components in the design of closed systems.

C. Engineering Models

In the category of engineering models, we consider models of all components except crops and humans. These might be limited to physical and chemical machines and processes; or they might also include biological agents in algal reactors and in waste processing, such as microbial reactors to convert cellulose wastes to usable glucose. Engineering models include all the physical devices to move materials to and from the crops and the humans.

For example, Blackwell and Blackwell[82] have used engineering models to examine the control of the thermal and fluid dynamics for an advanced crop growth research chamber under construction at NASA Ames Research Center. To perform research on crop growth in a closed environment, it is necessary to precisely control variables, such as lighting, temperature, oxygen, carbon dioxide, humidity, atmospheric pressure, and chemistry of the nutrient solution. The component devices for the atmospheric control system include the following devices in a closed loop around the plant growth chamber: heat exchangers, blowers, gas separators and intakes, valves, filters, and sample ports. In addition to the component devices, modeling studies during system development must take into account the measurement instruments and control algorithms that connect the measurements with the actuators of the component devices.

Blackwell and Blackwell[82] and Blackwell[83] describe the application of robust control theory to stabilizing the environment for the advanced crop growth chamber. Formal control procedures will be necessary if the system is to function with little or no human intervention and because special problems arise from the close coupling between the crops and the thermal and fluid parts of the chamber.

D. System Dynamics Models

System dynamics models of BLSSs explore how the entire system—humans, crops, waste processors, and all other components—behaves in time with explicit material cycles. Cycles of materials are crucial to the construction of these models. Note that cycles are neither inherent nor necessary to the nutritional or crop growth models, for these models are parts of the system dynamics models. Engineering models, when coupled with those for crop growth and nutrition, become system dynamics models.

Published studies of system dynamics in BLSSs include Averner,[84] Babcock et al.,[85] and Rummel and Volk.[86] These models consist of storage media for materials linked by processors, which move and transform materials between the storage areas. The Rummel and Volk BLSS model takes advantage of modular construction and has been adopted for further study and development by others at NASA.[87]

The general scheme for the flow of materials in the BLSS model is shown in Fig. 19. The model tracks carbon, hydrogen, oxygen, and nitrogen along pathways of chemical transformation that include 1) biosynthesis of protein, carbohydrate, fat, fiber, and lignin in the edible and inedible parts of plants; 2) food consumption and production of organic solids in human urine, feces, and wash water; and 3) operation of the waste processor. These pathways, as well as others involving water (such as crop transpiration, cooking, and human hygiene), drive mass flows of carbon dioxide, oxygen, water, and nitric acid to and from their individual storage medium or buffer reservoirs.

Experiments with the BLSS model have explored the effects of crop batch size and planting/harvesting schedules; mechanical failures of components, such as the waste processor; biological failures, such as crop disease; and variations in crew size. The model is an essential tool for understanding the behavior of the whole system in response to changes in designs and assumptions about the structure and behavior of the components. One example is shown in Fig. 20.

Figure 20 shows the BLSS model's output for the water in storage during three different possible scenarios for planting and harvesting. All three produce an average of about 800 grams of wheat per person per day (for six persons) and require a 55-day life cycle. One scenario harvests (and plants) a single large crop every 55 days. The other two scenarios have smaller plantings staged at intervals of 11 and 5 days. The oscillations in the water storage in the scenario with the 11-day harvests are about double the size of the oscillations with the 5-day harvests. This is not unexpected, since the growing crop accumulates water (basically in the edible tissues), depleting the water reservoir; and, when the crop is harvested, the inedible plant parts are sent to the waste pro-

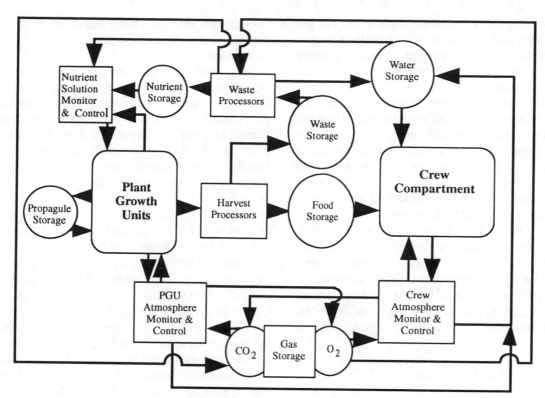

Fig. 19 Schematic of the BLSS model of Rummel and Volk.[86]

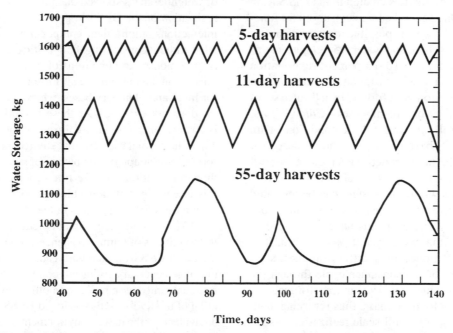

Time, days

Fig. 20 Output of the BLSS model for water storage as a function of different planting and harvesting schemes. All three cases have the same average daily food production, but harvesting schedule significantly affects the water mass in storage.

cessor, returning the water to storage.

The curve for the 55-day harvest scenario in Fig. 20 illustrates behavior that does not follow from this explanation of how water storage oscillates as a simple function of crop size and planting interval. The naive expectation would be for maximum and minimum water storage every 55 days. Instead, we find that every 55-day cycle has two maxima and two minima and a complicated shape compared to the simple cycles with the 11- or 5-day harvests. Understanding the results of the 55-day harvest requires an examination of all the contributing fluxes to and from water storage. Crop water uptake is governed by a nonlinear crop growth model (a logistic equation with rapid growth early in the life cycle and slower growth later). Water is supplied rapidly from the harvested waste of inedible biomass and more steadily from the stored food. The combination of these processes produces the complicated results shown.

This example is meant to convey a message beyond the mere analysis of water fluxes and water storage dynamics. We expect similar qualitative shifts in the behavior of the system with changes in design parameters in all aspects of a BLSS. Modeling such behavior is essential to the creation of control strategies.[82]

In addition to the system models described above, extensive mathematical modeling of biological systems of particular relevance to the BLSS have been carried out by Yu.M. Svirezhev (Svirezhev and Yelizarov,[88] Svirezhev and Logofet[62]). The subjects covered by Svirezhev include models in biogeocenology and the problem of optimal productivity of populations, "predator-prey" interactions, trophic structures, population age structures, the stability and reliability of biological communities, and artificial closed biological systems.

VII. Conclusion

1) The current state of BLSS development can be attributed mainly to research on models created in the U.S.S.R. in the 1970s and 1980s. One general conclusion about the functioning of such models is that it is possible to attain complete regeneration of the atmosphere and water, 95–99 percent utilization of carbon dioxide, and 10–26 percent regeneration of food. These models have demonstrated that humans can survive in an isolated environment formed by a limited set of plant organisms (including a one-member set—*Chlorella*) and their concomitant microflora. Under these conditions, with the exception of $O_2:CO_2$ balance, there is no evidence for lack of stationarity of the major functional characteristics of the models that would suggest any maximum duration of their existence. The processes within the system can be regulated through intrinsic regulation mechanisms with minimal control from without. Today, these models have accomplished virtually all of the tasks that were initially set for them. The next generation of BLSS models must differ from the first by virtue of greater closure of the substance cycle through the participation of heterotrophic organisms in transforming unused organic wastes into food biomass, thus returning them to the trophic chains of plants. Full-scale realization of such models will be most effective using all the experience that has been obtained to date within international programs.

2) The development of life support systems for space has also led to a new understanding of the potential relationship between biological and physical-chemical systems. For a long time, such systems were perceived as competitors, but there were no winners in this contest. The physical-chemical directions that previously seemed so promising have not yet led to the creation of even ground-based models that can fully regenerate the atmosphere and water without dead-end pro-

cesses. However, man-rated models of BLSSs, which perform a greater range of functions, have long been developed and tested.

As a result, the long-standing competition between physical-chemical and biological systems has inevitably been resolved through a natural compromise—acknowledgement of the need to create a life support system with parallel processes utilizing physical-chemical and biological technologies; i.e., the need to create a system that is neither exclusively physical-chemical nor biological. There is still no agreed-upon name for such systems; here, we call them mixed or hybrid.

3) The first official expression of this direction is the international CELSS Program (NASA, U.S.A.), with the goal of a life support system for Space Station and subsequent spacecraft. This program mandated the creation of just such a mixed system. Development of its biological components is currently in the phase of laboratory research.

However, the creation of mixed systems is virtually irrelevant to the main goal—modeling of BLSSs as relatively closed ecological systems—since mixed systems are controlled and monitored by external systems, instead of the mechanisms of internal self-control that are characteristic of biological systems at all hierarchical levels.

4) The first attempts to analyze the ecological consequences of weightlessness showed that they may act as barriers to the realization of the BLSS in general and, in particular, to the interactions among their components that have been postulated without considering the specific organisms involved and their responses to conditions of weightlessness. This pessimistic conclusion with regard to orbital flights is not valid for lunar and planetary bases, where the weightlessness factor does not exist. Under these conditions, altered gravity becomes, for terrestrial life forms, simply a quantitative variant of the normal gravitational environment, to which the life form can be adapted, first physiologically and then, possibly, though evolution. For the future, what is important is that this aspect of gravitational biology not be excluded from consideration in BLSS projects in the relatively near term.

5) The need to design and implement full-scale models of the conditions of human existence in complete isolation from the Earth's environment will lead, ultimately, to recognition that it is necessary to introduce this same "terrestrial environment" into these models. In other words, full-scale modeling of relatively well-developed BLSSs that are functional equivalents of the natural environment of humans are required. The interdisciplinary scale of this task has no analogs in the history of science—it is unprecedented. We have merely touched upon it in this chapter, neglecting problems of engineering and, partially, technology.

6) Today, no one nation possesses sufficient theoretical, scientific, biotechnological, and technical knowledge, not to mention experience with practical modeling of man-rated BLSSs, to reliably design second-generation BLSS models suitable for the manned space missions of the 21st century. It would seem to follow that reliable biomedical support of fu-

ture manned space programs can be most effective if based on the pooling of efforts and expertise acquired during the more than 30 years of work in creating models of biologically appropriate living environments for the extrabiospheric spacecraft of the future.

References

[1]Tsiolkovskiy, K.E. Exploration of outer space with jet rockets. *Collected Works*, vol. 2. Moscow, U.S.S.R. Academy of Sciences, pp. 128–130 (in Russian).

[2]Bowman, N.I. The food and atmosphere control problem in space vessels, Part II, The use of algae for food and atmosphere control. *Journal of the British Interplanetary Society*, 1953, no. 12, pp. 159–167.

[3]Burlew, I.S. *Algal Culture from Laboratory to Pilot Plant.* Washington, D.C., Carnegie Institute, 1953, p. 600.

[4]Myers, J. Basic remarks on the use of plants as biological gas exchangers in a closed system. *Journal of Aviation Medicine*, vol. 25, no. 4, 1954, pp. 407–412.

[5]Sisakyan, N.M.; Gazenko, O.G.; and Genin, A.M. Problems of space biology. In: Sisakyan, N.M., and Yazdovskiy, V.K., Eds. *Problems of Space Biology, Volume 1*, Moscow, U.S.S.R. Academy of Sciences, 1962, pp. 17–26 (in Russian).

[6]Sisakyan, N.M.; Parin, V.V.; Chernigovskiy, V.N.; and Yazdovskiy, V.K. Some problems in space research and exploration. In: Sisakyan, N.M., and Yazdovskiy, V.K., Eds. *Problems of Space Biology, Volume 1*, Moscow, U.S.S.R. Academy of Sciences, 1962, pp. 5–16 (in Russian).

[7]Semenenko, V.Ye.; Vladimirova, M.G.; and Nichiporovich, A.A. Intensification of photosynthetic productivity of a culture of one-celled algae. *Izvestiya AN SSSR, Seriya Biologicheskaya*, 1962, no. 2 (in Russian).

[8]Shepelev, Ye.Ya. The ecological system on space flights. *Aviatsiya i Kosmonavtika*, 1963, no. 1, pp. 20–25 (in Russian).

[9]Shepelev, Ye.Ya. Man-rated life support systems based on biological substance cycles in the cabins of spacecraft. In: Yazdovskiy, V.I., Ed. *Space Biology and Aerospace Medicine*. Moscow, Nauka, 1966, Chapter 14, pp. 330–362 (in Russian).

[10]Gaume, J.G. Plants as a means of balancing a closed ecological system. *Journal of Astronautics*, 1957, no. 4, pp. 72–75.

[11]Gafford, R.D., and Craf, C.E. A photosynthetic gas exchanger capable of providing for respiratory requirements of small animals. SAM 58-124, Randolph AFB, Tex., USAF School of Aviation Medicine, 1959, pp. 58–124.

[12]Myers, J.I. Study of photosynthetic regenerative systems on green algae. SAM 58-117, Randolph AFB, Tex., USAF School of Aviation Medicine Report, 1958, vol. 58, p. 117.

[13]Gazenko, O.G. Space biology. In: *Development of Biology in the U.S.S.R., Soviet Science and Technology after 50 Years, 1917–1967*, Moscow, Nauka, 1967, pp. 613–631 (in Russian).

[14]Bovee, H. H.; Christensen, G. M.; Zommers, I.; and Thompson, J. M. Life support parameters in the space environment. In: *Advances in Astronautical Science (Proceedings), Volume 9*, New York, 1963, pp. 336–344.

[15]Genin, A.M. Some principles underlying the formation of artificial living environments in the cabins of spacecraft. In: Sisakyan, N.M., and Yazdovskiy, V.I., Eds. *Problems of Space Biology, Volume 3*, Moscow, Nauka, 1964, pp. 59–65 (in Russian).

[16]Shepelev, Ye.Ya. Some problems in human ecology under conditions of closed substance cycle systems. In: Sisakyan, N.M., and Yazdovskiy, V.I., Eds. *Problems of Space Biology, Volume 4*, Moscow, Nauka, 1965, pp. 169–179 (in Russian).

[17]Gazenko, O.G., and Shepelev, Ye.Ya. Development of the ideas of K.E. Tsiolkovskiy on a biological method for supporting the habitability of spacecraft. In: *Proceedings of the 6th Lecture Series on Development of the Scientific Legacy of K.E. Tsiolkovskiy*, Moscow, U.S.S.R. Academy of Sciences, 1972, pp. 3–6 (in Russian).

[18]Shepelev, Ye.Ya. Biological life support systems. In: Calvin, M., and Gazenko, O.G., Eds. *Foundations of Space Biology and Medicine*, Washington, D.C., NASA Hq., vol. 3, chapter 10, pp. 274–308.

[19]Gazenko, O.G., and Shepelev, Ye.Ya. Long-term space flights and the human living environment. *Kosmicheskaya Biologiya i Aviakosmicheskaya Meditsina*, 1977, no. 1, p. 10 (in Russian).

[20]Gazenko, O.G.; Grigoryev, A.I.; Meleshko, G.I.; and Shepelev, Ye.Ya. Habitability and biological life support systems. *Kosmicheskaya Biologiya i Aviakosmicheskaya Meditsina*, 1990, no. 3, pp. 12–17 (in Russian).

[21]Vernadskiy, V.I. *Thoughts of a Naturalist*. Moscow, Nauka, 1977, p. 191 (in Russian).

[22]Telitchenko, M.M. Formation of biologically complete water by hydrobionts. In: *Biological Self-Purification and the Generation of Water Quality*, Moscow, Nauka, 1975, pp. 9–14 (in Russian).

[23]Kholodnyy, N.G. The biological significance of volatile organic substances emitted by plants. In: Kholodnyy, N.G. *Natural and Laboratory Environments*, Moscow, Moscow Society of Natural Scientists, 1949, pp. 156–173 (in Russian).

[24]Petryanov-Sokolov, I.V., and Sutugin, A.G. Aerosols in nature and industry. *Priroda*, 1933, no. 3, pp. 2–11 (in Russian).

[25]Bondaryov, L.G. The role of plants in the migration of mineral substances into the atmosphere. *Priroda*, 1981, no. 3, pp. 86–90 (in Russian).

[26]Bazilevich, N.I.; Rodin, L.Ye.; and Rozov, N.N. How much does the living substance of our planet weigh? *Priroda*, 1971, no. 1, pp. 46–53 (in Russian).

[27]Boychenko, M.M. On the formation of water quality by hydrobionts. *Nauchnyye Doklady Vysshey Shkoly, Biologicheskiye Nauki*, 1975, no. 4, pp. 74–77 (in Russian).

[28]Hoff, J.E.; Howe, J.M.; Mitchell, C.A.; and Carry, A. Nutritional and cultural aspects of plant species selection for

a regenerative life support system. NASA Contractor Report 166324, Moffett Field, CA, NASA Ames Research Center, 1982.

[29]Salisbury, F.B. Bioregenerative farming on the Moon. In: *Proceedings of the 8th International Academy of Astronautics (IAA) Man in Space Symposium*, Tashkent, U.S.S.R., Sept. 29–Oct. 4, 1989.

[30]Ashida, A.; Yoshioka, T.; Tanakura, S.; Takatski M.; Ysa, T.; Koisumi, M.; Oguchi, M.; and Nitta, K. Plant system for a lunar base. In: *Proceedings of the 8th IAA Man in Space Symposium*, Tashkent, U.S.S.R., Sept. 29–Oct. 4, 1989.

[31]Midorikawa, Y.; Fuji, T.; Terai, M.; Omasa, K.; and Nitta, K. A food/nutrient supply plant for lunar base CELSS. Paper presented at the 40th Congress of the International Astronautical Federation (IAF), Madrid, 1989.

[32]Bugbee, B., and Salisbury, F.B. Current and potential productivity of wheat for a controlled environment life support system. *Advances in Space Research*, vol. 9, no. 8, 1989, pp. 5–15.

[33]Lisovskiy, G.M., Ed. *A Closed Man-Higher Plants System. A 4-Month Experiment.* Novosibirsk, 1978, p. 138 (in Russian).

[34]Ivanova, I.Ye.; Derendyayeva, T.A.; Alekhina, T.P.; and Shaydorov, Yu.I. The higher plant component in man-rated biological life support systems. *Kosmicheskaya Biologiya i Aviakosmicheskaya Meditsina,* 1990, no. 4, pp. 40–43 (in Russian).

[35]Shepelev, Ye.Ya; Shaydorov, Yu.I.; and Popov, V.V. Reprocessing of plant wastes on a solid substrate for a man-rated biological life support system. *Kosmicheskaya Biologiya i Aviakosmicheskaya Meditsina,* 1983, no. 6, pp. 71–74 (in Russian).

[36]Yazdovskiy, V.I., and Ratner, G.S. Heterotrophic organisms—one of the sources for human nutrition on long-term space flights. In: Chernigovskiy, V.N., Ed. *Work Performance, Issues of Habitability and Biotechnology. Problems of Space Biology, Volume 7,* Moscow, Nauka, pp. 382–388 (in Russian).

[37]Antsyshkina, L.M.; Kirilenko, N.S.; Mamontov, V.Ya.; Melnikov, G.B.; and Ryabov, F.P. Experience maintaining fish in airtight aquaria with and without *Chlorella.* In: Sisakyan, N.M., and Yazdovskiy, V.I., Eds. *Problems of Space Biology, Volume 4,* Moscow, Nauka, 1965, pp. 646–654 (in Russian).

[38]Mironova, N.B. Comparative evaluation of the growth of Tilapia (*Tilapia massambica,* Peters) fed on *Chlorella* and other food. In: Chernigovskiy, V.N., Ed. *Work Performance, Issues of Habitability and Biotechnology. Problems of Space Biology, Volume 7,* Moscow, Nauka, 1967, pp. 505–512 (in Russian).

[39]Burenkov, M.SA., and Agre, A.L. Preliminary evaluation of the potential for using land molluscs as components of closed ecological systems. *Kosmicheskaya Biologiya i Aviakosmicheskaya Meditsina,* 1975, no. 4, pp. 90–91 (in Russian).

[40]Meleshko, G.I.; Shepelev, Ye.Ya.; Guryeva, T.S.; Bodya,

K.; and Sabo, V. Embryonal development of birds in weightlessness. *Kosmicheskaya Biologiya i Aviakosmicheskaya Meditsina,* 1991, no. 1, pp. 37–39 (in Russian).

[41]Takahashi, Y. Water oxidation waste management systems for a CELSS—the state of the art. *Biological Science in Space,* vol. 3., no. 1, 1989, pp. 45–54.

[42]Golubeva, Ye.G., and Yerofeyeva, T.V. Dynamics of growth of house fly larvae on wastes of a biological life support system. *Kosmicheskaya Biologiya i Aviakosmicheskaya Meditsina,* 1982, no. 6, pp. 74–76 (in Russian).

[43]Andre, M., and MacElroy, R.D. Plants and man in space. A new field in plant physiology. *Physiologist,* vol. 33, no. 1, (Suppl.), 1990, pp. S100–S101.

[44]MacElroy, R.D., and Smernoff, D.T., Eds. Controlled ecological life support systems. *Advances in Space Research,* vol. 7, no. 4, 1987, pp. 1–153.

[45]MacElroy, R.D.; Tibitts, T.W.; Thompson, B.G.; and Volk, T., Eds. Natural and artificial ecosystems. *Advances in Space Research,* vol. 9, no. 8, 1989, pp. 1–202.

[46]Dean, R.B.; Golub, M.A.; and Wydevan,T., Eds. Waste management in space. *Waste Management and Research,* vol. 9, no. 5, 1991, pp. 323–490 (whole issue).

[47]Takahashi, Y.; Wydevan, T.; and Koo, C. Subcritical and supercritical wet oxidation of CELSS model wastes. *Advances in Space Research,* vol. 9, no. 8, 1989, pp. 99–110.

[48]Wydevan, T.; Tremor, J.; Koo, C.; and Jacquez, R. Sources and processing of CELSS waste. *Advances in Space Research,* vol. 9, no. 8, 1989. pp. 85–97.

[49]Gitelzon, J.I.; Kovrov, B.G.; Lisovskiy, G.N.; Okladnikov, Yu.N.; Rerberg, M.S.; Sidko, F.Ya.; and Terskov, I.A. *Man-rated Experimental Ecological Systems. Problems of Space Biology, Volume 28,* Moscow, Nauka, 1975 (in Russian).

[50]Meleshko, G.I., and Shepelev, Ye.Ya. Biological life support systems. In: Gazenko, O.G., Ed. *Handbook of Physiology,* Moscow, Nauka, 1987, pp. 30–36 (in Russian).

[51]Meleshko, G.I., and Shepelev, Ye.Ya. Biological life support systems. In: *Kosmicheskaya Biologiya i Aviakosmicheskaya Meditsina,* vol. 22, no. 6, 1988, pp. 30–36 (in Russian).

[52]Sinyak, Yu.Ye. Water supply. In: Gazenko, O.G., Ed. *Handbook of Physiology,* Moscow, Nauka, 1987, pp. 340 (in Russian).

[53]Anisimov, B.V. Hygienic significance of ionization of the cabin atmosphere on manned spacecraft. In: Nefyodov, Y.G., Ed. *Sanitary, Hygienic, and Physiological Aspects of Inhabited Spacecraft. Problems of Space Biology,Volume 42,* Moscow, Nauka, 1980, pp. 68–79 (in Russian).

[54]Kondratyeva, Ye.M. Study of the group composition of concomitant microflora during long-term cultivation of *Chlorella* in a closed system. In: Gazenko, O.G., Ed. *Urgent Problems in Space Biology and Medicine,* Moscow, Institute of Biomedical Problems, 1975, pp. 112–113 (in Russian).

[55]Tirranen, L.S.; Gitelzon, J.I.; and Rerberg, M.S. Formation of the microflora component of higher plants in a man-rated closed ecological system. In: *Proceedings of 5th Con-*

gress of the All-Union Microbiological Association, Yerevan, 1975, p. 85 (in Russian).

[56]Yunusova, L.S.; Kondratyeva, Ye.M.; and Drova, N.A. Formation of a microbial cenosis of the photoautotrophic component in a man-rated biological life support system. In: Micro-organisms in Artificial Ecosystems, Novosibirsk, Nauka, 1985, pp. 143–146 (in Russian).

[57]Gitelzon, J.I.; Manudovskiy, N.S.; Pankova, I.M.; Posadskaya, M.N.; Somova, L.A.; and Tirranen, L.S. Microbiological Problems of Closed Ecological Systems, Novosibirsk, Nauka, 1981, p. 197 (in Russian).

[58]Zaloguyev, S.N.; Viktorov, A.N.; and Startseva, N.D. Sanitary-microbiological and epidemiological aspects of habitability. In: Nefyodov, Y.G., Ed. Sanitary, Hygienic, and Physiological Aspects of Inhabited Spacecraft, Problems of Space Biology, Volume 42, Moscow, Nauka, 1980, pp. 80–140 (in Russian).

[59]Drugova, N.A.; Chernova, L.S.; and Mashinskiy, A.L. Formation of a microbial cenosis of wheat plants under conditions of spacecraft habitability. Kosmicheskaya Biologiya i Aviakosmicheskaya Meditsina, 1989, no. 5, pp. 39–43 (in Russian).

[60]Viktorov, A.N., and Novikova, N.D. Characteristics of the formation of microflora on structural materials used in inhabited pressurized closed environments. Kosmicheskaya Biologiya i Aviakosmicheskaya Meditsina, 1985, no. 2, pp. 66–69 (in Russian).

[61]Kholodnyy, N.G. What's new in the aeroponic nutrition of plants. Priroda, 1951, no. 2 (in Russian).

[62]Svirezhev, Yu.M., and Logofet, D.O. The Stability of Biological Communities, Moscow, Nauka, 1978, p. 352 (in Russian).

[63]Shepelev, Ye.Ya., and Meleshko, G.I. Analysis of certain mechanisms underlying the stability of biological life support systems using the example of a culture of one-celled algae. In: Proceedings of the 8th Lecture Series Dedicated to Developing the Scientific Legacy and Ideas of K.E. Tsiolkovskiy, Kaluga, Sept. 14–17, 1973, Moscow, U.S.S.R. Academy of Sciences, 1974, pp. 76–84 (in Russian).

[64]Cook, J. Ecology of space flight. In: Odum, E.P., Ed. Fundamentals of Ecology, Philadelphia, W.B. Saunders, 1959, Chapter 20.

[65]Guryeva, T.S. Study of the potential for using leaf and stem mass of higher plants to obtain food products in a man-rated life support system. Thesis abstract, Moscow, Institute of Biomedical Problems, 1982, p. 37 (in Russian).

[66]Yunusova, L.S.; Kondratyeva, Ye.M.; and Drugova, N.A. Study of the microflora of the autotrophic component in a man-rated biological life support system. In: Proceedings of the 11th All-Union Working Meeting on the Substance Cycle in Closed Systems Based on Vital Activity of Lower Organisms, Kiev, Naukova Dumka, 1983, pp. 173–185 (in Russian).

[67]Kondratyev, Yu.I.; Bychkov, B.P.; Ushakov, A.S.; and Shepelev, Ye.Ya. The use of the biomass of one-celled algae to feed humans. In: Chernigovskiy, V.N., Ed. Work Performance, Issues of Habitability and Biotechnology. Problems of Space Biology, Volume 7, Moscow, Nauka, pp. 363–370 (in Russian).

[68]Parfenov, G.P. Weightlessness and Elementary Biological Processes. Problems of Space Biology. Volume 57, Moscow, Nauka, p. 272 (in Russian).

[69]Kordyum, G.P.; Polivoda, L.V.; and Mashinskiy, A.L. The effect of space flight conditions on micro-organisms. In: Dubinin, N.P., Ed. Gravity and the Organism. Problems of Space Biology, Volume 33, Moscow, Nauka, 1976, pp. 238–260 (in Russian).

[70]Meleshko, G.I.; Shepelev, Ye.Ya.; Kordyum, V.A.; Shetlik, I.; and Doukha, I. Weightlessness and its effect on micro-organisms and plants. One-celled algae. In: Gazenko, O.G., Ed. Results of Medical Research Performed on the Salyut-6–Soyuz Orbital Scientific Research Complex. Moscow, Nauka, 1986, pp. 369–380 (in Russian).

[71]Sychev, V.N.; Levinskikh, M.A.; and Livanskaya, O.G. Study of the growth and development of Chlorella exposed to space on Cosmos-1887. Kosmicheskaya Biologiya i Aviakosmicheskaya Meditsina, 1989, no. 5, pp. 35–39 (in Russian).

[72]Levinskikh, M.A., and Sychev, V.N. Growth and development of one-celled algae in space flight as part of an "algobacterial cenosis-fish" system. Kosmicheskaya Biologiya i Aviakosmicheskaya Meditsina, 1989, no. 5, pp. 32–35 (in Russian).

[73]Shepelev, Ye.Ya.; Bodya, K.; Mishchenko, V.F.; Fofanov, V.I.; Deshevaya, O.A.; Belak, M.; Sidorenko, L.A.; Peter, V.; et al. Outcome of an experiment on the incubation of quail eggs in weightlessness. In: Abstracts of Papers Presented at the 11th Meeting of the Working Group on Space Biology and Medicine, Intercosmos, Bucharest, 1982, pp. 121–122 (in Russian).

[74]Meleshko, G.I.; Shepelev, Ye.Ya.; Guryeva, T.S.; Bodya, K.; and Sabo, V. Embryonal development of birds in weightlessness. Kosmicheskaya Biologiya i Aviakosmicheskaya Meditsina, 1991, no. 1, pp. 37–39 (in Russian).

[75]Kokorin, I.I.; Pigareva, M.D.; Palmbakh, L.R.; Afanasyev, G.D.; and Mashinskiy, A.L. Embryonal development of quail in weightlessness. In: Dybinin, N.I., Ed. Biological Research on Salyut Space Stations, Moscow, Nauka, 1984, pp. 139–144 (in Russian).

[76]Serova, L.V.; Denisova, L.A.; Lavrova, Ye.A.; Makeyeva, V.F.; Natochin, Yu.V.; Pustynnikova, A.M.; and Shakhmatova, Ye.I. Parameters of reproductive functions of animals. Characteristics of embryos and placentae. In: Serova, L.V., Ed. Ontogenesis of Mammals in Weightlessness, Moscow, Nauka, 1988, pp. 72–79 (in Russian).

[77]Wade, R.C. Nutritional Models for a Controlled Ecological Life Support System (CELSS): Linear Mathematical Modeling. NASA CR 4229, Washington, D.C., NASA Hq., 1989.

[78]NASA. A diet expert subsystem program for the controlled ecological life support system. Contract NAS2-12991, Moffett Field, Calif., NASA Ames Research Center, 1990.

[79]Volk, T., and Bugbee, B. Effects of light and tempera-

ture on leaf emergence rate in wheat and barley crop. *Crop Science*, vol. 31, no. 5, 1991, pp. 1218–1224.

[80]Volk, T., and Rummel, J. D. Mass balances for a biological life support system simulation model. In: MacElroy, R.D., and Smernoff, D.T., Eds. *Controlled ecological life support systems,* NASA Conference Publication 2480, Moffett Field, Calif., NASA Ames Research Center, 1987, pp. 139–146.

[81]Volk, T., and Cullingford, H. Crop growth and associated life support for a lunar farm. In: Mendell, W., Ed. *Lunar Bases and Space Activities of the 21st Century*, Houston, Lunar and Planetary Institute, 1991.

[82]Blackwell, A. L., and Blackwell, C.C. A modeling system for control of the thermal and fluid dynamics of NASA CELSS Crop Growth Research Chamber. Paper presented at the 19th Intersociety Conference on Environmental Systems, San Diego, Calif., July 24–26, Society of Automotive Engineers (SAE) paper 89-1570, 1989.

[83]Blackwell, A. L. A perspective on CELSS control issues. In: MacElroy, R.D., Ed. *Controlled Ecological Life Support Systems: CELSS '89 Workshop*, NASA TM 102277, Moffett Field, Calif., NASA Ames Research Center, 1990, pp. 327–353.

[84]Averner, M. M. An approach to the mathematical modeling of a controlled ecological life support system. NASA-CR-166331, Moffett Field, Calif., NASA Ames Research Center, 1981.

[85]Babcock, P.S.; Auslander, D.M.; and Spear, R.C. Dynamic considerations of control of closed life support systems. *Advances in Space Research*, vol. 4, no. 12, pp. 263–270, 1984.

[86]Rummel, J. D., and Volk, T. A modular BLSS simulation model. In: MacElroy, R.D., and Smernoff, D.T., Eds. *Controlled Ecological Life Support System,* NASA Conference Publication 2480, Moffett Field, Calif., NASA Ames Research Center, pp. 56–66, 987.

[87]Cullingford, H. S. Development of the CELSS Emulator at NASA JSC, Controlled Ecological Life Support Systems. In: MacElroy, R.D., Ed. *Controlled Ecological Life Support Systems: CELSS '89 Workshop*, NASA TM 102277, Moffett Field, Calif., NASA Ames Research Center, pp. 319–325, 1990.

[88]Svirezhev, Yu.M., and Yelizarov, Ye.Y. *Mathematical Modeling of Biological Systems. Problems of Space Biology, Volume 20*, Moscow, Nauka, 1972 (in Russian).

[89]Gitelzon, I.I.; Terskov, I.A.; Kovrov, B.G.; Sidko, F.J.; Lisovskiy, G.M.; Okladnikov, Yu.N.; Belyanin, V.N.; Trubachov, I.N.; and Rerberg, M.S. Life support system with autonomous control employing plant photosynthesis. *Acta Astronautica,* 1976, vol. 3, no. 9–10, pp. 633–650.

[90]Gitelzon, I. I.; Terskov, I. A.; Kovrov, B. G.; Lisovskiy, G. M.; Sidko, F. J.; Okladnikov, Yu. N.; Trubachov, I. N.; Pankova, I. M.; Gribovskaya, I. V.; Denisov, G. V.; and Shilenko, M. P. Closed ecosystem as the means for outer space exploration by men. Preprint IAF-81-164, 1981, pp. 1–5.

[91]Lisovskiy, G.M.; Terskov, I.A.; Gitelzon, I.I.; Sidko, F.J.; Kovrov, B.G.; Shilenko, M.P.; Polonskiy, V.I.; and Ushakova, S.A. Experimental estimation of functional abilities of higher plants as medium regenerators in life-support systems. Preprint IAF-81-169, XXIIth IAF Congress, Rome, 1981, pp. 1–4.

Chapter 17

Life Support of Crewmembers After Unscheduled Landings in Unpopulated Areas or at Sea

V. G. Volovich

I. Introduction

When control systems fail or immediate descent becomes necessary because an emergency situation in a spacecraft cabin threatens the lives of the crew, the space vehicle may have to make an unscheduled landing in unpopulated, inaccessible regions, or in the ocean.

Search-and-rescue teams from the United States and the Russian Federation (formerly the Soviet Union) have all the necessary means to locate spacecraft and rescue their crews. However, when the landing site is far removed from the search-and-rescue base, when radio contact is not established, or if meteorological conditions around the landing (splashdown) site are very poor, the crewmembers may have to survive on their own.

After an unscheduled water landing, the period during which the crew will have to survive on their own will be relatively short. In 1975, Berry[1] reported that U.S. naval experience with recovery of downed aviators indicated that the longest recorded time before rescue was 24 h, 45 min. With the highly developed system for tracking the final stages of a spaceflight, it can be expected that space crews would be rescued relatively soon at sea. Rescue operations after a hard landing in an off-target area may require somewhat longer periods.

When the Voskhod 2 returned to Earth (because of failure of the solar orientation system), re-entry was ballistic with manual orientation control. As a result, the cosmonauts landed several thousand kilometers from the scheduled landing area, in a taiga region. Low air temperature, deep snow (greater than 1 m), and impenetrable forest complicated the task of the search-and-rescue group. The two crewmembers were compelled to survive on their own for a day and a half, during which they used their survival gear to protect themselves against temperatures of -40 °C, and to prepare meals, etc.

Long-term survival is especially difficult in regions with harsh climates (Arctic, desert). In addition to the adverse physiological effects of extreme environmental factors (high or low temperatures, intense solar radiation, etc.), many difficulties arise in meeting basic biological needs. Long-term survival of crews depends, first and foremost, on crewmembers' survival skills; that is, their ability to initiate sensible actions to protect their lives, health, and performance capacity.[2–4]

Many objective and subjective factors affect the process of long-term survival, either facilitating or impeding it; these are commonly termed "survival factors."[5,6] Survival factors may be classified as human, natural/environmental, resource/technical, and mixed[7] (see Fig. 1).

Human factors include the psychological and physical fitness of the individual to act under conditions of long-term survival, including physiological reserves and level of training.

Natural/environmental factors include ambient temperature and humidity, solar radiation, precipitation, barometric pressure, and wind. Terrain, water sources, flora and fauna, and photoperiod (polar day and night) are other examples of environmental parameters. The natural environment and its physical and geographical conditions have a strong influence on all human actions undertaken in conditions of long-term survival. Frequently these conditions are extreme; they can have very strong effects and "can disrupt the functional activity of the organism, pushing it to the verge of death."[8] The Arctic and tropics, mountains and desert, taiga and oceans each have their own peculiarities of climate, terrain, flora, and fauna. These in turn affect what specific actions humans must perform in order to survive: behavior, techniques for obtaining water and food, construction of shelters, measures to prevent diseases, etc. Humans can live under the most severe conditions for a long period of time; however, those who are unaccustomed to extremes of climate may be significantly less tolerant than acclimatized individuals.

The third group of factors, resource/technical, includes available survival gear, i.e., clothing, emergency gear, devices for signaling and communications, means for obtaining water, supplies of water and food, flotation devices, and materials at hand used for purposes of survival.

The fourth type of factor arises from interactions among the first three and may take on independent significance. Fac-

The author gratefully acknowledges the editorial contributions made to this chapter by Dr. Donald F. Stewart. This chapter was translated into English by Lydia Razran Stone.

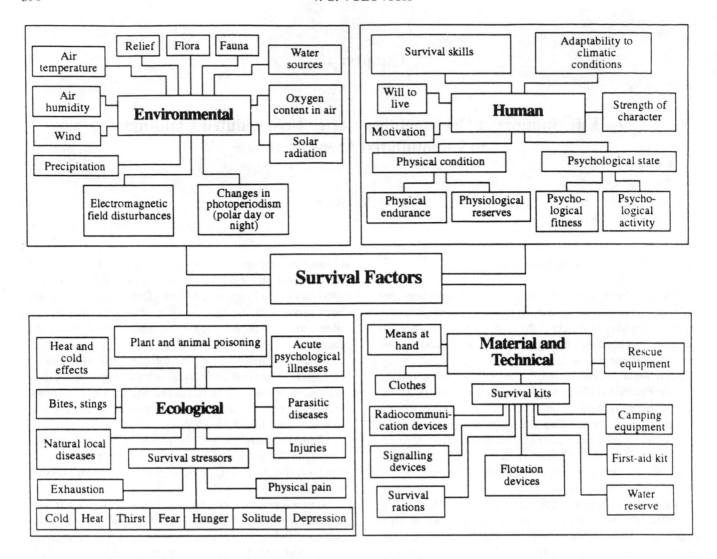

Fig. 1 Survival factors.

tors in this group include such things as poisoning by plant and animal toxins, infectious agents specific to certain geographic zones, altitude sickness, pathological effects of heat and cold, bites of poisonous animals and insects, parasitic diseases, and injuries from various causes. For example, according to data compiled by the NATO Advisory Group for Aerospace Research and Development (AGARD), after emergency landing of aircraft, approximately 70 percent of all individuals have sustained some level of injury, and after rescue by a search-and-rescue squad, almost 100 percent of crew and passengers are found to be suffering from injuries or diseases.[9,10] Because of this, the probability of survival decreases to 80 percent during the first 24 h after an emergency landing. In the absence of injury, the probability of survival after an emergency landing begins to decrease only on the third day. Factors of this type, referred to as "stressors of survival,"[2,4,6] also include cold, heat, hunger, thirst, exhaustion, isolation, physical pain, fear, and depression, all of which can be of great significance under certain circumstances.

It is well known that in extreme situations (shipwrecks,

aircraft crashes, fires, earthquakes, etc.) not everyone is capable of immediate, energetic, and effective action. Approximately 50–75 percent of victims react in a dysfunctional manner, termed a "panic response."[11] Such individuals may appear relatively calm. Another 12–25 percent display hysterical reactions, manifested in some individuals in strong motor excitement, tears, unconsciousness, and senseless random actions. Others may exhibit depression, deep prostration, indifference to events and surroundings, and inability to act. In such situations, only 12–25 percent of people retain control, rapidly assess conditions, and act decisively and rationally.[12] In most cases, after a period of time has elapsed, the majority of people calm down, adapt to the new, unfamiliar situation, and gradually begin to take the necessary steps to protect their lives and well-being.

One of the major reasons for the occurrence of dysfunctional states in response to emergency situations is fear. Under life-threatening conditions, feelings of fear may be associated with the uncertainty of the situation, one's own weakness, the anticipation of danger, etc. The emotion of fear is a natural reaction to danger and acts as a kind of warning system, signaling the need to take decisive measures to eliminate a threat to life.[13]

Since an individual's emotional reaction to danger depends to a great extent on his or her will, internal discipline, and "survival instinct," by learning to suppress and control fear, he/she can transform it into a kind of catalyst of energy and decisiveness. Here the emotion of fear is transformed into a sensation of readiness to combat danger.

After landing (splashdown) in an unscheduled region, a crewmember must solve a number of urgent problems. He must: 1) overcome the stress induced by the emergency situation; 2) provide first aid to the injured; 3) protect himself from the adverse effects of environmental factors (low or high temperatures, direct exposure to solar radiation, wind, etc.); 4) obtain water and food; 5) determine his location; and 6) establish radio contact and communication with the search-and-rescue team.

An emergency landing is a strong stressor and will affect emotional state. For this reason, before a plan of action is developed, time should be taken to allow all the crewmembers to calm down enough to evaluate rationally their circumstances. This may help them avoid errors and inappropriate decisions, which could have an adverse effect on the outcome of long-term survival situations.

II. Survival Kit

For use in case of emergency landings, spacecraft, as well as aircraft, carry kits containing various types of gear and supplies, typically referred to as "survival kits." These kits facilitate crew survival under adverse conditions and encourage crewmembers to attempt to overcome the difficulties that confront them.[14,15]

The many types of survival kits differ in design, size, and the gear and food products they contain. However, the contents of all of these kits can be subdivided into seven major categories:

1) Radio communications gear includes portable emergency shortwave or ultrashortwave radio sets, and radio beacons.

2) Visual signaling devices include mini-rockets, distress flares, smoke flares, signal lanterns, and dye powder.

3) Survival rations include canned or freeze-dried food products.

4) The emergency water gear includes a container, solar condensers, desalinating hardware (solar and chemical distillers), and a decontamination kit.

5) Camping gear typically includes a machete, a hunting knife, a compass, sunglasses, fire-starting devices, dry fuel, candles, a wire saw, fishing gear, an aluminized medical cape, mosquito netting, a flashlight, and foil.

6) Emergency flotation devices include such items as inflatable lifeboats and rafts, and an antiexposure dry suit.

7) The medical kit includes a tourniquet, bandages, iodine, antibiotics, antishock drugs, insect repellent, etc.

A. Radio Communications Devices

The survival kit includes small shortwave or medium-wave radio sets. There are many types of such sets, differing in design, size, range, and power source. For example, the survival kits of Russian spacecraft use the ultramicrowave R-855 and YuR-35 ultrashortwave radio sets, which provide reliable radio communications in telegraph and telephone modes with an aircraft flying at an altitude of 10 km at a range of more than 100 km.

The role of emergency radio equipment for locating and rescuing crews after emergency landings in inaccessible areas or on the water has been enhanced by the implementation of an international plan to use satellite systems to locate disaster victims. One U.S. design for a rescue homing system involves continuous tracking of emergency signals. Tests using LES-6 and ATS-3 satellites have demonstrated the potential of this system over an unlimited range. This idea was implemented in the 1980s in the KOSPAS-SARSAT project, with joint participation by scientists in the U.S.S.R., the United States, Canada, and France. [KOSPAS (acronym for the Russian words for "Space System for Search and Rescue of Vessels and Aircraft") is the part of the search system developed in the U.S.S.R. SARSAT (acronym for "Search and Rescue Satellite-Aided Tracking") is the part of the search system developed in the United States, Canada, and France.] The basis of the space search-and-rescue system will be several Russian and U.S. satellites in polar orbit at altitudes of 800–1000 km. A special small radio buoy on-board an aircraft or ship or in the pack of an expedition member will broadcast a distress signal every 50 s after activation. A satellite flying in the area will transmit the signals to the nearest information reception point. Ten such points have already been set up: four in the Russian Federation (in Arkhangelsk, Moscow, Novosibirsk, and Nakhodka), three in the United States (in Alaska, San Francisco, and Illinois), one in France (in Toulouse), one in Canada (in Ottawa), and one in Norway.

After they are processed, data obtained from the satellite make it possible to establish the coordinates of the disaster site and, on the basis of an identification code, to determine the nationality of the victims. For example, ships and aircraft of the U.S.S.R. were assigned code 221; United States, 111; Canada, 121; and France, 211. Between 1982 and 1988, this system aided in the timely rescue of 1131 individuals; 589 were in imminent danger of death due to air crashes, 495 were victims of shipwrecks, and 47 were victims of land disasters.[16]

B. Visual Signaling Devices

If radio contact fails, a search over a large area for a spacecraft or aircraft that has landed in an off-target site is very difficult. Harsh weather conditions and poor visibility, especially in the mountains, in forests, or on the ocean, can complicate the situation further. In such emergency situations, visual signaling devices, lamps, smoke flares, mini-rockets,

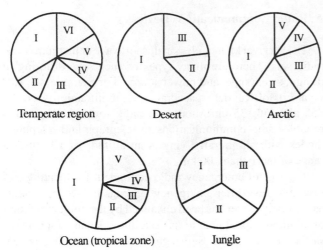

Fig. 2 Structure of mean daily weight loss in 3, 5 or 6 day experiments, during which subjects drank a controlled amount of water per day and consumed a subsistence diet. Each circle represents 100% of the total weight lost during the experiment. Each designated sector represents the weight lost during a single day of an exposure experiment in different climatic zones.

water dye powders, etc., can provide significant help in location of crews. For example, the orange smoke of the Russian PSND signal cartridge (analogous to the American MK-13 MOD-O) can be seen in the ocean at a distance of 2–4 km, and a bright crimson flame it produces can be seen at night at a distance of 10–12 km. Strobe beacons are also good signaling devices. A typical beacon made by the firm, Strobe Ident, is equipped with xenon lamps that periodically emit bright flashes that can be seen at night at a distance of up to 10 km. A very effective visual signaling device is the signal mirror. The brightness of the reflected light spot when the Sun is at an overhead angle of 130° is 4 million candles, and at a solar angle of 90°, it is 7 million candles. Flashes produced by the mirror can be detected from a search aircraft, at a distance of up to 24 km, long before the object itself can be seen.[17]

C. Emergency Rations

Humans can survive and maintain physical and mental activity for a relatively long period without food. When "fuel" is not received from without, the body will begin to utilize its own tissue stores. The human body possesses energy reserves equivalent to approximately 165,900 kcal.[18] Physiological data have demonstrated that 40–44 percent of these reserves may be consumed before a person dies.[19] If the daily energy expenditure of a human at rest is assumed to be 1800 kcal, tissue reserves would suffice for approximately 30–40 days of complete fasting. However, another significant factor, nitrogen loss, may become critical in long-term fasting. The body of a mature human being contains approximately 1000 grams of nitrogen as a component of protein, and losses of approximately 50 percent are sufficient to cause death.[20]

In subsistence on a low-calorie diet, as in total fasting, body weight gradually decreases. During the first day, weight loss is due to loss of fluid. When ambient temperatures are high, the rate of this process increases. As Fig. 2 shows, in the desert, two-thirds of all weight loss occurred during the first day of a 3 day experiment.[21]

Survival rations are used extensively in aviation and cosmonautics to provide carbohydrates, fats, and proteins for consumption in emergencies. The conditions under which emergency rations will be used impose a number of requirements on the products included in them. They must be usable without additional preparation, be readily assimilated, keep well under the most adverse climatic conditions, be filling, and facilitate fluid retention in the body. It is obvious that, with all these requirements, taste becomes a secondary concern.

In the opinion of the majority of experts, the survival rations must be balanced with respect to nutrients.[22] This principle has been followed in the development of survival rations for air and spacecraft crews in the United States and the U.S.S.R. Of course, under conditions of very-long-term survival, survival rations, no matter how rich and varied, can only partially meet physiological needs for energy and nutrients. However, their role remains very important, since the rations not only alleviate the fear of starvation, but also partially compensate for the loss of tissue reserves.[16,21,23,24] According to data obtained by American researchers, subjects surviving in the Arctic on emergency rations that compensated for only 10–15 percent of energy expended felt and performed better than a group fasting totally.[25]

Researchers have demonstrated that humans can live on rations containing 500 kcal/day for 2 weeks or longer without lasting damage to their health.[22] The sensation of hunger, occurring during the first 3–4 days, gradually diminishes. During the first 3–4 days of survival on a low-calorie diet, physical exercise evokes shortness of breath, accelerated development of fatigue, and slight vertigo; however, these symptoms are significantly less severe than in conditions of total fasting. In one experiment, physical and mental performance was found to be maintained at a rather high level over a number of days.[7,21]

Survival rations have been an integral part of survival kits since the first spaceflights. For the Vostok and Voskhod spacecraft, these rations consisted of freeze-dried products: meat, milk, cottage cheese, and cheese. In addition, the rations contained 300 grams of chocolate; 300 grams of sugar; and 18 grams of multivitamin capsules containing 1650 international units of vitamin A, 1 mg of vitamins B_1 and B_2, and 25 mg of vitamin C. The food was stored in plastic wrap and divided into portions for 3 days, each of which included breakfast, lunch, dinner, and supper. The rations for the 3-day period contained 241 grams of protein, 338 grams of fat, and 685 grams of carbohydrates, a total of 1450 grams and 6950 kcal.[26]

At the present time, the emergency rations utilized are intended for a single day and consist of freeze-dried cottage cheese with fruit puree, chocolate with a high melting point, prunes with walnuts, and pastry. The rations weigh 0.8 kg and contain 2800–3000 kcal.

Additional food sources may be found in the wild, including fish, reptiles, shellfish, etc. Various wild edible plants containing fats, proteins, carbohydrates, and minerals needed by the body may be especially important for supplementing survival rations if rescue does not occur prior to consumption of provisions.[27]

D. Water Supply

Loss of water from the body, even by only a few percentage points, leads to alteration of physiological processes; dehydration of over 10 percent significantly impairs the functioning of organs and systems, leading to death.

In areas with moderate temperatures in situations in which physical activity is relatively limited, humans need approximately 1.5–2.0 liters of water per day. This need increases significantly at high ambient temperatures, especially in the desert and tropics, reaching 4–6 liters and more per day. Conditions of long-term survival, especially in regions with high ambient temperatures and solar radiation, are conducive to rapid development of dehydration, so that water supply becomes an extremely critical problem.

In the Arctic, depending on season of the year, water sources may include desalinized ice, snow, and freshwater pools formed by snow melting on ice; in the tundra or forest, a wide variety of freshwater sources may exist, including lakes, rivers, and streams. In mountainous regions, water sources include rivers, brooks, mountain springs, and in snow-covered areas, Alpine lakes, glacier ice, and snow.

Water from moving sources, such as springs or mountain brooks, may be drunk with limited risk. Water from standing or slow-flowing bodies must be boiled or treated with special chemicals.

In a tropical forest, the need for water can be met not only from numerous moving and standing bodies of water, but also from so-called biological water sources—water-bearing plants such as liana, travellers' trees, bamboo, and baobabs.

Because of the limited number of water sources, water supply in the desert is a major problem.

A comprehensive set of measures to support water use and consumption during long-term survival can be derived from the following considerations:

1) Searching for water, especially in warm climates, is a highly critical activity.

2) If water sources are present, water should be consumed as desired; in hot climates, somewhat more water should be consumed than the minimum required to slake thirst.

3) When water supplies are limited, depending on circumstances, daily water consumption may have to be rationed and consumption of food inducing thirst should be curtailed.

4) Water obtained from standing and slow-moving bodies of water must be purified and disinfected.

5) Water may be obtained from dew, tree trunks, liana shoots, stalks of grass, etc.

6) Water may be obtained using solar condensers, polyethylene bags, and other devices.

7) Shelters (tents, canopies, etc.) provide protection from direct sunlight; clothing should be worn during the hot part of the day.

8) Activities at camp, marches, etc., should be scheduled to minimize heat production.

9) Consumption of seawater or other salty solutions, including urine, should be forbidden.

Containers made of nonoxidizing metal or special plastic with 1–1.5 liter capacity are used to store and transport emergency supplies of water. To ensure that the water remains potable, various special preservatives (e.g., silver) are used.

E. Emergency Medical Kit

The outcome of many injuries and acute conditions (snakebite, asphyxia, etc.) depends to a great extent on the timeliness and appropriateness of medical treatment. Under conditions of long-term survival, since the crew will have no one else to depend on, each crewmember must have the minimum medical knowledge needed to treat himself and others for bleeding, apnea, fractures, burns, food poisoning, etc., including knowledge of how to use the drugs and bandages in the emergency medical kit.

The medical kit is an integral part of the survival kit. It is difficult to stock the kit to deal specifically with everything that might occur. Since unscheduled crew landings may occur in diverse geographical regions under varying conditions, the contents of the medical kit must be multipurpose in nature. Here it is desirable to focus on problems that are most likely to occur under long-term survival conditions in general, with additional attention to conditions in specific geographical areas. For example, in case of a desert landing, the kit includes snakebite and spider-bite antitoxin, as well as sunscreen. For jungle survival, the kit should contain leech and flying insect repellent, a powder for fungal infections of the foot, an antimalaria drug, etc. In addition, the kit must contain the minimum drugs and bandages necessary for first aid for trauma, acute inflammatory conditions, and certain psychological states.

The following is an example of the possible contents of a medical kit for long-term survival:

1) For injuries, the kit may contain a rubber tourniquet, an individual bandage packet (no fewer than one per crewmember), sterile bandages and wipes, antiseptic bandages, adhesive tape, tincture of iodine, and medicinal distilled alcohol.

2) For shock, morphine solutions and vasoconstrictors may be included in the contents of the kit.

3) For infectious diseases of various kinds, including gastrointestinal and respiratory, the kit may contain broad spectrum antibiotics.

4) For acute cardiorespiratory disorders, the kit may contain nitroglycerine, corvallol (active ingredients: α-bromovaleric acid and phenobarbitol), obzidan (Inderal), caffeine solutions, and adrenaline and lobelin (synthetic version

of alkaloid present in lobelia plant, used to stimulate breathing) in ampules.

5) For burns and frostbite, synthomycin emulsion (D,L-treo-1-para-nitrophenyl-2-dichloracetyl amino-proprandiol-1,3) may be included for use as a topical antibiotic.

6) For inflammations of the eye, the kit may contain tetracycline ointment.

It would also be desirable for the kit to contain drugs that increase overall physiological tonus and performance [sidnocarb /N-phenylcarbamoyl-3-(B-phenylisopropyl)-sydnonimine/, a psychological stimulant, phenamine, cola, etc.], and alleviate the fear and psychological stress frequently occurring in individuals finding themselves in extreme situations. Some simple medical instruments are needed: pointed scissors, dressing forceps, a scalpel, and disposable hypodermics.

In addition to the drugs in the medical kit, it might be possible to use the fruit, leaves, roots, etc., of various wild medicinal plants for medical purposes. However, this would require that flight training include instruction in how to identify such plants and their medicinal properties and means of preparation.

III. Survival at High Latitudes

The vast 25 million km^2 polar region lying to the north of the 10° July isotherm is called the Arctic. It includes areas of Eurasia and the North American continent, as well as the Arctic Ocean with all its islands and archipelagos.

The major climatic characteristic of the Arctic is the long period of subfreezing temperatures. The mean annual temperature never exceeds 0 °C, and the mean monthly temperature during the winter drops to -24 to -50 °C.

The central portion of the Arctic is covered with ice throughout the year; the thickness of the ice reaches 2.5–3 m. Ice fields are in constant motion, and the rate fluctuates from several dozen meters to 40–50 km/day.[28] The general direction of ice movement is from east to west. In the summer, fog and rain take the place of cold and blizzards. Fog and cloudy skies impede astronomical determinations of location, as well as orientation and local movement. A unique characteristic of natural conditions in the Arctic is the altered photoperiodicity of the polar day and night. The period of the polar night has a particularly negative effect on the general behavior and status of humans. Its duration gradually increases with increasing latitude, reaching 175 days in the area of the North Pole.

In the Arctic, humans are subject to a multitude of adverse environmental factors. These may be divided into general and specific factors on the basis of their physical and chemical characteristics. The former include cold, harsh aerodynamic conditions, characteristics of nutrition, and other factors common to many areas. The latter category includes changes in photoperiodicity and electromagnetic factors, which affect various aspects of the physiological and psychological performance of humans at high latitudes.[29]

However, when measures are developed to ensure survival of spacecraft crews after landing in the Arctic, the greatest emphasis is placed on protection from the cold. The chilling effects of low temperatures increase with wind speed. Table 1 shows this function, the so-called windchill index.[30]

Clothing plays a crucial role in protecting humans from the cold. As Fig. 3 shows, duration of safe exposure to subfreezing temperatures is a direct function of temperature, type of activity, and the thermal insulating properties of clothing. The graph shows that at a temperature of -5 °C a person dressed in a flight suit will not remain in a state of thermal comfort for longer than half an hour (curve A). An individual can spend the same period at -30 °C if he/she wears woolen underwear and a quilted jacket (curve B), or at -50 °C in woolen underwear, a woolen sweater, and fur jacket and pants (curve C). If the jacket has a warm lining, and is made of water repellent fabric, the person will begin to get chilled only after 45–60 min.[30] Thus, even the warmest clothing can support positive thermal balance in subfreezing ambient temperatures for only a limited time. As soon as heat loss exceeds heat production, the body gradually gets chilled.[31]

To compute approximate duration of cold endurance in individuals wearing clothing with various insulating properties, V.I. Krichagin, V.I. Khrolenko, and A.I. Reznikov[32] constructed a special nomogram (Fig. 4) based on the formula

$$Q = \frac{0.18S(33 - t_B)}{I_{fact}}$$

where Q is the heat flow from the entire surface of the body in kilocalories per hour (kcal/h), S is the surface of the body in square meters (mean 1.6 m^2), I_{fact} the actual insulation of the clothing in "clo units", and t_B is the ambient temperature in degrees Celsius. (Clo is the amount of thermal insulation providing thermal comfort to humans at a state of rest with heat production of 50 cal/m^2·h; 1 clo = 0.18 °C/cal·m^2·h.)

The second (lower) portion of the nomogram enables derivation of the heat deficit in the body using the formula $D = Q - M$, where D is the heat deficit in the body (D = 80 kcal/h corresponds to transition to stage II discomfort; D = 180 kcal/h corresponds to the beginning of stage III discomfort); Q is the total heat loss (in kcal/h) by the body, determined in the upper portion of the nomogram; and M is the heat production of the body (in kcal/h).

Using this nomogram, one can predict approximate acceptable intervals of time for human cold exposure as long as the following initial parameters are known: 1) thermal insulating properties of the clothing, I_{fact} (at rest, with exertion, with or without wind); 2) air temperature (actual or hypothesized); 3) level of exertion; and 4) degree of discomfort deemed acceptable in the given situation. One can also estimate the value of energy expenditure required to prevent humans from freezing before rescue.

Space suits and pressure suits are not designed for prolonged human exposure to low temperatures. Thus, a temporary shelter is needed to provide protection from wind and

Table 1 Windchill index: the chilling capacity of the wind with respect to tissue, expressed as a temperature equivalent[1]

Estimated wind speed		Actual thermometer reading																							
		50		40.0		30.0		20.0		10.0		0		−10.0		−20		−30.0		−40		−50		−60	
		10		4.5		−1.1		−6.7		−12.2		−17.5		−23.3		−29		−34.5		−40		−46		−51	
mi/h	km/h	°F	°C	°F	°C	°F	°C	°F	°C	°F	°C	°F	°C	°F	°C	°F	°C	°F	°C	°F	°C	°F	°C	°F	°C
calm		50	10.0	40	4.5	30	−1.1	20	−6.7	10	−12.2	0	−17.5	−10	−23.3	−20	−29.0	−30	−34.5	−40	−40.0	−50	−46.0	−60	−51.0
5	8.05	48	8.9	37	2.8	27	−2.8	16	−8.9	6	−14.4	−5	−20.5	−15	−26.1	−26	−32.2	−36	−37.8	−47	−43.9	−57	−49.4	−68	−55.6
10	16.1	40	4.5	28	−2.2	16	−8.9	4	−15.6	−9	−22.8	−21	−29.4	−33	−36.1	−46	−43.2	−58	−50.0	−70	−56.7	−83	−63.4	−95	−70.6
15	24.1	36	2.2	22	−5.6	9	−12.8	−5	−20.5	−18	−27.8	−33	−36.1	−45	−42.8	−58	−50.0	−72	−57.8	−85	−65.0	−99	−72.8	−112	−80.0
20	32.2	32	0	18	−7.8	4	−15.6	−10	−23.3	−25	−31.8	−39	−39.4	−53	−47.2	−67	−55.0	−82	−63.3	−96	−71.1	−110	−78.9	−124	−86.7
25	40.2	30	−1.1	16	−8.9	−2	−17.5	−15	−26.1	−29	−33.8	−44	−42.2	−59	−50.6	−74	−58.9	−88	−66.7	−104	−75.6	−118	−83.3	−133	−91.7
30	48.3	28	−2.2	13	−10.6	−2	−19.0	−18	−27.8	−33	−36.1	−48	−44.4	−63	−52.8	−79	−61.7	−94	−70.0	−109	−78.3	−125	−87.2	−140	−95.6
35	56.3	27	−2.8	11	−11.7	−4	−20.0	−20	−28.9	−35	−37.2	−49	−45.0	−67	−55.0	−82	−63.3	−98	−72.2	−113	−80.6	−129	−89.4	−145	−98.3
40	64.4	26	−3.3	10	−12.2	−6	−21.1	−21	−29.4	−37	−38.5	−53	−47.2	−69	−56.1	−85	−65.0	−100	−73.3	−116	−82.2	−132	−91.1	−148	−100.0

Equivalent temperature

(Wind speeds greater than 64.4 km/h (40 mi/h) have little additional effect)

Little danger (for properly clothed person)

Increasing danger

Great danger

Danger from freezing of exposed flesh

Trenchfoot and immersion foot may occur at any point on this chart

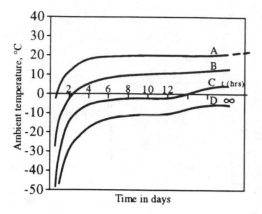

A – summer clothing

B – woolen underwear with cotton padded jacket

C – woolen underwear, woolen sweater, fur jacket and pants

D – same as C, but jacket has thermal lining and is covered with water repellant fabric.

Fig. 3 Endurance time of low temperatures as a function of thermal insulating properties of clothing in different temperature conditions and physical exertion.[30]

cold during the period before rescue. It is natural to use the cabin of the descent module as the first shelter. Field studies in the Arctic have shown that the air temperature in a mock-up of a descent module cabin, with outside air temperature at -30 °C, dropped to -14 °C over a period of 9 h. Rate of chilling of the cabin depends on a variety of factors: quality of external insulation provided by parachute cloth or snow blocks, operation of convective ventilation, frequency of opening of the exit hatch for ventilation and egress of crewmembers, orientation of the exit hatch with respect to the wind, etc.

However, it is impossible to avoid cooling of the cabin, since it has to be aired out periodically. If this is not done, the concentration of CO_2 will increase to the danger point.

Additional means of protection from the cold include the Forel dry suit, parachute cloth, and the metallized cape from the survival kit.[33] Longer periods of survival require a temporary shelter to be constructed from snow. Table 2 shows that air temperature in snow shelters inhabited by humans may exceed external temperatures by 15–20 °C. Even a short period of warming with a candle or dry fuel pellets can increase temperature from -25 to -27 °C outside to -2 to -3 °C inside.[21]

A reliable shelter that does not require a great deal of physical effort to construct makes use of the inflatable life raft,

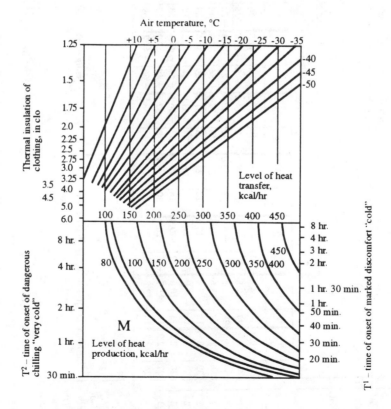

Fig. 4 Nomogram of cold endurance in humans as a function of thermal insulation of clothing, exertion, air temperature, and acceptable level of discomfort.[32]

Table 2   Air temperature in various types of shelters

Shelter type	External temperature, °C	Wind speed, m/s	Maximum temperature in shelter, °C	Maximum temperature during warming with dry fuel, °C	Duration of warming, h
KAPSh-1 tent (not insulated with snow)	- 40 to - 45 - 12	5–7 0	- 32 - 4	– 	–
KAPSh-1 tent (insulated with snow)	- 40	5–7	- 25	–	–
Snow burrow	- 25 to - 33	5–10	- 5	0	–
Snow cave	- 18 to - 27	0–1	- 5	0	3–4
Igloo	- 22 to - 27 - 35 to - 42	6–10 3–5	- 8 - 20	- 3 –	3–4 –
Snow hut insulated with parachute	- 22 to - 27	6–10	- 10	- 4	3–4

which is part of the emergency survival gear on U.S. spacecraft. Given the most modest means of warming (two candles), at a temperature 25 °C below zero, one can increase air temperature within the raft from -20 to +1 °C. Temperatures can be maintained at an even higher level if the raft is insulated with snow blocks.[34]

Many researchers have noted a significant increase in energy expenditure in the Arctic, induced not so much by the direct effects of the cold as by the wearing of heavy clothing and boots, high snow cover, and wind. For example, a change from intermediate weight to warm winter clothing increases energy expenditure by 16 percent, while the bulkiness of the clothing, which impedes movement, increases energy expenditure by another 15 percent.[35] Expenditure of energy in walking at rates of 4 and 4.5 km/h on level terrain in the temperate climatic band of the Arctic was 227 and 442 kcal/h, respectively.[36] This explains the very high caloric values of food rations for the Arctic and Antarctic. For example, daily caloric intake for wintering personnel at the ice stations North Pole-2 and North Pole-3 was 4500–5000 kcal.[37] The caloric value of the rations of wintering personnel at the U.S. Antarctic station reached 5994 kcal/day.[38] According to computations by K. Rodahl, to compensate for energy expended by military personnel in the U.S. Army in Arctic field conditions, rations would have to contain no fewer than 5500–6000 kcal.[39]

Survival rations for Arctic conditions must include the essential nutrients: fats, proteins, carbohydrates, and minerals. Because physiological requirements for vitamins in the Arctic are increased, their levels must also be increased: vitamin C to 150 mg, A to 2.5–3.0 mg, B_1 and B_2 to 5.0 mg, D to 1.25 mg, and nicotinic acid to 30–40 mg.

In Arctic conditions, despite the subfreezing ambient temperatures, water losses can be significant enough to cause dehydration. This danger results from perspiration during heavy physical work in warm clothing, the extreme dryness

and low temperature of inhaled air, and the loss of pulmonary heat and moisture to warm the inhaled air. Dehydration may also be facilitated by so-called cold diuresis, which causes urination frequency to increase to up to 10–15 times per day. This is induced by increased outflow of blood to the internal organs, and reabsorption of fluid in the kidneys.[37,40,41] However, attempts to arrest dehydration by increasing water intake are not always successful. This can be explained by the large quantity of sodium chloride in the urine, which causes a fluid-electrolyte imbalance and resultant fluid losses. To arrest this process, it is recommended that a daily dose of 0.5 gram soda (sodium bicarbonate) be ingested.[25] Daily consumption of water in the Arctic should be approximately 2–3 liters of water under conditions of moderate exertion[42] and 1.0–1.5 liters under conditions of light exertion.[4,43]

During the summer in the Central Polar Basin, the supply of fresh water can be supplemented from pools of melted snow formed on the surface of ice fields, from snow that has been desalinized over a period of many years, or from the outer layers of snow containing salt in quantities no greater than 7–10 mg percent. In the tundra, water can also be obtained from brooks and lakes.

The body is placed under particular stress traversing long distances in the Arctic. Low temperatures, wind, blinding blizzards, and other obstacles create problems that can be overcome only with a great deal of effort.

Expenditure of effort and energy when traversing terrain depends not only on rate of motion and weight of load carried, but also on the nature of the area and its terrain and soil. Energy expenditure while skiing on a smooth, level trail with a load of 15–35 kg at a rate of 3.7 km/h is 6.6 kcal/min. When the rate increases to 6.6 km/h, energy increases to 7.9 kcal/min, and at 10.5 km/h, it increases to 14.35 kcal/min.[44] The depth and density of snow cover have a major influence on the amount of energy expenditure. For example, walking at a rate of 2.4 km/h carrying a load of 9 kg through soft snow

g

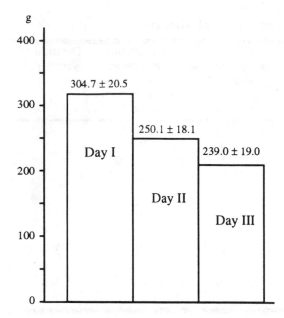

Fig. 5 Mean hourly water loss through sweating in a 3 day experiment involving desert exposure.[21]

with a depth of 10 cm, 20 cm, or 30 cm demands energy expenditures of 6.2, 9.3, and 12.4 kcal/min, respectively. If walking rate increases to 4 km/h, energy expended is 10.0, 13.0, and 16.0 kcal/min, respectively.

Bakhilly (fabric covers worn over footwear) are very effective in preventing boots from getting wet. Because of the air layer that forms on the boots' surfaces, temperatures remain relatively warm. The water vapor condenses on the inner surface of the bakhilly, which serves to dry the boots. It is recommended that plastic bags be put on over the socks, with a second pair of socks over the plastic. The "dead air" space formed provides reliable thermal insulation for the feet.

Keeping the head and face warm is especially important, since the heat emitted from these areas comprises 50–75 percent of the heat lost from the body.[45]

As was noted above, low temperatures combined with high wind speeds are particularly dangerous. In this situation, heat loss increases sharply, reaching extremes of 600–650 kcal/h. Heat generation cannot adequately compensate for this heat loss. As a result, the body loses heat and rapidly chills. Thus, body temperatures of subjects participating in a 40 h march through the tundra at an air temperature of -15 to -40 °C with wind reaching up to 20 m/s decreased from 3 to 35.4 °C.[37] In addition, when wind speed exceeds 10 m/s, normal respiration is disrupted since the airflow impedes inhalation and exhalation. Even more important, in such a blizzard people lose the ability to think logically, lose their sense of direction, and can easily freeze to death. "There can be no doubt," wrote the famous English polar explorer, Robert Scott, "that in a blizzard a man has not only to safeguard the circulation in his limbs, but struggle with a sluggishness of brain and an absence of reasoning power, which is far more likely to undo him."[46]

Long-term exposure of humans to low-temperature conditions, especially in windy weather, with inadequate clothing and no shelter or means for producing warmth may lead to hypothermia. Contributing factors may be exhaustion, lack of food, blood loss, etc.

Strenuous physical exertion in heavy clothing at low ambient temperatures is associated with copious perspiration. When perspiration soaks the clothing, the insulating properties of the clothing decrease. To prevent this, it is necessary to remove the outer clothing and ventilate the space beneath the clothing by unbuttoning the collar and cuffs. However, low temperatures, especially in the presence of wind, may lead to frostbite on the exposed areas of the body.

In the spring, individuals may suffer from snow blindness, which is burning of the conjunctiva and cornea by the Sun's ultraviolet rays reflected from snow crystals. Light-filtering sunglasses can provide reliable protection against snow blindness.

IV. Survival in the Desert

Deserts occupy one-fifth of the Earth's land mass.[47] Their climate is marked by high temperatures (up to 50–55 °C), high levels of solar radiation, and extremely low precipitation (not exceeding 100–120 ml per year).

Air temperature and direct and reflected solar radiation create high thermal loading on the human body, reaching 300 or more kcal/h.[48] Since the vital processes of humans and higher animals occur at a fixed, constant body temperature, even relatively slight shifts in either direction lead to changes in the processes of metabolism and the functional state of many organs and systems. When body temperature increases by a mere 2 °C, there are disruptions in the activity of the cardiovascular system, and work capacity diminishes. An increase of 4–5 °C or more is incompatible with life.

Either body temperature or the amount of excess heat per unit body surface can serve as the criterion for endurance of heat loads. A number of authors consider the critical body temperature to be 37.4–39.4 °C.[49–51]

The maximum endurable accumulation of heat in the body is 65–100 kcal/m². (See Refs. 50–53.) S. M. Gorodinskiy and coworkers have experimentally established that the maximum endurable thermal accumulation for conditions of rest is 89 ± 6 kcal/m². (See Ref. 54.)

Under ordinary conditions, excess heat is eliminated from the body in several ways: through convection, through radiation, through evaporation of water from the lungs, through heating of food and inspired air, by conduction through objects, and through perspiration. However, as ambient air temperature increases, perspiration becomes increasingly important. At temperatures of 34–35 °C, the evaporation of perspiration becomes the sole means through which the body can eliminate heat. Water has a high potential heat of evaporation. Thus, evaporation of 1 gram of water requires 50 kcal. Some of the water, approximately 250–1700 grams, is emitted directly from the surface of the body. This is the so-called "insensible perspiration" or "insensible weight loss." However, to combat serious hyperthermia, the body is equipped with a system of sweat glands. At an ambient temperature of 37–38 °C, loss of water through perspiration is approximately 300 grams/h; at temperatures of 42 °C and higher, it increases to 1–2 kg/h. Under short-term stress, the production of the sweat glands may reach 4.2 kg/h.[55] With heavy physical exertion in heat, humans may lose 10–12 kg of fluid per day.[48] It has been noted that as dehydration develops perspiration is inhibited. According to S. Robinson's data, at 3–4 percent dehydration, perspiration decreases by 15–20 percent.[56] As Fig. 5 shows, during their third day in a desert experiment, subjects' mean hourly perspiration decreased from 304.7 ± 20.5 to 239.0 ± 19.0 grams.[21]

Since sweat contains 0.2–0.4 percent sodium chloride, profuse perspiration may pose the threat of a salt deficit. When concentration of sodium chloride in sweat decreases to 0.1–0.15 percent, the body reacts by decreasing urination and increasing resorption of sodium in the renal tubules. Even given limited options under conditions of survival in the desert, the danger of pathological effects of heat can be minimized if individuals are sheltered from the effects of direct and reflected solar radiation, use the available water supply rationally, and limit physical activity during the hottest part of the day.

Reliable protection from solar radiation can be provided by a tent made of parachute cloth. Even the simplest shelter will decrease radiative heat transfer by 72–114 kcal/h, and convective heat transfer (from heated sand) by approximately 100 kcal/h.[48] Clothing plays an important protective role by preventing direct exposure of the skin to radiation, as well as preventing contact with convection heat from heated air.

The use of the spacecraft cabin as a temporary shelter is possible only if there is mechanical (forced) ventilation.

The decisive factor in desert survival is water. At air temperatures of 40–45 °C and with limited physical activity, approximately 4–5 liters/day are required. An experiment with night marches has shown the requirement to be no less than 7–8 liters of water under such conditions.[57] When water supplies are limited, the best procedure is to consume water in small portions, since in this way up to 80 percent of the water is used by the body as perspiration.

The sensation of thirst acts as a signal that the body needs water. However, thirst is slaked when only 60–80 percent of the deficit is compensated for. Thus, to compensate for true water loss, an additional 300–500 ml of water must be drunk. However, it should be remembered that when fluid loss amounts to 2–3 percent of body weight, it takes 5–6 h to compensate for the deficit, and when water loss is 5 percent, full compensation requires at least a day.[58]

Since physical work increases production of metabolic heat, it must be held to a minimum during the hottest portion of the day.

As noted above, water loss through perspiration is accompanied by loss of salt. However, additional intake of sodium chloride is advisable only for fluid losses greater than 3–5

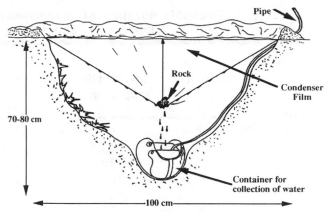

Fig. 6 Solar condenser.

liters.[59] Otherwise, intake of table salt may increase excretion of potassium and lead to a potassium deficit.[60] When the concentration of potassium in plasma drops below 1.5 mM/liter, cardiac activity may be disrupted. If potassium levels decrease further, the respiratory muscles may undergo paralysis.

Obtaining water in the desert is extremely difficult because of the scarcity of natural water sources. To obtain water, a polyethylene bag water collector is placed on plants and fastened at the bottom. Its productivity is up to 0.5–0.6 liters/day. Solar condensers (Fig. 6), which operate through absorption of moisture from the sand and subsequent condensation on the internal surface of a hydrophobic film, can also be used. One condenser may produce up to 1.5 liters of water per day.

Analyzing survival factors in the desert, one may conclude that duration of survival will depend primarily on daytime air temperatures and water supplies. This function is depicted in Table 3.

The incidence of diseases in the desert is mainly associated with the effects of high temperatures, solar radiation, and insufficient water consumption. Such diseases include heatstroke and sunstroke, dehydration, and salt depletion. Symptoms of these conditions and methods of treatment are described in various medical references and manuals.

Poisonous snakes present a real danger to human life and health in the desert. In case of snakebite, a cross-shaped cut 0.5–1.0 cm deep is made and the venom is sucked out by mouth if the mucous membrane of the mouth is unbroken, or with a special cupping glass with a rubber bulb. The cuts are rinsed with a weak solution of potassium manganate and hydrogen peroxide, and a sterile bandage is applied. The affected limb is immobilized using an immobilizing splint, as for a fracture. The victim must be given complete rest and must drink a great deal of fluid (tea, coffee, hot water). The most effective means of treatment is subcutaneous or intramuscular injection of a specific antitoxin in a dose of 500–1000 units in mild cases, up to 1500 units in moderately severe cases, and as much as 2000–2500 units in severe cases. It is categorically forbidden to put a tourniquet on the affected limb, give alcohol to the victim, cauterize the area of

Table 3   Probable duration of autonomous survival in the desert as a function of ambient temperature, supplies of water, and amount of activity

Amount of activity	Maximal daytime temp. in shade, °C	Supply of water per person, liters					
		0	1.14	2.27	4.45	11.35	22.72
		Probable duration of autonomous survival, days					
Remaining in tent	49	2	2	2	2.5	3	4.5
	43.3	3	3	3.5	4	5	7
	38	5	5.5	6	7	9.5	13.5
	26.5	7	7	7	10.5	15	23
	21	10	11	12	14	20.5	32
	15.5	10	11	12	14	21	32
	10	10	11	12	14	21	32
Marching at night	49	1	2	2	2.5	3	
	43	2	2	2.5	3	3.5	
	38	3	3.5	3.5	4.5	5.5	
	32	5	5.5	5.5	6.5	8	
	27	7	7.5	8.0	9.5	11.5	
	21	7.5	8.0	9	10.5	13.5	
	16	8	8.5	9	11	14	
	10	8	8.5	9	11	14	

the bite with heated metal, or sprinkle potassium manganate powder on the cut.[61]

Bites of poisonous arachnids and scorpions are also dangerous. Treatment with specific antitoxins is highly effective. One of the reliable means of treatment is cauterization of the wound with a match at the moment of inflammation. The poison thus brought to the surface is easily destroyed, decreasing subsequent poisoning.

V. Survival in the Tropics (Jungle)

All the characteristics of tropical climates are found in the jungle. The mean monthly temperature is 24–29 °C, with fluctuations over the course of a year not exceeding 1–6 °C. Annual total solar radiation reaches 80–100 kcal/cm,[2] which is almost twice as much as the average at latitudes of 40–50°. The air is saturated with water vapor, and thus the relative humidity is high: 80–90 percent. There is no shortage of precipitation in the tropics. Annual precipitation is 1500–12,000 mm.

The abundance and variety of tropical flora are unmatched in any other environment. According to data of the Danish botanist Varming, there may be over 400 species of trees in an area of 3 square miles and up to 30 species of epiphytes on every tree.

Tropical forests are divided into two groups: 1) primary, with a characteristic pluristratose configuration, but completely passable to humans; and 2) secondary, a chaotic mass of trees, bushes, bamboo, and high grass, through which movement is extremely difficult.

In the tropical forest more than other ecosystems, individuals who are unfamiliar with the environment tend to lose confidence in their ability to cope with their surroundings, resulting in depression and anxiety. The uniqueness and unfamiliarity of the environment, combined with the high temperature and humidity, affect the human psyche, leading to high levels of emotional tension, lethargy, and inappropriate behavior.

The combination of high temperature and high humidity in the tropics creates extremely adverse heat exchange conditions for humans. When high ambient temperatures makes heat elimination through convection and radiation impossible, evaporation of perspiration is the last available route through which the body can rid itself of excess heat. However if the air is saturated with moisture, evaporation will not occur. A state of hyperthermia may occur at temperatures of 30–31 °C if relative humidity is 85 percent. At a temperature of 45 °C and humidity of 65 percent, heat transfer ceases completely. The severity of the discomfort experienced depends upon the ability to perspire. When 75 percent of the sweat glands are operating, the sensation is described as "hot" and, when all glands are functioning, as "very hot."

V.I. Krichagin[62] developed a special chart to estimate the thermal status of the body as a function of stress on the perspiration system under conditions of high temperature and humidity. This chart visually represents human endurance of high ambient temperature (Fig. 7). In the first and second zones, thermal equilibrium is maintained without any special stress on the sweat glands, but even in the third zone, maintaining the body below the discomfort point requires constant, although moderate, stress on the perspiration system. In this zone, wearing of any clothing causes discomfort. In the fourth zone (zone of high perspiration rate), evaporation of sweat becomes insufficient to maintain normal thermal balance and the general state of the body gradually deteriorates. In the fifth zone, even maximal stress on the perspiration system cannot prevent accumulation of heat. Long-term exposure to these conditions inevitably leads to heatstroke. In the sixth zone, hyperthermia is inevitable if temperature increases by only 0.2–1.2 °C. Finally, in the seventh and most adverse zone, duration of exposure is limited to 1.5–2 h.

Profuse perspiration in response to thermal loading leads to loss of fluid. This has a negative effect on the cardiorespiratory system and also adversely influences muscle contractility. Muscle fatigue develops because of changes in the physical properties of colloids and their subsequent destruction.

To maintain positive fluid balance and support human thermal regulation in the tropics, lost fluid must continually be replaced. The quantity of fluid intake and the drinking schedule are extremely important, as is water temperature. The colder the water, the longer the endurance time in a hot environment. For example, drinking 3 liters of water at a temperature of 12 °C eliminates 75 kcal from the body. D. Gold,[31] who studied human heat exchange in a thermal chamber at temperatures of 54.4–71 °C, established that drinking water chilled to 1–2 °C increased endurance of these conditions by 50–100 percent. Decrease of temperature of drinking water to 7–15 °C was also effective.[63] In the tropics, profuse perspiration in response to physical exertion, along with dehydration, leads to significant salt loss. To prevent this, physiologists recommend, aside from abundant fluid intake, ingestion of sodium chloride. With fluid loss due to perspiration above 5.6 liters, salt may be ingested in the form of a powder, tablets, or a 0.1–0.2 percent solution in the amount of 2 grams/L of fluid.[64,65]

Food may be obtained by hunting, fishing, and foraging for wild edible plants. Many fruits, shoots, and roots of tropical plants (Table 4) contain virtually all the essential nutrients.[7]

Constant high temperature and humidity and the characteristics of the flora and fauna create conditions conducive to the development of a number of tropical diseases that can be a direct threat to the health of crewmembers. These conditions include heat exhaustion, heatstroke, bites of poisonous animals, ingestion of poisonous plants, infestation with worms indigenous to the soil and water, and finally, tropical diseases, such as malaria and yellow fever transmitted by vectors such as mosquitoes and midges.

Methods for preventing and treating tropical diseases are described in detail in special handbooks.[66,67] However, the importance of taking preventive measures against flying blood-feeding insects by the use of various repellents in the form of ointments and lotions should be emphasized. Wipes in the form of multilayers of gauze soaked in repellent in

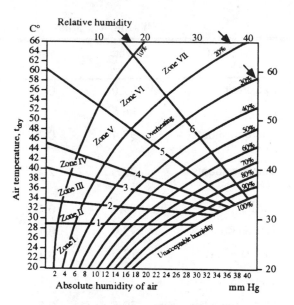

Fig. 7 Graph of endurance of high temperature and humidity.

hermetically sealed packets are particularly convenient. Such wipes can provide protection from insect bites for 3.5 h.[68]

VI. Survival in the Ocean

If a spacecraft splashes down in the open ocean, it will be recovered by sea and air rescue systems. Before rescue, the crew may remain in the descent module cabin. In calm conditions, this presents no problems, since the hatch may be left open, providing reliable ventilation. However, in a sea state of 3–4 or more, there is a risk that water will enter the cabin and impair stability and buoyancy. If the life support system has a reliable ventilation system, the crew may remain in the cabin with the hatch closed. However, if the life support system fails or the electrical power supply is interrupted, the cabin will begin to fill with carbon dioxide, and temperature and humidity will begin to exceed acceptable levels. If the cabin microclimate deteriorates, threatening the health of the cosmonauts, or if the buoyancy or stability of the descent module is impaired for any reason, the crew will be obliged to abandon the spacecraft and use the emergency flotation devices.

It is well known that the maximal temperatures of ocean surface waters do not exceed 29–30 °C. At the same time, even at water temperature as high as 33.3 °C, the human body begins to lose heat.[69] The lower the water temperature, the faster the process of chilling. For example, if the water temperature is 22 °C, the body loses 100 kcal every 4 min. As a result, body temperature eventually drops to life-threatening levels.

The period of time during which the human body can safely remain in the water is a function of water temperature. Even at a temperature of 24 °C, this period is only 7–9 h.[70] At 10–15 °C, the period is reduced to half. Water at a temperature of 2–3 °C leads to fatal hypothermia in 10–15 min, and at -2 °C,

Table 4   Food value (percentage) of wild edible plants [21]

Plant	Water	Fat	Protein	Carbohy-drates	Cellulose	Inorganic substance	Calories per 100 g
Breadfruit	87.0	0.2	0.6	10.3	1.2	0.2	44.0
Papaya	86.6	–	0.6	12.6	0.2	0.6	22.9
Bamboo shoots (fresh)	92.4	0.2	1.9	0.7	4.1	0.7	11.4
Bamboo shoots (dried)	22.6	2.1	22.7	13.8	30.8	8.0	115.6
Banana	89.4	0.1	0.6	7.1	1.3	1.5	30.7
Banana flower	92.0	0.1	1.4	4.5	0.6	1.1	24.8
Ku-may fruit (*Diocorea persimilis*)	73.0	0.1	1.1	24.0	1.6	0.2	96.5
Mong-nga tuber (*Angiopteris cohindunensis de Wrise Mon.*)	70.5	0.8	1.2	25.5	0.2	1.8	135.5
Guava	76.0	0.2	1.5	14.6	0.8	6.9	64.0
Dy-khy fruit (*Hodgsonia macrocarpa Cogniaux*)	5.6	62.1	1.3	31.0	–	–	710.0
Zy-gam fruit (*Gnetum formosum Mgf.*)	39.0	2.7	4.5	52.0	0.8	1.0	260.7
Dates	15.4	12.5	1.5	69.3	1.3	–	220.2
Coconut flesh	16.6	43.4	3.7	32.4	3.3	0.6	512.8
Mango	82.0	1.0	3.4	12.5	0.5	0.6	69.8
Cassava root	67.8	0.25	1.17	28.6	1.3	1.08	117.0

the survival period is reduced to 5–8 min.[24]

After disasters at sea in areas with water temperatures ranging from -1.1 to +9 °C, sailors and passengers began to die within 5–20 min.[71] According to other data, exposure to water temperatures of 0–10 °C leads to death in 20–40 min.[21,72] Most researchers have assumed that the cause of death in such a short period is hypothermia. However, Canadian scientists have demonstrated that even in icy water the rate of chilling of the core does not exceed 5.6–6 °C/h. Thus, fatal hypothermia would require at least 60–90 min.[73] Human death after shorter intervals evidently occurs as a result of cold shock induced by massive stimulation of the cold receptors of the skin,[74] a breathing disorder, or ventricular fibrillation.[72,75]

To ensure the safety of cosmonauts utilizing flotation devices, the survival kit on a Russian spacecraft contains the Forel antiexposure dry suit, consisting of an airtight shell, colored bright orange to facilitate detection, along with gloves and boots, all made of waterproof material. To increase Forel's thermal insulating properties of up to 3.5 clo, an antiexposure

thermal protection suit is included. Research performed in the Barents Sea has shown that the dry suit protects humans from hypothermia in icy water for more than 12 h. In tropical water, where water temperature reaches 29–30 °C, an individual may remain in the water for more than 3 days without experiencing cold.[30]

Medical aid to individuals rescued from cold water primarily involves active warming. The most effective warming technique is to immerse the victim in water with a temperature of 34–36 °C, which is gradually increased to 40°.[75] Hot water bottles may be applied to the sides of the chest cage and the groin.

American spacecraft that are scheduled to land in the water are provided with inflatable rafts as part of their survival kits. Research on tropical oceans has shown that although the microclimate of the area under the tent on SP-6 type rafts is harsher during the day than on an open boat, with higher temperature and humidity, subjects on the raft reported feeling significantly better than subjects on the boat. Their performance levels were higher, they experienced less thirst, and they felt better, despite some thermal discomfort. The subjects on the raft had somewhat lower sublingual temperature and less extra-renal fluid loss.

It is interesting that the simplest measures significantly diminish fluid loss, and increase safe survival duration. For example, subjects unremittingly exposed to the sun lost 420 ± 15 ml of water per hour. However, simply wetting the undershirt with water from the sea decreased water loss to 170 ± 13 ml/h.[37] Survival rations, particularly those high in carbohydrates, are a recommended food supply during long-term survival at sea. Research performed in the Black Sea in the late 1970s showed that, among rations equal in caloric value (400 kcal/day), pure carbohydrates caused the least amount of renal fluid loss; furthermore, subjects felt better.[21]

An important problem for survival at sea is supply of fresh water. Aside from water supplies in the survival kit, fresh water may be obtained from seawater by using various types of distilling devices. Drinking untreated seawater has been categorically forbidden since 1959 by the World Health Organization,[76] since seawater induces profound disturbances in the function of a number of organs and systems. As numerous investigations in the United States, England, and the Soviet Union have shown, daily ingestion of 500 ml of fresh water supports life in the tropics. Simple measures, such as staying in the shade, wetting the clothes with seawater, and limiting physical activity during the hottest part of the day, significantly decrease water loss due to perspiration, further reducing the threat of dehydration.

Thus, if a spacecraft crew acts appropriately during an unscheduled splashdown and uses the survival gear and material at hand correctly, the chances of survival will be greatly increased in any geographic region of the globe.

VII. Survival Training of Crewmembers

There is only a small probability that today's spacecraft will land in an unpopulated area. This is especially true of the Shuttle, which can land only in specially equipped airfields, and it is virtually impossible to abandon ship in space. Nevertheless, even if the possibility is small, the crews of spacecraft must be trained for survival. To be prepared for spacecraft landing in an unscheduled area in an inaccessible location or for splashdown in the ocean, the crew not only must have access to emergency equipment, but also must possess special knowledge and skills essential for protecting themselves from adverse, sometimes extreme, climatic conditions and for obtaining food and water until they are rescued. For this reason, survival training is one of the most important components of space crew training programs. Such training in the classroom focuses on general issues of long-term survival in an unpopulated area, the physical geographical regions of a possible landing site, and the use of emergency equipment. Crewmembers also develop orientation skills and learn to use standard and available means for signaling, to construct temporary shelters out of various materials at hand

(snow, branches, parachute cloth, etc.), and to establish radio communications using the emergency radio set. During the final stage of training, crewmembers go out in the field in conditions simulating those of long-term survival in an unpopulated area under various physical/geographical conditions.[33,77,78] For example, at Perrin Air Base (Texas), American astronauts studied survival skills for 5 days.[79] During a 3 day training session in Stend Air Force Base (Nevada), they mastered the construction of shelters made of snow and branches, and were taught techniques for orientation in the taiga, etc.[80,81] The training program also included 12 h on a life raft.[82] The success of teaching survival procedures depends on providing students with clear ideas of how to act in actual conditions.[81] An important aspect is teaching crewmembers how to see objects in the environment from the point of view of their use in survival: for example, a tree as a source of shade or material for a fire, an anthill for determining which way is north, a watch glass for starting a fire, and pins to be bent into fish hooks.

However, it is even more important to prepare members of space crews psychologically for survival. This will build self-confidence and help them develop a kind of natural resistance to stress situations. It will also reinforce the major postulate of survival: that one can and will maintain one's life and health in the harshest physical/geographical conditions if one knows how to use everything provided by the natural environment. Training also imparts tenacity, willpower, steadfastness, and ingenuity.

References

[1]Berry, C. Descent and landing of space crews and survival in an unpopulated area. In: Calvin, M., and Gazenko, O.G., Eds. *Foundations of Space Biology and Medicine*, Washington D.C., NASA Hq., 1975, Vol. III, pp. 345–372.

[2]Volovich, V.G. *One on One With Nature*. Moscow, Voyenizdat, 1989 (in Russian).

[3]U.S.S.R. State Standard Long-term survival and rescue of aircraft crews after forced landing or splashdown. GOST 24 215-80, Moscow, U.S.S.R. State Commission on Standards, 1980 (in Russian).

[4]Nicholson, J.E. Survival stress. *Flying*, 1968, vol. 83, pp. 46–47.

[5]Thyurst, J.S. Individual reactions to community disaster. The natural history of psychiatric phenomena. *American Journal of Psychiatry,* 1951, vol. 107, pp. 764–769.

[6]McLaughlin, D.R. Survival: Thinking cool. *Aerospace Safety*, 1981, vol. 36, no. 2, pp. 16–19.

[7]Volovich, V.G. Survival medicine: Tasks and prospects. *Journal of Wilderness Medicine*, 1992, no. 3, pp. 256–259.

[8]Korolenko, Ts.P. *Human Psychology in Extreme Conditions*. Leningrad, Nauka, 1978 (in Russian).

[9]Verheij, T. *Medical Aspects of Survival*. Oslo, Loughton, 1983.

[10]Singer, T.J. An introduction to disaster: Some considerations of a psychological nature. *Aviation, Space and Envi-*

ronmental Medicine, 1982, vol. 53, no. 3, pp. 245–250.

[11]Deaton, J.E. The psychology of survival. *Approach,* 1981, vol. 27, pp. 3–8.

[12]Tucker, G.J. Psychological aspects of sea survival. *Approach,* 1966, vol. 7, no. 9, pp 26–30.

[13]Simonov, P.V. Emotional reactions of humans to extreme factors. In: *Physiology of Extreme States and Individual Protection Measures,* Moscow, Meditsina, 1982, pp. 7–8 (in Russian).

[14]Kitayev-Smyk, L.A. *The Psychology of Stress.* Moscow, Nauka, 1983 (in Russian).

[15]Maniguet, X. *Survivre.* Paris, Albin Michel, 1988.

[16]Martinez, M. To save a life. *Airman,* 1968, vol. 12, no. 4, pp. 34–37.

[17]Gilbert, W.W. Life successfully ejected over water. What next? *Proceedings of the Annual Symposium of Survival and Flight Equipment Association,* San Diego, Calif., 1968, pp. 17–33.

[18]Cahill, G.F. Starvation in man. *New England Journal of Medicine,* 1970, vol. 282, pp. 668–675.

[19]Nikolayev, Yu.S. Development of the ideas of therapeutic fasting. In: *Problems of Therapeutic Fasting,* Moscow, Medgiz, 1969, pp, 19–48 (in Russian).

[20]Young, V.R., and Scrimshaw, N. The physiology of starvation. *Scientific American,* 1971, vol. 225, no. 4, pp. 14–21.

[21]Volovich, V.G. *Man in Extreme Environmental Conditions.* Moscow, Mysl, 1983 (in Russian).

[22]Pokrovskiy, A.A. *Discussions on Nutrition.* Moscow, Medgiz, 1964 (in Russian).

[23]Whittingam, R.G. Factors affecting the survival of man in hostile environments. In: *Textbook of Aviation Physiology,* 1965, pp. 479–507.

[24]Weis, I. Survival - Fakten und Daten aus klimatologischer Sicht. *Truppen-Praxis,* 1974, no. 3, pp. 205–210.

[25]Rogers, T.A., and Eksnis, E.G. Studies on Arctic survival. *Proceedings of the XVIIIth National Congress on Aviation and Space Medicine,* Oslo, 1969, pp. 236–240.

[26]Bychkov, V.N.; Ushakov, A.S.; Kondratyev, Yu.I.; and Kasatkina, A.G. Survival rations of dry products in polymer packets. *Voyenno-Meditsinskiy Zhurnal,* 1963, no. 10, pp. 70–73 (in Russian).

[27]Koshcheyev, A.K. *Wild Edible Plants.* Moscow, Pishchevaya Promyshlennost, 1980 (in Russian).

[28]Vize, V.Yu. *The Seas of the Soviet Arctic.* Leningrad, Glavsevmorputi, 1948 (in Russian).

[29]Kaznacheyev, V.N. *Contemporary Aspects of Adaptation.* Novosibirsk, Nauka, 1980 (in Russian).

[30]Nesbitt, P.H.; Pond, A.W.; and Allen, W.H. *The Survival Book.* New York, 1959.

[31]Gold, J. Calorie neutralization during thermal stress. *Aerospace Medicine,* Nov. 1960, vol. 31, no. 11.

[32]Krichagin, V.I.; Khrolenko V.M.; and Reznikov, A.I. Cold endurance as a function of the protective properties of clothing. *Voyenno-Meditsinskiy Zhurnal,* 1968, no. 10, pp. 54–58 (in Russian).

[33]Volovich, V.G. Crew behavior in contingency landings. In: Gazenko, O.G., Ed. *Space Biology and Medicine,* Moscow, Nauka, 1987, pp, 194–228 (in Russian).

[34]Westergaard, F.G. Dingy on the ice cap. *The MAC Flyer,* 1972, Vol. 19, no. 8, pp. 19–22.

[35]Goldman, R.F., and Teitlebaum, A. Increased energy cost and multiple clothing layers. *Journal of Applied Physiology,* 1972, vol. 33, pp. 181–182.

[36]Boriskin, V.V. *Human Life in the Arctic and Antarctic,* Leningrad, Meditsina, 1973 (in Russian).

[37]Volovich, V.G. *Life Support of Crews of Flight Vehicles After Forced Landings and Splashdowns,* Moscow, Nauka, 1976 (in Russian).

[38]Milan, F.A., and Rodahl, K. Caloric requirements of man in the Antarctic. *Journal of Nutrition,* 1961, vol. 75, no. 2, pp. 152–156.

[39]Rodahl, K. Nutritional requirements in cold climates. *Journal of Nutrition,* 1954, no. 53, pp. 575–588.

[40]Paleyev, N.R. On physiological shifts in the human body under conditions of work on drifting stations. In: *Issues of Acclimatization of the Population in the Arctic,* 1959, vol. 92, pp. 242–244.

[41]Rogers, T.A.; Setlif, J.A.; and Buck, A.S. Minimal rations for Arctic survival. *Aerospace Medicine,* 1968, vol. 39, no. 6, pp. 585–587.

[42]Kandror, I.S. Physiological shifts in the human body during acclimatization in the Far North. In: *Human Health in the Far North,* Moscow, Medgiz, 1963, pp. 13–27 (in Russian).

[43]Hawkins, M.F. Problems of survival resulting from passenger aircraft accidents in the Arctic. *Proceedings of XVIIIth National Congress on Aviation and Space Medicine,* Oslo, 1969, Aug., p. 81.

[44]Soul, R.G, and Goldman, R.F. Terrain coefficients for energy cost predictions. *Journal of Applied Physiology,* 1972, vol. 32, 15, pp. 706–708.

[45]Petykowski, J.L. Down in cold weather. *Aerospace Safety,* 1978, vol. 34, no. 2, pp. 10–13.

[46]Scott, R.F. *Scott's Last Expedition,* London, Smith, Elder & Co., 1913, p. 343.

[47]Babayev, A.G.; Drozdov, N.N.; Zonn, I.S.; and Freykin, Z.G. *Deserts.* Moscow, Mysl, 1986 (in Russian).

[48]Adolf, E. *Physiology of Man in the Desert,* Moscow, Inostrannaya Literatura, 1952 (translated into Russian).

[49]Afanesyeva, R.F.; Dedenko, N.I.; and Okunev, S.G. On certain indications characterizing the limits of human endurance of heat loading. *Kosmicheskaya Biologiya i Meditsina,* 1970, no. 4, pp. 48–51 (in Russian).

[50]Hall, J.F., and Polte, J.W. Physiological index of strain and body heat storage in hyperthermia. *Journal of Applied Physiology,* 1960, vol. 15, pp. 1027–1030.

[51]Azhayev, A.N. *Physiological and Hygienic Aspects of the Effects of High and Low Temperatures,* Moscow, Nauka, 1979 (in Russian).

[52]Webb, P. Temperature stress. In: Armstrong H.G., Ed., *Aerospace Medicine,* Baltimore, Williams and Wilkins, 1961,

pp. 633–640.

[53]Kaufman, W.C. Human tolerance limits for some thermal environments of aerospace. *Aerospace Medicine*, 1963, vol. 34, no. 10, pp. 889–896.

[54]Gorodinskiy, S.M.; Bovro, G.V.; Perfilova, Ye.M.; Pletenskiy, Yu.G.; and Salivon, S.G. On the dynamics of thermal stress and the human endurance limits for thermal loading. *Kosmicheskaya Biologiya*, 1968, no. 1, vol. 73–81 (in Russian).

[55]Machle, C.W., and Hatch, T.F. Heat: Man's exchanges and physiological responses. *Physiological Review*, 1947, vol. 27, no. 2, pp. 200–228.

[56]Robinson, S. Temperature regulation in exercise. *Pediatrics*, 1963, no. 32, pp. 691–702.

[57]Kondratenko, N.N. Across Karakum. *Prostor*, 1987, no. 1, pp. 118–148 (in Russian).

[58]Yunusov, A.Yu. *High Temperature and Fluid-Electrolyte Metabolism*. Tashkent, Soviet Academy of Sciences, 1969 (in Russian).

[59]Dmitriyev, M.V. Drinking schedules in high ambient temperatures. In: *Physiology of Heat Exchange and Hygiene of Industrial Climate*, Moscow, Nauka, 1961, pp. 286–299 (in Russian).

[60]Boaz, T.D. Some comments on water and salt. *Military Medicine*, 1969, vol. 134, pp. 413–415.

[61]Sultanov, M.N. *Poisonous Animal Bites*, Moscow, Medgiz, 1963 (in Russian).

[62]Krichagin, V.I. Devices and methods for estimating endurance of high and low ambient temperatures. *Voyenno-Meditsinskiy Zhurnal*, 1965, no. 10, pp. 30–38 (in Russian).

[63]McPherson, R.K. *Physiological Responses to Hot Environments*, London, Her Majesty's Stationery Office, 1960.

[64]Silchenko, K.K. Acclimatization of personnel to hot climates. *Voyenno-Meditsinskiy Zhurnal*, 1974, no. 5, pp. 52–54 (in Russian).

[65]Malhotra, M. S.; Sridharan, K.; and Venkaswamy, J. Potassium losses in sweat under heat stress. *Aviation Space and Environmental Medicine*, 1976, vol. 47, no. 5, pp. 503–508.

[66]Moshkovskiy, Sh.D., and Plotnikov, N.N. *A Short Handbook on Infectious and Parasitic Diseases of Hot Climates*, Moscow, Medgiz, 1957 (in Russian).

[67]Kassirskiy, I.A., and Plotnikov, N.N. *Diseases of Hot Climates*, Moscow, Medgiz, 1964 (in Russian).

[68]Shtunderenko, G.V.; Burykina A.P.; and Kharitonova, S.I. Efficacy of repellent wipes in field conditions. *Voyenno-Meditsinskiy Zhurnal*, 1976, no. 6, p. 76 (in Russian).

[69]Joiner, W.C. Cold water immersion. *Aerospace Safety*, 1978, vol. 34, no. 1, pp. 6–7.

[70]Carlson, L.D.; Hsien, A.C.L.; Fullington, F.; and Eisner, R.W. Immersion in cold water and body tissue insulation. *Journal of Aviation Medicine*, 1958, vol. 29, pp. 145–152.

[71]McCance, R.A.; Unglay, C.C.; Crosfill, J.W.L.; and Widdowson, E.M. The hazards to men in ships lost at sea, 1940-1944. Medical Research Council, Special Report Series, no. 291, London, Her Majesty's Stationery Office, 1956.

[72]Keating, W.R. *Survival In Cold Water*, Oxford, England, Blackwell Scientific Publication, 1969.

[73]Hayward, J.S., and Eckerson, J.D. Physiological responses and survival time predictions for humans in ice-water. *Aviation, Space and Environmental Medicine*, 1984, vol. 55, no. 3, pp. 106–122.

[74]Beckman, E.L.; Reeves, E.; and Goldman, R.F. Current concepts and practices applicable to the control of body heat loss in aircrew subjected to water immersion. *Aerospace Medicine*, 1966, vol. 37, pp. 348–357.

[75]Harnett, R.M.; Pruitt, J.R.; and Sias, F.R. A review of the literature concerning resuscitation from hyperthermia. Part II - Selected rewarming protocols. *Aviation, Space and Environmental Medicine*, 1983, vol. 54, no. 6, pp. 487–495.

[76]The danger of drinking sea water. *WHO Chronicle*, 1962, vol. 16, no. 9, pp. 343–345.

[77]Beregovoy, G.T.; Yaropolov V.I.; and Baranetskiy I.I. *Handbook on Space Flight Safety*, Moscow, Mashinostroyeniye, 1989, p. 336 (in Russian).

[78]*Air Force Times*. 1968, vol. 29, no. 6, p. 30.

[79]Cosmonaut training. *Kosmicheskaya Biologiya i Aviakosmicheskaya Meditsina*, 1968, no. 7, p. 58 (in Russian).

[80]Scientists, engineers seek roles in space. *Aviation Week and Space Technology,* 1964, vol. 81, no. 21, pp. 48–49.

[81]Colin, J. Man in space. *Kosmicheskaya Biologiya i Aviakosmicheskaya Meditsina*, 1968, no. 7, pp. 4–24.

[82]Slayton, D. Astronaut training and preflight preparations. *Proceedings of the Conference on the Results of the First U.S. Manned Suborbital Flight,* Jun. 6, 1961.

[83]Korobeynikov, M.P. *Modern Warfare and Psychological Problems*, Moscow, 1972, p. 132.

Appendix: Units of Measurement

International System of Units (SI)

Quantity	Unit	Symbol International	Russian	
		International	Russian	
1. Basic Units				
Length	meter	m	м	
Mass	kilogram	kg	кг	
Time	second	s	с	
Electric current	ampere	A	а	
Temperature	degree Kelvin	K	К	
Luminous intensity	candela	cd	кд	
Quantity of substance		mol	мол	
2. Supplementary Units				
Plane angle	radian	rad	рад.	
Solid angle	steradian	sr	ср	
3. Derived Units in Volume II				
Force	newton	N	Н	$kg \cdot m \cdot s^{-2}$
Pressure	pascal (N/m^2)	Pa	Па	$kg \cdot m^{-1} \cdot s^{-2}$
Work, energy, quantity of heat	joule	J	Дж	$kg \cdot m^2 \cdot s^{-2}$
Power	watt	W	вт	$kg \cdot m^2 \cdot s^{-3}$
Luminous flux	lumen	lm	лм	$cd \cdot sr$
Illumination	lux	lx	лк	$Lm \cdot m^{-2}$

Measures of Length

	inch	foot	yard	mile	centimeter	meter	kilometer
inch	1	0.083	$2.78 \cdot 10^{-2}$	$1.58 \cdot 10^{-5}$	2.54	$2.54 \cdot 10^{-2}$	$2.54 \cdot 10^{-5}$
foot	12	1	0.333	$1.89 \cdot 10^{-4}$	30.5	0.305	$3.05 \cdot 10^{-4}$
yard	36	3	1	$5.68 \cdot 10^{-4}$	91.44	0.914	$9.1 \cdot 10^{-4}$
mile	$6.34 \cdot 10^4$	5280	1760	1	$1.61 \cdot 10^5$	1609	1.609
centimeter	0.394	$3.28 \cdot 10^{-2}$	$1.09 \cdot 10^{-2}$	$6.21 \cdot 10^{-6}$	1	0.01	10^{-5}
meter	39.4	3.28	1.094	$6.21 \cdot 10^{-4}$	100	1	.001
kilometer	$3.94 \cdot 10^4$	3280	1094	0.621	10^5	1000	1

Measures of Mass

	ounce	pound	gram	kilogram	metric tonne
ounce	1	.0625	28.3	$28.3 \cdot 10^{-2}$	$2.83 \cdot 10^{-5}$
pound	16	1	453	0.453	$4.53 \cdot 10^{-4}$
gram	0.035	$2.204 \cdot 10^{-3}$	1	10^{-3}	10^{-6}
kilogram	35	2.204	1000	1	10^{-3}
metric tone	$3.5 \cdot 10^4$	2204	10^6	1000	1

Units of Pressure

	atm	Pa	bar	kgf/cm^2	cm H$_2$O	mm Hg	psi
atm	1	$1.013 \cdot 10^5$	1.013	1.033	1033	760	14.70
Pa	$9.869 \cdot 10^{-6}$	1	10^{-5}	$1.02 \cdot 10^{-5}$	0.0102	0.0075	$1.451 \cdot 10^{-4}$
bar	0.9869	10^5	1	1.02	1020	750	14.51
kgf/cm^2	0.9681	98,066	.9807	1	1000	735	14.22
cm H$_2$O	$9.68 \cdot 10^{-4}$	98.07	$9.807 \cdot 10^{-4}$	0.001	1	0.735	.01422
mm Hg	0.001316	133.3	0.00133	0.00136	1.36	1	0.01934
psi	0.06804	6895	0.06895	.0703	70.323	51.70	1

Units of Power

	W	J/min	kgf·m/min	kcal/min	Btu/min
W	1	60	6.12	$1.43 \cdot 10^{-2}$	$5.693 \cdot 10^{-2}$
J/min	0.0167	1	0.1019	$2.39 \cdot 10^{-4}$	$9.47 \cdot 10^{-4}$
kgf·m/min	0.164	9.81	1	$2.34 \cdot 10^{-3}$	$9.30 \cdot 10^{-3}$
kcal/min	69.7	4187	427.0	1	3.968
Btu/min	17.56	1055.6	107.6	0.252	1

$1 \text{ kgf} = 9.811 \text{ kg·m/sec}^2$ (weight of 1 kg mass)

Units of Temperature

$$°C = 5/9 \, (°F - 32) \qquad °F = 9/5 \, °C + 32$$

Addresses of Contributors to Volume II

U.S. Contributors

Averner, Maurice M., Ph.D.
Life and Biomedical Sciences and Applications Division
Code ULM
NASA Headquarters
Washington, DC 20546

Coleman, Martin E., Ph.D.
Biomedical Operations and Research Division
Space Life Sciences Directorate, Code SD411
NASA Johnson Space Center
Houston, TX 77058

Evanich, Peggy L.
Office of Advanced Concepts and Technology, Code CD
NASA Headquarters
Washington, DC 20546

Grounds, Phylis F.
Man-Systems Division, Code SP
NASA Johnson Space Center
Houston, TX 77058

Humphries, William R., Ph.D.
Code EP1
NASA Marshall Flight Center
Huntsville, AL 35812

James, John T., Ph.D.
Biomedical Operations and Research Branch, Code SD4
NASA Johnson Space Center
Houston, TX 77058

Koros, Anton S.
Lockheed Engineering & Sciences Company, Code C95
2400 NASA Road 1
Houston, TX 77058

Lane, Helen D., Ph.D.
Biomedical Operations and
Research Branch, Code SD4
NASA Johnson Space Center
Houston, TX 77058

Langdoc, William A., Ph.D.
Chief, Facilities Operations Branch
Man-Systems Division, Code SP5
NASA Johnson Space Center
Houston, TX 77058

Lengel, Robert C., Jr., Ph.D.
Tracor Applied Sciences
6500 Tracor Lane
Austin, TX 78725

McBarron, James W., II
Chief, EVA Branch, Code EC611
NASA Johnson Space Center
Houston, TX 77058

McGinnis, Michael R., Ph.D.
Department of Pathology
University of Texas Medical Branch
Galveston, TX 77550

Murray, Robert W.
Box 551
Onalaska, TX 77360

Perner, Chris D., Ph.D.
Man-Systems Division, Code SP
NASA Johnson Space Center
Houston, TX 77058

Pierson, Duane L., Ph.D.
Biomedical Operations and Research Branch, Code SD4
NASA Johnson Space Center
Houston, TX 77058

Sauer, Richard L., P.E.
Biomedical Operations and Research Branch, Code SD411
NASA Johnson Space Center
Houston, TX 77058

Seshan, Panchalam K., Ph.D.
Code 125-112
Jet Propulsion Laboratory
Pasadena, CA 91109

Sulzman, Frank M.
Chief, Research Programs Branch
Life and Biomedical Sciences and Applications Division,
Code ULM
NASA Headquarters
Washington, DC 20546

Villarreal, Jennifer D.
Man-Systems Division, Code SP
NASA Johnson Space Center
Houston, TX 77058

Volk, Tyler, Ph.D.
Earth Systems Group
Department of Applied Science
26 Stuyvesant Street
New York, NY 10003

Waligora, James
Space Biomedical Research Institute, Code SD5
NASA Johnson Space Center
Houston, TX 77058

Wheelwright, Charles D.
Lockheed Engineering & Sciences Company, Code C44
2400 NASA Road 1
Houston, TX 77058-3711

Whitsett, Charles E. (deceased)

Russian Contributors

Abramov, Isaak Pavolvich
NPO "Zvezda"
39 Ulitsa Gogolya
Tomolino, Moskovskaya oblast 140070
Russia

Azhayev, Aleksandr Nikolayevich
Institute of Aeronautics and Space Medicine
12 Petrovsko-Razumovskaya alleya
Moscow 125083
Russia

Berlin, Anatoliy Arkadevich
Institute of Biomedical Problems
76a Khoroshevskoye shosse
D-7 Moscow 123007
Russia

Bychkov, Valentin Panfilovich
Institute of Biomedical Problems
76a Khoroshevskoye shosse
D-7 Moscow 123007
Russia

Gaydadymov, Viktor Borisovich
Institute of Biomedical Problems
76a Khoroshevskoye shosse
D-7 Moscow 123007
Russia

Genin, Avram Moiseyevich
Institute of Biomedical Problems
76a Khoroshevskoye shosse
D-7 Moscow 123007
Russia

Guzenberg, Arkadiy Samuilovich
NPO "Energiya"
Kaliningrad
141070 Moskovskaya oblast
Russia

Malkin, Viktor Borisovich
State Central Institute of Physical Culture
4 Sirenevyy Bulvar
Moscow 105483
Russia

Meleshko, Ganna Iosifovna
Institute of Biomedical Problems
76a Khoroshevskoye shosse
D-7 Moscow 123007
Russia

Popov, Igor Gennadiyevich
Institute of Biomedical Problems
76a Khoroshevskoye shosse
D-7 Moscow 123007
Russia

Popov, Vasiliy Vasilevich
Institute of Biomedical Problems
76a Khoroshevskoye shosse
D-7 Moscow 123007
Russia

Severin, Guy Ilyich
NPO "Zvezda"
39 Ulitsa Gogolya
Tomolino, Moskovskaya oblast 140070
Russia

Shepelev, Yevgeniy Yakovlevich
Institute of Biomedical Problems
76a Khoroshevskoye shosse
D-7 Moscow 123007
Russia

Shumilina, Galina Arkadevna
Institute of Biomedical Problems
76a Khoroshevskoye shosse
D-7 Moscow 123007
Russia

Sinyak, Yuriy Yemelyanovich
Institute of Biomedical Problems
76a Khoroshevskoye shosse
D-7 Moscow 123007
Russia

Skuratov, Vladimir Mikhaylovich
Institute of Biomedical Problems
76a Khoroshevskoye shosse
D-7 Moscow 123007
Russia

Viktorov, Aleksandr Nesterovich
Institute of Biomedical Problems
76a Khoroshevskoye shosse
D-7 Moscow 123007
Russia

Volovich, Vitaliy Georgiyevich
Institute of Biomedical Problems
76a Khoroshevskoye shosse
D-7 Moscow 123007
Russia

Index

419